Cardiopulmonary cerebral resuscitation

W9-BXZ-869

International Resuscitation Guidelines

Prepared for the *World Federation of Societies of Anaesthesiologists* Committee on Cardiopulmonary Resuscitation and Critical Care

Peter Baskett (*Chairman*) (UK)
Nicholas G. Bircher (USA)
Nancy Caroline (USA, Israel, Kenya)
Tess Cramond (Australia)
Elena Damir (USSR)
Wolfgang Dick (W. Germany)
Tatsushi Fujita (Japan)

Ex officio (WFSA)
Say Wan Lim (Malaysia)
Jose R. Nocite (Brazil)
Carlos Parsloe (Brazil)
John S.M. Zorab (UK)

With input from the *European Academy of Anaesthesiology* Committee on Cardiopulmonary Resuscitation:

J. Crul (*Chairman*) (Netherlands)
P. Baskett (UK)
W. Dick (W. Germany)
S. Fitzal (Austria)
J.C. Otteni (France)
W. Roese (E. Germany)
D. Scheidegger (Switzerland)

Written for physicians of all disciplines, and other health professionals, to enhance their ability to resuscitate; and for physician and nonphysician resuscitation instructors and organizers.

Cardiopulmonary Cerebral Resuscitation

BASIC AND ADVANCED CARDIAC AND TRAUMA LIFE SUPPORT

An Introduction to Resuscitation Medicine
Third Edition

Peter Safar and Nicholas G. Bircher

From the International Resuscitation Research Center, the Department of Anesthesiology and Critical Care Medicine, and the Presbyterian-University Hospital, University of Pittsburgh, USA

W.B. Saunders Company Ltd   London   Philadelphia   Toronto   Sydney   Tokyo

W B Saunders Company Ltd 24–28 Oval Road
Baillière Tindall London NW1 7DX UK
West Washington Square
Philadelphia, PA 19105
1 Goldthorne Avenue
Toronto, Ontario M8Z 5T9
Harcourt Brace Jovanovich Group
(Australia) Pty Ltd
Post Office Box 300
North Ryde, NSW 2113, Australia
Harcourt Brace Jovanovich Japan Inc.
Ichibancho Central Building, 22–1 Ichibancho
Chiyoda-ku, Tokyo 102, Japan

Dr Bircher's opinions expressed in this book are his and are not to be construed as reflecting the views of the Navy Department, or the Naval Service at large, or the Department of Defense.

First edition by P. Safar; published by Laerdal Medical, 1968
Second edition by P. Safar; published by Laerdal Medical, 1981
Third edition by P. Safar & N. Bircher; published by W. B. Saunders Company Limited in association with Laerdal Medical, 1988

 Laerdal Medical

Readers interested in translated editions of this work should contact Laerdal Medical, PO Box 377, N-4001 Stavanger, Norway.

British Library Cataloguing in Publication Data
Safar, Peter
Cardiopulmonary cerebral resuscitation:
an introduction to resuscitation
medicine.
1. Cardiac resuscitation
I. Title II. Bircher, Nicholas G.
III. World Federation of Societies
of Anaesthesiologists
616.1′290252 RC682

ISBN 0-7216-2156-2

Typeset and printed in Great Britain by the Alden Press, Oxford

Contents

Foreword to Second Edition *R. Frey* xiii
Foreword to Third Edition *P. Baskett and J. Crul* xiv
Preface xv
Acknowledgments xvii
Introduction (Figures 1 & 2; Table 1) 1
History 7
Phases and Steps of Cardiopulmonary Cerebral Resuscitation 9
    American Heart Association CPR standards of 1985 11

PHASE I: BASIC LIFE SUPPORT—Emergency
    Oxygenation 13

Chapter 1A   Step A: Airway Control (Figures 3–20; Table 2) 15

Causes of Airway Obstruction 15
Recognition of Airway Obstruction 16
Emergency Airway Control Measures 16
  1) Backward tilt of head (Figs. 3 & 4) 17
  2) Positive pressure inflation attempts (Fig. 5) 20
  3) Triple airway maneuver (head-tilt, mouth open, jaw-thrust)
     (Fig. 6) 22
  4) Manual clearing of the airway (Figs. 7–10) 25
  5) Clearing the airway by suction(Fig. 11) 32
  6) Pharyngeal intubation (Fig. 12) 34
  7) Esophageal obturator airway insertion (Fig. 13) 37
  8) Tracheal intubation (Figs. 14–16; Table 2) 40
  9) Alternatives to tracheal intubation (Figs. 17 & 18) 59
  10) Other steps of airway control (Figs. 19 & 20) 62

Chapter 1B   Step B: Breathing Support (Emergency Artificial
    Ventilation and Oxygenation) (Figures 21–28; Table 3) 68

Ventilation Patterns (Fig. 21) 68
  Positive end-expiratory pressure 69
Spontaneous Breathing of Oxygen with Positive Airway Pressure
    (Fig. 22) 72
Direct Mouth-to-Mouth and Mouth-to-Nose Ventilation (Fig. 23) 75
Mouth-to-Adjunct Ventilation 79
  Mouth-to-airway (Fig. 12-c) 79
  Mouth-to-mask with oxygen (Fig. 24) 79
Bag–Valve–Mask with Oxygen (Fig. 25) 83

Manually Triggered Oxygen-Powered Ventilators (Fig. 26)   86
Automatic Ventilators   88
Translaryngeal Oxygen Jet Ventilation   89
High-Frequency Jet Ventilation (Fig. 27)   89
Oxygen Delivery Systems (Fig. 28)   92
Selecting Ventilation and Oxygenation Techniques (Table 3)   94

Chapter 1C   Step C: Circulation Support (Cardiac Resuscitation) (Figures 29–36)   98

Causes of Cardiac Arrest   98
Recognition of Cardiac Arrest (Fig. 29)   99
Closed-Chest Cardiopulmonary Resuscitation (Figs. 30–33)   101
Combinations of Ventilation and Cardiac (Chest) Compressions for
    Standard External CPR (Figs. 32 & 33)   107
    One-operator CPR (Fig. 32)   107
    Two-operator CPR (Fig. 33)   107
    Simplified technique of external CPR basic life support   113
Transition from One to Two Operators   113
Switching between Two Operators   113
Monitoring the Effectiveness of CPR   114
Simultaneous Ventilation–Compression CPR   114
CPR Outside the Hospital   116
External CPR Machines (Chest Thumpers)   117
The C–A–B Sequence Controversy   117
Emergency Management of (Traumatic) Hemorrhage (Figs. 34 & 35)   119
    Life-supporting first aid   119
    Advanced trauma life support   119
Extrication and Positioning for Shock (Fig. 36)   122
Primary and Secondary Survey of Trauma Cases   124

PHASE II: ADVANCED LIFE SUPPORT—Restoration of
    Spontaneous Circulation   127

Chapter 2D   Step D: Drugs and Fluids (Figures 37–41)   129

Routes for Drugs and Fluids   129
    Peripheral intravenous route (Fig. 37)   129
    Intrapulmonary route   132
    Intracardiac route   132
    Intramuscular route   132
    Central venous route (Fig. 38)   132
    Monitoring pulmonary artery catheterization (Fig. 38)   134
    Arterial puncture   136
    Radial artery catheterization   136
    Femoral artery catheterization (Fig. 39)   137

Laboratory Measurement of Blood Gases and pH (Fig. 40)   138
Other Respiratory Monitoring Methods   139
   Continuous end-tidal carbon dioxide monitoring (capnography)   139
   Mass spectrometry   141
   Noninvasive (pulse) oximetry   141
   Transcutaneous PO_2 and PCO_2 analyses   141
   Emergency spirometry   142
Arterial Pressure Monitoring   143
Drugs   145
   Principal drugs during CPR Steps A–B–C   145
   Epinephrine (adrenaline)   149
   Sodium bicarbonate   150
   Tris buffer (THAM)   152
   Lidocaine (lignocaine)   152
   Procaine, procainamide   153
   Bretylium   153
   Cardiovascular stimulants   154
   Norepinephrine (noradrenaline)   155
   Dopamine   156
   Dobutamine   157
   Amrinone   157
   Metaraminol   157
   Ephredrine   158
   Isoproterenol   158
   Atropine   159
   Calcium   159
   Calcium entry blockers   160
   Digitalis   162
   Corticosteroids   163
   Vasodilators   163
   Nitroprusside   164
   Nitroglycerin   164
   Propranolol   165
   Narcotic analgesics   165
   Diuretics   166
   Barbiturates   166
   Diazepam (Valium)   167
   Phenytoin (Diphenylhydantoin, Dilantin)   167
   Muscle relaxants   168
   Miscellaneous drugs   169
Fluids   171
   Infusion strategies and hypovolemia   171
   Choice of intravenous fluids   173
   Oral fluid therapy   176
   Conclusion   177

Chapter 2E   Step E: Electrocardiographic Diagnosis
      (Recognition and Treatment of Dysrhythmias)
      (Figures 42–46)   178
Techniques of Electrocardiography   178
ECG Patterns of Cardiac Arrest (Fig. 42)   181
   Ventricular fibrillation   181
   Electromechanical dissociation and asystole   181
Life-Threatening Dysrhythmias (Figs. 43–46)   183
   Sinus tachycardia and sinus bradycardia (Fig. 43)   183
   Paroxysmal supraventricular tachycardia (Fig. 43)   183
   Premature atrial complexes (Fig. 43)   186
   Atrial fibrillation (Fig. 44)   186
   Junctional (nodal) rhythms (Fig. 44)   186
   Atrioventricular blocks (Fig. 45)   187
   Premature ventricular complexes (Fig. 46)   193
   Ventricular tachycardia (Fig. 46)   193
   Ventricular fibrillation (Fig. 46)   197
   Electromechanical dissociation and asystole (Fig. 46)   198

Chapter 2F   Step F: Fibrillation Treatment (Defibrillation)
      (Figures 47–53)   199
Introduction (Figs. 47–50)   199
Techniques for Electric Defibrillation   202
   Defibrillators   203
   Techniques (Fig. 49)   204
   Empirical countershock   207
   Synchronized cardioversion   209
Automatic External Electric Defibrillation (Fig. 50)   209
Automatic Internal (Implanted) Defibrillation   210
Emergency Cardiac Pacing   211
Open-Chest Cardiopulmonary Resuscitation (Figs. 51 & 52)   212
   Evaluation of open-chest CPR   217
Extracorporeal Oxygenation and Circulation (Fig. 53)   219
   Emergency cardiopulmonary bypass   219
   Intra-aortic balloon counterpulsation   222
   Extracorporeal membrane oxygenation   222
   Extracorporeal lung assist   223
Concluding Comments on Advanced Life Support   225

PHASE III: PROLONGED LIFE SUPPORT—Post-Resus-
      citative Brain-Oriented Therapy, Cerebral Resuscitation 227

Chapter 3   (Figures 54–56; Tables 4–12)   229
Introduction   229

Post-Resuscitation Syndrome (Figs. 54–56)   232
Stabilization of Extracerebral Organ Function   238
  Pulmonary support (Table 4)   239
  Arterial blood gases and acid–base status   240
  Cardiovascular support (Fig. 40)   241
  Other organ system support (Table 5)   243
Standard Brain-Oriented Intensive Therapy (Table 6)   245
  Extracranial homeostasis measures   245
  Intracranial homeostasis and pressure control   247
Special Brain Resuscitation Potentials (Table 7)   251
  1) General brain-oriented intensive therapy by protocol   252
  2) Promotion of reperfusion (Fig. 55)   252
  3) Barbiturates   254
  4) Calcium entry blockers   256
  5) Free radical scavengers   257
  6) Etiology-specific combined therapies   258
  Miscellaneous brain resuscitation measures   259
Evaluating Insult, Progress and Outcome (Tables 8–10)   261
  Evaluating insult (Table 8)   261
  Evaluating progress and coma (Table 9)   263
  Predicting outcome   266
  Evaluating outcome (Table 10)   266
Starting and Terminating Emergency Resuscitation   269
  When not to undertake emergency resuscitation   269
  When to terminate emergency resuscitation   269
  Cardiac death (irreversible cardiac arrest)   269
  Apparent brain death during emergency resuscitation   270
Terminating Long-Term Resuscitation   272
  Brain death determination and certification (Table 11)   272
  Critical care triage (Table 12)   276
  Letting die   276

Chapter 4   Special Considerations (Figures 57–58; Table 13)   279

Introduction   279
Special Technical Considerations   279
  Pediatric cardiopulmonary resuscitation (Fig. 57)   279
  Neonatal resuscitation by Peter Safar and Ian Holzman (Table 13)   286
  Witnessed arrest (cough CPR and Precordial thump) (Fig. 58)   291
  Complications and pitfalls of CPR   294
Special Dying Mechanisms   296
  Sudden cardiac death, myocardial ischemia and infarction   296
  Alveolar anoxia   299
  Asphyxia   300
  Exsanguination cardiac arrest   302

Hypoglycemia 303
Hypothermia 304
Hyperthermia 306
Electrolyte and acid–base derangements 307
Special Emergencies 308
  Electric Shock 308
  Drowning 310
  Acute Pulmonary Edema 312
  Pulmonary Embolism 314
  Status Asthmaticus 315
  Carbon Monoxide Poisoning 316
  Anesthesia-Related Cardiac Arrest 317
  Drugs and Poisons 318
  Anaphylaxis 319
Advanced Trauma Life Support 320
  Introduction and patient assessment 320
  Severe polytrauma 324
  Circulatory shock 325
  Burns 327
  Radiation injuries 329
  Cerebral trauma 331
  Spinal cord trauma 333
  Thoracic trauma 333
  Abdominal trauma 335
  Extremity trauma 337
  Anesthesia in disasters 337

Chapter 5   Teaching of First Aid and Resuscitation (Figure 59; Tables 14–20) 339

What to Teach to Whom (Table 14) 339
How to Teach and Test Resuscitation Skills 343
  Teaching the lay public 343
  Teaching health care personnel 344
  Teaching methodology (Table 15; Fig. 59) 345
Teaching CPR Basic Life Support Without Equipment 350
  Mouth-to-mouth risks to trainee rescuers 350
Teaching CPR Basic Life Support With Equipment 351
Teaching Proficiency in Endotracheal Intubation 353
Teaching Advanced Life Support and Prolonged Life Support 353
Testing (Tables 16–20) 354

Chapter 6   Organization (Table 21) 360

Hospital-Wide Organization 360

Community-Wide Organization (Table 21)   362
Ambulances   363
Hospitals   365
Advanced Life Support Units   366
   Equipment: Advanced life support stations   367
Legal Considerations   369
Disaster Resuscitology   371
   Dying processes in disasters   373
   Resuscitation potentials in disasters   374
   National disaster medical systems   375
   Local disaster medical systems   377
   Nuclear disasters   377
   Nuclear war   378

Chapter 7 Philosophical-Ethical Conclusions   379
   By Peter Safar and Nancy Caroline

Delivery of Cardiopulmonary Cerebral Resuscitation   379
Ethical Questions in the Future   380
Near-Death Experiences   382
Resuscitation and the Evolution of Man   383

References   385

Glossary   429

Suggested case report form for CPCR attempt (Table 22)   440

Instruction card 'Life Supporting First Aid—CPR' (Fig. 60)   442

Index   445

Foreword to the Second Edition

One of the most important goals of the World Federation of Societies of Anaesthesiologists (WFSA) is the progress of the methods of resuscitation throughout the world. For this reason the Committee on Cardiopulmonary Resuscitation (CPR) of the World Federation of Societies of Anaesthesiologists in 1965 asked a world pioneer of resuscitation, Peter Safar, Professor of Anesthesiology at the University of Pittsburgh, Pennsylvania, to write a manual on CPR.

A generous grant from the Asmund Laerdal Company, which also printed the manual, led to its worldwide distribution, starting with the WFSA Congress in London in September 1968. Between 1968 and 1978 about 250 000 copies were distributed gratis or sold at cost throughout the world. These copies were printed in 15 languages.

At the WFSA meeting in Kyoto in 1972 the manual was praised as a major contribution of WFSA, and Peter Safar deserves great credit for its success.

The impact of the simplicity of modern CPR as presented in the manual's first edition is retained in the second edition, but the need for many advances beyond basic life support, particularly the logical expansion of CPR to cardiopulmonary-cerebral resuscitation (CPCR) has necessitated an entirely new manual for the 1980s.

In the second edition the author, Peter Safar, has synthesized accepted and proven techniques, his own clinical teaching and research experiences in resuscitation over 30 years, together with new concepts and possibilities.

Anesthesiologists have pioneered much of the initiating research, training mechanisms and delivery programs of CPR since the 1950s. CPCR, which represents the acute phase of critical care medicine (intensive therapy), should, however, be pursued with multidisciplinary participation and contribution.

It is hoped that anesthesiologists will retain and expand their roles as initiators, teachers, leaders and team members in resuscitation around the world.

Rudolf Frey✠
Dr. med., FFARCS
Mainz 1981

Chairman of the Committee
on Cardiopulmonary
Resuscitation,
World Federation of Societies
of Anaesthesiologists

Professor of Anaesthesiology
Johannes Gutenberg-University
D-6500 Mainz
F.R. Germany
✠Professor Frey died
on 23 December 1981

Foreword to the Third Edition

The Committees on Cardiopulmonary Resuscitation of the World Federation of Societies of Anaesthesiologists and the European Academy of Anaesthesiology are once again grateful to that pioneer, Peter Safar, and now to his co-author, Nicholas Bircher, for preparing on their behalf the third edition of this extremely popular publication. This latest version has been substantially revised and expanded where necessary in response to modern developments in the subject, many of which have emanated from the International Resuscitation Research Center in Pittsburgh. This edition has been written and produced with the utmost speed to ensure that the contents are right up to date at the time of publication. This has meant that the authors have consumed a considerable amount of midnight oil and that the publishers have given of their very best.

Resuscitation is currently enjoying a renaissance of interest worldwide, thanks to a greater appreciation of its potential. The wish of the late Rudolf Frey that anesthesiologists everywhere will expand their interest and participation in the subject, which he expressed in his foreword of the second edition in 1981, has largely been realized. This step forward is due in no small part to the quality of Peter Safar's authorship and the efficiency and generosity of the Laerdal Corporation, mediated through Asmund's son, Tore, who arranged for the supply and distribution of many free copies of the first and second editions to deserving causes.

There is little doubt that this edition will uphold the reputation of this book as one of the most important contributions to the subject yet produced. Both CPR Committees are extremely pleased to be associated with this work, which has undoubtedly been instrumental in saving very many valuable lives, throughout the world. The third edition will continue this tradition.

Chairman of the Committee
on Cardiopulmonary Resuscitation
World Federation of Societies of
Anaesthesiologists

Peter J.F. Baskett BA, MB BCh, BAO, FFARCS
Consultant Anaesthetist, Frenchay Hospital
and The Royal Infirmary, Bristol,
United Kingdom

Chairman of the Committee on
Cardiopulmonary Resuscitation
European Academy of
Anaesthesiology

Professor Jan F. Crul, MD, FFARCS
Chairman Institut voor Anestesiologie Nijmegen,
Netherlands

Preface

The first modern resuscitation manuals, written in the 1950s, were on rescue breathing; those written in the 1960s were on cardiopulmonary resuscitation (CPR). The latter included the *first* edition of this teaching text, a 48-page manual solicited by the World Federation of Societies of Anaesthesiologists' (WFSA) CPR Committee, authored by PS and published in 1968 by Asmund S. Laerdal. About 250 000 copies in 15 languages were distributed gratis or sold at cost worldwide.

The *second* edition of this text, also authored by PS, and published by Asmund S. Laerdal in 1981, was a new book of 240 pages, with 45 figures and 19 tables. About 100 000 copies in 12 languages were distributed gratis or sold worldwide. It addressed the demand for more sophisticated knowledge, increased opportunities for reversing dying processes, increasingly complex methods, and expansion of CPR to cardiopulmonary cerebral resuscitation (CPCR). Because good patient outcome often depends not only on the speed and quality of emergency resuscitation, but also on long-term resuscitation (intensive care), the author added a brief review of post-resuscitative life support. This included support of recovery of the target organ, the brain.

The present *third* edition, published in 1988 by Saunders and Laerdal jointly, represents a revision and expansion of the technique-oriented book to an 'Introduction to Resuscitation Medicine' of about 450 pages, with 60 figures and 22 tables. It includes the important changes to previous US national guidelines and standards introduced by the American Heart Association's (AHA) 1985 National Conference on CPR and Emergency Cardiac Care (ECC), to which the senior author of this book has contributed since the 1950s. New sections or new emphases taking this book beyond AHA standards include open-chest CPR, emergency cardiopulmonary bypass, automatic defibrillation, fluid resuscitation, pathophysiology of the post-resuscitation syndrome, cerebral resuscitation, prolonged life support, over thirty special dying processes, advanced trauma life support, disaster medicine, and ethical-philosophical considerations.

The objective of this book is to convey the knowledge that should be acquired before skill practice, resuscitation attempts on patients, and the organization and conduct of training programs in basic, advanced and prolonged life support. A book cannot teach vital skills. These can be acquired only through practice—on manikins, on other trainees and on patients. This book is primarily for physicians of all disciplines and for nonphysician instructors of resuscitation. It is impossible to obtain an international or even a national consensus on what to teach to whom and how, because this field is complex and constantly changing. Recommendations on resuscitation have been developed by national and international groups since the 1960s. For basic life support by lay persons, we consider *standards* desirable. It is important that teaching materials be kept simple and uniform within each country, to avoid confusion and hesitation in actual situations. For life support by medical personnel, however, we prefer flexible *guidelines* rather than rigid standards. These guidelines should not hinder innovation. Prompt changes should be possible when documentation of life-saving or teaching advantages of new techniques has been provided. Rigid standards imply that they are based on hard data, which is usually not the case, and suggest punitive action for noncompliance, which is inappropriate. This book reflects majority agreement by the members of the WFSA CPR Committee. Most of the techniques taught have been incorporated into recommendations by the American Heart Association, the National Research Council (USA), and several countries' national and international Red Cross societies.

It is important that medical personnel maintain sufficient flexibility regarding guidelines to take into account the differing resources, priorities and cultural constraints in various countries. Thus, resuscitation leaders in each country should feel free to modify the contents of this book to improve the acceptability and implementation of resuscitation services in their environment.

The science of reanimatology (a term introduced by Vladimir Negovsky), and the CPCR delivery mechanisms of emergency and critical care medicine (intensive therapy) are multidisciplinary endeavors. Some anesthesiologists were initiators of modern resuscitation. The present and future involvement of anesthesiologists as researchers, clinical leaders, team members, consultants or teachers will depend on personal interest, availability and competence, and on local circumstances. We hope that this manual will help all types of professionals to skilfully reverse, either personally or indirectly, acute dying processes in patients whose time to die has not yet come. Our goal, of course, is to restore life with quality, including human mentation.

Peter Safar
Nicholas G. Bircher

Pittsburgh, 1987

Acknowledgements

For the ability and opportunity to contribute to resuscitation medicine, I am grateful to my parents, teachers, colleagues, students, and friends, and the University of Pittsburgh. For support and for maintaining our home and tolerating a 'workaholic', I thank my wife Eva and my sons Philip and Paul. For help with completion of this book, my thanks go to the staff of the International Resuscitation Research Center, University of Pittsburgh, in particular to Gale Foster and Fran Mistrick; to the Anesthesiology department's editor Lisa Cohn; to H. Eikeland and the Laerdal Company for the superb illustrations; to the W.B. Saunders Company, London, for rapid printing; and to the World Federation of Societies of Anaesthesiologists (WFSA) Committee on Cardiopulmonary Resuscitation (CPR) for sponsorship. I thank Drs N. Abramson, P. Baskett, P. Berkebile, A. Grenvik, I. Holzman, J. Lane, B. Lind, A. Meisel, and the late J. Redding for their suggestions; Drs R. Albarran, J. Donegan, and W. Montgomery of the American Heart Association CPR-ECC Committee for their cooperation; and Drs P. Baskett, N. Caroline and J. Zorab for valuable editorial help. I am grateful to Dr Peter Winter, chairman of the Department of Anesthesiology, University of Pittsburgh, for his friendship and his support of resuscitation research. I thank my friend and associate since 1978, N. Bircher, for having agreed to co-author this book and to update it in years to come.

The resuscitation research over the past 30 years by me and my collaborators has been supported by the US Army's Surgeon General, the National Institutes of Health (USA), the Pennsylvania Department of Health, the Asmund S. Laerdal Foundation, and grants from other sources. The authors of this book are deeply indebted to all the coinvestigators, consultants, research fellows, and technicians of the multidisciplinary International Resuscitation Research Center at the University of Pittsburgh for their input.

Special credit goes to the late Asmund Laerdal of Stavanger, Norway, who, since we first met in 1958, has helped bring about modern resuscitation—as a pioneer, as an inventor, designer and manufacturer of resuscitation teaching materials, equipment and supplies, and as a patron of resuscitation research, symposia and guidelines. He persuaded me to write the 1968 and 1981 WFSA CPR manuals. His death in 1981 was a great loss for resuscitation medicine. Our deepest gratitude goes to his son, Tore Laerdal, director of Laerdal Medical and the Laerdal Foundation since 1981. His dedication and wisdom are helping CPR move into the computer age. He has helped the global spread of resuscitation by arranging many translations of the 1981 edition. By having persuaded me and W.B. Saunders, London, to embark on this third edition, he has enabled the WFSA to continue contributing to resuscitation medicine worldwide.

Peter Safar, Pittsburgh 1987

xvii

To
the memory of
Elizabeth and Hanni
who needed and taught
resuscitation

Introduction

Potentially reversible airway obstruction, hypoventilation, apnea (respiratory arrest), blood loss, pulselessness (cardiac arrest) and brain injury are among the leading causes of death resulting from heart attacks, accidents and other medical emergencies[236, 736a, 783] (Fig. 1). The leading causes of preventable or reversible sudden death before old age are ventricular fibrillation from ischemic heart disease (with or without myocardial infarction); coma causing airway obstruction, hypoventilation and apnea; exsanguination; nontraumatic accidents (e.g. drowning, poisoning); and trauma with exsanguination or severe brain injury, caused by violence, human error, failure of technology and natural disasters[751–756].

Irreversible brain damage may occur when very low oxygen transport (e.g. very severe shock or hypoxemia) or no oxygen transport (cessation of circulation, i.e. cardiac arrest = clinical death) lasts longer than a few minutes. The precise time limits are currently under reinvestigation. The immediate application of modern resuscitation is often capable of reversing clinical death and thereby preventing brain death, vegetative survival and panorganic (biologic) death; and of reducing cerebral and overall crippling in survivors (Fig. 1). Resuscitative measures can be initiated anywhere, without the use of equipment, by trained individuals, ranging from the lay public to physician specialists. In some cases only brief basic life support is needed to achieve prompt complete recovery. In others, advanced life support and sophisticated prolonged life support must follow to give the patient an appropriate chance.

Resuscitation medicine is based on an understanding of the pathophysiology of acute dying processes (Fig. 1)[736a] and knowledge of resuscitation methods (Fig. 2)[23a, b, 720]. The biologic limits and therapeutic potentials of reversing terminal states and clinical death, as well as methods by which outcome could be reliably predicted early post-insult, are under intensive investigation (Table 1).

Definitions are listed in the Glossary. Briefly, apnea is 'absence of breathing movements'. Cardiac arrest is 'the clinical picture of overall cessation of circulation', which includes 'unconsciousness, apnea or gasping, pulselessness in large arteries, and death-like appearance'. 'Clinical death' is coma, apnea and pulselessness (cessation of all blood flow), with cerebral failure still potentially reversible.

Cardiac arrest may be *primary*, as in sudden ventricular fibrillation (common) or primary asystole (less common). Some cerebral neurons can survive ischemic periods of up to 20 minutes[28], perhaps even 60 minutes[357]. At this time (1987), however, resuscitability of the entire organism with human mentation has been very rare after primary normothermic cardiac

1

arrest of over 5 minutes, due to the numerous factors in addition to anoxia, which before, during and after the arrest can reduce the chance for a good outcome[745]. As our understanding and control of post-arrest derangements improves, occasional good recovery after up to 10–20 min of normothermic cardiac arrest has been seen in animals[760a] and patients[760b].

Cardiac arrest may also be *secondary*, as it occurs over minutes in alveolar anoxia, asphyxia, or exsanguinating hemorrhage; or as it occurs over hours, in severe hypoxemia due to pulmonary edema or pneumonia, shock due to trauma (hypovolemia), sepsis, cardiac failure or obstruction of flow (e.g. massive pulmonary embolism), or in acute intracranial pathology (Fig. 1)[736a, 749]. In such secondary cardiac arrests, permanent brain damage sometimes follows CPR attempts after less than 5 minutes of no blood flow due to tissue hypoxia before the onset of arrest. For pathophysiologic mechanisms, see relevant reviews[72a, 163, 736a].

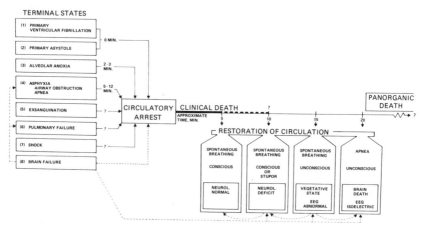

Fig. 1. Flowchart illustrating diagrammatically the development of circulatory arrest— suddenly (Terminal States 1, ventricular fibrillation; or 2, primary asystole); over minutes (Terminal States 3–5); or protracted (Terminal States 6–8). Clinical death is 'total circulatory arrest with potential reversibility to complete recovery, including brain function'. Duration of reversible clinical death depends on terminal state, resuscitation and post-resuscitation syndrome. After restoration of circulation, various possible outcomes. (From Safar P, chapter 1. In: *Principles and Practice of Emergency Medicine.* G Schwartz, P Safar, J Stone et al. (Eds). Philadelphia, W.B. Saunders, 1986.)

Table 1. Phases, steps and measures of cardiopulmonary cerebral resuscitation.

Phases	Steps	Measures performed	

Establish unresponsiveness—Activate EMS system

Phases	Steps	*Without* equipment	*With* equipment
I **Basic life support** (BLS) (Emergency oxygenation)	Airway control	(1)*Backward tilt of head *Supine aligned position *Stable side position (2)*Lung inflation attempts (3)*Triple airway maneuver (jaw-thrust, open mouth) (4)*Manual clearing of mouth and throat Back blows— manual thrusts	(5) Pharyngeal suctioning (6) Pharyngeal intubation (7) Esophageal obturator airway insertion (8) Endotracheal intubation Tracheobronchial suctioning (9) Cricothyrotomy Translaryngeal O_2 jet insufflation (10) Tracheotomy Bronchoscopy Bronchodilation Pleural drainage
	Breathing support	*Mouth-to-mouth (nose) ventilation	Mouth-to-adjunct with or without O_2 Manual bag-mask (tube) ventilation with or without O_2 Hand-triggered O_2 ventilation Mechanical ventilation
	Circulation support	*Control of external hemorrhage *Position for shock Pulse checking Manual chest compressions	Mechanical chest compressions Open chest direct cardiac compressions Pressure pants (MAST) for shock
II **Advanced life support** (ALS) (Restoration of spontaneous circulation)	Drugs and fluids		i.v. lifeline
	Electrocardiography		ECG monitoring
	Fibrillation treatment		Defibrillation
III **Prolonged life support** (PLS) (Cerebral resuscitation and post-resuscitation Intensive therapy)	Gauging		Determine and treat cause of demise Determine salvageability
	Human mentation		Cerebral resuscitation
	Intensive care		Multiple organ support

* Life-supporting first aid.

CARDIOPULMONARY – CEREBRAL RESUSCITATION

PHASE ONE **BASIC LIFE SUPPORT**
Emergency Oxygenation

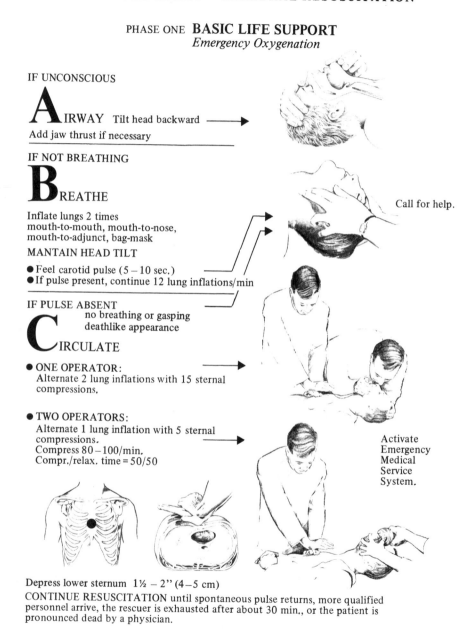

IF UNCONSCIOUS

AIRWAY Tilt head backward ⟶
Add jaw thrust if necessary

IF NOT BREATHING

BREATHE

Inflate lungs 2 times
mouth-to-mouth, mouth-to-nose,
mouth-to-adjunct, bag-mask

MANTAIN HEAD TILT

● Feel carotid pulse (5 – 10 sec.)
● If pulse present, continue 12 lung inflations/min

Call for help.

IF PULSE ABSENT
C no breathing or gasping
deathlike appearance
IRCULATE

● ONE OPERATOR: ⟶
Alternate 2 lung inflations with 15 sternal
compressions.

● TWO OPERATORS:
Alternate 1 lung inflation with 5 sternal
compressions. ⟶
Compress 80 – 100/min.
Compr./relax. time = 50/50

Activate
Emergency
Medical
Service
System.

Depress lower sternum 1½ – 2" (4–5 cm)
CONTINUE RESUSCITATION until spontaneous pulse returns, more qualified
personnel arrive, the rescuer is exhausted after about 30 min., or the patient is
pronounced dead by a physician.

Fig. 2. Phases and steps of cardiopulmonary cerebral resuscitation (CPCR). Basic life
support (Steps A–B–C). See text.

PHASE TWO **ADVANCED LIFE SUPPORT**
Restoration of Spontaneous Circulation

DO NOT INTERRUPT CARDIAC COMPRESSIONS AND LUNG VENTILATION
INTUBATE TRACHEA WHEN POSSIBLE

DRUGS AND FLUIDS, I.V. LIFELINE

EPINEPHRINE (ADRENALINE)
0.5 - 1.0 mg I.V. repeat every 5 min. until spontaneous pulse returns

SODIUM BICARBONATE
1 mEq/kg I.V. if arrest over 5 min.
Monitor and normalize arterial pH and blood gases

I.V. FLUIDS as indicated

E.K.G.   Ventricular fibrillation ? Asystole ? Bizarre complexes ?

FIBRILLATION TREATMENT

IMMEDIATE EXTERNAL DEFIBRILLATION
D.C. 200-300-360 Joules
Repeat shock as necessary
LIDOCAINE (LIGNOCAINE)
1–2 mg/kg I.V. if necessary
continue I.V. infusion

IF ASYSTOLE
repeat Epinephrine every 5 min. Vasopressors as needed.

CONTINUE RESUSCITATION until good pulse.
Restore normotension promptly

D.C. 200-360 J

PHASE THREE **PROLONGED LIFE SUPPORT**
Post-Resuscitative Brain-Oriented Therapy

GAUGING   Determine and treat cause of arrest
Determine salvageability

HUMAN MENTATION - -   CEREBRAL RESUSCITATION

INTENSIVE CARE

Immediately after restoration of spontaneous circulation and throughout coma - -
Ameliorate post-anoxic encephalopathy:
Monitoring (CV, art, (PA), bladder catheters; EKG)
Normotension. Oxygenation. Controlled Ventilation. Blood Variables. Temperature.
Relaxation. Sedation. Fluids. Electrolytes. Glucose. Alimentation. Drugs. (ICP)
(For Innovative Therapy see Chapter III)

Fig. 2 *(cont.).* Phases and steps of cardiopulmonary cerebral resuscitation (CPCR).
Advanced life support (Steps D–E–F) and prolonged life support (Steps G–H–I). See
text.

History

In 1985, modern cardiopulmonary resuscitation (CPR) was 25 years old[23a, 429, 699, 720]. There were few immediately applicable effective emergency resuscitation techniques available before the 1950s. Modern respiratory resuscitation was pioneered in the 1950s[220, 699, 704]; external cardiac resuscitation in the 1960s[699]; and cerebral resuscitation after cardiac arrest in the 1970s when CPR was extended to cardiopulmonary cerebral resuscitation (CPCR)[720, 734a, 759]. Modern fluid resuscitation for circulatory shock was pioneered in the 1930s (Blalock, 1940[89]). Intensive therapy (long-term resuscitation), essential in many cases for optimal outcome after emergency resuscitation, was initiated in the 1950s in Scandinavia (Nilsson, 1951[150, 590]; Ibsen, 1952[364]; Holmdahl, 1962[352]; Norlander, 1965[594, 595]), and in Baltimore, USA (Safar, 1958[711]), and was developed by several groups around the world in the 1960s[66, 238, 408, 436, 448, 630, 833, 849]. Pediatric ICUs also followed in the 1960s[44, 395]. Modern CPCR is based on ideas conceived or accidentally discovered over at least four centuries. They have been rediscovered, re-explored, and put together into an effective resuscitation system in the 1950s and 1960s.

The *early history* of CPR includes: rescue breathing on a child by Elijah (*The Bible*, 1 Kings 17:17–22); controlled intermittent positive pressure ventilation (IPPV) by Vesalius (1543)[921]; mouth-to-mouth ventilation of an adult by Tossach (1771)[898]; jaw thrust for airway control by Esmarch (1878)[233] and Heiberg (1874)[333]; successful open-chest CPR in animals by Boehm (1878)[93] and Schiff (1882)[318, 773]; and in patients first by Igelsrud (1900)[852], Keen[401] and Zesas[988]; successful open-chest defibrillation in animals by Prevost and Battelli (1899)[638], Hooker (1933)[353] and Wiggers (1940)[963] and in patients first by Beck (1947)[61]; successful external CPR in animals by Boehm (1878)[93], Guthrie (1920)[625, 856] and Gurvich (1946)[312], and in patients by Maass (1892)[498]; successful external defibrillation in animals by Prevost and Battelli (1899)[639], Hooker (1933)[353] and Gurvich (1946)[312]; brain-oriented resuscitation attempts (Stewart and Guthrie, 1906)[856]; and pathophysiologic research on dying and resuscitation (Negovsky, 1940s)[577]. Translaryngeal tracheal intubation was introduced almost simultaneously by many (Macewen, 1880[499]; Chaillou, 1895[136]; Kirstein, 1895[413]; Dorrance, 1910[203]; Kuhn, 1911[437]; Jackson, 1913[369]; Macintosh, 1920[500]; Rowbothan and Magill, 1921[504, 686]; Waters, 1933[935]).

The *recent history* of modern CPR shows a series of landmark developments during the past 30 years: proof that ventilation with the operator's exhaled air is physiologically sound (Elam, 1954[220]); proof in curarized adult human volunteers without tracheal tube of the ventilatory superiority of mouth-to-mouth (nose) ventilation over the manual chest-pressure arm-lift

7

methods (Safar, 1958[699]); studies showing why and how soft-tissue obstruction of the upper airway in unconscious patients can be prevented or corrected, by backward tilt of the head, forward displacement of the mandible, and opening of the mouth (Safar, 1958, 1959[700, 704]); proof of the ventilatory superiority of mouth-to-mouth ventilation over the manual chest-pressure arm-lift methods in children (Gordon, 1958[289]); rediscovery, laboratory documentation and the first clinical proof of efficacy of external cardiac (chest) compressions (Kouwenhoven, 1960[429]); combining steps A (head-tilt, jaw-thrust), B (positive pressure ventilation), and C (external cardiac compressions) (Safar, 1961[709a]); the first successful electric defibrillation of a human heart via thoracotomy (Beck, 1947[61]); the first successful external electric defibrillations and pacings of human hearts (Zoll, 1956[996]); the concept of 'the heart too good to die' (reversible sudden cardiac death) (Beck, 1960[7, 62]); the concept of 'the brain too good to die' (Safar, 1970[734a, 759]); and the development of cardiac arrest-CPR animal models (Negovsky and associates in the 1940s[577–580]; Safar and associates in the 1950s[736a, 745]).

Important for implementation of CPCR were the following: proof of the feasibility of teaching CPR to the lay public (Safar, 1958[700]; Lind, 1961[471]; Elam, 1961[223]; Winchell, 1966[967]; Berkebile, 1973[73]); proof that lay people in the field will perform direct mouth-to-mouth breathing (Elam, 1961[223]; Lind, 1963[472]) and CPR (Lund, 1976[492]; Cobb, 1980[153]); creation of realistic training aids (Laerdal, 1958[720]); and agreements on details of techniques and teaching methods through many national committees and organizations, and the international resuscitation symposia of Stavanger in 1961 (Poulsen, 1962[631]) and Oslo in 1967 (Lund, 1968[491]). In the USA, the Wolf Creek CPR researchers' symposia, started in 1975, are being held every five years[606, 660 734], preceding the American Heart Association CPR Standards Conferences[23a, b].

The early sparks of resuscitation failed to benefit patients over several centuries, probably because the following three events did not come about until the 1950s or 1960s: (1) communication and collaboration between laboratory researchers, clinicians and field rescuers; (2) scientific proof of the efficacy of each one of the steps A through I of CPCR (Fig. 2; Table 1); and (3) combining steps A through I into a clinically feasible and effective system, and delivering it as a continuum from the scene via transportation into the hospital[23a, 720]. Thus, over the past 30 years, old techniques have been refashioned into new systems. CPCR works, and thousands of lives could be saved each year if enough individuals were properly trained in resuscitation. Clinical results depend heavily, however, upon initiating properly performed resuscitation techniques at the earliest possible moment.

Phases and Steps of Cardiopulmonary Cerebral Resuscitation

In 1961, for didactic purposes, Safar divided cardiopulmonary cerebral resuscitation (CPCR) into three phases[715, 720]: I, basic life support; II, advanced life support; III, prolonged life support; and into nine steps, using the letters of the alphabet from A through I (Fig. 2; Table 1). (Since the introduction of CPR in 1960, Safar has used the term 'basic life support' for Steps A, B and C; 'advanced life support' for Steps D, E and F; and 'prolonged life support' for Steps G, H and I—irrespective of the use of equipment. The American Heart Association, on the other hand, uses the term 'basic life support' for Steps A, B and C without the use of equipment; and the term 'advanced life support' for Steps A, B and C with the use of equipment, plus all other steps.)

Phase I, *basic life support* (BLS), is emergency oxygenation. It consists of Steps A, Airway control; B, Breathing support, i.e. emergency artificial ventilation and oxygenation of the lungs; and C, Circulation support, i.e. recognition of pulselessness, emergency artificial circulation by cardiac (chest) compressions, control of hemorrhage and positioning for shock.

As soon as feasible after initiation of Phase I, call for help, without interrupting resuscitation, and activate the community's Emergency Medical Services (EMS) system (inside hospitals, the CPR team response). Ask a helper to call your community's emergency phone number for an ambulance. Make sure you know this number. Say it is a resuscitation case. If you are alone, use your best judgment when to call, with minimal interruption of resuscitation. If no phone and no helper are available, continue resuscitation for at least 30 min (if you consider the patient salvable) or until medical personnel take over.

Phase II, *advanced life support* (ALS), is restoration of spontaneous circulation and stabilization of the cardiopulmonary system, by restoring adequate arteriovenous perfusion pressure and near-normal arterial oxygen transport (i.e. arterial oxygen content times cardiac output). Phase II consists of Steps D, Drugs and fluids via intravenous infusion; E, Electrocardiography; and F, Fibrillation treatment, usually by electric countershock.

The sequential actions in performing Phases I and II, which lead to the establishment of adequate spontaneous circulation, should be as rapid as possible. External chest (cardiac) compressions produce very low perfusion pressures, cardiac output and cerebral and coronary blood flows[82b, 757]— particularly if not started immediately upon onset of pulselessness—but it can be initiated immediately, even by lay persons. Open chest cardiac

9

compressions are more effective and produce near-normal perfusion pressures, cardiac output and cerebral and coronary blood flows[82a, 758], and can be initiated within one minute, but must be performed by a trained physician. Emergency cardiopulmonary bypass permits full control over flow, pressure, and composition and temperature of blood[758], but must be performed by a specially trained medical team and requires several minutes to be initiated.

Phase III, *prolonged life support* (PLS), is post-resuscitative brain-oriented intensive therapy. It consists of steps G, Gauging, i.e. determining and treating the cause of the arrest and deciding whether to continue; H, Human mentation, to be restored hopefully by new cerebral resuscitation measures; and I, intensive care (long-term resuscitation), for multiple organ failure in the post-resuscitative period[759]. Phase III should be continued until the patient regains consciousness and extracerebral organ functions have been stabilized, or brain death has been certified, or the underlying disease makes further resuscitation efforts senseless.

Life-supporting first aid (LSFA) comprises basic measures without the use of equipment, to be learned by the general public[81, 107, 234, 443, 444, 676, 744]. LSFA should include basic cardiac life support (BCLS) (CPR steps A, B and C without equipment) plus basic trauma life support (BTLS). This combination is essentially eight steps (Fig. 60): (1) control of external hemorrhage by compression and elevation; (2) positioning of the conscious victim in shock (horizontal, legs up); (3) opening the airway of the unconscious victim by head-tilt, jaw-thrust and mouth-open; (4) clearing mouth and pharynx manually; (5) rescue breathing by mouth-to-mouth (nose); (6) determining carotid pulselessness and performing external CPR-BLS; (7) positioning the unconscious, adequately breathing victim on his/her side, with the head tilted backward; and (8) moving the victim to safety by rescue pull, with head, neck and chest supported in the aligned position.

Trauma-oriented CPCR includes 'basic trauma life support' (BTLS = LSFA above) and 'advanced trauma life support' (ATLS), as it is taught, for example, by the American College of Surgeons[22b]. We consider as 'trauma-oriented CPCR' the Steps A–I (Fig. 2; Table 1) with several differences in emphases. For Step A, maximal backward tilt of the head is changed to moderate backward tilt, with jaw-thrust and open mouth added, to avoid adding possible cervical spinal cord injury; in head-injured patients, tracheal intubation must avoid coughing and straining. For Step B, oxygenation is more often needed than artificial ventilation, since apnea is rare in trauma, while hypoxemia is common. Chest injury requires one to consider the constant risks of airway obstruction, tension pneumothorax, open pneumothorax, massive hemothorax, flail chest, and cardiac injury and tamponade. For Step C, control of hemorrhage is most important, while cardiac (chest) compressions in the exsanguinated person are useless without massive i.v. infusions. For step D, fluids are more important than drugs, utilizing large-bore i.v. lifelines and other measures for treating traumatic hypovolemic shock. Steps E and F must be available for trauma cases, but are rarely needed except for cases of chest injury. Phase III is of paramount importance in ATLS, particularly after polytrauma including head and chest injury.

ATLS procedures include use of military (medical) antishock trousers (MAST), tracheal intubation, and percutaneous invasive methods such as i.v. infusions, cricothyrotomy, pleural drainage and pericardial drainage— all to be performed by physicians. Several ATLS measures are considered by some to be suitable for performance by specially trained paramedics. Resuscitative surgery for control of intracranial hematoma or exsanguinating intrathoracic or intra-abdominal hemorrhage requires an experienced surgical (physician) trauma team and hospital or mobile operating room. Airway obstruction, exsanguinating external and internal hemorrhage and potentially noncrippling brain injury are the principal causes of preventable mortality from trauma. Rapid surgical control of intracranial, intrathoracic and intra-abdominal hemorrhage requires skillfully rapidly employed surgical procedures. Resuscitative anesthesia and surgery are presently not considered as part of ATLS, but rather as definitive surgical care in hospitals. We recommend that emergency thoracotomy and recognition and drainage of an epidural hematoma be included in ATLS courses for physicians.

American Heart Association CPR Standards of 1985

The above summarized Phases and Steps A–I (Table 1, Fig. 2) include and go beyond the 1985 American Heart Association (AHA) standards. The latter[23a, b] represent the following changes over the AHA standards of 1980[606, 660, 734].

For *basic life support* (BLS), backward tilt of the head by chin support is favored over neck lift, although the latter remains acceptable. The triple airway maneuver (moderate backward tilt of the head, plus mouth open, plus jaw-thrust) is stressed, particularly for victims of trauma, in whom maximal backward tilt of the head is warned against. The only CPR Steps ABC combination to be taught to laymen is the one rescuer technique—two lung inflations alternated with 15 sternal compressions (2:15 ratio), with compressions at a rate of 80–100 per minute. The two rescuer technique should not be taught to laymen, but should be taught (in addition to the one rescuer technique) to health professionals. It should start with two lung inflations. This should be followed by a compression:ventilation ratio of 5:1, with a brief pause for every ventilation after every fifth sternal compression. Each inflation should take 1–2 seconds, to minimize high airway pressures which can inflate the stomach. Passive exhalations should be complete. Health professionals may be taught cricoid pressure to counteract gastric insufflation. Back blows have been eliminated and the abdominal thrusts (Heimlich maneuver) have been recommended by the AHA as the principle measure for treating acute asphyxiation from foreign body obstruction. (See Chapter 1A/4 for opposing international recommendations, which retain back blows and finger sweeps, and place less confidence in abdominal thrusts.) The AHA further stresses the near-zero risk of transmitting AIDS, hepatitis, or herpes by mouth-to-mouth manikin practice, or actual performance on victims. Details on manikin hygiene are included in the standards. First responders and health professionals are encouraged to use exhaled air ventilation adjuncts (e.g. masks, airways).

For *advanced life support* (ALS), the 1985 AHA standards stress early defibrillation by emergency medical technicians. Automatic external defibrillation is recommended for clinical trials. Several new drugs have been described. Calcium and isoproterenol have been essentially eliminated from the recommendations. Epinephrine remains the most important resuscitation drug. The value of intratracheal administration of epinephrine has been re-emphasized. Sodium bicarbonate i.v. should not be used routinely, and in cases of prolonged arrest should be used sparingly, to avoid severe alkalemia and transient hypercarbia during the low flow state of CPR. Sodium bicarbonate is recommended, however, as needed (and if possible titrated according to arterial pH and base deficit), to counteract the profound acidemia early after restoration of spontaneous circulation, when massive washout of acid occurs; this should be combined with controlled hyperventilation. The venous lifeline should be via arm or central venous catheter, rather than via leg vein. Hypothermic cardiac arrest and resuscitation in children and neonates are treated with special considerations. For *prolonged life support* (PLS) with cerebral resuscitation, there are no new recommendations or guidelines except for brain-oriented intensive care life support control of some key extracerebral variables. These topics are treated extensively in the international guidelines of this book and in the literature[759].

PHASE I:

BASIC LIFE SUPPORT
Emergency Oxygenation

Chapter 1A

Step A: Airway Control

Cause of Airway Obstruction

The most common site of airway obstruction in comatose patients is hypopharyngeal, occurring when the relaxed tongue and neck muscles fail to lift the base of the tongue and epiglottis from the posterior pharyngeal wall, when the patient's head is in the flexed or mid-position (Fig. 3-A)[704]. Holding the head tilted backward is therefore the most important first measure in resuscitation, since this maneuver stretches the anterior neck structures and thereby lifts the base of the tongue from the posterior pharyngeal wall[561, 704–706] and the epiglottis from the laryngeal entrance[94]. Sometimes additional forward displacement of the mandible[233, 333] is required to produce this stretch, particularly when nasal obstruction necessitates opening of the mouth, which in turn reduces the stretch on anterior neck structures. The combination of backward tilt of the head, forward displacement of the mandible and opening of the mouth constitutes the 'triple airway maneuver'[561, 704, 732], also known as the 'jaw-thrust maneuver'. In about one-third of unconscious patients the nasal passage is obstructed during exhalation, because of a valve-like behavior of the soft palate[705, 718]. Moreover, the nose may be blocked by congestion, blood or mucus. Inspiratory efforts may suck the base of the tongue[310] and the epiglottis[94, 772] into obstructing positions. Airway obstruction by the base of the tongue depends on the position of the head and jaw and can occur regardless of whether the patient is lateral, supine or prone[34, 704]. Although gravity may aid in the drainage of liquid foreign matter, it does not relieve hypopharyngeal soft tissue obstruction, and backward tilt of the head or jaw-thrust or both are required.

Another cause of airway obstruction is the presence in the upper airway of foreign matter such as vomitus or blood, which the unconscious patient cannot eliminate by swallowing or coughing. Laryngospasm is usually caused by upper airway stimulation in the stuporous or lightly comatose patient. The larynx can close actively through spasm, or passively like a ball valve[240]. Lower airway obstruction may be the result of bronchospasm, bronchial secretions, mucosal edema, and inhaled gastric contents or foreign matter.

Airway obstruction may be complete or partial. Complete obstruction is silent and leads to asphyxia (hypoxemia plus hypercarbia), apnea and cardiac arrest (if not corrected) within 5–10 minutes. Partial obstruction is noisy and must also be promptly corrected as it can result in cerebral or pulmonary edema, exhaustion, secondary apnea, cardiac arrest and hypoxic brain damage.

Recognition of Airway Obstruction

Complete airway obstruction is recognized when one cannot hear or feel air flow at the mouth or nose. When there are spontaneous breathing movements, the presence of inspiratory retraction of supraclavicular and intercostal areas and absent chest expansion with inhalations provide additional clues. During apnea, when such spontaneous breathing movements are absent, *complete* airway obstruction can be recognized by the difficulty encountered in inflating the lungs when attempting to ventilate the patient with positive pressure. *Partial* airway obstruction is recognized by noisy air flow, which, during spontaneous breathing, may be accompanied by retraction of the intercostal muscles and suprasternal area. *Snoring* suggests that the partial obstruction is hypopharyngeal, due to the base of the tongue; *crowing* suggests laryngospasm; *gurgling* points to the presence of foreign matter; and *wheezing* signals bronchial narrowing.

The immediate sequelae of airway obstruction may also be suspected on clinical grounds. Hypercarbia, for example, is suspected when there is somnolence and is confirmed by measurement of increased arterial PCO_2. Hypoxemia is suspected when there is tachycardia, restlessness, sweating or cyanosis, and is confirmed by measurement of decreased arterial PO_2. Absence of cyanosis, however, does not rule out severe hypoxemia. Needless to say, during acute airway obstruction, attempts at clearing the airway and reoxygenation have absolute priority over arterial blood gas determinations.

Emergency Airway Control Measures (Table 1)

Emergency oxygenation of the nonintubated patient is an art that is best acquired through guided clinical experience. Measures for emergency airway control are being improved continuously. Nonetheless, those described here have withstood the test of time. These measures should be practiced to perfection on manikins; it is then desirable to also practice on unconscious (anesthetized) patients under the direction of an experienced anesthesiologist. Recognition of acute airway obstruction must go hand in hand with therapeutic action, step by step. The airway control measures (Table 1) are intended primarily for the *unconscious* patient whose treatment requires rapid stepwise progression until the obstruction is controlled. Airway control measures 4, 5, 8 and 10 (Table 1) may also be required for selected *conscious* patients.

1) Backward tilt of head[704] (Fig. 3)

If the victim is unconscious, backward tilt of the head, forward displacement of the mandible, or both, prevents hypopharyngeal obstruction by the base of the tongue (Figs 3–5)[704]. Chin support (chin lift) (Fig. 3-B)[222, 310, 689, 704] is to prevent sagging of the chin and to maintain the mouth slightly open. Chin support does not displace the mandible forward, as does jaw thrust. Head-tilt by chin support (Fig. 3-B) may be used interchangeably with head-tilt by neck lift (Fig. 3-C), both methods being acceptable[562, 689]. If only one method is taught to the lay public, head-tilt by chin support is preferred. If with head-tilt alone airway obstruction persists, the mandible should be displaced forward (jaw-thrust) and the mouth held slightly open (triple airway maneuver) (Fig. 6).

In the trauma victim, moving the cervical spine may add injury to the spinal cord. Do not turn the trauma victim's head to the side, do not flex it (bend the neck forward) and do not maximally tilt the head backward. Instead, use moderate backward tilt of the head, ask an assistant to maintain in-line traction on the head and if necessary add jaw-thrust and open the mouth. Airway maintenance takes precedence over cervical trauma.

If dentures are firmly in place, leave them in position, as they maintain the contour of the mouth and make artificial ventilation somewhat easier; if they are loose, remove them.

Technique of head-tilt (Fig. 3)

If you suspect that the victim is *unconscious*—

Establish his/her unresponsiveness (tap or gently shake the victim and shout).

Tilt the head backward maximally, using chin support (chin lift) (Fig. 3-B). With one hand at the forehead apply firm backward pressure to tilt the head backward, and with the fingers of your other hand support the chin to provide stretch of the anterior neck structures, but at the same time keeping the mouth slightly open. Do not compress the neck under the chin, as this may cause obstruction.

As an alternative method, use head-tilt by neck lift, i.e. with one hand under the neck and the other at the forehead (Fig. 3-C). This usually results in slight opening of the mouth, but may cause sagging of the chin.

If you suspect neck trauma, tilt the head backward only moderately and add jaw-thrust and open the mouth if necessary (Fig. 6).

Call for help. Stay with the patient.

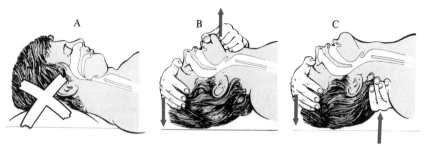

Fig. 3. Backward tilt of head. (A) In the comatose patient, with head in mid-position or flexed, there is hypopharyngeal obstruction by the tongue and laryngeal obstruction by the epiglottis. (B, C) Backward tilt of the head stretches anterior neck structures and lifts the base of the tongue off the posterior pharyngeal wall and the epiglottis off the larynx entrance. (B) Head tilt by chin support (chin lift) maneuver (preferred method). Stretch the neck and hold the mouth slightly open. (C) Head tilt by neck lift maneuver (alternative method).

Fig. 4. Positioning of the unconscious patient. (A) If in need of resuscitation, use supported supine (face-up) position with head–neck–chest aligned. (B) If not in need of resuscitation (breathing spontaneously), use stable side position.
(A) Supported supine aligned position—for resuscitation. Hold the head, neck and chest aligned with slight traction. With both your hands at the sides of the face, provide moderate backward tilt of the head and jaw-thrust and open the mouth. Prevent flexion and rotation of the head.

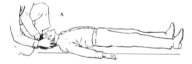

(B) Stable side position—for spontaneously breathing unconscious patient.

(1) Flex the leg closest to you.

(2) Put the hand closest to you under the buttocks.

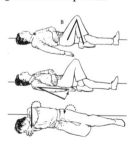

(3) Gently roll onto his/her side.

(4) Tilt the head backward and keep the face low. Put the upper hand under the lower cheek to maintain head-tilt and to prevent the patient from rolling onto his/her face. The lower arm behind the back prevents him/her from rolling backward.

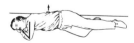

Positioning (Fig. 4)

The unconscious patient should be placed horizontally, supine (face up) as long as he/she needs resuscitation. Only when clearing the airway is required may transient head-down tilt be used for gravity drainage of liquid foreign matter. Avoid the prone (face-down) position, because it makes the face inaccessible, produces mechanical obstruction and reduces thoracic[704, 707] and pulmonary[791] compliance. When the unconscious patient is breathing adequately, the stable side position is preferred, particularly when the head cannot be continuously held and airway control provided by a rescuer on a 1:1 basis, as in mass casualties. Some teach the stable side position as the first step after having determined unconsciousness, for airway clearing, to be followed by turning supine (face up) if artificial ventilation is needed.

Techniques for positioning (Fig. 4)

If the victim is comatose and not breathing adequately—

Place him/her in the 'supported supine aligned position' and position yourself first at the top of the head (vertex) (Fig. 4-A).
Elevate the shoulders slightly by a pillow or folded towel to facilitate holding the head tilted backward. Do not place a pillow under the unsupported head of an unconscious patient, as it flexes the neck forward, causing hypopharyngeal obstruction (except when the trachea is intubated).

If you suspect neck trauma—

Hold the patient's head, neck and chest aligned and provide only moderate (not maximal) backward tilt (Fig. 4-A). Add jaw thrust and open the mouth if necessary (Fig. 6). Do not turn the head laterally. Do not flex the head forward. When he/she must be turned in order to clear the airway, hold the head–neck–chest aligned while another rescuer turns him/her.

If the victim is comatose and *breathing adequately* spontaneously—

Place him/her in the 'stable side position' with the head tilted backward and the mouth slightly downward to promote gravity drainage of liquid foreign matter from the mouth (Fig. 4-B). Support the head when you turn him/her, so as not to aggravate a cervical spine injury. Some teach the stable side position as the first step after having determined unconsciousness, for airway clearing, to be followed by turning supine if artificial ventilation is needed.

2) Positive pressure inflation attempts (Fig. 5)[220, 699, 921]

Emergency ventilation and oxygenation attempts in the unconscious patient should start with backward tilt of the head (and in addition, if necessary, jaw thrust and opening of the mouth). If the airway remains obstructed—with or without spontaneous breathing efforts evident—add positive pressure inflation attempts (Chapter 1B).

For the first few inflations, positive end-expiratory pressure (PEEP) (staircase ventilation) is no longer recommended, as the need for it has not been documented, a sustained rise in intrathoracic pressure can stop a feebly beating heart and pharyngeal pressures which exceed 20–25 cm H_2O can insufflate the stomach[630] and thereby promote regurgitation. Therefore, ventilation of the nonintubated patient should be done with moderate airway pressure and inflation rate[528].

In the relaxed comatose patient, a helper may counteract gastric insufflation and regurgitation by holding the cricoid cartilage of the larynx pressed backward to occlude the esophagus. Cricoid pressure[403, 763, 785, 855] is presently recommended only for use by trained health professionals, not by lay people, as knowledge of anatomy is needed to perform it safely. When high inflation pressures are needed, tracheal intubation is desirable (see below).

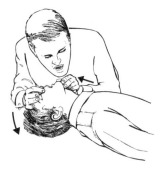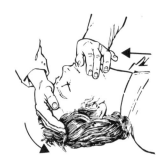

Fig. 5. Techniques for backward tilt of the head. Backward tilt of the head by chin support, plus positive pressure inflation with mouth-to-mouth (left) or mouth-to-nose (right) exhaled air inflations. During mouth-to-nose ventilation, close the mouth for each inflation and slightly open the mouth for each exhalation.

Techniques of inflation attempts (Fig. 5)

If the victim is unconscious, tilt his/her head backward. If you cannot *hear* and *feel* air flow at the mouth or nose or cannot see the chest rise—
   Assess airway patency by lung inflation attempts with intermittent positive pressure ventilation (IPPV).
   Use exhaled air (e.g. mouth-to-mouth, mouth-to-nose, mouth-to-adjunct) (Fig. 5); air (e.g. self-refilling bag–valve–mask unit); or oxygen-enriched air (e.g. mouth-to-mask with oxygen, bag–valve–mask with oxygen). Inflate slowly (1–2 seconds per inflation). Try to overcome airway obstruction and lung–chest resistance. The chest must rise with each inflation attempt. When it rises, let the victim exhale passively. Adapt inflation patterns (pressure, volume, rate and rhythm) to airway–lung–chest resistances, gas leaks and the victim's own breathing efforts.
   Initiate ventilation with two inflations. If apnea continues, control ventilation with about one inflation every 5 seconds in adults and large children, one every 3 seconds in small children and infants.
   If he/she shows spontaneous breathing movements, assist (augment) ventilation by intermittent positive pressure breathing (IPPB) (i.e. assisted ventilation, AV); or by intermittent mandatory ventilation (IMV). After tracheal intubation, continuous positive pressure ventilation (CPPV) may be indicated (Chapter 1B).

3) Triple airway maneuver (head-tilt, mouth open, jaw-thrust)[562, 704, 732] (Fig. 6)

In about 20% of unconscious patients, backward tilting of the head is not by itself sufficient to open the air passage[718]. In such circumstances, additional forward displacement of the mandible[233, 333] can establish a patent airway[224a, 704, 718]. Even using these two maneuvers together, expiratory nasopharyngeal obstruction may occur in about 30% of unconscious patients when the mouth is closed[718]. For this reason, the mouth should be held slightly open, i.e. the lower lip retracted. In this regard, it is important to note that when the mouth is wide open some stretch of the neck is lost, with consequent return of partial or complete hypopharyngeal obstruction. The necessary degree of stretch can, however, be regained by forward displacement of the mandible (jaw thrust)[562, 704]. The foregoing observations led to the development of the 'triple airway maneuver'—the combination of: (1) backward tilt of the head; (2) opening of the mouth; and (3) forward displacement of the mandible (jaw-thrust)—as the ideal manual method for producing supralaryngeal upper airway patency[704] (Fig. 6). Despite the fact that this maneuver is technically difficult, studies have shown that it can be taught to and mastered by lay personnel[107, 234, 744].

This procedure is mildly painful and, for that reason, not only provides a patent airway but also serves as a useful test for the depth of unconsciousness and arouses protective airway reflexes in the lightly comatose patient. The patient who makes no purposeful response to the maneuver can safely be assumed to be in coma. In patients with suspected neck injury, *maximal* backward tilt of the head might aggravate a spinal cord injury. (Flexion and rotation of the head are absolutely contraindicated.) In such cases, *moderate* backward tilt of the head plus open mouth plus jaw-thrust (triple airway maneuver) is the best method of airway control, short of endotracheal intubation.

Backward tilt of the head, jaw thrust and opening of the mouth can be practiced on manikins, anesthetized or comatose patients, and coworkers.

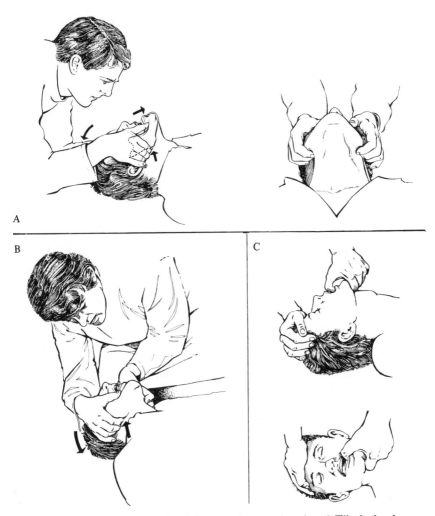

Fig. 6. Triple airway maneuver (head tilt + mouth open + jaw thrust) Tilt the head backward, open the mouth (and keep it open), and displace the mandible forward. (A) With the operator at the patient's vertex, for spontaneously breathing patient. See text. (B) With the operator at the side of the patient, for direct mouth-to-mouth ventilation. Seal the nose with your cheek for mouth-to-mouth breathing. Seal the mouth with your other cheek for mouth-to-nose breathing. (C) Modified triple airway maneuver by thumb-jaw lift method (for a relaxed patient only).

Technique of triple airway (jaw-thrust) maneuver (Fig. 6)

If the victim is *unconscious* and not breathing adequately with backward tilt of the head alone (or when apneic, not easily ventilated with head-tilt alone)—

Add jaw-thrust and slight opening of the mouth.

Grasp the ascending rami of the mandible in front of the ear lobes, using fingers 2–5 (or 2–4) of both hands and pull forcibly upwards (forwards), displacing the mandible so that the lower teeth jut out in front of the upper teeth (two-handed jaw lift; jaw-thrust). Retract the lower lip with your thumbs. Do not grasp the horizontal ramus of the mandible as this may close the mouth.

If the victim is breathing spontaneously, position yourself at the vertex (Fig. 6-A).

If he/she is hypoventilating or not breathing and you intend to use mouth-to-mouth ventilation, position yourself at the side of the head (Fig. 6-B). Readjust your hands to a comfortable position (e.g. your elbows resting on the ground). Encircle the mouth widely with your lips, and occlude the nose with your cheek when blowing. For mouth-to-nose ventilation, encircle the nose with your lips, and occlude the mouth with your other cheek or your thumb.

If he/she is relaxed, you can also provide head-tilt plus open mouth plus jaw thrust effectively by displacing the mandible forward with your thumb in the mouth (thumb jaw lift) (Fig. 6-C). Do not use this method if the patient is responsive, as he/she may bite your thumb. During mouth-to-mouth breathing, blow while sealing your lips around your thumb and the mouth.

4) Manual clearing of the airway[700, 720] (Fig. 7)

When positive pressure inflation attempts meet obstruction in spite of having tried repositioning backward tilt of the head, opening of the mouth and jaw-thrust—or when vomit or other foreign matter appears in the mouth—you should suspect upper airway obstruction by foreign matter. This calls for forcing open the mouth (Fig. 7-A) and clearing foreign material from the mouth and pharynx by finger sweep (Fig. 7), back blows and abdominal or chest thrusts (Figs. 8–10), until suctioning (Fig. 11) and pharyngolaryngoscopy, suctioning and extraction under vision, and tracheal intubation are possible.

Techniques of manual airway clearing (Fig. 7)

If you suspect foreign matter in the mouth or throat and cannot ventilate the lungs—

Force the mouth open, using one of the following three maneuvers:

1. The 'crossed-finger maneuver' (Fig. 7-A) for the moderately relaxed jaw[700, 720]. Position yourself at the top or the side of the patient's head. Insert your index finger into the corner of the mouth, and press your index finger against the upper teeth; then press your thumb, crossed over your index finger, against the lower teeth, thereby forcing the mouth open. To leave ample room for instrumentation, be sure to insert your fingers into the far corner of the patient's mouth.
2. The 'finger behind teeth maneuver' (Fig. 7-B) for the tight jaw[697]. Insert one index finger between the patient's cheek and teeth and wedge the tip of your index finger behind the last molar teeth.
3. The 'tongue–jaw–lift maneuver' (Fig. 7-C) for the fully relaxed jaw[291]. Insert your thumb into the patient's mouth and throat, and with the tip of your thumb lift the base of the tongue. The other fingers grasp the mandible at the chin and lift anteriorly.

The above maneuvers for forcing the mouth open may also be needed for suctioning, or insertion of airway or laryngoscope.

Sweep one or two *fingers* (perhaps covered with a piece of cloth) through the mouth and pharynx for clearing (Fig. 7-A). Wipe out liquid foreign matter with the index and middle fingers. Try to extract solid foreign matter from the pharynx with your hooked index finger or using your index plus middle fingers like tweezers (Fig. 7-C).

Drain liquid foreign matter by turning the head to the side. In accident victims, turning the head to the side or flexing it forward must be avoided since this may aggravate a spinal cord injury. If head turning is necessary in accident victims, the entire patient should be turned as a unit, with an assistant holding the head, neck and chest in alignment (Fig. 4).

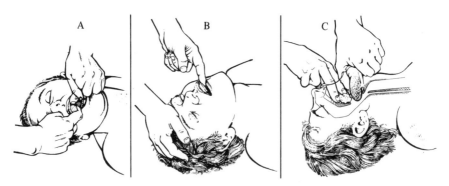

Fig. 7. Three methods to force the mouth open for clearing, finger sweeping, suctioning and inserting of airways or laryngoscope: (A) 'crossed-finger' maneuver for the moderately relaxed jaw; (B) 'finger behind teeth' maneuver for the tight jaw; (C) 'tongue-jaw-lift' maneuver for the very relaxed jaw.

Thrusts and back blows for foreign body obstruction[23b, 183, 183a, 290, 311, 334, 335, 658, 691] (Figs. 8–10)

Finger sweeping (Fig. 7) should be tried first when upper airway obstruction by *liquid* or semi-solid matter is suspected at any time during resuscitation of the patient without tracheal tube. In witnessed inhalation of *solid* foreign matter (e.g. food), however, thrusts and blows are recommended first (in conscious patients) and in addition to finger sweep (in unconscious patients).

Thrusts and back blows are controversial techniques[23b, 658]. The estimated death rate from inhaled or swallowed objects in the USA is 3000 cases per year, but the incidence seems less in other countries. Since few of these cases have had autopsy proof of foreign body obstruction, sudden cardiac death may be the cause of many of these deaths. True foreign body obstruction occurs particularly with food during meals (café coronary)[328]. The obstructing inhaled object which the patient cannot spit out is impacted in the hypopharynx over the laryngeal entrance. Objects which have entered through the larynx into the tracheobronchial tree can cause severe symptoms, but rarely complete airway obstruction, since the major bronchi are wider than the larynx entrance.

In witnessed foreign body aspiration, when the patient is *conscious* and *partially* obstructed (can talk), he/she should be encouraged to take deep breaths and cough and spit it out. Digital probing, thrusts and back blows should be avoided, as such maneuvers may aggravate the obstruction. The patient should be entered into the EMS system and taken rapidly to the nearest hospital or physician by ambulance, with oxygen inhalation en route.

In witnessed foreign body aspiration, when the patient is *conscious* or unconscious, but *completely* obstructed, with cyanosis, ineffective cough, or unable to talk or cough, any possibly effective measure is justified as an act of desperation. No single method should be taught to the exclusion of others. Sudden complete obstruction can cause unconsciousness from hypoxemia within 1–2 minutes.

Severe foreign body obstruction is *suspected*: (1) in the *conscious* patient who is suddenly unable to speak, breathe or cough and/or uses the distress signal for choking (i.e. clutching his neck) (Fig. 8); (2) in the *unconscious* patient when in spite of upper airway control the lungs cannot be inflated; and (3) when foreign body inhalation has been witnessed.

The most effective and *definitive* methods for relieving airway obstruction due to aspiration of foreign material require adjunctive equipment and special training: (1) use of a laryngoscope or tongue blade and flashlight for visualization of the mouth, pharynx and larynx entrance; (2) extraction of the foreign material under direct vision by Kelly clamp, Magill forceps or suction; and (3) if complete obstruction persists, endotracheal intubation (Figs. 14–16), cricothyrotomy (Fig. 17), or translaryngeal jet insufflation (Fig. 18). Such equipment should be employed only by health care professionals trained in its use.

Blind extraction attempts with instruments are hazardous. There are no data to support the use of devices for foreign body extraction without visualization, such as the 'Choke Saver' or 'Throat-E-Vac'.

For use by *lay personnel* in cases of solid foreign material obstruction, abdominal thrusts[334, 335], chest thrusts[311] and back blows[290] have been recommended for some time, in attempts to loosen the object impacted in the upper airway. Data about all these indirect maneuvers are controversial and mainly anecdotal[334, 335, 658].

Subdiaphragmatic abdominal thrusts, also called the Heimlich maneuver, have been promoted by the originator[334, 335] and others[615]. The American Heart Association and the American Red Cross have not only added it to the sequence for treatment of foreign body obstruction but also replaced back blows with abdominal thrusts[25]. In contrast, the League of Red Cross Societies and the World Federation of Societies of Anaesthesiologists guidelines do not recommend teaching the Heimlich maneuver because of its dubious efficacy and notable risks[126]. Recommendations are based mainly on anecdotal evidence from conscious patients with sudden complete foreign body obstruction who ejected the foreign body (maybe spontaneously) when abdominal thrusts were used[334, 335, 615]. There is also anecdotal evidence of failures with this technique[658], and evidence of possible complications caused by it, such as gastric rupture[172, 922], pneumomediastinum, aortic injury[141], liver rupture[658, 889], other injuries[607] and regurgitation[658].

The rationale for the use of subdiaphragmatic abdominal thrust is that it pushes the diaphragm upward and thereby creates an artificial cough to expel an obstructing foreign body. Physiologic evidence indicates that abdominal thrusts produce very weak increases in airway pressure when the airway is closed and very low airflow rates when the airway is open[290, 691].

In summary, neither abdominal thrusts nor chest thrusts nor back blows produce pressures or flows as effective as those created by natural cough[290, 311, 691]. This difference may be accentuated in the choking patient who obstructs, after a coughing spell, with a low residual lung volume.

Chest thrusts, which are essentially the same as external cardiac compressions, may be safer in the unconscious patient. Chest thrusts may induce ventricular fibrillation in the beating but hypoxic heart. They likewise produce pressures and flows lower than those produced by active coughing[311].

Back blows produce higher airway pressures than thrusts when the airway is closed[290], but might either loosen the object[290] or impact it further into the standing or sitting victim[183a, b].

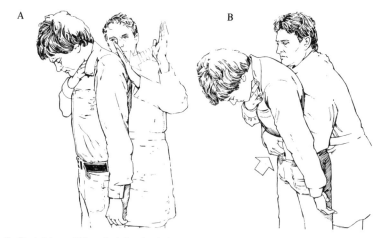

Fig. 8. Back blows (A) and abdominal thrusts (B) for complete foreign body obstruction in the *conscious* standing or sitting victim. For back blows deliver a series of 3–5 sharp blows with the heel of your hand over the victim's spine between the shoulder blades. If possible lower the head below the chest to utilize gravity. For abdominal thrusts observe the choking signal (victim clutching neck). Ask the victim to cough and spit it out. Apply abdominal thrusts by standing behind the victim. Wrap your arms around his/her waist, make a fist with one hand, place the thumb side of your fist against the abdomen in the midline slightly above the navel, below the xiphoid process. Grasp your fist with your other hand. Press your fist into the abdomen with a quick upward thrust. Repeat thrusts, each being a distinct, separate movement.

In advanced pregnancy or marked obesity, use chest thrusts (not shown). Stand behind the victim, encircle the chest, place the thumb side of your fist on the middle of the sternum, avoiding the xiphoid process and ribs. Grab your fist with your other hand and perform backward thrusts.

Be prepared to catch the victim when he/she collapses. If this occurs, gently lower him/her to the floor and put him/her horizontal, face up. Continue as shown in Fig. 9.

Because of the uncertainties about back blows and the need for simplicity in teaching, the American Heart Association decided in 1986 not to teach them any more[23b]. The League of Red Cross Societies decided to teach them[126]. Because anything is worth trying in a degenerating situation, we (WFSA) suggest teaching any improvised sequence of finger sweep, abdominal or chest thrusts, back blows, ventilation attempts, finger sweep, etc.! The American Heart Association does recommend back blows for infants and small children.

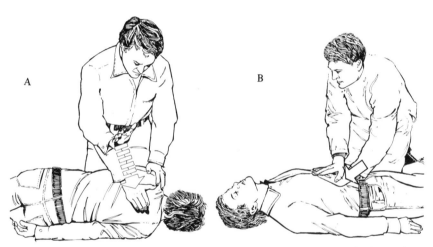

Fig. 9. Back blows (A) and abdominal thrusts (B) for complete foreign body obstruction in the *unconscious*, lying (horizontal) victim. For back blows roll the victim on his/her side facing you, with the chest against your knees; deliver 3–5 sharp blows with the heel of your hand over the victim's spine, between the shoulder blades. For abdominal thrusts, if the victim is unconscious and you suspect foreign body obstruction, place him/her supine, horizontal, face up. Use finger sweep, trying to remove the foreign object manually (Fig. 7) and try to ventilate. If unsuccessful, apply subdiaphragmatic abdominal thrusts. Kneel at the side of the abdomen or straddling it (astride the thighs). Place the heel of one hand against the abdomen, in the midline, slightly above the navel and below the xiphoid process. Place your second hand directly on top of your first hand. Press into the abdomen with a quick upward thrust in the midline. Do not press to the right or left of the midline.

In advanced pregnancy, marked obesity, infants and small children, use chest thrusts (not shown). These are performed like external cardiac compressions, i.e., in the adult, with the heel of the hand on the lower half of the sternum.

Perform up to 6–10 abdominal (or chest) thrusts, followed by finger sweep and ventilation attempt; and repeat 6–10 thrusts, etc., until you can ventilate him/her or a helper arrives who is trained and equipped to extract the foreign body under direct vision.

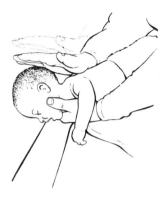

Fig. 10. Back blows in infants and small children. Hold the child face down, supporting chin and neck with your knee and one hand, and apply gentle back blows between the shoulder blades. For chest thrusts (not shown), place the child face up on your forearm, lower the head, and apply chest thrusts gently with two fingers, as in external cardiac compressions. If the child's airway is only partially obstructed and he/she is conscious and able to breathe in the upright position, do not turn him/her head down. *Do not* use abdominal thrusts in infants and small children.

Techniques for foreign body clearing (Figs. 8–10)

The *sequences* recommended by the authors for use in victims with suspected foreign body obstruction are as follows:

(1) If the victim is *conscious*, ask if he/she is choking, and encourage him/her to expel the foreign body by coughing and spitting it out. Apply abdominal thrusts until the foreign body is expelled or the patient becomes unconscious.

(2) If the victim is *unconscious*, place him/her in a horizontal position. If you suspect a foreign body, force the mouth open and perform the finger sweep (manual clearing of mouth and pharynx) (Fig. 7). Then attempt to ventilate the lungs. Slow forceful inflations can often force air around the foreign body. During ventilation attempts, try to alleviate the obstruction by widening the hypopharynx with jaw thrust.

If unable to ventilate, perform up to 6–10 abdominal or chest thrusts, followed by finger sweep and ventilation attempts. If unsuccessful, turn the patient on his/her side and try 3–5 back blows, followed by finger sweep and ventilation attempts. If unsuccessful, again try abdominal thrusts–sweep–ventilate–back blows–sweep–ventilate, as long as necessary.

Ask a second person to activate the EMS system. Call trained personnel with laryngoscope, forceps and suction for extraction of the foreign body under direct vision (Figs. 14–16).

If the patient can be ventilated and is pulseless, add chest compressions (CPR).

In infants and small children, the markedly obese or pregnant women, do *not* use abdominal thrusts and back blows. Use chest thrusts performed like external heart compressions.

As a final measure, use tracheal intubation, cricothyrotomy (Fig. 17) or translaryngeal oxygen jet insufflation (Fig. 18), if you are a trained health professional and equipment is available.

5) Clearing the airway by suction[679] (Fig. 11)

Suction has not been listed together with manual clearing because it requires equipment. Suction devices include a vacuum source, a yoke with a control valve, a nonbreakable collection bottle, a large-bore, nonkinking connecting tube, sterile suction tips and catheters of various sizes, water for rinsing and a suction trap (Fig. 11). Wall suction or portable suction pumps used for pharyngeal suctioning should be powerful enough to clear semisolid foreign matter. Ideally, it should produce a negative gauge pressure of at least 300 mmHg when the tube is occluded, and air flow of at least 30 l/min when the tube is open[679]. Less vacuum is required for tracheobronchial suction in adults and even less for pharyngeal and tracheobronchial suction in children and infants. For tracheobronchial suction, the vacuum should be variable to avoid lung injury and asphyxia from lung collapse.

Blind nasotracheal suction attempts in the nonintubated conscious patient call for the sitting sniffing position with raised occiput, head tilted backward and leaning forward. After topical anesthesia of the nasal passage, a well lubricated, curved-tip catheter is inserted during a deep inhalation, while the tongue is pulled forward with a piece of dry gauze. This technique is safe only in the cooperative patient. In stupor or coma it may produce intractable laryngospasm, vomiting with aspiration, and asphyxial or reflex cardiac arrest.

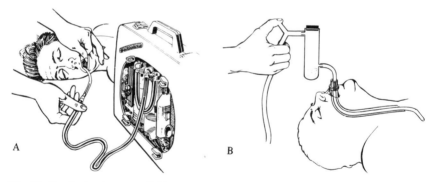

A

B

Fig. 11. Suctioning by controllable wall suction or portable suction (A) of oropharynx with rigid tonsil suction tip; (B) of nasopharynx or tracheobronchial tree with curved-tip soft catheter. (B) also shows suction trap for collection of suctioned material for examination. Finger tip on–off control of pharyngeal suction tip (A: thumb on orifice) and catheter (B: thumb on Y connector).

Technique of suctioning (Fig. 11)

For suction of *mouth and oropharynx* of the unconscious patient, use a tonsil suction device (Fig. 11-A). This is a rigid (metal or plastic) suction tip with multiple holes at the end. Force the mouth open with any of the maneuvers shown in Fig. 7, and sweep the suction tip through the mouth and pharynx. Suction each nostril separately while occluding the other nostril.

For suction of the *tracheobronchial* tree and *nasopharynx*, use a well lubricated, soft, curved-tip catheter (Fig. 11-B). The curved tip permits deliberate insertion into one or other main bronchus, whereas straight catheters usually pass only into the right main bronchus because of its smaller angle to the trachea. Insertion via tracheal or tracheostomy tube into the left main bronchus can also be enhanced by turning the head to the right. Choose a tracheobronchial suction catheter of a diameter which leaves room between the suction catheter and the wall of the tracheal tube through which it is inserted, so that air can enter the lungs during suctioning. Use tracheal suction tubes with a T or Y tube or lateral opening for on–off control. For tracheobronchial and nasal suctioning insert the catheter without suction and withdraw with rotation.

For suction with need for inspection and examination of the suctioned material, use a suction trap (Fig. 11-B). When suctioning the tracheobronchial tree after suspected aspiration, examine the suctioned material's color, consistency and pH (with litmus paper), and send a sample for bacterial smear, culture and antibiotic sensitivity tests.

6) Pharyngeal intubation[698] (Fig. 12)

Nasopharyngeal and oropharyngeal tubes (Guedel), commonly known as 'airways', hold the base of the tongue forward and counter obstruction by the lips and teeth. Thus, they can be substituted for two components of the triple airway maneuver—jaw thrust and opening of the mouth—which are not easily maintained over long periods. Even with a pharyngeal tube in place, however, the third component of the triple airway maneuver— backward tilt of the head—is still required. This is because, with flexion of the neck, the tip of the tube may become partially withdrawn and the base of the tongue is pressed against the posterior pharyngeal wall between the tip of the tube and the laryngeal entrance. An occasional patient may also require jaw-thrust in spite of the pharyngeal tube.

Airways should be inserted into comatose patients only, as these devices may provoke laryngospasm or vomiting in persons with intact upper airway reflexes. Shortened airways, however, can be improvised to serve as mouth props (bite blocks) in conscious or stuporous patients. Nasopharyngeal tubes can cause epistaxis, which can however be minimized by use of a soft tube and correct technique. Advantages of the nasopharyngeal over the oropharyngeal tube also include the ability to insert the tube in patients with trismus or clenched jaws and better tolerance even in the marginally stuporous patient. The oropharyngeal tube provides a wider airway.

With the present fear of becoming infected by the patient's saliva, there may be a recurrence of mouth-to-mouth adjuncts such as the S-tube[698, 699] and masks[220, 729]. New designs should have a valve, which prevents exhaled air from blowing into the rescuer's face, and a nipple for oxygen insufflation.

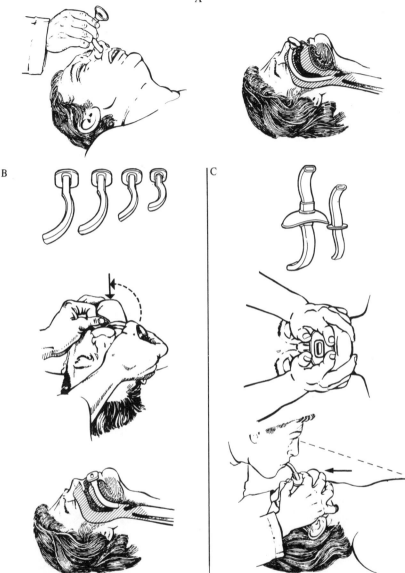

Fig. 12. Nasopharyngeal and oropharyngeal tubes (airways). (A) Nasopharyngeal tube. Insert the well lubricated tube into the patent nasal passage (parallel to palate) until the tip rests in the hypopharynx (indicated by good air flow). (B) Regular oropharyngeal tubes. Insert only if the jaw is moderately relaxed. Force the mouth open and insert the tube *over* the tongue with 180° rotation, without pushing the base of the tongue backward. Preferably use the tongue blade without turning the airway. The tip should lie in the hypopharynx. (C) S-shaped mouth-to-airway oropharyngeal tubes (adult–child size; child–infant size). Insert like a regular oropharyngeal tube. Seal the flange and nose. Tilt the head backward. Inflate the lungs as described in Chapter 1B.

Techniques of pharyngeal tube insertion (Fig. 12)

If head-tilt, open mouth and jaw-thrust (Fig. 6) fail to open the airway, or if long-term jaw-thrust becomes too tedious, insert a pharyngeal tube.

Nasopharyngeal tubes should be of very soft rubber or plastic (Fig. 12-A). Insert the tube (well lubricated, preferably with anesthetic water-soluble lubricant) until you feel the 'give' when the tube passes the posterior wall of the nasopharynx. Then advance the tube until air flow is optimal. Too deep insertion may cause laryngospasm or entry into the upper esophagus. Check the air flow before securing the tube with tape.

Oropharyngeal tubes are of the Guedel type (Fig. 12-B). They come in several sizes (large adult, adult, child, infant, newborn) and are made of rubber, plastic or metal. For resuscitation, at least three sizes (adult, child, infant) should be on hand. For insertion, first force the mouth open with the crossed-finger, tongue-jaw-lift or finger-behind-teeth maneuver (Fig. 7). Then insert the tube over the tongue (Fig. 12-B). This can be accomplished either by first inserting the tube into the mouth with the curve reversed (convexity caudad) and then rotating it into its proper position, or preferably under direct vision by using a tongue blade to lift the base of the tongue while the tube is slid past it. Incorrect placement of an oropharyngeal tube can push the tongue back into the pharynx and produce airway obstruction. Forceful insertion of a pharyngeal tube must also be avoided. Teeth can easily be damaged. Lips should not be caught between the teeth and the tube.

S-tubes are S-shaped mouth-to-airway ventilation adjuncts which can be reversed to provide two sizes each (Fig. 12-C).[698,699] New designs with one-way valves are recommended. Prevent leakage of air with both your thumbs (or thenar eminences) pinching the nose, the tips of both thumbs and index fingers pressing the flange over the mouth, and fingers 2–5 pulling on the ascending rami of the mandible. An alternative method (not shown in Fig. 12) is one hand pinching the nose and your other hand, with its palm pulling the chin up and the head tilted backward, pressing the flange against the lips with the fingers.

7) Esophageal obturator airway insertion[200, 201] (Fig. 13)

The esophageal obturator airway[201] is a tube meant to be passed blindly into the esophagus of relaxed, comatose, apneic patients—by personnel unable to, not permitted to, or not trained to intubate the trachea. The cuff of the esophageal tube is used to prevent gastric regurgitation and reduce gastric insufflation during positive pressure artificial ventilation without endotracheal tube.

The esophageal obturator airway is a large-bore tube, approximately the size of a tracheal tube, with a rounded closed tip distally, a cuff to be inflated in the esophagus, and multiple openings at the hypopharyngeal level through which air or oxygen is delivered by intermittent positive pressure to enter the larynx and trachea, while a face mask prevents leaks through the mouth and nose[201].

A modification, the esophageal gastric tube airway[291] uses the lumen of the tube for insertion of a thinner gastric tube for gastric drainage. It is therefore without openings at the pharyngeal level and provides ventilation through an additional port in the mask, utilizing the natural nasal passage (which may be obstructed). A valve prevents reflux of gastric contents.

Physicians and nurses working in Emergency Departments must be familiar with the esophageal obturator airway and the proper timing and technique of its removal. Experience with this is most easily gained in the operating room during routine extubation after general anesthesia.

The esophageal obturator airway does not in any way provide definitive control over or protection of the airway[38]. Thus, it should not be considered a substitute for endotracheal intubation, but rather viewed as an alternative to a simple mask device. Because its insertion is relatively easy and does not require visualization of the larynx, it has been used by paramedics in large series of cardiac arrest cases outside hospitals[291, 775, 822]. However, its clinical performance is inferior to endotracheal intubation[323, 520, 792]. The main drawbacks to its use are difficulty in providing a tight mask fit, and inability to control laryngospasm, suction of the tracheobronchial tree, or protect the lungs against aspiration of foreign matter or blood from the upper airway.

Complications of esophageal obturator airway insertion have occurred primarily in spontaneously breathing patients who were not deeply comatose. Injuries encountered include esophageal laceration and perforation, asphyxia from inadvertent tracheal intubation (which may occur in up to 10% of cases, but is of no consequence if immediately recognized), and provocation of laryngospasm, vomiting and aspiration[23, 323]. Use of the device should be restricted to adequately trained personnel. For paramedics, endotracheal intubation should be a mandatory skill, and esophageal obturator airway insertion only an optional skill[23, 126].

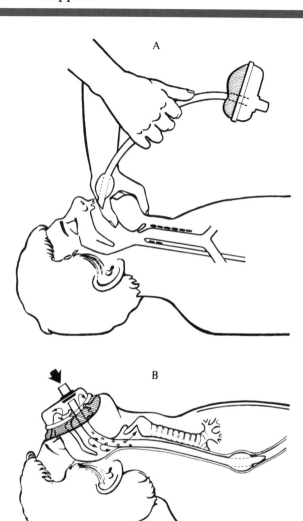

Fig. 13. Esophageal obturator airway, for insertion only into relaxed, comatose apneic adult patients, by personnel unable to perform tracheal intubation. Do not use in comatose spontaneously breathing patients. (A) Blind insertion via the mouth into the esophagus. For insertion keep the neck in the mid-position or slightly flexed and use the tongue–jaw lift maneuver (Fig. 7). Do not use force during insertion. (B) Correct position for intermittent positive pressure ventilation. For ventilation keep the head tilted backward. Leave in place for only a short time. See text.

Technique of esophageal obturator airway insertion (Fig. 13)

Insert an esophageal obturator airway only into the deeply comatose apneic patient, e.g. the patient in cardiac arrest. Its use is contraindicated in children under 16 years, in patients who have swallowed caustic agents, and in patients with any known history of esophageal disease.

Attach the mask to the proximal end of the tube. Open the patient's mouth and hold the mandible and tongue forward with your thumb (Fig. 13-A). Insert the esophageal obturator airway through the patient's mouth into the esophagus while the patient's head is held in mid-position. Confirm correct positioning of the tube and inflate the esophageal cuff. Seal the mask against the patient's face and ventilate by mouth-to-tube or bag–valve unit (Fig. 13-B). During ventilation hold the head tilted backward.

When a patient is delivered to the Emergency Department with an esophageal obturator airway in place and is deeply comatose, intubate the trachea with a cuffed tube *prior* to removal of the esophageal obturator airway. Deflate the esophageal cuff and withdraw the tube. Be prepared to suction regurgitated material which appears immediately upon removal of the esophageal obturator airway.

If the patient is recovering reflexes, leave the esophageal obturator airway in place until he/she is conscious and breathing spontaneously or at least has recovered protective upper airway reflexes, since removal may be followed by massive regurgitation.

Do *not* insert an esophageal obturator airway into the comatose spontaneously breathing patient with *head injury*, as reacting on the tube may cause laryngospasm and active vomiting, and straining can increase intracranial bleeding and pressure. Instead, use the triple airway maneuver (Fig. 6), pharyngeal tube (Fig. 12) and oxygen by mask until tracheal intubation with relaxant, by an expert, is possible.

8) Tracheal intubation (Figs. 14–16, Table 2)

An endotracheal tube can isolate the airway, keep it patent, prevent aspiration, and facilitate ventilation, oxygenation and suctioning. During CPR, since high pharyngeal pressures can cause gastric insufflation and regurgitation, trained personnel should intubate the trachea with a cuffed tube as soon as possible. The person conducting emergency intubation must be highly trained and use intubation frequently or be regularly retrained. Patients with acute intracranial pathology (e.g. head injury) and others with potentially difficult intubation problems when managed in the field by those who are not experts in intubation should receive oxygenation and assisted ventilation by mouth-mask-oxygen or bag-mask-oxygen as long as feasible, since tracheal intubation—the desired ultimate step in the airway management of these cases—must be performed following hyperventilation and without coughing, i.e. if necessary with paralysis by succinylcholine. This difficult technique must be perfected through operating room intubation practice. It is dangerous in the hands of a person who can intubate but is not trained in intubating the paralyzed patient in the anesthesia setting.

The technique of translaryngeal endotracheal intubation by direct laryngoscopy with cuffed tubes, which revolutionized anesthesia and resuscitation, was pioneered by many (see historic introduction to this book). By the 1950s, N.A. Gillespie[274], P. Flagg[243]; V. Apgar (neonatal resuscitation); and D. Leigh, R. Stephen, R. Smith and M. Deming (pediatric endotracheal anesthesia) had helped to bring about modern endotracheal techniques for resuscitation.

In the *unconscious* patient, endotracheal intubation is the definitive means of emergency airway control. It is indicated in most comatose patients unless the upper airway reflexes are intact, coma is expected to be brief in duration and the patient is attended continuously by personnel experienced with airway control in the unintubated patient. As a guide, the patient who tolerates an intubation attempt needs a tracheal tube.

In the *conscious* patient, endotracheal intubation is also indicated when there is: (1) inadequate spontaneous clearing of the tracheobronchial tree; (2) suspected aspiration; (3) absence of laryngeal reflexes; or (4) need for prolonged mechanical ventilation. After 7–10 days, and earlier in selected cases, a switch to tracheotomy should be considered.

Since the 1960s, the introduction of improved cuffs and tubes has minimized laryngotracheal damage[128, 129, 309, 330, 331, 475, 476, 712]. Thus, in comatose patients, tracheotomy may be delayed if extubation is expected to be possible in 1–2 weeks. Selected conscious patients in need of prolonged ventilation, however, may be more comfortable and be given the opportunity to talk if the switch to tracheotomy is performed earlier.

Manual airway control, ventilation and oxygenation attempts without equipment or with simple adjuncts should always precede attempts at tracheal intubation. *During CPR*, however, lung inflations accompanying heart compressions require high pharyngeal pressures which may cause gastric insufflation. This can promote regurgitation and aspiration. Therefore, during CPR, the trachea should be intubated as soon as possible, but only after adequate preoxygenation and without interrupting cardiac compressions for more than 15 seconds at a time. Once the tracheal tube has been inserted, lung inflations do not have to be synchronized with chest compressions. Lung inflations that fall between chest compressions may give better oxygenation; those that fall simultaneously with chest compressions may give better blood flow (Chapter 1C). After *trauma*, in the comatose patient, safe tracheal intubation may require use of a paralyzing drug, and must therefore be performed by skilled personnel (see Rapid sequence intubation, below).

Tracheal intubation may be performed through the mouth or through the nose. Orotracheal intubation under direct vision is preferable in an emergency situation, since it can be accomplished more rapidly and with less trauma than nasotracheal intubation.

Equipment for tracheal intubation (Fig. 14, Table 2)

The equipment needed for laryngoscopy, extraction of foreign bodies and tracheal intubation should be in every prehospital life-support station, ambulance, emergency department and ICU, and in other selected hospital locations (Fig. 14). Details depend on individual preference, but certain basic elements must be present at all locations. Immediate readiness is important. All equipment should be checked daily for patency of tracheal tube, cuffs, adequacy of laryngoscopy batteries, etc.

Most endotracheal tubes as supplied are longer than necessary and should be cut (Table 2-A). The length of tube needed can be estimated by placing it alongside the patient's face and neck, with the bifurcation of the trachea being at the manubriosternal junction. The appropriate tube diameters are critical, particularly in selecting tubes for children (Table 2-A), but can be estimated from the diameter of the child's little finger. For resuscitation trays an assortment from 2.5 to 9 mm inside diameter in 0.5 mm increments is adequate. Most endotracheal tubes have one curve which tends to make the tube press on the posterior aspects of the laryngeal entrance. To minimize this pressure, Macintosh and Lindholm have designed an S-shaped tube[331]. This, however, is more difficult to insert than the regular tube, and must be inserted with the use of a stylet.

Anesthesiologists, critical care physicians, emergency physicians and ambulance personnel should be able to intubate the trachea with the straight blade (Jackson–Wisconsin, Magill or Flagg type), the straight flat blade with curved tip (Miller type), and the curved blade (Macintosh type) (Fig. 14). The straight blades are designed to pick up the epiglottis directly (Fig. 15), while the curved blade, which slips into the vallecula just above the epiglottis, lifts the epiglottis off the larynx indirectly by pulling on the

Table 2-A. Approximate sizes of endotracheal and tracheostomy tubes.

		Orotracheal Tubes*				Length of tube (cm)**		Suction catheters (French sizes)	Adapters (ID) (mm)†	Tracheostomy tubes			
Approx. age	Weight (kg)	Inside diameter (ID) (mm)	Outside diameter (OD) (mm)†	French size (circumference)	Magill sizes	OT	NT			Shiley	Aberdeen	Hollinger	Approx. length (mm)
Adult male	8.0–10.0		14.0	42		22–26	29	14					60
			13.3	40									
			13.0	39									
(French 34–40)			12.7	38	10								
			12.3	37									
			12.0	36									
Adult female	7.5–9.0		11.7	35	9	20–24	27	12					
			11.3	34									
(French 32–36)			11.0	33	8	20–24	27	12					60
			10.7	32									
16–21 yrs	7.5		10.7	32	8	19	25	10	9	6	7.0	6	60
			10.3	31	7	19	25	10	9	6	7.0	6	
14–16 yrs	7.0		10.0	30	6	18	24	10	9	6	6.0	6	60
			9.7	29		18	24	10	9	6	6.0	6	
10–14 yrs	6.5		9.3	28	5½	17	22½	10	8	4	6.0	5	55
			9.0	27	5	17	22½	10	8	4	6.0	5	
8–10 yrs	6.0		8.7	26	4½	15	22	10	7	4	5.0	4	55
			8.3	25	4	15	22	10	7	4	5.0	4	
6–8 yrs	16–20	5.5	8.0	24	3½	14	18½	10	7	4	5.0	4	50
			7.7	23	3	14	18½	8	7	4	5.0	4	
5–6 yrs	11–15	5.0	7.3	22	2½	13	17	8	6	4	5.0	4	50
			7.0	21	2	13	17	8	6	4	5.0	4	
3–5 yrs	9–11	4.5	6.7	20	1½	12	15½	8	6	3	5.0	3	45
			6.3	19	1	12	15½	8	6	3	5.0	3	
18 mos–3 yrs	5–9	4.0	6.0	18		11	14	8	5	2	4.5	3	45
			5.7	17		10	12½	6	5	1	4.0	2	
6–18 mos	2.5–5	3.5	5.3	16	0	10	12	6	5	0	3.5	1	40
			5.0	15		10	11½	6	4	0	3.5	1	
Newborn–6 mos	2–2.5	3.0	4.7	14	00	9½	10½	6	4	0	3.5	0	30
			4.3	13		8	9	6	3	0	3.5	0	
Premature	1–2	2.5	4.0	12		8	9	6	3	00		00	<30
			3.7	11		8	9	6	2	00		00	

* For adults and large children, tubes with large-volume soft cuffs are recommended; for children under 6 years of age, uncuffed tubes. For nasotracheal tubes select 1 mm outside diameter (2–3 French size) smaller than for orotracheal intubation.

** Lengths: orotracheal tubes given here are short, to be used with the adapter just outside the mouth. They may be used longer. OT = orotracheal, NT = nasotracheal. NT = OT + 2–3 cm. Length in cm < 14 yrs age = age in yrs/2. Distance from upper teeth to carina averages 28 cm in men, 24 cm in women, 17 cm in children (age 6 yrs), 13 cm in infants; from upper teeth to the tip of the tube should be 4–6 cm shorter in adults (e.g. 22 cm in men, 19 cm in women).

† Inside diameter (ID) is 1–4 mm less than outside diameter (OD), depending on the wall thickness of the tube. French size = outside diameter in mm × 3

Table 2-B. Laryngoscope blades.

Size	Straight blade		Curved blade	
	Length (mm)	Example	Length (mm)	Example
Adult (large)	190	Flagg No. 4	158	Macintosh No. 4
Adult (medium)	160	Flagg No. 3	130	Macintosh No. 3
Child (2–9 yrs)	133	Flagg No. 2	108	Macintosh No. 2
Child (3 mos–2 yrs)	115	Wis-Hipple No. $1\frac{1}{2}$	100	Macintosh No. 1
Infant (under 3 mos)	102	Flagg No. 1, Miller Infant No. 1		
Premature	75	Miller Premature No. 0		

Table 2-C. Rigid tube bronchoscopes (use ventilation attachment).

Age	Inside diameter (mm)	Length (cm)
Adult (large)	9	40
Adult (medium)	7	40
Child (5–8 yrs)	5	30–33
Child (1–4 yrs)	4	26
Infant (under 1 yr.)	3	26

glosso-epiglottic frenulum. The curved blade does not touch the larynx itself and therefore probably produces less trauma and less reflex stimulation; it also permits more room for viewing and for tube insertion (Fig. 16). The choice of blade is influenced by personal preference. All blades come in several adult, child and infant sizes (Table 2-B).

Tubes with large-volume, low-pressure soft cuffs are recommended for adults and children over 5 years of age. For infants and small children, cuffed tubes are usually not necessary because the narrow subglottic diameter provides an adequate seal. Narrow small-volume, high-pressure cuffs should not be used because they may cause necrosis of the tracheal mucosa[330]. Overinflation of the cuff can be avoided by monitoring intracuff pressure (which in large soft cuffs equals airway and tracheal wall pressure)[128, 129] or by use of a pressure-limiting balloon. Large-volume low-pressure soft cuffs[712], if inflated just to the point of abolishing audible leak (+ 1–2 ml), exert lateral tracheal wall pressures of 5–25 mmHg during IPPV[128, 129], which are less likely to produce ischemia of the mucosa and tracheal dilatation than the previously used small-volume, stiff high-pressure cuffs. The foam rubber cuff is another safe version[390]. The tubes should be made of nonirritating plastic. Those reinforced with coiled wire are less likely to kink or be compressed, but are more difficult to insert and require a stylet for insertion. All tubes must have standard 15 mm male fittings.

A blunt-tipped malleable metal *stylet* makes the curvature of the tube controllable. When used it should not protrude beyond the distal end of the tube. Use of a straight stylet, bent 45° at the distal fifth of its length (hockey stick configuration), together with a curved laryngoscope blade facilitates intubation under difficult circumstances, even when only the rim of the epiglottis or the arytenoids can be visualized.

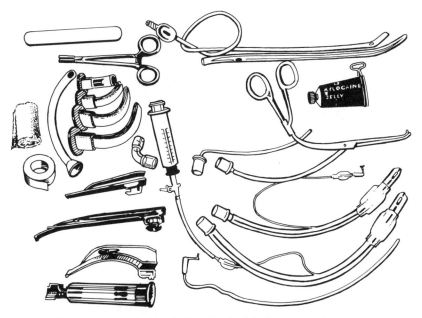

Fig. 14. Equipment for tracheal intubation. On the left, from top to bottom: tongue blade, clamp for cuff, bite block, tape to secure the tracheal tube, nasopharyngeal tube, oropharyngeal tubes, curved connector, laryngoscope handle with adult curved and straight blades and child straight blade. At the right, from top to bottom: curved-tip tracheal suction catheter, pharyngeal rigid suction tip, lidocaine water-soluble jelly, Magill forceps, three-way stopcock (or built-in ball valve) and syringe for cuff inflation, assortment of tracheal tubes, sizes infant French 12 (2.5 mm ID) to large adult French 38 (9.0 mm ID); stylet. (See text.)

ANATOMY

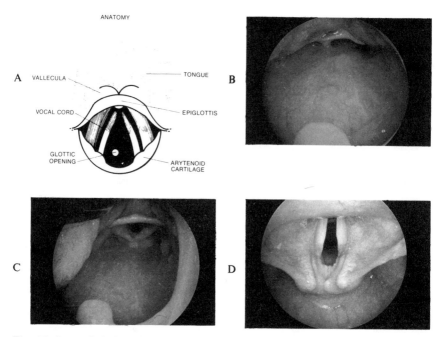

Fig. 15. Anatomical views for endotracheal intubation. (A) Diagram of the anatomy of the laryngeal entrance exposed by direct laryngoscopy. (From American Heart Association Advanced Life Support Slide Series, 1976.) (B) First direct laryngoscopic view during tracheal intubation; exposure of uvula and epiglottis. (C) Second direct laryngoscopic view during tracheal intubation; exposure of arytenoids. (D) Third direct laryngoscopic view during tracheal intubation; exposure of glottis. The anterior commissure is not fully seen. The posterior commissure is below. (Views B, C and D are from C.E. Lindholm.)

Fig. 16 (opposite). Technique of orotracheal intubation. (A) Laryngoscopy for endotracheal intubation with straight laryngoscope blade. Left, insertion of blade; right, larynx exposed. Note the elevated occiput with the head tilted backward (sniffing position), and the direct elevation of the epiglottis with the tip of the blade. Do not use the teeth as a fulcrum. Keep pressure off the upper teeth and lip! See text.
(B) Laryngoscopy for endotracheal intubation with curved laryngoscope blade. Left, insertion of blade; right, larynx exposed. Note the indirect elevation of the epiglottis by the tip of the blade elevating the base of the tongue. Note also the direction of lift, which is anteriorly and inferiorly at 45° to the vertical (coronal) plane. See text. (C) Exposure of the larynx with a curved blade and insertion of a cuffed tube through the right corner of the mouth, while looking along the laryngoscope blade. See text.

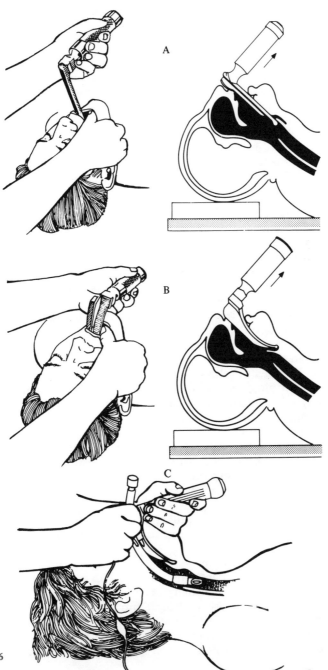

Figure 16

Technique of orotracheal intubation (Figs. 15, 16)

Learn orotracheal intubation by observing and practicing under expert guidance, first on adult and infant intubation manikins, then on anesthetized patients in the nonemergency setting.

Pay attention not only to insertion of the tube into the trachea, but also the many ancillary steps before and after intubation.

Become skilled with the techniques of your personal preference, and perform in an orderly, systematic and well rehearsed way.

Consider the following recommended sequence of action (based on the authors' experience) and learn it from supervised practice to perfection.

1. Have an experienced assistant available if possible.
2. Select, prepare and check the equipment (Fig. 14). Do not depend on others.

   (a) Select the appropriate size tracheal tube (Table 2-A) and spare tubes one size smaller and one size larger.

   (b) Select the appropriate size and type of laryngoscope (Table 2-B). Check the laryngoscope light.

   (c) Lubricate the tracheal tube with a water-soluble anesthetic jelly, e.g. lidocaine (lignocaine, Xylocaine).

   (d) Check the cuff by inflation with syringe via stopcock or one-way valve and cuff pilot tube, and deflate the cuff.

3. Have the patient in the supine position, with the occiput elevated and the head tilted backward at the atlanto-occipital joint (sniffing position), to bring the laryngoscope blade and trachea into a straight line (alignment of oral, pharyngeal and laryngeal axes) (Fig. 16).

4. Oxygenate the patient, preferably with 100% O_2, for at least 2 minutes (e.g. with bag–valve–mask oxygen) if feasible. In the relaxed (apneic) patient, have your assistant prevent gastric insufflation and regurgitation by pressing the cricoid backward. In the not relaxed (spontaneously breathing) patient, cricoid pressure might cause laryngospasm.

5. Interrupt ventilation for intubation. When intubating an apneic patient, hold your own breath and stop the intubation attempt when you become short of breath.

6. For insertion of the tube:

   (a) First force the patient's mouth open with your right hand (e.g. with the crossed-finger maneuver) (Fig. 7).

   (b) Grasp the laryngoscope handle firmly with the left hand and insert the blade from the right corner of the patient's mouth, pushing the tongue to the left so as not to have the view obscured by the tongue bulging over the open side of the laryngoscope blade

(Figs. 15 and 16). Protect the lips from being injured between the teeth and the blade.

(c) Gently move the laryngoscope blade toward the midline and visualize the patient's mouth, uvula, pharynx and epiglottis (Fig. 15-B), while moving your right hand to the patient's forehead or occiput to hold the head tilted backward.

(d) Lift the epiglottis directly with the straight blade (Fig. 16-A) or indirectly with the curved blade (Fig. 16-B). Visualize the arytenoids and the midline (the most important landmarks) (Fig. 15-C), and finally the vocal cords (desirable but not essential) (Fig. 15-D).

(e) Expose the larynx by pulling the laryngoscope handle upward (forward) at a right angle to the blade. Do not use the upper teeth as a fulcrum. Do not rotate the laryngoscope blade at the wrist, as this moves the larynx anteriorly and out of view. When using the curved blade, insertion too deep will push the epiglottis downward, whereas a too superficial insertion will make the base of the tongue bulge and obscure the vision of the larynx. Using the straight blade, insertion too deeply into the esophagus will lift the entire larynx out of view. These mistakes can be avoided by recognition of the arytenoid cartilages (Fig. 15-C).

(f) If necessary, ask an assistant to push on the neck to move the larynx backwards or to one side for a better view (Fig. 15-D), and to retract the right corner of the mouth to gain space for tube insertion.

(g) Insert the tracheal tube (with your right hand) through the right corner of the patient's mouth, while looking through the laryngoscope blade (Fig. 16-C). Twist the tube if necessary. Observe the tip of the tube and the cuff as they pass into the larynx entrance. If you use a stylet, have the assistant withdraw it while you hold the tube with its tip engaged in the larynx. Advance the tube so the cuff is placed just below the vocal cords. This correct placement will in the majority of average-sized adults put the tube length marker of 21 ± 2 cm at the upper teeth.

(h) Ask the assistant to hold the tube in place against the corner of the patient's mouth. If the jaw is relaxed, remove the laryngoscope blade; if not, fold the handle and leave the blade temporarily as a bite block.

7. Inflate the cuff temporarily to achieve a seal during IPPV and protect against aspiration.

8. Immediately ventilate and oxygenate by a self-refilling bag–valve–oxygen unit or an anesthesia circuit, and switch to a mechanical ventilator if desired, but only after the position of the tube and ability to ventilate have been ascertained by manual lung inflations. Auscultate chest.

9. Turn ventilation and oxygenation over to your assistant.

10. Remove the laryngoscope blade and insert an oropharyngeal tube or bite block.

11. Have the tube positioned to avoid bronchial intubation by having watched the cuff go through the larynx, retained the correct depth of tube insertion by marking the tube length at the level of the upper teeth, and by observing both sides of the chest expand with IPPV.

Auscultate both lungs to rule out bronchial (usually right bronchial) intubation and to determine the need for suctioning.

An optional method for proper tube placement is to press with one finger into the suprasternal notch and feel for the tip of the tube, and then to advance the tube with the other hand 2 cm further. Again, retain the correct depth of tube insertion.

12. Tape the tube securely to the patient's face. When the cheeks are unshaven or moist, a dry, broad, loose tape can be placed around the neck and both cheeks first and the tube taped to it; or an umbilical tape placed loosely around the neck can be tied to the tube.

13. While applying continuous positive pressure, deflate and then reinflate the cuff permanently, but only to the point of abolishing audible leaks. Inflate large low-pressure cuffs to 15–20 cmH$_2$O intracuff pressure between lung inflations.

14. Suction the tracheobronchial tree if necessary. If aspiration is suspected, use a suction trap for inspection and examination of the material removed (Fig. 11-B).

15. Establish nonkinking, nonslipping connections to the ventilation–oxygenation device.

16. In a patient with deep coma or gastric distension, insert a gastric tube, preferably through the nose—if this proves impossible, through the mouth (see below).

17. During anesthesia, insert an esophageal stethoscope for monitoring of heart and breath sounds.

18. Deliver oxygen via a heated humidifier or nebulizer and use atraumatic aseptic suctioning as needed.

Rapid sequence intubation[763, 785, 855]

The patient with a full stomach who is in need of general anesthesia or the patient who is in coma from head injury and needs respiratory resuscitation may require rapid sequence endotracheal intubation with preoxygenation, paralysis and apnea. This technique may be life saving if performed by experts in anesthesiology, but is dangerous (can result in asphyxiation) if performed by unskilled personnel. Be prepared with suction in case of regurgitation. The choice between the supine and the semi-sitting position is controversial. The supine position (particularly if the head is lowered) may counteract aspiration, while the semi-sitting position may discourage possible regurgitation.

After preoxygenation, preferably with 100% oxygen without positive pressure, or with positive pressure plus an assistant pressing on the cricoid backward to occlude the esophagus, induce anesthesia with pentothal (or ketamine if desired). Immediately paralyze the patient with succinylcholine 1–2 mg/kg i.v. Intubate swiftly.

The comatose patient after *head injury*, in need of respiratory resuscitation from asphyxiation due to convulsions, vomiting, trismus, laryngospasm and coughing, is the most challenging example. Anesthesia induction is not necessary, but the use of i.v. thiopental and/or i.v. lidocaine can be useful in blocking the reflex arterial and intracranial hypertension caused by upper airway stimulation, even in coma. The patient may have to be intubated with a muscle relaxant, since coughing and straining in the presence of brain contusion can cause additional cerebral edema and hemorrhage. The arterial PCO_2 should be kept low and arterial PO_2 high. Excessive movement of the head may aggravate a neck injury. Nasotracheal intubation is uncertain and may aggravate a basal skull fracture. Thus, emergency orotracheal intubation under paralysis should be performed by an expert team, as loss of the airway and asphyxial death may result. The procedure includes hyperventilation with 100% O_2 by mask under full paralysis with succinylcholine and cricoid pressure, using curved laryngoscope blade, stylet, and immobilization of the head–neck–chest in aligned mid-position by an assistant.

Intubating the awake patient

Endotracheal intubation of the awake patient is occasionally indicated prior to general anesthesia in aspiration risks, when a difficult intubation is anticipated, or in cases of severe pulmonary insufficiency; for upper airway and laryngoscopic procedures; and in selected cases for prolonged mechanical ventilation, as in patients with severe chest injury.

Tracheal intubation of the conscious patient is difficult and requires skill, experience and artistry. Topical anesthesia of the upper airway mucosa is provided by spraying a topical anesthetic, e.g. 4% lidocaine from a nebulizer, first onto the tongue and oropharyngeal mucosa, then under direct vision, with a partially inserted laryngoscope blade, onto the hypopharynx and supraglottic laryngeal mucosa, avoiding stimulation of the gag reflex.

The tracheal mucosa is then sprayed with 2–3 ml of 4% lidocaine either by instillation through the glottis into the tracheal lumen using a cannula with multiple holes, or by translaryngeal injection through the cricothyroid membrane into the tracheal lumen, using a thin (e.g. 22 gauge) needle. If the indication for awake intubation is a full stomach, the tracheal mucosa should not be anesthetized.

The procedure may be facilitated by small doses of a sedative or analgesic by i.v. titration, e.g. diazepam, morphine or meperidine (pethidine, Demerol). (Fentanyl, an excellent narcotic adjuvant for balanced anesthesia of the intubated patient, can produce apnea and chest wall spasm in the spontaneously breathing patient.) Take care not to abolish the response to verbal command. Suction should be ready to cope with regurgitation. For intubation, the laryngoscope blade and tracheal tube must be handled securely, gently applying pressure only when and where absolutely necessary. The operator's reassuring voice is most important. Should the patient regurgitate or vomit before the tube is inserted, suctioning and coaching cough can help clearing.

Technique of nasotracheal intubation

Nasotracheal intubation is more difficult, more time-consuming and potentially more traumatic (epistaxis) than orotracheal intubation. The blind nasotracheal technique is less predictable. Furthermore the technique carries the risk of introducing nasal bacteria into the trachea and sometimes into the bloodstream. It is not a suitable procedure for emergency airway control in the asphyxiating patient. However, in several circumstances in which the patient is breathing spontaneously and is not asphyxiating and time permits, nasotracheal intubation may be considered for cases of tight jaw (trismus) or inability to tilt the head backward (suspected neck fracture). It is also thought by some that nasotracheal tubes are more suitable for long-term intubation, as they are better tolerated than oral tubes. There are, however, problems with damage to the nasal mucosa and with pain and infection of the paranasal sinuses. Nasotracheal intubation is contraindicated in head injury with possible basal skull fracture.

Technique of nasotracheal intubation

For intubating through the patient's nose select the patient's more patent nasal passage by checking his ability to sniff through each nostril separately.

For intubating the *conscious* patient, apply a nasal vasoconstrictor (e.g. phenylephrine drops or spray) to dilate the nasal air passage, together with a topical anesthetic, e.g. 4% lidocaine to minimize discomfort. Alternatively, cocaine 1–2% may be used in small amounts, as it is both a potent topical vasoconstrictor and a topical anesthetic. Apply topical anesthesia to hypopharynx, larynx and trachea as described above.

Use a soft, well curved, cuffed nasotracheal tube and lubricate it well. In adults, use about one size (1 mm diameter) smaller than you would use for orotracheal intubation (Table 2-A).

Insert the tube through the more patent nostril, parallel to the palate. Ideally the tube's bevel should face the nasal septum to avoid damaging the turbinates. Tilt the patient's head backwards moderately and elevate the occiput (sniffing position). Advance the tube beyond the 'give' of the posterior wall of the nasopharynx.

For *blind* nasotracheal intubation, maneuver the tip of the tube laterally by twisting it, and maneuver it anteriorly or posteriorly by extending or flexing the head (not in suspected neck injury!).

Advance the tube during inhalations, listening for air flow or coughing that indicate entry into the larynx. Maintain pressure on the cricoid cartilage with the index finger and thumb, as this favors the tube entering the larynx and helps the operator recognize the tip of the tube in the vallecula or either pyriform fossa.

If the conscious or unconscious patient's mouth can be opened, facilitate nasotracheal intubation by visualizing the larynx. In this case hold the laryngoscope in your left hand, direct the tube with Magill's forceps or a large Kelly clamp in your right hand, grasp the tube and guide it under direct vision into the larynx—while your assistant advances the tube through the nose.

Difficult intubation

Intubation attempts may fail when there is inadequate muscular relaxation, poor technique or anatomic abnormality. Difficulty with intubation can be anticipated, for example, when the patient has taut neck tissues, a short thick neck, receding jaw, protruding jaw, inability to tilt the head backward, a narrow oral cavity or a large tongue. In such patients, intubation should be attempted by the most skilled anesthesiologist immediately available, with skillful oxygenation by mask between intubation attempts. He will first attempt the regular method (Figs. 14–16), and if this fails consider tactile transillumination, fiberoptic laryngoscopic versions of intubation, or other special approaches[542, 633, 642, 859, 861, 923]. In desperation, he should resort early enough to cricothyrotomy (Fig. 17).

Tactile digital orotracheal intubation

This technique, performed without the use of a laryngoscope, was practiced widely by pediatricians during the early 1900s for choking victims of diphtheria, and is now being revived. It can be practiced on cadavers. It is applied clinically: (1) in the deeply comatose patient when a laryngoscope is not available; (2) when cervical spine injury is suspected and orotracheal intubation by laryngoscope is not possible because of no maximal head tilt being allowed; and (3) because of secretions. Tactile orotracheal intubation is an alternative to blind nasotracheal intubation, which is difficult to learn, is unreliable, and is endowed with its own complications.

Use a lubricated tube with stylet bent into a J-shaped orotracheal tube. Hold the tube in your right hand and stand at the right side of the patient, facing his/her right shoulder. After preoxygenation, insert the index and middle fingers of your left hand into the mouth, and while depressing the tongue reach with your fingertip for the epiglottis. Guide the tube along your fingers toward the palpated epiglottis. If your fingers seem too short, go in via the corner of the mouth. With your fingers, pull the base of the tongue and the rim of the epiglottis forward, while maneuvering the tip of the tube into the larynx entrance with your right hand. Withdraw the stylet and advance the tube further, to 21 ± 2 cm from the upper teeth in an average adult.

Transillumination orotracheal intubation[923]

This technique utilizes a lighted stylet (Flexilum, Concept Corp.) and was first recommended by Berkebile of Pittsburgh for blind orotracheal intubation in the operating room. The method has been used recently with considerable success even in the prehospital setting by physician-guided paramedics.

Insert the flexible light into a regular orotracheal tube to illuminate its tip. Bend the tube slightly more than 90°. Grasp the patient's tongue with gauze and pull it forward. Slide the tube in, toward the larynx, and pick up the epiglottis. Observe its correct passage in the midline by watching the light on the skin of the neck. Lateral illumination indicates wrong position into the piriform fossa; subdued light, esophageal placement; and bright light in the midline, correct position. Engage the larynx with the tip of the tube. Withdraw the stylet while pressing the tube against the tongue. Advance the tube into the proper position.

For difficult emergency intubation attempts, combining the tactile technique with use of the illuminated stylet proved quite effective.

Fiberoptic laryngoscopic intubation[642]

When difficult intubation is anticipated or encountered and the patient is breathing spontaneously (and therefore intubation need not be performed within seconds), use of a flexible fiberoptic laryngoscope (fiberscope) is another possibility. A well lubricated fiberscope or pediatric fiberoptic bronchoscope of 3–4.3 mm outside diameter is passed through a tracheal tube with at least 5 mm internal diameter. Use topical anesthesia if appropriate. Fiberoptic laryngoscopy is not easy and calls for midline landmarks to be observed. It takes too long to be reliable for emergency intubation and reoxygenation in the asphyxiating patient.

For nasotracheal fiberoptic intubation, pass the nasotracheal tube through the naris into the oropharynx. Assist ventilation with oxygen via a special curved adapter with suction port. Insert the fiberscope through the suction port and advance it through the nasopharyngeal tube until you see the epiglottis. Pass the fiberscope between the cords. Advance the nasotracheal tube over the fiberscope into the trachea. Position the tip of the tube under vision.

For orotracheal fiberoptic intubation, either hold the tongue forward with your fingers and guide the fiberscope behind the base of the tongue, then look for epiglottis and cords; or use a laryngoscope to approach the epiglottis; or use a wide-bore oropharyngeal airway or mouth prop (oral airway intubator) and look for the epiglottis and cords. Insert the fiberscope and advance the orotracheal tube, which has been previously threaded over the fiberscope, over it into the trachea.

Tracheal intubation in infants and small children (see also Chapter 4)

When intubating the trachea in infants and small children, the operator must keep in mind that the infant's larynx in relation to that of the adult is located higher in the neck and more anteriorly, has a floppy U-shaped epiglottis, and is funnel-shaped, with the narrowest diameter at the level of the cricoid ring. Selecting a tube with too large a diameter can cause croup with asphyxia from reactive narrowing at the cricoid level following extubation.

For intubation in infants, particularly in newborns, a straight blade (e.g. a Miller blade) is more satisfactory than the curved laryngoscope blade (Table 2-B). Since the small dimensions of the infant make accidental bronchial intubation more likely, carefully place the tip of the endotracheal tube just beyond the vocal cords, into the upper trachea. For long-term use in infants, regular plastic tubes without shoulders are less injurious. Selecting the tube with the optimal diameter and length (Table 2-A), use of perfectly atraumatic techniques and attention to details are important (see pediatric anesthesiology textbooks).

Extubation

Extubation is potentially hazardous, and its safe execution depends on special knowledge and skills. At the end of general anesthesia in the healthy person the endotracheal tube is removed either under sufficient depth of anesthesia to obviate postextubation laryngospasm, or when the patient has recovered upper airway reflexes and responds to command. Respiratory insufficiency (hypoxemia, hypercarbia), acute acid–base abnormalities and circulatory derangements should all be ruled out prior to extubation. Ideally, to avoid progressive atelectasis after extubation, the patient should be conscious, hemodynamically stable, and able to achieve upon command an inspiratory capacity ('sighing volume') of at least 15 ml/kg or a negative inspiratory force of at least 25 cmH$_2$O on airway obstruction of 15 seconds. Other signs of recovered muscular power include ability to squeeze your hand, raising the head on command, and the absence of chest retraction during spontaneous breathing. Also, the stomach should not be distended. If a gastric tube is in place, it must be suctioned before extubation.

Technique for extubation

Have an assistant help you.
 Suction the patient's mouth, oropharynx and nasopharynx.
 Allow the patient to breathe 100% oxygen for 2–3 minutes. If chest auscultation reveals noise, suction the tracheobronchial tree with a separate, sterile, curved-tip catheter. After suctioning, again allow the patient to breathe 100% oxygen.
 While you apply sustained positive pressure into the trachea by bag compression, instruct your assistant to deflate the cuff of the endotracheal tube; the positive pressure helps to exsufflate secretions, which have accumulated above and below the cuff. Suction the pharynx promptly.
 Having deflated the cuff, remove the tube gently while maintaining positive pressure with 100% O$_2$ in the trachea. Do not continue tracheal suction during withdrawal of the tracheal tube, as this can empty the lungs and cause severe hypoxemia. After removal of the tube, continue oxygenation by mask, using approximately 50% oxygen.
 Be prepared to treat postextubation laryngospasm with oxygen by positive pressure and, if necessary, with a relaxant (succinylcholine) and reintubation. Be prepared to treat vomiting with forceful suction and aspiration with reintubation. For extubation of patients with upper airway problems, have cricothyrotomy equipment ready.

Complications of tracheal intubation[112, 209, 542, 861]

Attempts at endotracheal intubation can injure the lips, tongue, teeth, pharynx, tonsils and larynx. Nasotracheal intubation can cause epistaxis and, in addition, injure the nasal mucosa and the adenoids. Undetected, inadvertent intubation of the esophagus is the most dangerous complication of orotracheal and nasotracheal intubation attempts. Esophageal intubation may go unnoticed unless one listens carefully for breath sounds over both sides of the chest and over the epigastrium. Other potential complications include: tube obstruction by compression, kinking, obstructing secretions, biting, a bulging cuff, an uneven too narrow lumen, or obstructing adapters; accidental bronchial intubation; too shallow tube insertion with cuff above cords; and accidental tube dislodgment. Nonkinking nonslipping connections are important[231]. Persistent coughing (bucking, chest wall spasm) calls for positive pressure inflation with oxygen, and may require sedation, anesthesia, or even paralysis (succinylcholine) to facilitate oxygenation and prevent asphyxia.

Long-term complications following extubation may include aphonia, sore throat, ulcers and granulomas of the larynx, and dilation, rupture and stenosis of the trachea at the levels of the tube tip of the cuff.

In spite of these possible complications, correct use of tracheal intubation has become the cornerstone of emergency resuscitation and long-term airway control in the critically ill patient.

Gastric intubation

In the conscious patient, gastric intubation usually presents little difficulty if the patient can assist by swallowing. In comatose patients, however, gastric intubation may be more difficult. Most comatose patients, particularly CPR cases, should have a nasogastric tube passed, but *after* tracheal intubation. In stupor and coma, it is not advisable to attempt gastric intubation before the airway has been secured with a cuffed tracheal tube, since the gastric tube can provoke vomiting or passive regurgitation and aspiration. The tube renders the esophageal sphincters incompetent. This caveat applies to insertion of both small-bore tubes and large-bore tubes (commonly used for gastric lavage). Furthermore, ventilation–oxygenation and chest compressions should not be interrupted during gastric intubation. During CPR-ALS, do not disturb efforts to restart spontaneous circulation by attempts at gastric intubation, which can wait unless there is severe distension of the abdomen.

Technique of gastric intubation

Insert a nasogastric tube in the relaxed comatose patient, facilitated by use of ample (water-soluble) lubricant and giving the tube's tip a slight bend.

Insert the tube through the more patent nasal passage, with the bend pointing anteriorly, and feel the 'give' of the posterior wall of the nasopharynx.

Turn the bent tip posteriorly and use your other hand to lift the larynx forward to open the upper esophageal sphincter; do this by grasping the larynx from the outside, pressing your thumb on one side and your middle finger on the other side behind the larynx. Now advance the gastric tube to engage into the upper esophagus and feed it into the stomach.

If necessary, insert your index finger into the hypopharynx for palpation, straightening and bimanual advancement of the tube. Occasionally a laryngoscope may be helpful so that the tube may be directed into the esophagus under direct vision using Magill's forceps.

9) Alternatives to tracheal intubation

Cricothyroid membrane puncture (cricothyrotomy) and translaryngeal oxygen jet insufflation are alternative steps of last resort when endotracheal intubation is impossible in an asphyxiating patient and necessary equipment for these alternative techniques is immediately available. During the procedure, a helper should try to oxygenate the patient by mask. These two alternative measures are rarely needed, but should be part of the therapeutic repertoire of trained professionals involved in emergency resuscitation. Both measures are part of advanced trauma life support (Chapter 4).

Cricothyrotomy is preferable to translaryngeal jet ventilation in the spontaneously breathing patient and in complete airway obstruction. Translaryngeal oxygen jet ventilation, which requires compressed oxygen delivered at high pressure and the necessary connections for intratracheal insufflation, is preferred over cricothyrotomy as an elective procedure for anesthesia in patients undergoing operations on the upper airway in the presence of laryngeal or supralaryngeal obstruction.

Cricothyrotomy[101, 719] (Fig. 17)

This technique is for spontaneous breathing of air or oxygen, artificial ventilation and suctioning. The procedure must be performed only by those who have practiced it under guidance on an animal, cadaver, or manikin. Particularly when performed in children, there is a risk of producing subglottic stenosis. Cricothyrotomy calls for the largest available cannula that does not cause injury to the larynx, i.e. in the adult 6 mm and the large child 3 mm outside diameter. Merely cutting through the cricothyroid space with a penknife does not establish an airway. The opening must be kept patent, and a standard adapter must permit connection of ventilation equipment.

Cricothyrotomy should be with a skin incision and piercing of the membrane under vision. Blind (percutaneous) automatic cricothyrotomy techniques (e.g. with 'tracheotome') are hazardous and therefore not recommended. The presently recommended methods for adults are: (1) 'cut and poke' method[719], using a pointed curved uncuffed metal cannula with standard 15 mm male adapter; and (2) pushing through the cut a cuffed tracheal or tracheostomy tube of 5 mm internal diameter.

Translaryngeal oxygen jet insufflation[371, 372, 415, 811, 823, 835] (Fig. 18)

This technique consists of insertion of a 12–16 gauge over-the-needle catheter through the cricothyroid membrane, and intermittent insufflation of oxygen. A high-pressure source (30–60 psi, i.e. 2–4 atmospheres) of oxygen is required to overcome the resistance of the system. The chest must be carefully observed and the valve must be turned off the moment the chest rises to prevent lung rupture.

Passive exhalation is achieved through the upper airway, which *must* be at least partially open, to avoid lung rupture. In cases of complete upper airway obstruction, a second large-bore tracheal catheter needle, perhaps with intermittent suction, should be inserted to accommodate exhalations. Inflation starts with some air entrainment and ends with upward leakage through the larynx. The most life-threatening possible complication (which can be avoided with proper technique) is interstitial oxygen insufflation from lung rupture or from accidental insertion of the catheter into tissue spaces instead of into the tracheal lumen. This tracheal insufflation technique can exsufflate upper airway secretions but does not allow suctioning of the tracheobronchial tree, as is possible via endotracheal or cricothyrotomy tube. For translaryngeal high-frequency ventilation, see Chapter 1B.

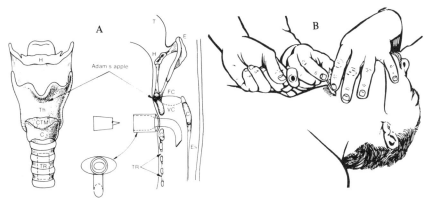

Fig. 17. Cricothyrotomy. (A) Anatomy with cannula in place. H, hyoid bone; Th, thyroid cartilage; C, cricoid cartilage; TR, trachea; CTM, cricothyroid membrane; E, epiglottis; T, tongue; FC, false cords; VC, vocal cords; Es, esophagus. Beveled curved cannula with knife blade (with handle rubber stopper, to be carried safely within the 15 mm slip joint of the cannula) (Safar and Penninckx). The cannula shown can be made from curved endotracheal tube slip joints (6 mm outside diameter for adults; 3 mm outside diameter for large children), with a 15 mm male adapter to connect the ventilation equipment. A special cannula is not essential. Regular small-bore cuffed endotracheal or tracheostomy tubes with 6 mm outside diameter are satisfactory in adults. For small children and infants use the smallest size uncuffed endotracheal or tracheostomy tube (Table 2) or, as a compromise, large (e.g. 12–14 gauge) catheter-outside-needle from i.v. supplies. (B) Technique of cricothyroid membrane puncture via small horizontal skin incision (see text).[719]

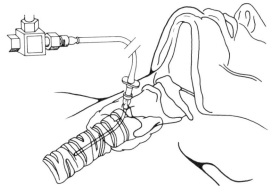

Fig. 18. Translaryngeal oxygen jet insufflation. Prepare the necessary equipment assembly, consisting of a 30–60 psi (2–4 atm.) oxygen source, high-pressure tubing, valve (three-way stopcock or push-button release valve), extension tubing and 14–16 gauge over-the-needle catheter. Hold the head tilted backward, hold the larynx between your thumb and middle finger, and identify the cricothyroid membrane with your index finger. Insert the catheter needle through the cricothyroid space into the tracheal lumen, pointing downward. Ensure correct catheter placement by free aspiration of air. Connect the extension tube equipment assembly. Inflate the lungs by turning the valve or stopcock until the chest moves; then turn the valve off and let the patient exhale passively through the mouth and nose. (From the American Heart Association Advanced Life Support Slide Series, 1976).

10) Other steps of airway control

Tracheotomy, bronchoscopy, bronchodilation and pleural drainage all are elective (though sometimes urgent) procedures, which are adjunctive to the steps of emergency airway control described so far.

Tracheotomy[836] (Fig. 19)

This is for long-term airway management and, ideally, should be done under conditions of optimal lighting and sterility in the operating room. In acute emergencies, the skilled operator can perform endotracheal intubation or cricothyroid membrane puncture more rapidly than tracheotomy. (The resulting opening in the tracheal wall is called 'tracheostomy'; the opening which results from suturing the entire lumen of the trachea into the skin after laryngectomy is called 'tracheostoma'.)

A switch from tracheal tube to tracheostomy tube should be considered when tracheal cannulation is expected to be needed longer than 7–10 days, or when the patient is conscious and wishes to talk during prolonged artificial ventilation. This is possible with the use of an uncuffed tube, a cuffed tube with deliberate minimal cuff leak[712], or a 'speaking tracheostomy tube'[731], but not with a translaryngeal tube. Whenever possible tracheotomy should be done as an elective procedure and in the oxygenated, well ventilated patient, if necessary with a tracheal tube in place[836].

Indications for tracheostomy include acute upper airway inflammation. *Laryngotracheobronchitis* may benefit transiently from racemic epinephrine (adrenaline) aerosol administered into the upper airways via nebulizer. *Epiglottis* with asphyxia, however, calls for endotracheal intubation by an expert, or tracheotomy.

Bronchoscopy[365, 836]

This is needed to clear the tracheobronchial tree after aspiration of solid foreign matter or obstruction by thick mucus or blood. For tracheobronchial clearing, the rigid tube bronchoscope is more effective than bronchoscopy with the flexible fiberoptic bronchoscope, which has only a narrow lumen for suctioning. Bronchoscopy in critically ill patients (conscious or unconscious) should be undertaken during spontaneous breathing with oxygenation and assisted ventilation, using jet insufflation or a ventilating bronchoscope[565, 702]. In massive aspiration of solid foreign matter, ventilation bronchoscopy can be a life-saving resuscitative measure.

The flexible fiberoptic bronchoscope[365] has advantages for examination and for removing mucous plugs from smaller bronchi, particularly in the upper lobes. Lung rupture is possible during fiberoptic bronchoscopy through an endotracheal tube with IPPV if exhalation is impaired by the scope diameter within the tube.

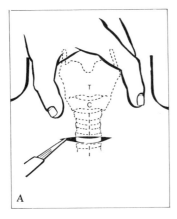
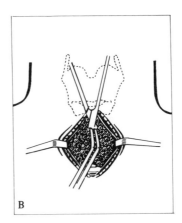
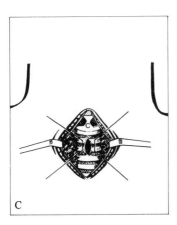
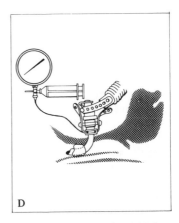

Fig. 19. Technique of tracheotomy. (A) Make a horizontal or vertical skin incision.
(B) Ligate and divide the thyroid isthmus if necessary, and expose tracheal rings 1–4.
(C) Ask an assistant to withdraw the translaryngeal (endotracheal) tube partially, with the
tip remaining in the larynx. Place stay sutures through tracheal rings 2 and 3 on both
sides of the anticipated opening for immediate access to the tracheal lumen in case of tube
dislodgment later. Make a midline incision of tracheal rings 2 and 3 (an oval-shaped or
inverted V-shaped excision in adults). (D) Quickly insert an appropriate size tracheostomy
tube (Table 2-A) with a large soft cuff. Inflate the cuff to abolish audible leak. Connect
via a nonslip swivel adapter to the ventilation–oxygenation device. Remove the
translaryngeal (endotracheal) tube only after adequate ventilation via tracheostomy tube
has been confirmed.

Bronchodilation and clearing[736c]

These are important in the management of status asthmaticus, bronchitis with asphyxiation, near-drowning and aspiration. An example of lower airway control is the following combination recommended for an asthmatic crisis: (1) titrated positive pressure ventilation with oxygen (assisted IPPB by mouth piece or mask; controlled IPPV, CPPV or IMV via endotracheal tube); (2) humidification to promote mucociliary escalator clearing; (3) bronchodilation by metaproterenol aerosol plus aminophylline i.v.; (4) shrinkage of the mucosa by a sympathetic alpha-receptor stimulator aerosol; (5) arterial pH normalization with $NaHCO_3$ or THAM i.v., and hyperventilation[394]; (6) a steroid in high doses (methylprednisolone or dexamethasone i.v.); and (7) paralysis (curarization) and sedation for full ventilatory control with slow flow rates and 100% O_2 via tracheal tube, and tracheobronchial suctioning. Steroids even when given i.v. begin to help control acute asthma attacks only after a few hours[394]. Nonabsorbable beclomethasone aerosol is for maintenance asthma therapy, not for status asthmaticus (Chapter 4). Water, isotonic saline or drug aerosol therapy, useful in a variety of acute upper and lower airway problems, can be administered with spontaneous[545], manually assisted[538] or controlled ventilation[736c]. Add hydration i.v.

Pleural drainage[22] (Fig. 20)

Emergency pleural drainage is required when air, fluid or blood collects in the pleural cavity with such rapidity or in such volume that ventilation is progressively impaired. Perhaps the most acute such emergency is *tension pneumothorax*, in which a leak in the lung parenchyma, acting as a one-way valve, results in increasing compression of lung, airways and vena cava. Tension pneumothorax can asphyxiate the patient rapidly by lung collapse and bronchial kinking and compression due to mediastinal displacement.

Suspect tension pneumothorax when there is tracheal deviation from the midline on neck palpation, progressive inability of the chest to deflate, deterioration of the pulse, unilateral distension of the chest, distension of the abdomen from inversion of the diaphragm and pneumoperitoneum, tympanism on percussion, mediastinal shift on percussion and/or interstitial emphysema with subcutaneous crepitation at the neck (from interstitial alveolar rupture). Auscultation can be deceptive, but absence of breath sounds on one side is highly suggestive.

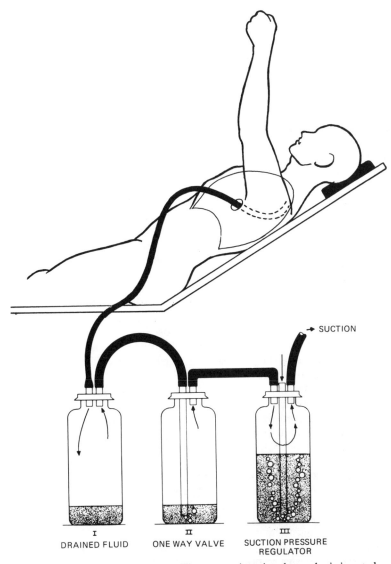

Fig. 20. Technique of pleural drainage. The appropriate size chest tube is inserted through a stab incision in the skin and into the pleural cavity, with the open technique (blunt Kelly clamp pierced through the intercostal space and pried open for tube insertion) or the closed technique (using a trocar). The latter technique requires greater skill to avoid complications. One lateral-to-posterior chest tube, with multiple holes, is usually sufficient. The tube is connected to the bottle system consisting of bottle I for collection of fluids; bottle II, a one-way valve; and bottle III to keep a constant controllable negative pressure. For transportation a one-way valve instead of the three-bottle system is used. In hospitals the three-bottle system may be replaced by a chest suction device (e.g. Pleurevac) provided it permits control of negative pressure and a high flow rate.

Figure labels:

SUCTION

I — DRAINED FLUID
II — ONE WAY VALVE
III — SUCTION PRESSURE REGULATOR

Technique of pleural drainage (Fig. 20)

For emergency pleural drainage in suspected pneumothorax, first perform a diagnostic tap of the suspected pleural space with a needle in the second intercostal space, midclavicular line, in the supine or semi-sitting position. If air escapes, insert a large-bore chest tube and connect it to a one-way valve or drainage system serving the same purpose. As a temporary measure, several large-bore catheter needles can be inserted.

For draining blood or fluid, a large chest tube is needed from the start.

For trauma with suspected hemopneumothorax, insert one large-bore tube with multiple holes for drainage of air plus fluid inserted via the 5th or 6th intercostal space at the midaxillary line. Insert this lateral chest tube toward the posterior aspects of the thoracic cavity, and advance the tip of the tube toward the apex of the hemithorax.

Perhaps the safest technique for chest tube placement involves *blunt puncture* with a Kelly clamp. Make an incision through the skin wheal and place a stitch for securing the catheter. With a Kelly clamp, blunt dissection is carried down to the rib. The pleura is penetrated just above the rib with the tip of the closed Kelly clamp, and the thoracostomy tube, with one end clamped off, is then rapidly introduced between the spread jaws of the clamp. The tube is then secured as previously described.

The *Argyle* plastic thoracostomy tube with enclosed trocar is much simpler to use than the trocar and plastic catheter, but it requires meticulous care lest overzealous attempts to penetrate the chest wall lead to parenchymal lung damage. As in the previously described technique, make a small incision in the anesthetized skin and place a stitch. Advance the Argyle catheter through the incision, at right angles to the skin, just superior to the rib. When the sharp inner trocar enters the pleural space, advance the tube over it to the previously placed silk suture marker. After the tube has been secured to the skin, place a Kelly clamp between the skin and the tip of the trocar and remove the trocar.

Whatever system is used, certain general principles apply to the care of all patients connected to water-seal drainage:

1. Each thoracostomy tube requires a separate closed drainage system.
2. All connections between chest tubes and drainage tubing should be securely taped.
3. The water level in the water-seal bottle must be closely monitored.
4. The water-seal bottle should be placed at least 50 cm below the

patient's chest, lest the negative pressure generated during deep inhalation pulls air from the bottle into the chest.

5. The water level in the suction control bottle must also be closely monitored and adjusted to provide the desired amount of negative pressure.

6. Thoracostomy tubes should be secured in a manner to prevent kinking and traction. Connecting tubing should be long enough to permit the patient to sit up or turn 180° laterally.

7. Tubing and bottles must be checked frequently for patency; the water column in the water-seal tube should oscillate with ventilation.

8. Kelly clamps should always be immediately available at the bedside, in case of inadvertent disconnection of any part of the system.

Chapter 1B

Step B: Breathing Support (Emergency Artificial Ventilation and Oxygenation)

Ventilation Patterns (Fig. 21)

Current methods of artificial ventilation are based on intermittent inflation of the lungs with positive pressure applied to the airway, followed by passive exhalation at atmospheric airway pressure (Fig. 21-A). The forces that must be overcome with IPPV in order to achieve lung inflation are primarily the elastic resistance of the lungs and thorax and the airway resistance. Thus, intermittent positive pressure (controlled) ventilation (IPPV) is the basic artificial ventilation pattern. Research in the 1950s on emergency artificial ventilation without equipment proved the superiority of IPPV with exhaled air (mouth-to-mouth/nose ventilation) over the back-pressure and chest-pressure arm-lift maneuvers then in vogue[699]. The latter techniques failed to ventilate the lungs of curarized human volunteers without tracheal tubes because of inadequate force of inflation and inability of the operator to control the patient's airway. Therefore, the back-pressure arm-lift (prone) method (Holger-Nielsen), chest-pressure arm-lift (supine) method (Silvester) and other 'push-pull' methods of emergency artificial ventilation[157, 288, 591] have become obsolete and are now recommended only when mouth-to-mouth ventilation is impossible, e.g. in cases of severe facial trauma.

Shallow spontaneous breaths may be augmented with assisted ventilation (patient-triggered, operator- or ventilator-augmented breaths)[544, 718] (Fig. 21-A) or with intermittent mandatory ventilation (IMV) (spontaneous breathing with operator- or ventilator-controlled inflations at a superimposed slower rate)[206] (Fig. 21-B). All these methods may be performed with exhaled air, air or oxygen.

During controlled, assisted or intermittent mandatory ventilation, positive end-expiratory pressure (PEEP) is used to open and stabilize collapsed or fluid-filled alveoli. Expiratory retardation is used to prevent intrapulmonary airway collapse during exhalation in conditions which narrow or soften bronchi (e.g. asthma, emphysema[736c]). Negative pressure in the airway (PNPV) can enhance venous return of blood into the heart in hypovolemia, but is not recommended because it can enhance intrapulmonary airway collapse and pulmonary edema.

Most of the airway pressure patterns of assisted and controlled positive pressure ventilation (Fig. 21) can be provided either without equipment or with only portable equipment, although some would require at least homemade improvisations of customary portable equipment. However, artificial ventilation with expiratory retardation, PEEP, IMV and assist/control mode is easier and better performed with mechanical ventilation (MV), using a wide variety of ventilators[166, 228, 408, 552, 568, 630, 736c, 799, 836]. Intermittent deep lung inflations (sighing) to counteract atelectasis[66], with about 15 ml/kg tidal volumes, is best performed spontaneously in the conscious patient, and by bag–valve unit via cuffed tracheal tube in the unconscious patient.

Prolonged mechanical positive pressure ventilation of any kind is better performed via an endotracheal tube or tracheostomy tube. Without the use of a tracheal tube, gastric insufflation frequently occurs when pharyngeal pressures exceed 20 cmH_2O[690].

Lung rupture due to positive airway pressure is related to lung pathology (such as bullous emphysema) and alveolar distension. To deliver adequate tidal volumes, peak airway pressures of 30 cmH_2O or less are usually adequate. Some patients with partial airway obstruction or stiff lungs or chest (low compliance), however, may require up to 70 cmH_2O peak inspiratory pressures. Lung rupture may be prevented by avoiding overdistension, keeping PEEP as low as possible and allowing full passive exhalations. This may require a relatively slow ventilation rate.

Circulatory depression from increased airway pressure is related to high mean intrathoracic pressure and is more likely to occur in patients with normal (compliant) lungs and low blood volume[162]. In patients with fairly normal lungs, IPPV will depress cardiac output least if each positive airway pressure inflation phase is followed by twice as long an exhalation phase at atmospheric pressure which lets the heart fill with blood (1:2 ratio; 'waltz rhythm')[162]. Patients with sick lungs who need high airway pressures are fortunately less likely to develop hypotension from reduced venous return, as the stiff lungs transmit less alveolar pressure to the pleural space and mediastinum. Moreover, in cardiogenic shock, IPPV and even better systole-synchronized IPPV enhances cardiac output[626, 627].

Indications for mechanical ventilation include: (1) inability of the patient to maintain a normal arterial PCO_2; (2) excessive work of breathing; (3) metabolic acidemia when the patient cannot hyperventilate enough spontaneously to normalize arterial pH without becoming exhausted; and (4) severe flailing of the chest wall.

Positive end-expiratory pressure[407, 622, 736c] (Fig. 21)

When *hypoxemia* persists during mechanical ventilation with IPPV, the addition of PEEP is desirable. PEEP allows an abrupt decrease of airway pressure to a sustained elevated plateau. IPPV plus PEEP is CPPV. This is indicated when the patient demonstrates an inability to maintain arterial PO_2 above 60 mmHg with an inhaled oxygen concentration of 100% $(FIO_2 = 1.0)$ short-term, or 50% $(FIO_2 = 0.5)$ long-term. Thus, the switch from spontaneous breathing (SB) of oxygen to mechanical ventilation with CPPV and oxygen is indicated primarily when a further increase in arterial PO_2 without invoking toxic FIO_2 (over 0.5 long-term) is needed, and when hypoxemia occurs in the unconscious, confused, or otherwise uncooperative patient who requires a tracheal or tracheostomy tube. PEEP is produced by attaching a threshold resistance to the expiratory port of the non-rebreathing valve of the manual or mechanical ventilator. The level of PEEP must be selected carefully and adjusted to an optimal range in a titrated fashion:

1. Prophylactic PEEP (1–5 cmH₂O) is used to prevent atelectasis and increase FRC above closing volume.
2. Conventional PEEP (5–20 cmH₂O) is indicated if an FIO_2 of 0.6 cannot maintain PaO_2 at or above 60 mmHg. PEEP over 10 cmH₂O requires a tracheal tube.
3. High PEEP (over 20 cmH₂O) is employed in extreme hypoxemia and only by intensive care experts for prolonged mechanical ventilation. High PEEP is *not* for emergency resuscitation[407].
4. Optimal PEEP, which may, depending upon circumstances, fall anywhere along the above spectrum, needs to be titrated[303, 871].

In examining the concept of optimal PEEP, it is important to understand that arterial PO_2 reflects only the lung's ability to oxygenate arterial blood. Since the ultimate goal is adequate tissue oxygenation, a more sensitive guide for the adjustment of PEEP may be to monitor not only arterial PO_2, but also changes in mixed venous PO_2 (pulmonary artery or superior vena cava PO_2). In general, CPPV increases arterial PO_2 with each increment of PEEP. However, when high levels of PEEP are needed for maximal reduction in shunting, by opening closed or fluid-filled alveoli, a concomitant reduction in cardiac output may occur. Furthermore, when excessive PEEP decreases systemic arterial pressure, coronary and cerebral blood flow may decrease and the resulting myocardial ischemia may reduce cardiac output further. This untoward effect can be at least in part counteracted by blood volume expansion, together with the use of a cardiac inotropic agent (e.g. dopamine) to maximize pulmonary flow of unshunted blood and maintain arterial perfusion pressure.

Fortunately, the stiffer the lungs, the lower the positive airway pressure transmitted to the pulmonary circulation and venae cavae. Thus, in patients who truly need PEEP, higher levels of PEEP are less likely to decrease cardiac output, to increase pulmonary vascular resistance and to reduce venous return. When PEEP is used, there should always be pleural drainage 'standby', and personnel must be alert to recognize and promptly treat tension pneumothorax by insertion of a chest tube and reduction in airway

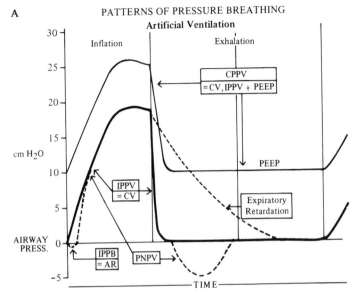

A   PATTERNS OF PRESSURE BREATHING

Artificial Ventilation

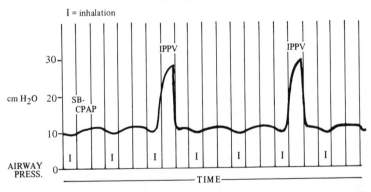

B   Intermittent Mandatory Ventilation

$$IMV = \begin{array}{c} SB\text{-}Atm.\,P. \\ or \\ SB\text{-}CPAP \end{array} + IPPV\ (slow\ rate)$$

I = inhalation

Fig. 21. Airway pressure patterns of assisted and controlled positive pressure ventilation. (A) IPPV, intermittent positive pressure (controlled) ventilation; CV, controlled ventilation; IPPB, intermittent positive pressure (assisted) breathing; AR, assisted respiration; PEEP, positive end-expiratory pressure (for alveolar recruitment); CPPV, continuous positive pressure ventilation, i.e. IPPV plus PEEP; expiratory retardation, for splinting airways in emphysema. PNPV, positive–negative pressure (controlled) ventilation. (B) Airway pressure with intermittent mandatory ventilation (IMV), i.e. spontaneous breathing (SB) with continuous positive airway pressure (CPAP) and manual or mechanically controlled lung inflations (IPPV) superimposed (see text). I, spontaneous inhalations. IMV requires a special ventilator. MV = mechanical ventilation.

pressure. Weaning from and discontinuance of mechanical ventilation should ideally be accomplished before removal of the chest tube. Advanced respiratory intensive care[736c, 799] should be based on respiratory pathophysiology[66, 596].

Spontaneous Breathing of Oxygen with Positive Airway Pressure[50, 297, 301, 304] (Fig. 22)

During normal breathing, there is slight negative airway pressure during inhalation and slight positive airway pressure during exhalation. PEEP is commonly used to refer to airway pressure maintained above atmospheric during the expiratory phase of the breathing cycle; however, PEEP is primarily applied to mechanical (artificial) ventilation (MV), and when it is added to IPPV it becomes CPPV (Fig. 21). Spontaneous breathing with positive airway pressure (SB-PAP) (Fig. 22) does not require a ventilator. SB-CPAP up to 10–15 cmH$_2$O can be applied to conscious cooperative patients via mouthpiece, mask, nasal mask, nasal prongs, pharyngeal tube or head box (in babies); or with higher pressures or in coma via endotracheal tube or tracheostomy tube. In contrast, IPPV or CPPV by MV usually requires an endotracheal or tracheostomy tube.

The *function* of SB-PAP is to increase the pressure gradient between alveoli and pleura (transpulmonary pressure), i.e. the pressure tending to distend alveoli with a method simpler than MV. SB-PAP with oxygen plays a major role in the treatment of hypoxemia due to reduced FRC, usually from collapsed or fluid-filled alveoli. It increases the number of functioning alveoli (recruitment) and serves as a splint (preventing collapse), thereby maintaining an increased volume of gas in the lungs. Through this increase in FRC and the attendant reduction in shunting, the arterial PO$_2$ in hypoxemic patients is increased[622, 736c]. Furthermore, a continuous slight increase in airway pressure, by stabilizing alveoli and their perfusion, may promote regeneration of surfactant[149].

Acute pulmonary edema, for example, when it has not yet progressed to the stage at which tracheal intubation is required, may benefit from SB-PAP with 100% O$_2$ without tracheal tube. In respiratory care for neonates with respiratory distress syndrome SB-PAP with carefully controlled FIO$_2$ (to prevent blindness from retrolental fibroplasia due to high arterial PO$_2$) has become the most effective method, used via nasal prongs, head box or endotracheal tube, and has replaced MV as the initial life-support method.

SB-PAP (primarily during expiration, EPAP) was used long ago in adults with pulmonary edema[50], but later abandoned. When in 1970 SB-PAP was introduced into neonatal respiratory care[301], one of us (PS) reintroduced it with continuous positive airway pressure (SB-CPAP) by mask or tracheal tube into adult respiratory care[301]. We hoped to avoid the need for cuffed tracheal tubes with their associated complications. The simplicity of SB-

CPAP with FIO_2 0.5–1.0 without endotracheal intubation should be explored for oxygenation of mass casualties of toxic gases and vapors or smoke inhalation, which kill via pulmonary consolidation and progressive hypoxemia (e.g. the disaster of Bhopal, India, 1985). Tracheal intubation and mechanical ventilation of hundreds of victims at once would not be feasible.

Prerequisites for use of SB-PAP without tracheal tube include: (1) a conscious, cooperative patient with intact upper airway reflexes; (2) a high gradient between PaO_2 and FIO_2; (3) adequate spontaneous tidal volumes of at least 10 ml/kg; and (4) normal or low $PaCO_2$.

The required *assembly* (Fig. 22) includes a threshold resistance in the form of a PEEP valve, which may be a simple water bubbler, a compact mushroom spring or magnetic valve, a floating ball valve (held vertically), a Laerdal PEEP valve, or an Ambu PEEP valve. In general, threshold resistor-type PEEP and 'pop-off' valves are less likely to result in dangerous airway pressure build-up and pulmonary barotrauma than the previously used flow resistor-type valves. During SB-CPAP, the level of expiratory PAP (EPAP) is determined by the PEEP value; and of inspiratory PAP by the pressure in the circuit when inspiration is begun, and by the relationship between gas flow from the source and the patient's peak inspiratory flow rate. SB-CPAP short-term (e.g. in acute pulmonary edema) can be given with a high continuous inflow of 100% O_2 (at least 30 l/min). For prolonged use, ideally the gas from the source should be FIO_2-controlled (oxygen–air mixer), humidified (heated humidifier) and—at least in adults—passed through an elastic reservoir bag. The high inspiratory flow rate required for SB-CPAP can be obtained via an air–oxygen mixer or a Venturi air entrainment system (Vital Signs, Inc.). Finally, the equipment includes a transparent tight-sealing face mask (e.g. Laerdal cushion mask, new anatomic mask or pocket mask) which should be fastened to the patient's face via a head strap or elastic head net (used for wound dressings), a nasal mask or—in the very cooperative patient—a mouthpiece.

Most conscious patients receiving SB-CPAP without tracheal tube benefit from it and tolerate prophylactic peak pressures of 3–5 cmH_2O. Pressures may be increased to 10–15 cmH_2O if the patient tolerates it; a gastric tube is advisable. Higher pressures should be administered only via tracheal or tracheostomy tube, since esophageal opening pressure is 15–25 cmH_2O[690] and higher pressures can cause dyspnea, hypoventilation, gas swallowing and gastric distension. For adjusting SB-PAP, one should monitor patient comfort, respiratory frequency and effort (to estimate the work of breathing), airway pressure and (ideally) also $PaCO_2$.

Advantages of SB-PAP over other oxygen administration techniques are: (1) the iatrogenic infection often associated with tracheal intubation may be avoided; (2) FRC is increased (shunting decreased) over that obtained with SB at atmospheric pressure; (3) ventilation–perfusion matching and cardiac output may be better than during MV with PEEP (CPPV) because of lower mean intrathoracic pressure (which also requires less fluid loading to maintain cardiac output); (4) patients tolerate SB-PAP better than they do MV (CPPV) and thus require less sedation; (5) less risk of barotrauma; and (6) simplicity and low cost (disasters).

Disadvantages of SB-PAP in comparison with intratracheal CPPV include: (1) the patient must cooperate (which is not always possible in critical illness); (2) risk of gastric distension and aspiration, even in the cooperative patient; (3) facial ischemia from mask trauma; (4) otitis media due to increased nasopharyngeal pressure; and (5) increased work of breathing to the point of dyspnea and CO_2 retention, requiring a switch to CPPV. The technique is contraindicated in patients with stupor–coma, nausea or vomiting, small spontaneous tidal volumes, circulatory instability, or cerebrospinal fluid (CSF) leak (basal skull fracture).

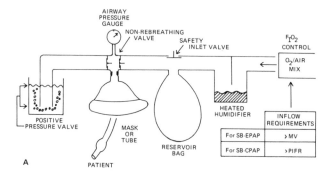

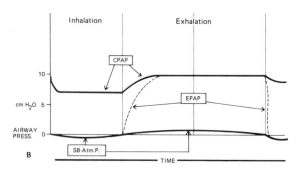

Fig. 22. Spontaneous positive pressure breathing. (A) Oxygen setup via mask, tracheal tube or tracheostomy tube. For spontaneous breathing (SB) with expiratory positive airway pressure (EPAP), the continuous inflow rate of oxygen–air mixture must at least equal minute volume; for SB with continuous positive airway pressure (CPAP), it must be at least peak inspiratory flow rate (more than 25 l/min during quiet breathing). The bubble PEEP valve at the left could be replaced with 'dry' valves (mushroom, magnetic, ball or other). (B) Airway pressure patterns achieved with the equipment outlined in A.

Direct Mouth-to-Mouth and Mouth-to-Nose Ventilation[220, 221, 289, 699, 700, 703–706] (Fig. 23)

Exhaled air, which contains 16–18% oxygen, has been found to be an adequate resuscitative gas, provided that the patient's lungs are normal and the operator uses about twice normal tidal volumes, of about 1.0 l in the average adult[220]. This usually results in arterial PCO_2 values of 20–30 mmHg in the rescuer and 30–40 mmHg in the patient; and in arterial PO_2 values of over 75 mmHg (oxygen saturation over 90%) in the patient with normal lungs.

Thus, emergency artificial ventilation should not be delayed by attempts to find and apply adjuncts. Direct exhaled air ventilation—also called 'rescue breathing'—is always readily available. In acute apnea, exhaled air immediately does more good than air or oxygen minutes later.

Whenever adequate ventilation (as judged by intermittent chest expansion and escape of exhaled air) cannot be achieved with equipment used for providing IPPV with air or oxygen, immediate return to IPPV by mouth-to-mouth (or nose) ventilation is indicated.

The process of blowing air into the patient's mouth or nose not only inflates the lungs but may also force air into the *stomach*, particularly when the air passage is obstructed or the inflation pressure excessive—in the relaxed victims 15–25 cmH₂O or higher[690]. Although usually some air blown into the stomach is harmless, it can be minimized by blowing slowly (1–2 seconds per inflation), and only until the chest rises. A health professional, as a helper who knows anatomy, may prevent air from entering the stomach by pressing the cricoid cartilage backward to occlude the esophagus. Occasionally, inflation of the stomach may make lung inflations more difficult and provoke regurgitation and aspiration. Therefore, if the patient's stomach bulges markedly, to the extent that it interferes with ventilation, press with your hand briefly over the epigastrium (between sternum and umbilicus). This will force air out of the stomach. Since this maneuver may also cause regurgitation, tilt the patient's head down if possible, and turn the head and shoulders to one side and be prepared to clear the pharynx. As soon as possible after suspected aspiration, intubate and suction the trachea, and drain the stomach via a nasogastric tube.

Ensure adequate ventilation by observing the patient's chest to determine whether it rises and falls, feeling air moving from you into him/her, and hearing and feeling air escape during exhalations. This usually results in the average adult in the desired tidal volumes of 0.8–1.2 liters.

Some individuals may find it easier to overcome their hesitations regarding direct mouth-to-mouth contact by blowing through a handkerchief (or saliva filter) placed over the patient's mouth and nose.

In unconscious victims of *trauma*, for spontaneous and/or mouth-to-mouth breathing, have a helper apply gentle axial traction, tilt the head backward only moderately (not maximally), and, if necessary, displace the mandible forward (jaw-thrust) and retract the lower lip (mouth open). Flexion (chin on chest) and lateral turning of the head and neck must be avoided in patients with suspected neck injury. Nevertheless, the airway has precedence over the cervical spine.

In the *tracheotomized* patient or *laryngectomee*, perform direct mouth-to-tracheostomy tube or mouth-to-stoma inflations[23b, 701]. Improvise control of leaks between tube and skin. Persons who have undergone a laryngectomy (surgical removal of the larynx) have a permanent stoma (opening) that connects the trachea directly to the skin. When such an individual requires direct mouth-to-stoma ventilation, seal your mouth around his stoma and blow air into his stoma until the chest rises. Other persons may have a temporary tracheostomy tube. To ventilate, mouth and nose must usually be sealed by the rescuer's hand to prevent leakage. This problem is alleviated when the tracheostomy tube has a cuff.

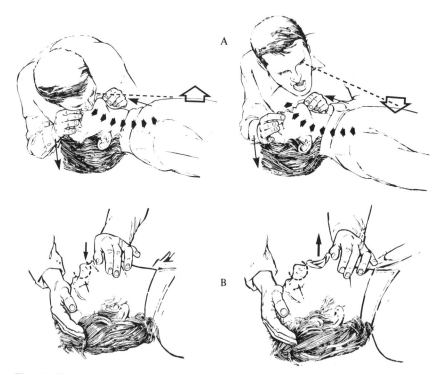

Fig. 23. Direct exhaled air ventilation (see text). (A) Mouth-to-mouth ventilation (with head tilt by chin support). Inflation (left) with nose held closed, and passive exhalation (right) through mouth held open. (B) Mouth-to-nose ventilation (with head tilt by chin support). Inflation (left) with mouth held closed, and passive exhalation (right) through mouth held open.

In *small children and infants*, exhaled air ventilation is performed with the same technique, but cover both the mouth and the nose of the child with your mouth and use small breaths of less volume to inflate the lungs at a more rapid rate. In newborn babies, the volume between your cheeks is adequate, i.e. ventilate with 'puffs'. Backward tilt of the head should not be exaggerated, since the infant's trachea may be occluded by excessive hyperextension.

Technique of mouth-to-mouth ventilation[699] (Fig. 23-A)

1. If the victim is unconscious, tilt his/her head backward using chin support—with one hand on the forehead and the other hand holding the chin, preventing it from sagging and holding the mouth slightly open (Fig. 3-B). Head-tilt by neck lift (Fig. 3-C) is an alternative method.
2. If the patient is not breathing (you cannot hear or feel airflow at the mouth or nose or cannot see the chest rise and fall), pinch the nose with one hand, take a deep breath, seal your mouth around the mouth (mouth plus nose in infants and small children) with a wide open circle, and blow until the chest rises. While blowing, watch the chest to see whether it rises with your inflation. (Blow gently into children; use only puffs for infants to avoid lung rupture.)
   As an alternative method for preventing air leakage through the nose, press your cheek against the nostrils while blowing.
   Minimize blowing air into the stomach by making each inflation 1–2 seconds long. If high inflation pressure seems required, have an assistant (health professional only) press on the cricoid cartilage (just below the Adam's apple) to occlude the esophagus.
3. When you see the chest rise, stop inflation, release the seal of your mouth against the patient's mouth, turn your face to the side, and allow him/her to exhale passively completely.
4. When exhalation is finished, give the next lung inflation. Volume is more important than rhythm. Give two initial lung inflations, each over 1–2 seconds, each followed by complete passive exhalation. Then check the carotid pulse. If the pulse is present, repeat inflations—in adults about one every 5 seconds (12 per minute); in children about one every 4 seconds (15 per minute); in infants about one every 3 seconds (20 per minute)—until the patient starts breathing adequately spontaneously.
   If the pulse is absent, start with heart (chest) compressions (Step C), about 15 compressions at a rate of 80–100 per minute (slightly slower than 2 compressions per second). Again give two lung inflations as before and continue 15 compressions until the carotid pulse returns

(check every 1–2 minutes). Continue inflating the lungs until he/she starts breathing adequately.

5. If you cannot inflate the lungs, readjust head-tilt and chin support and blow again. If you still fail, add jaw-thrust and open the mouth (Fig. 6) and blow again. If you still fail, use finger sweep (Fig. 7), abdominal thrusts and back blows (Figs. 9 and 10).

Technique of mouth-to-nose ventilation[224] (Fig. 23-B)

When it is impossible to open the victim's mouth (trismus), as during seizures, when blowing into the mouth meets obstruction, or when the mouth is not easily accessible as with resuscitation started in water, use mouth-to-nose ventilation.

1. Use head-tilt and chin support as with mouth-to-mouth ventilation. Cup one hand under the chin and close the mouth with your thumb.

2. Take a deep breath; encircle the nose with your mouth (avoid pinching the nose with your lips) and blow until the chest rises. Open the mouth for exhalation, as the patient may have expiratory nasopharyngeal obstruction (encountered in about one-third of comatose patients, due to a valve-like behavior of the soft palate).

In most countries mouth-to-mouth ventilation is taught as a first step, with mouth-to-nose as an alternative. In some countries, mouth-to-nose is the preferred method. Both methods should be taught to all personnel.

Mouth-to-Adjunct Ventilation[220, 698] (Fig. 12-C, 24)

Since the development of mouth-to-mouth ventilation, the first adjuncts recommended for exhaled air ventilation were masks[220] and special pharyngeal tubes[698]. However, the lay public should not be taught the use of adjuncts in preference to direct mouth-to-mouth. Exhaled air ventilation adjuncts should ideally have one-way valves, which close during positive pressure inflation and open during exhalation, venting the victims exhaled air (which some fear might contain infectious organisms) away from the operator. These adjuncts should also have a valved port (nipple) for adding a continuous flow of oxygen. During *direct* mouth-to-mouth ventilation prevention of infection via saliva by use of a *filter cloth*, and *oxygen enrichment* of the operator's exhaled air[341], are possible.

Mouth-to-airway[698, 699] (Fig. 12-C)

The S-tube, a double Guedel airway, overcomes the aesthetic objection to direct mouth-to-mouth contact, keeps the victim's mouth open, and assists in maintaining a patent airway. Like all pharyngeal tubes, however, it may induce gagging, laryngospasm or vomiting if inserted into the conscious or merely stuporous patient. Shortened S-tubes or mouth props obviate upper airway stimulation, but may cause problems with air leakage and obstruction. The Brooke Airway is a modified S-tube incorporating a separate exhalation valve. Hospital and ambulance personnel have used S-tubes and regular pharyngeal tubes effectively.

Mouth-to-mask with oxygen[729] (Fig. 24)

The Laerdal pocket mask can be used safely by trained lay personnel, but does not improve ventilation efficacy over direct mouth-to-mouth[107, 234]. One advantage of the pocket mask is its oxygen inlet nipple[729]. It provides an inspired oxygen concentration of 50–80% during spontaneous breathing and 50–100% during artificial ventilation with delivered continuous inflow rates of 15 l/min.

All types of trained personnel attempting to ventilate manikins and patients seem to be more effective with the mouth-to-mask than with the bag–valve–mask technique[340, 379]. The latter leaves only one hand free for support of mask fit and head tilt (which closes the mouth under the mask), does not usually permit jaw thrust during IPPV by one operator, and often provides less than 1 liter inflation volume, which is hardly enough to overcome the leakage with a poor mask fit. In contrast, the pocket mask provides up to 4 liters reserve volume (the rescuer's vital capacity) to overcome leakage, and keeps both hands free to provide mask fit and jaw-thrust. When jaw-thrust is required, mouth-to-mask ventilation is more easily performed than mouth-to-mouth, since the operator can remain positioned at the patient's vertex. It has been strongly recommended (AHA) that in emergency resuscitation prior to endotracheal intubation, mouth–mask–oxygen is preferred over the use of bag–valve–mask devices, except for personnel extensively trained in the use of bag–valve–mask devices, such as anesthesiologists.

Masks should be transparent to permit recognition of cyanosis, vomitus, mucus and blood, and clouding with spontaneous exhalations for monitoring. They should provide an effective seal on the face, an oxygen insufflation nipple, a breathing port with a standard 15/22 mm connector, and a head strap to hold the mask loosely on the patient's face during spontaneous breathing and one-operator CPR, when continuous holding of the mask is not possible. The masks should fit adults, children and infants. The adult pocket masks can fit all ages; for infants it should cover the entire face and should be applied upside down, with the nose part of the mask over the chin.

Recent studies in Norway[107] and the USA[234] indicate that use of the pocket mask helps lay persons to learn the technique of exhaled air ventilation on each other without manikins, and encourages learning to displace the mandible forward (jaw thrust). The latter is particularly desirable for use in accident victims in lieu of maximal backward tilt of the head.

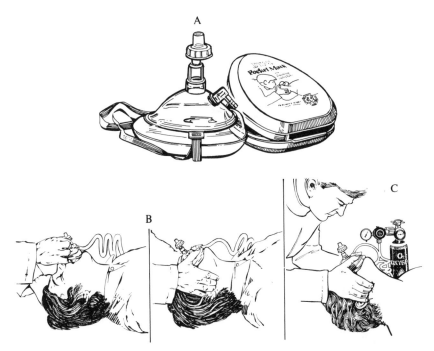

Fig. 24. Pocket mask with oxygen insufflation nipple for mouth-to-mask ventilation with oxygen, and for spontaneous inhalation of oxygen[729]. (A) Laerdal pocket transparent folding mask with 15 mm male breathing port, oxygen insufflation nipple, inflated cushion, head strap and IPPV non-breathing valve to divert the patient's exhaled air away from the rescuer's face. (B) In the comatose patient, tilt the head backward. Open the mouth by retracting the lower lip, and apply the rim of the mask over the chin to keep the mouth open. Apply the entire mask over the mouth and nose. (C) Clamp the mask to the face with both thumbs (thenar eminences) on top of the mask and fingers 2–5 of both hands grasping both ascending rami of mandible in front of the earlobes. Pull forcefully upward (forward) so that the lower teeth are in front of the upper teeth and chin juts out. The mouth should remain open under the mask. The front of the neck must be maximally stretched. Do not pull on the chin as this tends to close the mouth. Take a deep breath, blow into the port of the mask until the chest moves, remove your mouth and let the patient exhale passively through the valve. Sustain this maneuver as long as the patient is unconscious or until a pharyngeal or endotracheal tube can be inserted. For long-term ventilation, a pharyngeal tube is helpful because it can usually replace jaw thrust.

In infants apply the mask upside down and cover the entire face. Use only puffs from your cheeks.

When oxygen is available, deliver it via the nipple of the mask. Oxygen at 10–15 l/min continuous flow results in about 50% oxygen inhaled. With higher flows, artificial ventilation with 100% oxygen is possible by intermittently occluding the breathing port with your tongue and opening it when the chest rises to permit exhalation.

For use during CPR or in the spontaneously breathing patient, when continuous manual support of mask fit is not possible, strap the mask to the face loosely.

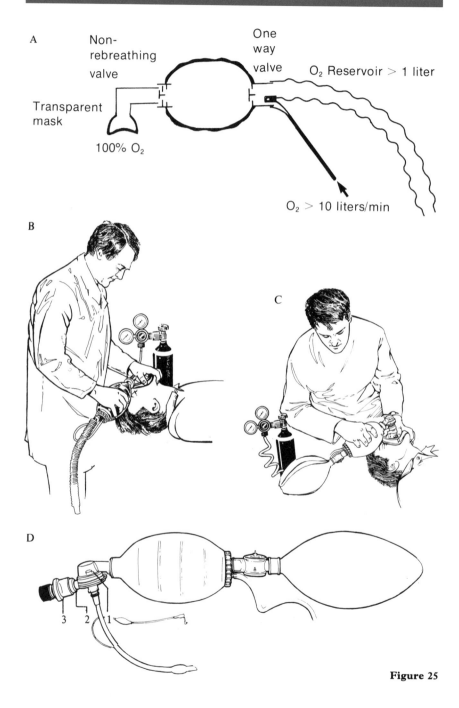

A

Non-rebreathing valve

One way valve

O_2 Reservoir > 1 liter

Transparent mask

100% O_2

O_2 > 10 liters/min

B

C

D

3 2 1

Figure 25

Bag–Valve–Mask with Oxygen[688, 732] (Fig. 25)

The development of the self-refilling bag–valve–mask unit by Ruben[688] followed the bellows–valve–mask devices of the Oxford[501] and Kreiselman[433] types used during World War II and emergency anesthesia bag–mask units[347, 501, 542]. The self-refilling bag–valve unit may be used with mask, endotracheal tube, esophageal obturator airway or tracheostomy tube. It is not easy to use with a mask, but is particularly valuable and effective for ventilation and oxygenation of the intubated patient, which can easily be mastered by nonphysicians. Its 1–1.5 liter bag provides less reserve gas volume in case of leakage than does mouth–mask–oxygen, and does not leave both hands free to provide jaw thrust. Therefore the operator must be prepared to insert a pharyngeal tube, must be able to provide a tight fit with one hand, and must be experienced with and skillful in the use of these devices.

The recommended bag–valve–mask units must permit delivery of oxygen during both spontaneous and artificial ventilation (Fig. 25-A)[762]. They must be easily cleaned and sterilized. They should consist of a self-refilling bag with an inlet valve to which an oxygen reservoir tube (Fig. 25-B) or reservoir bag (Fig. 25-C) may be attached, and a nonrebreathing valve at the mask or tracheal tube. To deliver 100% oxygen, the reservoir must be at least as large as the bag volume and the oxygen inflow rate must at least equal the minute volume. The nonrebreathing valve must have an expiratory valve to permit delivery of the gas mixture from the bag during spontaneous breathing. The device should have a nonsticking valve that does not permit backward leak, and that does not lock in the inflation position during delivery of oxygen. A pop-off valve which can be closed is desirable. There should be transparent, well fitting face masks of various sizes, and standard 15/22 mm fittings. It should be impossible to assemble the components of the bag–valve–mask unit incorrectly. It should be available in adult and pediatric sizes, perform under extremes of environmental temperature and be suitable for practice on manikins. Although the main advantage of the bag–valve–mask unit constructed as described above is its ability to deliver 100% oxygen, in some

Fig. 25 (opposite). Self-refilling bag–valve–mask unit with oxygen. (A) Diagram of a self-refilling bag with inlet valve, oxygen tube reservoir and nonrebreathing valve, Ruben-Ambu[688]. (B) *Laerdal* Silicon Resuscitator with large-bore tube oxygen reservoir. (C) *Laerdal* Silicon Resuscitator with bag oxygen reservoir (with safety inlet and overflow valves). A continuous flow of oxygen is delivered into the reservoir at atmospheric pressure. (There are other acceptable bag–valve–mask units, such as the *Ambu* Resuscitator and the *Puritan* (Bennett) Resuscitator PMR-2.)

Clamp the mask to the patient's face with a regular grip (C) or, an improved method (B).

(D) Bag–valve–tube unit for IPPV with PEEP and 100% oxygen. 1, Nonrebreathing valve (Laerdal) with (2) expiration diverter. 3, Separate PEEP valve (Ambu) mounted on the expiration port of the standard Laerdal nonrebreathing valve.

examples an excessive oxygen flow rate with slow bag release may cause the valve to lock in the inspiratory position and cause lung rupture. For the same reason oxygen must never be delivered under pressure directly into the self-refilling bag. Among the commercially available units, the Laerdal Silicon Resuscitator fulfills the above requirements (Fig. 25)[732].

Holding the mask and the head with one hand and providing additional jaw-thrust is difficult for the inexperienced (Fig. 25). Since use of the bag–valve–mask unit usually closes the mouth under the mask, some unconscious patients require an oropharyngeal or nasopharyngeal tube to overcome nasal obstruction. You may use your knee(s) or hip for reinforcing head-tilt and your chin for reinforcing mask fit. If you must use both hands for providing mask fit and jaw-thrust, ask your assistant to squeeze the bag. You also can squeeze the bag between your arm (elbow) and your waist, if you use an extension tube between nonrebreathing valve and bag.

With an oxygen flow of over 10 l/min into the reservoir at the bag intake valve, the inhaled oxygen concentration in adults is 80–100% when using a reservoir; and 30–50% without a reservoir.

Modifications of the self-refilling bag–valve–mask unit permit special uses:

1. IPPV with 100% oxygen plus adjustable PEEP, with a modified Laerdal or Ambu unit (Fig. 25-D)[194, 732] may be lifesaving in pulmonary edema, aspiration, near-drowning or other conditions associated with increased pulmonary shunting.
2. For anesthesia with minimal equipment for field conditions in poor developing countries or in disasters[383, 391,501a, 616, 710], a draw-over (mainstream) volatile anesthetic vaporizer (e.g. Penlon, halothane; Macintosh, ether vaporizer) is inserted between the oxygen reservoir and self-refilling bag. This unit is only to be used by those with training in anesthesia.
3. Bronchodilator aerosol administration with a nebulizer interposed between the nonrebreathing valve and the patient permits the patient to augment his/her inhalations (via mouthpiece or mask) by synchronized bag squeezing[538].

Spontaneous breathing with positive airway pressure (SB-PAP) requires a different equipment assembly (Fig. 22). Most self-refilling bag–valve–mask units cannot be used safely for SB-PAP, as sustained positive pressure can lock the nonrebreathing valve in the inflation position and cause lung rupture.

Technique of bag–valve–mask ventilation and oxygenation (Fig. 25)

1. Position yourself at the patient's vertex. Tilt the head backward. If the patient is comatose, insert an oropharyngeal or nasopharyngeal tube.
2. *Spread* the mask, *mold* it over the mouth and nose, *clamp* it to the face with one hand, *tilt* the head backward, and *squeeze* the bag until the chest rises.
3. Release the bag to allow for complete passive exhalation. Abrupt bag release is necessary for proper valve function.

For *clamping the mask* to the patient's face use one of the following two maneuvers:

1. Press with your thumb over the superior (over the nose) part of the mask, with your index finger over the inferior part, and use your middle, ring and little fingers to pull the chin upward and backward (Fig. 25-C). If necessary press chin on mask.
2. With a flat mask, hook your fingers around the patient's chin and apply pressure on the top of the mask with the palm of your hand, always maintaining backward tilt (Fig. 25-B).

Manually Triggered Oxygen-Powered Ventilators[592] (Fig. 26)

Oxygen-powered manually and demand triggered ventilation devices (e.g. Elder, Robertshaw, Isaacson, Emerson valves) permit instantaneous manual initiation and termination of positive pressure inflation with oxygen via mask, esophageal obturator airway, endotracheal tube or tracheostomy tube. They are powered by a high pressure (50 psi) oxygen source. Recommended units should do the following[592]: (1) deliver 100% oxygen; (2) provide an instantaneous and constant flow rate of 40 l/min for adults (with lower adjustable flow rates for infants and children); (3) have the manual trigger positioned so that both hands of the operator can hold the mask and provide head-tilt and jaw-thrust, while triggering inflations; (4) have a safety valve to pop off at about 60 cmH$_2$O for adults (with a switch to 30 cmH$_2$O for infants and children) with an audio alarm to detect high resistance to inflation; (5) have standard 15/22 fittings; (6) be rugged and function in extreme environmental temperatures; and (7) function as a demand oxygen inhalation device for spontaneous breathing.

In the past, very high instantaneous flow rates have been recommended to enable lung inflations between uninterrupted chest compressions. Devices delivering high flow rates may cause high pharyngeal pressures and gastric distension and should therefore be used with cricoid pressure or via tracheal tube. Recent recommendations[23b] call for lower flow rates and for briefly interrupting chest compressions during CPR for lung inflations.

The principal *disadvantages* of oxygen-powered manually triggered ventilation devices, in comparison with the bag–valve–mask and mouth-to-mask techniques, are their dependence on compressed gas; the inability of the operator to feel resistance during inflation; unchecked peak inflation pressures, which are able to cause gastric insufflation, regurgitation, lung rupture and tension pneumothorax; inability to deliver humidified oxygen; and need for additional training.

Manually triggered oxygen-powered ventilators should be used only by trained and experienced personnel, and only on adult patients. Do not use these devices in children and infants.

The *technique* is as follows: tilt the head back, insert a pharyngeal tube if it is tolerated, apply the mask firmly with both hands, push the trigger, watch the chest move and release the trigger for complete passive exhalation. Add jaw-thrust if necessary.

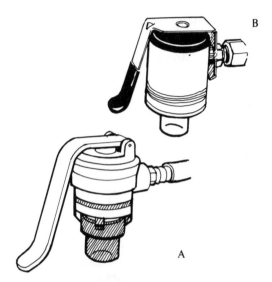

Fig. 26. Ventilation-demand inhalation valves of several manually triggered oxygen-powered resuscitators, to be attached to a mask or tracheal tube: (A) Elder valve, (B) Robertshaw valve.

Automatic Ventilators[408, 568, 736c]

For *emergency artificial ventilation* without a tracheal tube most oxygen-powered, time cycled, pressure-limited ventilators (resuscitators) used in the past in ambulances are *not* recommended. The reasons that such devices are not in favor is that the fixed cycling pressure does not permit adaptation of inflation volume, pressure, flow and rhythm to changing mask leakage, lung–thorax compliance, airway resistance and spontaneous breathing efforts. In addition, 'suck-and-blow' units interfere with passive exhalation. During external chest compressions, because of widely fluctuating airway pressure, these devices tend to cycle prematurely into exhalation. Their heavy weight, complexity and cost are added disadvantages. Many of them cannot be adapted for optimal continuous oxygen flow (demand valve for spontaneous breathing).

Some new *adjustable-pressure* oxygen-powered automatic ventilators, such as the Bird Mark VIII are exceptions. Some are small and portable and can provide many of the required ventilation patterns (Fig. 21). They have been used successfully for ventilating intubated patients with near-normal lungs, not only in hospitals but also in ambulances. Volume-set, time-cycled ventilators are preferred. Rugged field ventilators, such as the Pneupac, offer a useful alternative[5].

Historically, prolonged mechanical ventilation before the 1950s was usually provided by *tank ventilators* (body box, iron lung). It ventilates by intermittent negative pressure around the body, with the airway exposed to atmospheric pressure. This ventilation approach is *not* recommended, even for prolonged ventilation, as it provides inadequate ventilation power, adjustability and airway control, and makes the patient inaccessible and immobile[364, 712]. The only possible usefulness of tank or body cuirass ventilators is for weaning or assisting nonintubated paralyzed (neurologic) patients.

For *prolonged mechanical ventilation* of the intubated patient with abnormal lungs in the hospital, a great variety of suitable automatic ventilators with adjustable and readable airway pressure, tidal volume, flow rate and cycling rate could be recommended. These ventilators should be capable of producing IPPV, with or without PEEP, and intermittent mandatory ventilation or assisted ventilation (Fig. 21), with controllable inhaled oxygen concentrations and capability of delivering drug aerosols and warm humidity. Most *motor-powered* mechanical ventilators, favored in intensive care units because of their reliability, are not suitable for emergency artificial ventilation or long-term ventilation in ambulances, as they are not portable and depend on electric line current.

The desired criteria for the functioning of an '*ideal*' *mechanical ventilator* for sophisticated intensive care we consider to be the following[736c] (Figs. 21, 22):

1. (volume set) tidal volumes between 0 and 2 liters;

2. inflation frequencies between 0 and 40 per minute (optional up to 100 per minute for high frequency IPPV without jetting, see below);
3. airway pressures between 0 and 70 cmH$_2$O;
4. an end-inspiratory pause;
5. PEEP of 0–20 cmH$_2$O (optional to 50 cmH$_2$O);
6. adjustable time and flow rates during inflation and exhalation;
7. assistor, controller, mixed and IMV modes;
8. an SB-CPAP/EPAP mode for IMV;
9. an automatic sighing mechanism (optional);
10. an adjustable safety pop-off pressure valve;
11. controllability of inhaled oxygen and carbon dioxide concentrations (ideally through servo control);
12. an optional negative end-expiratory pressure (NEEP) mode;
13. a heated humidifier with airway temperature and humidity controls;
14. a drug aerosol nebulizer;
15. a device to permit drainage of condensed water in tubings;
16. an air intake bacterial filter;
17. an exhaled air scavenger or bacterial air filter;
18. lightweight, nonslipping, nonkinking connections to the patient;
19. an alarm to indicate volume, pressure or cycling failure, extremes of gas temperature and disconnection;
20. a reliable inexpensive power source;
21. readable tidal volumes, rates, minute volumes, airway pressures and FIO_2 (for monitoring).

None of the existing ventilators have all these characteristics incorporated, but some come close to it.

Translaryngeal Oxygen Jet Ventilation[371, 372, 417, 835]

This method is ready for clinical trials in emergency resuscitation including CPR[99, 416]. Its basic mode is with regular ventilation rates. Although an invasive method, it may simplify emergency ventilation and oxygenation in the hands of specially trained personnel. For technique see Fig. 18.

High-Frequency Jet Ventilation[417]

This is a novel method for the delivery of oxygen which challenges established concepts of physiologic dead space and alveolar ventilation[415–417]. It is an alternative to conventional automatic ventilation, but not a panacea. There are three modes developed in the laboratory and presently under clinical trial:

1. high-frequency IPPV with rates up to 100 per minute via tracheal

tube[812]: estimated tidal volumes are near or greater than the dead space;
2. high-frequency jet ventilation (HFJV) via small-gauge catheter inserted into the trachea percutaneously (via the cricothyroid membrane) or via tracheal or tracheostomy tube, with frequencies of 100–500 per minute and tidal volumes smaller than the dead space[415] (Fig. 27);
3. high-frequency oscillations with frequencies of 500–3000 per minute via open, valveless tracheal tube[496].

These high cycling rates are produced by portable jet ventilators with fluidic or electric valves. They produce mean airway pressures of 2–7 cmH_2O provided the upper airway is open. High-frequency ventilation with tidal volumes at or below dead space volume can maintain normal arterial PO_2 and PCO_2, probably through flow- and diffusion-enhanced gas mixing in the airways, which permits use of very small tidal volumes of bulk movement of gas.

Advantages, according to Klain[417], include: (1) low airway pressure (less pulmonary barotrauma); (2) no need for synchronization with spontaneous breathing; (3) less injury to the tracheal mucosa when used with a translaryngeal catheter; and (4) the ability to counteract aspiration and soft tissue obstruction. In dogs with normal lungs during CPR from ventricular fibrillation or asphyxial cardiac arrest, HFJV reoxygenated the arterial blood as readily as did IPPV[99].

Disadvantages include: (1) inability to suction the tracheobronchial tree; (2) percutaneous cannulation; (3) risk of tissue insufflation; (4) dependence on special equipment; and (5) requirement of an at least partially open upper airway for exhalations. High-frequency ventilation can eliminate carbon dioxide, but it cannot reliably reverse pulmonary shunting (recruit alveoli) in pulmonary edema and consolidation (ARDS)[777], at least not as effectively as periodic deep lung inflations (sighs) and IPPV plus optimal PEEP. Of course, HFJV can be used with PEEP and intermittent sighs may be added. In lung failure, both IPPV and HFJV need to be used with the same PEEP level. The only difference is gas delivery via a thin catheter and the fact that each inflation is not a sigh, as in IPPV.

Fig. 27 (opposite). High-frequency jet ventilation. (A) Basic setup requires a 50 psi air and/or oxygen source. A blender allows adjustment of the appropriate concentration of oxygen for both jet ventilator and entrainment circuit. A jet cannula (e.g. 14b Angiocath) is inserted into the endotracheal tube through the wall or through a T-connector attached to it. A special 'Hi-Lo' jet tube with a jet channel built into its wall can also be used. Humidification is added directly to the jet through a Y-connector by an infusion pump. (B) Diagram of the system for transtracheal high-frequency jet ventilation. A blender provides mixing of high pressure (50 psi) oxygen and air for the ventilator. A jet cannula is inserted by cricothyroid membrane puncture and attached to the ventilator. If ventilatory support longer than 1 hour is anticipated, humidification is achieved by infusing water through a Y-connector in the jet tubing, usually at the rate of 10 ml/h. This connector can also be used for administering drugs directly into the jet stream for intrapulmonary application. (From M. Klain: *Prospectives in High-Frequency Jet Ventilation*, courtesy of Martinus Nijhoff Publishers, The Hague, Netherlands).

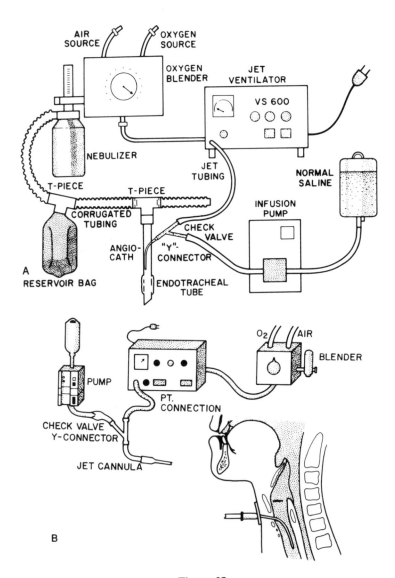

Figure 27

Oxygen Delivery Systems[736c] (Fig. 28)

During emergency resuscitation, additional oxygen (50–100% inhaled oxygen) should be introduced as soon as it becomes available, in order to increase oxygen delivery. While healthy lungs permit full oxygenation of arterial blood with use of exhaled air or air, most patients requiring resuscitation have abnormal lungs. This includes some alveoli unventilated because of being collapsed or fluid-filled (intrapulmonary right-to-left shunting), others less ventilated than perfused (ventilation–perfusion mismatching), and others ventilated but not perfused (physiologic dead space). Thus optimal resuscitation requires a higher inspired oxygen concentration than that provided in exhaled air or air. Supplemental oxygen should also be used for critically ill patients without respiratory or cardiac arrest, as for those with suspected myocardial infarction, polytrauma or coma of any cause.

For CPR, use 100% oxygen first if available. Inhalation of 100% oxygen is safe for at least 6 hours, but the concentration should be reduced to about 50% within about 6–12 hours if arterial PO_2 permits, to avoid pulmonary damage due to high alveolar PO_2. This occurs after about 48 hours of 100% oxygen inhalation[156]. Fifty per cent oxygen appears to be safe for unlimited long-term use. Sick lungs with shunting increase the tolerance of greater than 50% oxygen inhaled[51, 969, 970].

Oxygen administration by any method requires an oxygen source, such as a portable small cylinder; a movable large oxygen cylinder as found on emergency vehicles and in hospitals; or piped wall oxygen (Fig. 28). Appropriate yoke, valve, flowmeter, humidifier and connecting tubing to the patient's oxygen administration equipment are as important as the oxygen cylinder and the mask. This equipment must be understood by all health care personnel involved in resuscitation and intensive care. Oxygen sources must be capable of delivering oxygen at a pressure of 30–60 psi (2–4 atmospheres) to resuscitators and mechanical ventilators and be available to deliver oxygen at near atmospheric pressure at controllable flow rates for mask and bag–valve units. For emergency resuscitation, exact oxygen concentrations are not necessary. For evaluation of arterial PO_2 values, however, and for long-term respiratory care, knowing the exact delivered oxygen concentration is facilitated with use of air–oxygen mixers and a leak-free system.

Dry air or oxygen inhaled for prolonged periods stops ciliary clearing of the tracheobronchial mucosa and promotes pulmonary infection. Adequate natural humidification is possible only when breathing through the nose. For long-term oxygen inhalation through the mouth, endotracheal tube or tracheostomy tube, the oxygen must be humidified and ideally also warmed to about body temperature. Cold bubble humidifiers are inadequate for long-term use. Warmed bubble or surface humidifiers are preferred over nebulizers, since the latter offer a greater risk of droplet-mediated iatrogenic infection.

Recommended for emergency resuscitation cases with spontaneous breathing is oxygen administration via a simple versatile (pocket) mask (Fig. 24) or a self-refilling bag–valve–mask unit (Fig. 25).

For spontaneous breathing of humidified oxygen via tracheal tube, the patient is best connected to a large-bore valveless T-tube (with a short tail). Customary flow rates (e.g. 10 l/min) will provide inhaled oxygen concentrations lower than those delivered because air is entrained as well. Inhaled oxygen concentrations, however, will equal delivered concentrations with the use of the T-tube when inflow rates exceed average peak inspiratory flow rates (approx. 20–25 l/min in the adult). Artificial ventilation is possible by intermittently occluding the tail of the T-tube. The chest must be watched to prevent lung rupture.

During spontaneous breathing (SB) of 50–100% oxygen (via strapped-on mask, mouthpiece or tracheal tube), arterial PO_2 can often be raised further in the presence of reversible shunting (e.g. pulmonary edema) by adding continuous positive airway pressure (SB-CPAP) of 5–15 cmH_2O. This can be provided with equipment assembled from available components (Fig. 22)[736c].

Not recommended for emergency resuscitation cases are the oxygen delivery systems commonly used for conscious patients, e.g. semi-open valveless oronasal masks with or without bags; the aerosol oxygen mask; the

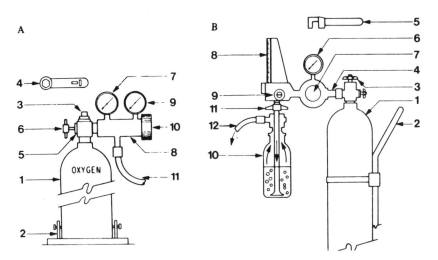

Fig. 28. (A) Portable oxygen delivery system: 1, small cylinder; 2, stand; 3, cylinder valve; 4, wrench; 5, yoke; 6, yoke handle; 7, cylinder pressure gauge; 8, reducing valve; 9, flow meter; 10, needle valve; and 11, delivery tube. (B) Moveable oxygen delivery system: 1, large cylinder; 2, movable cart; 3, cylinder valve; 4, yoke; 5, wrench for fastening yoke; 6, cylinder pressure gauge; 7, reducing valve; 8, flow meter; 9, needle valve; 10, bubble humidifier; 11, wing nut for humidifier; and 12, delivery tube.

nasal cannula; the nasopharyngeal oxygen catheter (obsolete); the Venturi mask; and the oxygen tent.

The *Venturi mask* is a semi-open oronasal mask delivering known inhaled oxygen concentrations of 24–40%. It is recommended for stable chronic obstructive pulmonary disease (emphysema) patients without shunting, who may hypoventilate when given high concentrations of oxygen to breathe. If acutely decompensated or in need of resuscitation, these patients should be given higher concentrations of oxygen, but their ventilation should be assisted or controlled or spontaneous breathing continuously verbally coached. Under no circumstances should 100% oxygen be withheld from a clinically hypoxemic (cyanotic) patient.

Selecting Ventilation and Oxygenation Techniques[630, 736c, 836] (Table 3, Figs. 21, 22)

Emergency resuscitation should begin with hyperventilation by IPPV, using 100% oxygen if available (Fig. 21). After re-oxygenation, tidal volume and rate requirements vary greatly between patients and disease states. Proof of the adequacy of *alveolar ventilation* is an arterial PCO_2 of 35–45 mmHg; and proof of the adequacy of *oxygenation* is an arterial PO_2 of at least 80 mmHg. The acid–base status is reflected in arterial pH and base excess (Fig. 41) (Chapter 2).

Arterial blood gas determinations should ideally be available to guide emergency artificial ventilation, but are not available at all hospitals. Where arterial blood gas determinations are not available, clinical judgment should be used to suspect hypercarbia (somnolence, poor chest movements) and hypoxemia (restlessness, tachycardia, cyanosis). Absence of cyanosis does not rule out hypoxemia. When in doubt, give oxygen and assist or control ventilation.

For post-resuscitative intensive care, arterial catheterization for blood gas determinations are highly desirable. The required skills and equipment should be provided in every emergency hospital (Chapter 2).

When, after cardiac arrest and restoration of spontaneous circulation, the patient resumes spontaneous breathing, it is desirable to continue intermittent mandatory ventilation with 50–100% oxygen as long as he/she is unconscious. When the patient recovers consciousness, inhalation of oxygen should be continued at least until hospital admission, when care will be assumed by personnel experienced in advanced respiratory therapy and further adjustments made. Even if the patient did not receive CPR and is breathing spontaneously, he/she should, if cyanotic or dyspneic, inhale 50–100% oxygen during transportation.

For *controlled ventilation* of the comatose patient in the absence of blood gas determinations, ventilate with 50% oxygen using tidal volumes of approximately 15 ml/kg body weight (1000 ml/70 kg), approximately 12 times per minute (one inflation every 5 seconds). In the absence of lung changes this will maintain arterial PCO_2 at 25–35 mmHg and arterial PO_2 over 100 mmHg in most cases.

Subsequent adjustment of artificial ventilation must take into account at least the following: (1) peak inspiratory airway pressure; (2) tidal volume; (3) rate; and (4) inhaled oxygen concentration. Additional considerations include PEEP, inspiratory flow rate and expiratory flow rate.

Most patients with near-normal lungs can be ventilated adequately with any simple, inexpensive ventilator. Patients with abnormal lungs may require expensive volume-set ventilators with multiple adjustments; if such apparatus is not available, manual IPPV with bag–valve unit or an anesthesia circuit can provide most of the patterns shown in Fig. 21.

Oxygenation of arterial blood will require one or more of the following measures:

1. Provision of ventilation volumes and rates adequate to keep arterial PCO_2 at normal or moderately low levels.
2. Increase of inhaled oxygen to about 50%. If the lungs are healthy, exhaled air or air is adequate. However, augmentation of inspired oxygen concentration to about 50% is needed when some lung areas are relatively less ventilated than perfused.
3. Increase of inhaled oxygen to 50–100% and addition of some form of continuous positive pressure for alveolar recruitment (SB-CPAP; IPPV + PEEP = CPPV). This is needed when there is alveolar shunting (some blood flowing through nonventilated alveoli).
4. Optimization of cardiac output (blood volume and pressure, and heart pumping action). Low cardiac output in the presence of shunting reduces arterial PO_2.

Arterial oxygen transport to the organism is blood flow (cardiac output) times arterial oxygen content. Arterial oxygen transport requires not only an adequate arterial PO_2, but also an adequate hemoglobin concentration (hematocrit of 30–40%) and adequate blood flow (which in turn requires adequate blood volume, arterial pressure and cardiac pumping action).

For failure of ventilation, a systematic progression of measures from spontaneous via assisted to controlled ventilation is recommended (Table 3-A).

For failure of oxygenation, a stepwise increase in the complexity of positive pressure techniques and other measures is recommended (Table 3-B). The objective of these measures will be to maintain near-normal levels of arterial PCO_2, PO_2 and pH.

To guide oxygenation therapies, changes in arterial PO_2 during inhalation of a known oxygen concentration should be observed (alveolar-arterial PO_2 gradient). When recording arterial PO_2 values, inhaled oxygen concentration of 21–100% (FIO_2 0·21–1·0) and ventilatory pattern (SB; IPPV; CPPV; AV; MV) must be stated to make the PO_2 value meaningful.

The 100% oxygen test[736c] (recommended for guiding the therapies of Table 3-B)

Test 1—Determine the arterial PO_2 during breathing of air at atmospheric pressure at least 5 minutes. (This step should be omitted when the patient requires oxygen, which is usually the case during emergency resuscitation.) If arterial PO_2 is less than 80 mmHg, go to Test 2.

Test 2—Determine the arterial PO_2 after at least 5 minutes of 100% oxygen breathing at atmospheric pressure (spontaneous breathing), for instance by bag–valve–mask unit. With normal lungs the arterial PO_2 should be 500–600 mmHg. If arterial PO_2 is 100 mmHg, a 20% shunt is estimated; if 50 mmHg, a 50% shunt. Precise determination of shunt is complicated and usually not necessary. If arterial PO_2 is less than about 200 mmHg, go to Test 3.

Test 3—Determine the arterial PO_2 after at least 5 minutes of some form of positive pressure ventilation with 100% oxygen (SB-PAP; CPPV). This reveals whether the shunting found in Test 2 is partially reversible by positive airway pressure, and which form of therapy is most effective. Bring the arterial PO_2 to at least 60 mmHg in the conscious patient, or at least 100 mmHg in the unconscious patient, by following the steps of Table 3-B.

During controlled ventilation, PEEP can be optimized by monitoring changes in mixed venous PO_2 (PvO_2) (i.e. pulmonary artery or, as a compromise, superior vena cava PO_2[871]. PvO_2 would drop below about 35 mmHg when blood flow is reduced, as in shock or with excessive PEEP. Optimizing PEEP is also possible by monitoring airway pressure fluctuations required for a given tidal volume (compliance); the pressure should be minimized (compliance optimized).

When the patient recovers consciousness, weaning from controlled via intermittent mandatory (or assisted) ventilation to spontaneous breathing should be with oxygen enrichment (e.g. $FIO_2 = 0.5$). Weaning should be guided not only by blood gas values and other measurements, but also by clinical judgment, common sense and how the conscious patient feels and cooperates.

Safe indications and techniques for *oxygen administration* in abnormal pressure conditions need special physiologic knowledge and logistic considerations. These conditions include *high altitude*[716] and *hyperbarism* (diving, high pressure chamber)[161, 969, 970]. *Hyperbaric oxygenation* needs reinvestigation for use in prolonged resuscitation.

Important: Successful resuscitation requires more than ventilation and oxygenation. Oxygen and substrate delivery to tissues depends on tissue perfusion and arterial oxygen content. Tissue perfusion depends on cardiac output, which in turn is governed by venous return, cardiac pumping action and peripheral resistance. Arterial oxygen content depends on the arterial PO_2 and hemoglobin content. Blood flow equals pressure gradient divided by resistance. Peripheral resistance varies between and within different vascular beds; it is increased where there is vasospasm, tissue edema, blood sludging or clotting. Thus, the measures described in Chapters 1C, 2 and 3 are important for tissue oxygenation.

Table 3. Stepwise selection of ventilation patterns (see Fig. 20).

(A) Failure of ventilation (airway, muscle or CNS dysfunction)

Indications: $PaCO_2 > 45$ mmHg
Inspiratory capacity ('sigh') < 15 ml/kg body weight

Treatment: Use FIO_2 30–50%
Airway pressure at end-exhalation is 0–5 cmH$_2$O for Steps 1–4

Steps
1. Spontaneous breathing
2. Assisted ventilation or IMV
3. IPPV (controlled ventilation)
4. IPPV with expiratory retardation to minimize wheezing

(B) Failure of oxygenation (alveolar dysfunction)

Indications: $PaO_2 < 100$ mmHg $(FIO_2$ 50%)

Treatment: Use FIO_2 50–100% (100% less than 6 hours)
Airway pressure at end-exhalation is 5– > 20 cmH$_2$O (titrated) for Steps 1–5

Steps
1. Spontaneous breathing
2. Spontaneous breathing with CPAP
3. IMV
4. IPPV without PEEP
with low PEEP 5–10 cmH$_2$O
with high PEEP 10–20 cmH$_2$O
with 'super PEEP' greater than 20 cmH$_2$O
5. Improve circulation, metabolism, colloid osmotic pressure, osmolality, fluids, electrolytes, renal function (diuretic, dialysis)

For weaning, use the sequence of steps in reverse.

For abbreviations, see glossary.

Chapter 1C

Step C: Circulation Support (Cardiac Resuscitation)

Causes of Cardiac Arrest (Fig. 1)

Cardiac arrest may be primary or secondary[736a]. The most common cause of *primary* cardiac arrest is ventricular fibrillation from (transient) focal myocardial ischemia. Other causes of primary cardiac arrest include ventricular fibrillation and asystole from acute myocardial infarction, heart block, electric shock or certain drugs. *Secondary* cardiac arrest is most commonly caused by asphyxia or exsanguination, and can develop rapidly or slowly. Examples of *rapid* secondary cardiac arrest include asphyxia from airway obstruction or apnea, rapid blood loss and alveolar anoxia (from acute pulmonary edema or inhalation of oxygen-free gas). Examples of *slow* secondary cardiac arrest include severe hypoxemia (from pneumonia or pulmonary edema and consolidation, i.e. shock lung); oligemic or distributive (septic) type shock; electromechanical dissociation (EMD) in end-stage cardiogenic shock; and acute brain insults (leading to medullary failure and severe intractable hypotension and apnea). Primary mechanical asystole (pulselessness) with EMD, resulting in electric asystole as caused by hypoxemia, asphyxia or exsanguination, in previously healthy hearts, can often be easily reversed to spontaneous normotension using CPR Steps A–B–C, epinephrine and rapid restoration of blood volume. If heart disease causes prolonged ventricular fibrillation, which gets weaker and becomes electric asystole as pulselessness without CPR progresses, or if defibrillation leads to secondary EMD and electric asystole, spontaneous normotension is very difficult to achieve with CPR advanced life support.

Sudden complete cessation of circulation, from whatever cause, results usually in unconsciousness within about 15 seconds[683]; an isoelectric electroencephalogram (EEG) in 15–30 seconds[581]; agonal gasping; and apnea and maximal pupillary dilation starting at 30–60 seconds. When no blood flow lasts 5 minutes or more, restoration of normal perfusion pressure is followed by the post-resuscitation syndrome (Chapter 3)[580, 749, 759]. Thus, irrespective of the cause of cardiac arrest, if irreversible cerebral damage or death is to be prevented, CPR must be started immediately. For if, in primary cardiac arrest, the onset of reoxygenation by CPR is delayed beyond about 5 minutes, the chances of recovery without brain damage are small unless special, still in part experimental, brain resuscitation measures

98

are employed (Chapter 3). This critical time interval may be longer in hypothermic patients, those who have taken certain drugs, and in young children.

Recognition of Cardiac Arrest (Fig. 29)

Reversible cardiac arrest is defined as 'the clinical picture of overall cessation of circulation'. Cessation of circulation is diagnosed when all the following conditions are present: *unconsciousness; apnea or gasps; death-like appearance* (cyanosis or pallor); and *absence of pulse in large arteries* (e.g. carotid or femoral). Pulselessness of the carotid artery is the most important of these signs (Fig. 29) and is to be favored over absence of heart sounds, an unreliable sign. Notably, peripheral pulses may be absent in spite of the presence of the carotid pulse, particularly in hypovolemia. Palpation of the femoral artery, however, is an acceptable means of checking for the presence or absence of pulses. As a general rule, if the radial pulse is palpable, the systolic blood pressure is greater than 80 mmHg; if the femoral pulse is palpable, the systolic pressure is greater than 70 mmHg; and if the carotid pulse is palpable, the systolic pressure is greater than 60 mmHg.

In *infants* and *small children*, the carotid pulse may also be felt, but this easily compresses the airway or causes laryngospasm. Thus, determination of pulselessness by feeling the brachial or femoral artery or the abdominal

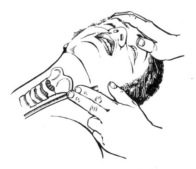

Fig. 29. Feeling for the carotid pulse to determine pulselessness. Maintain backward tilt of the head with one hand, while feeling for the patient's carotid pulse with your other hand. Check the side of the patient's neck closest to you; do not reach over the neck, as this maneuver is awkward and may also occlude the patient's airway. Feel for the pulse by placing your index and middle fingers gently on the patient's larynx (Adam's apple); then slide your fingers off to the side and press gently backward on the neck. Palpate with the flat portion of your fingers, rather than with the tips. If you do this correctly, the carotid artery should lie beneath your fingers. When feeling the artery, take care not to occlude it. Palpate long enough (5–10 seconds) to ensure that you do not miss a slow heart rate. Practice on normal patients.

aorta is recommended. In large children, feeling the carotid pulse is preferred.

Although dilated pupils are sometimes listed as an additional sign, one should not wait for pupils to dilate, since this may take more than 1 minute after cessation of circulation to occur. In some patients in cardiac arrest the pupils never dilate at all[266]. Drugs may alter pupil size and reaction. Relative changes in pupil size are of little value during CPR. Pupillary reactivity can, however, be valuable as its recovery during CPR indicates effectiveness of artificial circulation, and after restoration of normotension indicates neurologic improvement.

Closed-Chest Cardiopulmonary Resuscitation (Fig. 30, 31, 32 and 33)[23, 252, 385, 429, 498, 709, 720]

The rediscovery of *external cardiac (chest) compressions* (Step C)[384, 429] and their combination with airway control (Step A) and artificial ventilation (Step B)[326, 709a, b] have made it possible for any trained person to promptly initiate attempts at reversal of clinical death, even outside the hospital.

Artificial circulation seems most readily produced by intermittent chest compressions[429]. Blood flows are low, are improved by 50:50 compression: relaxation ratio, and little influenced by rates of 40–120 per minute[883]. Since the heart occupies most of the space between the sternum and the spine in the lower chest (Fig. 30) intermittently depressing the sternum was favored in patient trials[384]. Laboratory workers since the late 1800s have effectively treated pulselessness from anesthetic overdose in animals with lateral chest compressions (see all historic references).

The *mechanism* by which external chest compressions move blood has recently been reinvestigated. Intermittently pressing the sternum downward (backward) may produce some systemic and pulmonary blood flow by variable combinations of the following two mechanisms: (1) squeezing the heart between the sternum and spine (heart pump mechanism), particularly when the heart is large and the chest is compliant as in children and small broad-chested dogs[42, 189, 429]; and (2) overall intrathoracic pressure fluctuations (chest pump mechanism), particularly when the chest is large as in large keel-chested dogs[693, 950]. A diffuse rise in intrathoracic pressure can force blood out of heart, lungs and great vessels due to valving of the great veins at the thorax inlet[171, 242]. When sternal pressure is released, the elasticity of the chest wall causes the heart and thorax to expand and refill with blood (thoracic diastole). Meanwhile the blood is oxygenated in the lungs. Functional valving of large veins at the thoracic inlet[242] and diaphragm[459] has been demonstrated. Historically, Waters in the 1920s suggested producing some blood flow with forceful IPPV without sternal compressions[934]. Redding in 1958 tried and abandoned this approach, as it produced only a trickle of blood flow in dogs with cardiac arrest. Sternal compressions can produce systolic aortic pressure peaks of 100 mmHg and more, but the diastolic pressure produced may be as low as 10 mmHg without, and somewhat higher with, epinephrine. The systolic central venous, right atrial, jugular venous and intracranial pressures are increased almost as much as arterial pressure, which leads to only minimal perfusion pressures[78, 79, 502, 674a]. Without coronary and cerebral arteriovenous perfusion pressures of at least 30–40 mmHg, the chances to sustain viability of the brain and to restore spontaneous heart action are small[169, 198, 625, 657, 875]. The low perfusion pressures produced by standard external CPR result in a cardiac output, carotid artery blood flow and cerebral blood flow of usually less than 30% of normal flow, sometimes less than 10% of normal[16, 78, 79, 118, 185, 325, 326, 337, 423, 456, 489, 502, 650, 876].

Cerebral blood flow during external CPR can sometimes be near zero after arrest times (without CPR) of 2–5 minutes or longer[456]. This is probably due to blood thickened by stasis and low pressure due to vasoparalysis. Cerebral blood flow (CBF) must be at least 50% of normal to maintain or restore consciousness[431] and at least 20% of normal to maintain cell viability[875]. CBF less than 10% normal may be worse than no flow[662] and CBF 10–20% normal may be better than no flow[841].

Coronary perfusion pressures and blood flows are extremely low (sometimes zero) during external CPR, due to the high right atrial pressure peaks[198, 586]. This explains the difficulties in restoring spontaneous cardiac contractions after prolonged external CPR.

Attempts at augmenting the blood flows produced by standard external CPR rely on augmenting intrathoracic pressure fluctuations. Simultaneous ventilation–compression (SVC) CPR (high airway pressure IPPV simultaneous with chest compressions and abdominal binding)[139] had been studied and abandoned in the 1960s[77, 325, 965]. Detailed recent reinvestigation of these methods showed variable results depending on experimental conditions[84] (see below). Briefly, these and other 'pneumatic' modifications of standard external CPR sometimes augmented extracerebral blood flow and even cerebral blood flow, but not coronary flow[423, 489], and in other experiments increased cerebral venous pressure and intracranial pressure to the point of reducing cerebral perfusion pressure and oxygenation[79]. Epinephrine or fluid load i.v. can more reliably augment diastolic arterial and perfusion pressures and blood flow during external CPR[23b, 657]. During open-chest direct cardiac compressions or emergency cardiopulmonary bypass, venous pressures are not increased and perfusion pressures and blood flows through myocardium and brain can be restored to and maintained at near normal levels (Chapter 2). These invasive methods, however, must be performed by physicians and cannot be started as promptly as external CPR.

To *conclude*: Optimally performed standard external CPR can be initiated by anyone. It often produces blood flows through heart and brain sufficient to sustain tissue viability if started instantaneously upon onset of pulselessness. If delayed, external CPR produces minimal, unpredictable, borderline blood flows. It therefore represents only a stop gap holding maneuver until restoration of normal spontaneous blood pressure either occurs spontaneously (as sometimes in asphyxia) or is accomplished with the use of electric defibrillation and/or drugs. In witnessed cardiac arrest, immediate defibrillating countershock should precede CPR. If pulselessness persists or a defibrillator is not immediately available, CPR Steps A–B–C must not be drawn out, but attempts at restoration of spontaneous circulation pursued as vigorously as possible from the start (Chapter 2).

The recommended *technique* of emergency artificial circulation by sternal compressions, to be effective and to avoid injury, calls for pressure at exactly the lower half of the sternum (Figs. 30 and 31)[23b]. The layman can be taught to recognize the sternum by feeling the abdomen (which is soft) and the sternum (which is hard). The pressure point is identified by feeling for the base of the xiphoid process (where the lower margins of the rib cage meet in the midline) and by placing two fingers just above this point on the lower portion of the sternum and the heel of the other hand adjacent to the two fingers; this identifies the lower half of the sternum as the correct point for applying pressure (Fig. 31-A).

An alternative method is feeling for the base of the xiphoid process (lower end of the sternum) and suprasternal notch (upper end of the sternum) with both hands, dividing in half the distance between them, and pressing on the lower half of the sternum (Fig. 31-B).

Compression of the sternum should be forceful enough to produce a good artificial carotid or femoral pulse. One must bear in mind, however, that the strength of the artificial pulse one feels does not necessarily reflect the degree of blood flow. Another member of the team should monitor the pulse produced. Sternal compressions should be regular, smooth and uninter-

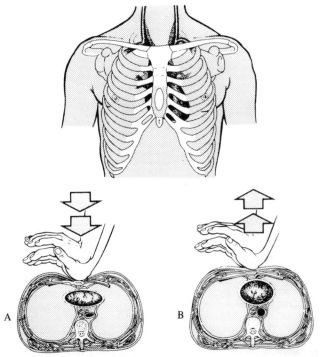

Fig. 30. External chest (cardiac) compressions. Top: the correct place for application of the hands, i.e. the lower half of the sternum. Bottom: (A) Compression of the chest cavity between the sternum and the spine with the heel of hand applied to the sternum, and the second hand applied on top of the first hand. (B) Release of pressure to let chest fill. Compress and release for 50% of each cycle. Maintain contact between your hand and the sternum.

rupted. The operator's arms should be vertical with the elbows locked. In adults, compression should be applied using the entire body weight with arms straight, rather than arm muscles alone, to avoid fatigue. One should not lift one's hands from the sternum between compressions, but release pressure completely, since venous return may be impeded by residual elevation of intrathoracic pressure. Compression should be with the heels of one's hands, keeping the fingers raised to avoid producing rib fracture by pressing against the lateral aspects of the thorax. Pressing below the xiphoid may cause regurgitation or rupture of the liver, pressing too high may fracture the sternum.

The patient must be in the horizontal position to permit venous return, which may be promoted by raising the legs. The patient must also be on a firm surface (ground, floor, hard litter, spine board or—in the hospital—a cardiac arrest bed board). Cardiac compressions should not be delayed when such hard support is not immediately available. If the patient is in bed, one should not waste time moving him to the floor, but slip a bed board or tray between his thorax and the mattress. Ideally, chest boards for CPR should elevate the shoulders to maintain the head tilted backward even when unsupported.

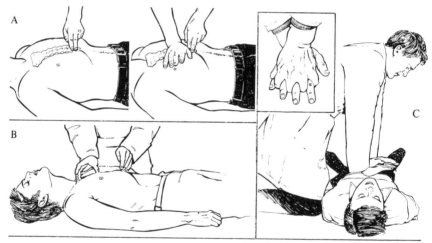

Fig. 31. Technique of external chest (cardiac) compressions. (A) Identification of the correct point for external chest compressions, i.e. by feeling (with your hand nearest the feet) for the base of the xiphoid (where the rib margins meet), and measuring two fingers cephalad (upward); then applying the heel of your other hand over the lower half of the sternum. (B) Identification of the correct pressure point by an alternative method, i.e. by feeling for the suprasternal notch with one hand and for the base of the xiphoid with the other hand, measuring one-half of this distance, and compressing the lower half of the sternum. (C) Body and hand position for external chest compressions. Compress straight downward on the sternum, using part of your body weight. Keep your arms straight and your hands off the ribs. Inset: alternative method for performing external chest compressions with the heel of your lower hand, by locking the fingers of both hands.

Technique of external chest (cardiac) compressions for adults and large children (Figs. 30, 31)

1. Position yourself at either side of the patient, who is supine (face up), horizontal, on a hard surface.
2. Locate the lower margins of the rib cage and where they meet at the midline (xiphoid–sternal junction).
3. Place two fingers over the lower end of the sternum (breast bone) and place the heel of one hand next to the two fingers, over the pressure point at the lower half of the sternum. Place the heel of your other hand on top of your first hand (Fig. 31-A).
    An alternative method is to identify the lower half of the sternum with two hands identifying the upper and lower end of the sternum and its midpoint, as shown in Fig. 31-B.
4. Push the sternum downward toward the spine about 1.5–2 inches (4–5 cm). The force required varies and should not be more than necessary for sternal displacement.
5. Hold the sternum down for 50% of the cycle, to push blood out of the heart (chest) (artificial systole). Then release rapidly and wait for the other 50% of the cycle, to let the heart (chest) fill with blood (artificial diastole)[883].
6. Reapply pressure at a rate of 80–100 per minute (slightly slower than two compressions per second).
7. Alternate two lung inflations with 15 sternal compressions. If you are two health professionals you may alternate 1 lung inflation with five sternal compressions. In either case, briefly interrupt sternal compressions for lung inflations.
8. Never interrupt compressions except for a few seconds since, even when optimally performed, external CPR produces only borderline circulation.

Technique **of external chest (cardiac) compressions for small children and infants** (Chapter 4)

1. The heart in infants and small children also lies under the lower half of the sternum, as in adults, but the danger of injuring the liver is greater[889]. Apply cardiac compressions one finger breadth below the midpoint where (usually) the line between the nipples crosses the sternum[23b], i.e. compress the lower half of the sternum. In small children, compress the lower half of the sternum with one hand only; in infants with the tips of two fingers.

An alternative technique of external cardiac compressions in infants is for the rescuer to encircle the infant's chest with both hands and to compress the midsternum with both thumbs.

2. Press on the sternum downward, with less force than in adults, namely only 1–1.5 inches (2.5–4 cm) in small children; and about 0.5 inch (1–2 cm) in infants.

3. Compress in children at a rate of 80–100 per minute as in adults; in infants at a rate of at least 100 per minute (about two compressions per second).

4. Since backward tilt of the infant's head lifts the back, support the back by one of your hands, a folded blanket or other support, or ask a helper to support the shoulders and chest. Most infants have an open airway with the head in the neutral position.

Combinations of Ventilation and Chest (Cardiac) Compressions for Standard External CPR (Figs. 32, 33)

Chest compressions alone[429] cannot provide ventilation of the lungs and must therefore be combined with intermittent positive pressure ventilation IPPV[709a, b]. There is nothing sacrosanct about presently recommended rates and ratios of ventilation and sternal compressions. They are a compromise based on experimental data[326] and practical feasibility[384]. There has to date been no systematic evaluation of the influence of rate and ratio of ventilations and chest compressions on outcome of patients after CPR.

One-operator CPR (Fig. 32)[23b, 326]

It is important to teach this technique to the public, i.e. to all persons over 10–12 years of age in all countries of the world. Rarely will there be more than one skilled bystander—lay person or health professional—present at the scene at first. The presently recommended compromise for combining ventilations and sternal compressions for use by the lay public continues to be two lung inflations alternated with 15 sternal compressions[326]. The new recommendations[23b] call for all ventilations to be moderately slow (1–2 seconds for each inflation, followed by complete passive exhalations) to minimize gastric insufflation and regurgitation (provoked by high pharyngeal pressures) and deep (0.8–1.0 liters per tidal volume in adults); for initiation of CPR with two lung inflations; and for all sternal compressions to be faster than 1 per second, i.e. 80–100 per minute, to guarantee at least 60 compressions per minute in spite of the necessary pauses for ventilations.

Ideally the patient's head should be held tilted backward for airway control, not only while ventilating but also when compressing the chest. This would require a second operator to hold the head during chest compressions, or raising the shoulders with a rolled blanket or hard object, such as a special molded CPR board.

Two-operator CPR (Fig. 33)[23b, 326]

The newly recommended technique[23b] consists of chest compressions at a rate of 80–100 compressions per minute, with a brief pause after every fifth compression to allow for one lung inflation to be interposed (1–2 seconds per inflation, followed by complete passive exhalations). This author (P.S.) has researched and taught this combination since 1960[326, 697, 709], since we found interposing lung inflations in less than 1 second between uninterrupted chest compressions to be very difficult, if not impossible, in the nonintubated patient without creating pharyngeal pressures above gastric inflation pressures.

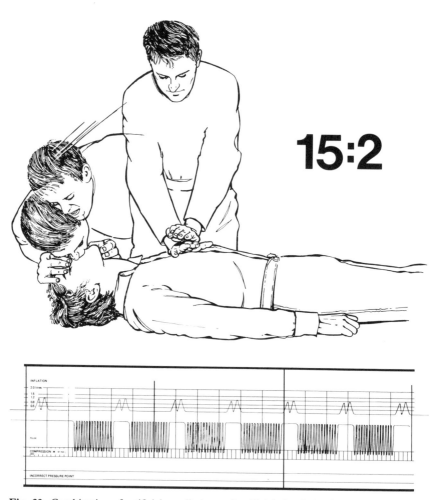

Fig. 32. Combination of artificial ventilation and artificial circulation by a single operator without equipment using external CPR. This is the only CPR basic life support steps A–B–C combination recommended for use by laymen. The authors recommend it for use by any rescuer for any nonintubated patient. Performance (top) and recording manikin printout (bottom). Note: two lung inflations (each inflation 1–2 seconds, followed by complete passive exhalation), pulse feeling, and, if no pulse, alternating 15 chest compressions at a rate of 80–100 per minute with two lung inflations, and continue alternating 15:2.

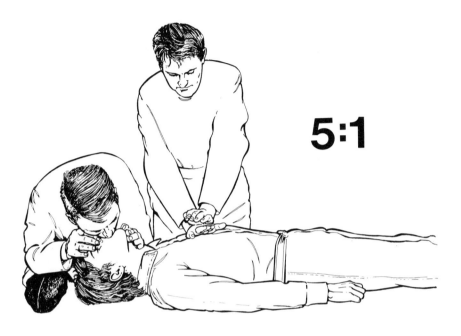

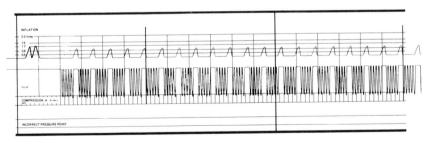

Fig. 33. Combination of artificial ventilation and artificial circulation by two operators without equipment. This combination is recommended only for use by CPR-trained health care providers. Performance (top) and recording manikin printout (bottom). Note: two lung inflations (each inflation 1–2 seconds, followed by complete passive exhalation), pulse feeling, and, if no pulse, alternating 5 chest compressions at a rate of 80–100 per minute, and brief interruption after every fifth compression with one lung inflation, and continue alternating 5:1. The rescuers should be on opposite sides of the victim.

The two-operator CPR method of alternating five compressions with one ventilation is recommended by the American Heart Association for use by health professionals. Lay persons should be taught only the one-operator technique of 15:2[23b]. We recommend the 15:2 technique for all patients without endotracheal tubes, for use by any type and number of personnel. This is because alternating 5:1 seems difficult to teach, because there is no physiologic advantage of one over the other, and because simplicity of what to teach to whom is important.

After endotracheal intubation, lung inflations may be *nonsynchronous* with sternal compressions. Inflations which happen to occur interposed will favor lung expansion[326], while inflations which happen to occur simultaneous with chest compressions may augment blood flow[139, 326, 693, 965]. However, ventilations performed simultaneously with compressions require high airway pressures, which can be safely performed only via endotracheal tube.

The two operators should position themselves on opposite sides of the patient, which permits easy changing of position without interruption of the rhythm. Alternating between ventilation and sternal compressions should be rapid. When ventilating by mouth-to-mask or bag–valve–mask, the mask should be strapped to the patient's face to avoid delays caused by frequent reapplications of the mask. The ventilating operator is best positioned at the side of the patient's head for direct mouth-to-mouth ventilation, and at the patient's vertex for use of equipment.

Technique of external CPR basic life support: *one-operator CPR* (Figs. 29–32)[23b]

(Recommended by the American Heart Association as the only technique recommended for use by the lay public. Recommended by the authors for use by one or more operators, lay or health professional, on any *non*intubated patient.)

Kneel or stand at the victim's side.

1. If the victim is unconscious, tilt the head backward maximally, using chin support to hold the mouth slightly open. Add jaw-thrust if necessary. If you suspect spinal injury, use moderate backward tilt only until the airway is open. Check for breathing (listen and feel for air flow at the mouth/nose, look for chest rise and fall).

2. If the victim is not breathing, give two deep lung inflations (make the chest rise). Inflate moderately slowly by taking 1–2 seconds per inflation, followed by complete passive exhalation.

3. Feel for the carotid pulse (5–10 seconds) (Fig. 29). If the pulse is present, continue ventilations at an approximate rate of 12 per minute in adults (one every 5 seconds), 15 per minute in children (one every 4 seconds), 20 per minute in infants (one every 3 seconds).

4. If the pulse is absent, start chest compressions with recommended technique (Fig. 32): give 15 sternal compressions at a rate of 80–100 per minute (i.e. slightly slower than two compressions per second). After 15 compressions, pause briefly to give two more lung inflations. Continue to alternate 15 compressions and two inflations. Give each sternal compression over 50% of the cycle, and release the sternum for the other 50%.

Compress the sternum about 1.5–2 inches (4–5 cm) in adults, 1–1.5 inches (2.5–4 cm) in small children, and 0.5 inch (1–2 cm) in infants. Check for return of a spontaneous pulse every 1–2 minutes. Continue Steps A–B–C until spontaneous pulse returns, Steps A and B until adequate spontaneous breathing returns; and Step A until the victim regains consciousness.

Technique of external CPR basic life support: *two-operator* CPR (Fig. 33)[23b]

(Recommended by the American Heart Association for use by health professionals only, on nonintubated patients.)

Operators 1 and 2, position yourselves on opposite sides of the victim for easy switching of roles. (In Fig. 33, for purposes of clarity of illustration, both rescuers are shown on the same side of the patient.)

1. If the victim is unconscious, ventilating operator 1 tilt the head backward.
2. If the victim is not breathing, give two deep lung inflations.
3. Feel for the carotid pulse (Fig. 29).
4. If the victim is pulseless, tell circulating operator 2 to start sternal compressions. Operator 2 compress the sternum at a rate of 80–100 per minute. Ventilating operator 1 give the victim one deep lung inflation after every fifth sternal compression, while circulating operator 2 interrupts sternal compressions briefly to let you inflate the victim's lungs (Fig. 33). Continue alternating five sternal compressions and pause with one lung inflation until a spontaneous pulse returns.

Technique of external CPR Steps A–B–C for use by health professionals on *intubated* patients

1. Ventilating operator 1, position yourself at the patient's vertex. Inflate the lungs with IPPV at a rate of approximately 12 per minute (15 per minute in small children; 20 per minute in infants), without synchronizing the chest compressions during CPR. You thus randomly interpose ventilations between or superimpose them on chest compressions.
2. Circulating operator 2, position yourself at the patient's side. Compress the sternum uninterrupted at a rate of 80–100 per minute (in infants at least 100 per minute).
3. Ventilating operator 1, monitor intermittently the artificial carotid pulse, or ask a third operator to monitor the femoral pulse. Check for return of spontaneous pulse during brief interruptions of chest compressions.
4. Initiate earliest possible defibrillation, epinephrine i.v., and restoration of spontaneous normotension.

Simplified technique of external CPR basic life support

The effort in 1985 by the American Heart Association CPR Committee toward simplifying CPR-BLS could be taken further by local or state agencies or teachers in other countries. We suggest the following for use by *any* types and numbers of operators on *any* pulseless patient of *any* age who are not intubated. 'Remember, we have *two* hands and *ten* fingers' (Ormato):

1. If the patient is *unconscious*, tilt the head backward, open the mouth slightly, and add jaw-thrust if necessary.
2. If he/she is *not breathing*, give him two lung inflations, each inflation over about 2 seconds, followed by complete passive exhalation.
3. Feel for the carotid pulse (about 2 × 2 seconds). If the pulse is present, continue lung inflations, one about every 2 seconds in and 2 seconds out (i.e. 15 per minute). If the pulse is absent, give about 10 sternal compressions at a rate of about two compressions per second (i.e. 120 compressions per minute). Compress the sternum in adults about 2 inches. Continue alternating about two lung inflations with 10 sternal compressions. Check for spontaneous pulse about every 2 minutes.
4. Make every possible effort primarily to defibrillate within about 20 seconds of collapse, to start CPR within about 2 minutes of pulselessness, and secondarily to defibrillate and restore spontaneous normotension within about 10 minutes of CPR. If unresponsiveness lasts beyond about 10 hours, prognosis is guarded; if it lasts beyond about 10 days, prognosis is poor.

Transition from One to Two Operators[23b]

After operator 1 has begun Steps A and B and determined pulselessness, he/she initiates one-operator CPR with the ratio of 15 compressions followed by two inflations. Operator 2, on arrival, should identify him/herself as being trained in CPR and ask if operator 1 wants help. After operator 1 has finished 15 compressions followed by two lung inflations, he stays at the head of the patient and checks the carotid pulse. Operator 2, meanwhile, locates the landmarks and gets in position to deliver chest compressions. After the 5-second pulse check, if operator 1 reports 'no pulse', he gives one ventilation and then operator 2 commences chest compressions. Compressions and ventilations then continue with a ratio of 5 : 1, with a compression rate of 80–100 per minute, and a brief pause after every fifth compression for a 1–2 second inflation followed by passive exhalation.

Switching between Two Operators[23b]

The two operators are on opposite sides of the patient, operator 1 ventilating and operator 2 performing sternal compressions. When operator 2 gets tired, he says 'switch' during the pause for ventilation. Immediately after the ventilation of the next cycle, operator 2 moves to the head and checks for a pulse. Meanwhile, operator 1 moves to the chest and locates the landmarks for chest compressions. If operator 2 finds no pulse, he/she gives a ventilation, and reports 'no pulse—resume CPR'. Operator 1 then resumes chest compressions at a rate of 80–100 per minute. Operator 2 should monitor sternal compressions by palpating the carotid artery.

Monitoring the Effectiveness of CPR

The ventilating operator should do this by (1) intermittently palpating the carotid pulse; and (2) by checking whether a spontaneous pulse has returned, at first after 1 minute of CPR and every 2–5 minutes thereafter, during brief interruptions of sternal compressions. The pupils should also be examined periodically, as constriction and return of reaction to light suggest improvement of cerebral blood flow, whereas fixed dilated pupils are an equivocal sign as to the brain's status and the efficacy of CPR.

During CPR Steps A–B–C, earliest possible attempts at electric defibrillation, endotracheal intubation and epinephrine i.v. or intratracheally should be carried out (Chapter 2). CPR should be continued until a spontaneous pulse is restored. While in ventricular fibrillation a spontaneous pulse is not expected to return until successful defibrillation, in asphyxial cardiac arrest a spontaneous pulse may return rapidly without defibrillation after a few minutes of effective CPR. Artificial ventilation (with oxygen if available) should be continued for the duration of coma (at least several hours), eventually by mechanical ventilation via endotracheal tube, in an ICU setting, until monitored, titrated weaning to spontaneous breathing is possible.

Sternal compressions are an effective method of *mechanical pacing*, making the well oxygenated heart contract spontaneously in patients with heart block with severe bradycardia or asystole. However, since external cardiac compressions are painful, the conscious person with severe bradycardia is better treated with repetitive chest thumping (Chapter 4) while waiting for the appropriate drugs and pacemaker insertion.

Simultaneous Ventilation–Compression CPR

SVC-CPR[139, 693, 950] evolved from studies in the 1960s[326, 965] and recent studies showing the chest pump mechanism of CPR as a possibility [139, 171, 693, 950, 954]. It is an attempt to improve blood flow over that produced by standard external CPR and consists of one positive pressure lung inflation simultaneously with each chest compression at a rate of 40 per minute (compression:relaxation time ratio 60:40%) plus continuous abdominal binding[140, 140a]. SVC-CPR attempts had been abandoned earlier because of the need for high inflation pressures, the difficulty in synchronization and the risk of liver rupture[325, 326, 965]. Compared with standard external CPR, SVC-CPR can augment common carotid artery blood flow[139, 326, 693, 965] and unpredictably improve cerebral blood flow[423, 489], but—if compared in broad-chested dogs with optimal standard external CPR—can also increase intracranial pressure, and thereby worsen cerebral perfusion pressure, blood flow and oxygenation[79]. SVC-CPR as compared to SECPR did not improve outcome in dogs[83, 406b, 659]. SVC-CPR requires an endotracheal tube, since airway pressure peaks may be over 100 cmH$_2$O, and require special apparatus, since manual synchronization is difficult. Thus, SVC-CPR is *not* a basic life support method; nor is the use of abdominal binders[23b, 140, 587]; nor are the much more effective methods for augmenting the borderline blood flow produced by external CPR of intravenous or intratracheal epinephrine[109, 143, 225, 325, 424, 588, 653] or augmentation of circulating blood volume[325]. SVC-CPR as part of prolonged advanced cardiac life support in the field has been investigated in a randomized clinical study; no improvement in outcome has been demonstrated so far (Weisfeldt, unpublished). Research into improvement of myocardial and cerebral blood flow by *basic* external CPR, without the need for equipment, for use by the lay public, should continue. High-impulse sternal compressions at a high rate[23b, 506] and intermittent sternal and alternating abdominal compressions[599, 643, 676, 925] do not require a tracheal tube, but do not convincingly improve myocardial and cerebral blood flow and can cause trauma.

More important than complex equipment-dependent techniques, which would provide only slight improvements of blood flow over that produced by external CPR, is rapid restoration of adequate spontaneous circulation by defibrillation, fluids and drugs; or, where this is not promptly possible, the initiation of optimal artificial reperfusion by open-chest CPR or emergency cardiopulmonary bypass (Chapter 2).

Attempts at increasing blood flow during standard external CPR by *restraining the abdomen* (without SVC) by hand on abdomen[325, 655] or by military (medical) anti-shock trousers (MAST) inflated from the legs to the costal margin[16a, 78] have resulted in slight augmentation of common carotid blood flow. This, however, also resulted in decreased cerebral oxygenation (increased venous and intracranial pressure), increased acidemia, decreased lung–chest compliance, hypoxemia, and damage to liver and other organs[16a, 78]. The leg portion of the MAST during CPR, however, is safe and may or may not be helpful by producing increased vascular resistance and autotransfusion[125a]. During cardiac arrest in experimental animals, intermittent overall chest compressions, particularly if performed mechanically ('vest-CPR'), and particularly if combined with intermittent simultaneous abdominal compressions, with various ventilation patterns superimposed, have resulted in near-normal perfusion pressures and blood flows, but only if there was near zero arrest time (no flow time) and epinephrine was used to raise the diastolic aortic pressure[140a, 589a].

High-frequency oxygen jet ventilation during external CPR makes synchronization of ventilation with chest compressions unnecessary, and in dog experiments resulted in blood gas and carotid flow values comparable to those produced by IPPV[99]. In the weakly beating heart during cardiogenic shock, systole-synchronized high-frequency (high intratracheal pressure) IPPV by jet ventilation can augment cardiac output[626, 627].

CPR Outside the Hospital

Ventilation and cardiac compressions should be established by the manual technique before the victim is moved with manual or mechanical CPR. It is desirable that spontaneous circulation be restored at the scene before moving the patient, but this depends on the availability of defibrillator, drugs, other equipment and personnel trained in advanced life support. Ideally, early defibrillation should be provided in the field by all ambulance services, and hopefully in the future also by lay persons using 'smart' automatic external defibrillators[176b]. Early pre-hospital defibrillation in sudden cardiac death demonstrably improves neurological outcome in patients[153, 216a, 869, 939]. If the patient must be moved for restoration of spontaneous circulation, a spontaneous pulse does not return with CPR alone, and a defibrillator is not available, CPR must be continued without interruption during transport. This may prove difficult.

When moving the patient with manual CPR, the ventilating operator works from the head end of the stretcher, while the operator compressing the chest works from the side, and three or more bystanders carry the stretcher. The most experienced person present should act as team leader and coach the others. When moving the patient over narrow stairways and other difficult routes, manual CPR will have to be improvised, but should not be interrupted for more than about 15 seconds at a time. A wooden backboard recommended for cases of suspected spine injury is also useful for transport of patients with CPR, provided the patient is strapped securely to the board. Mechanical CPR devices also considerably facilitate transport.

Artificial circulation with the patient in the *upright position* (e.g. sitting, standing, hanging) is ineffective as the chest does not fill with blood. Electric linemen who suffer cardiac arrest on the *poletop* should be lowered as quickly as possible without delay by CPR attempts (except head tilt), and effective CPR should be performed on the ground. In many awkward situations, CPR Steps A–B–C must be carried out with ad hoc improvisation during rescue.

In the ambulance, for one-operator CPR, the operator kneels on a pillow near the side of the patient's head and chest, keeping the head tilted backward with a roll under the shoulder or by use of a special backboard, which keeps the head tilted backward. A pharyngeal tube may be inserted and a transparent mask strapped loosely to the patient's face to avoid delays from frequent reapplications of the mask. The 2:15 ratio is used by the single operator, remaining at the side also for ventilation. For the operator performing CPR in the ambulance, the astride position may offer advantages over the conventional position. The single operator, facing cephalad toward the patient's face, sits on a bench placed over the patient's hips or astride the patient. For ventilation, the operator improvises by pushing the chin upward (backward) to maintain head tilt when giving lung inflations via mask from a hand-triggered oxygen-powered ventilator or an improvised mouth–tube–valve–mask assembly. For chest compressions he/she is in an optimal position. Early endotracheal intubation (Chapter 1A) is highly desirable as it greatly facilitates CPR-BLS and ALS during transport.

External CPR Machines

CPR machines (chest thumpers)[592, 884] with mechanical ventilators attached are of value during difficult transport situations inside and outside hospitals. These machines provide more consistent CPR than the manual technique, and about the same amount of blood flow. They cannot 'feel' like the operator's hand can and, therefore, if not ideally adjusted and constantly monitored may cause internal injuries. When CPR machines are used, manual CPR must be started first. 'Thumpers' should be used only by personnel expertly trained in both manual and mechanical CPR, and who have practiced the change over from manual CPR to use of the mechanical device. Read the manufacturer's instructions carefully[592].

These chest thumpers should provide an adjustable stroke of 1.5–2 inches, be applied rapidly without interruption of manual CPR for more than 5 seconds at a time and support backward tilt of the head. The operator must do this; the machine cannot. When a mechanical device for ventilation is incorporated, it should be a volume- or time-cycled, not a pressure-cycled, ventilator. These devices are best employed with a cuffed endotracheal tube, since their ventilators do not adapt to the changing leaks and resistances usually encountered with ventilation by mask. Presently available chest thumpers are not suitable for infants and children. A rescuer must remain at the patient's head all the time to monitor plunger action and ventilation and to check the pulse.

The C–A–B Sequence Controversy[174, 460]

Some CPR educators in Europe recommend teaching two sequences: (1) Steps A–B–C as described in this manual, for secondary cardiac arrest (e.g. asphyxia); and (2) Steps C–A–B for witnessed primary cardiac arrest (e.g. sudden cardiac death)[174]. The latter recommendation is based on the likelihood that in sudden cardiac arrest the arterial blood remains oxygenated for many minutes; it therefore could, according to this line of reasoning, be circulated with external cardiac compressions for the first 30–60 seconds, without delaying blood flow by Steps A and B. This method offers no clear physiological advantage[460], since deoxygenation during Step C is rapid.

In the meantime, a majority of existing guidelines continue to recommend the simple A–B–C sequence for both primary and secondary arrest, to avoid confusion[460]. The difference between the two techniques may be more apparent than real, for in sudden cardiac arrest the patient continues gasping for 0.5–1 minute. This is a sign of brain stem perfusion and in itself might promote some blood flow. In such cases the need for Steps A and B is obviated and the rescuer may proceed immediately to feeling the pulse and (if the pulse is absent) start external cardiac compressions. After 15 sternal compressions, the operator should ventilate two times and continue CPR.

Comment: When after initiation of closed-chest CPR you cannot restore spontaneous circulation within a few minutes (with or without defibrillating countershocks), try to augment cerebral and coronary blood flow during CPR with epinephrine given i.v. or intratracheally. If you are a physician trained in the method, do not hesitate to switch to open-chest CPR, which is physiologically superior to any closed-chest method (Chapter 2). CPR via thoractomy requires CPPV via endotracheal tube and should only be performed by a physician.

Emergency Management of (Traumatic) Hemorrhage (Figs. 34, 35)[22b, 25, 902]

Step C of CPCR, Circulation support, as part of basic and advanced *trauma* life support (BTLS, ATLS), includes primarily emergency treatment of the bleeding patient who may be hypotensive, but has a spontaneous pulse. BTLS is life-supporting first aid (LSFA), which must start with control of external hemorrhage and airway control.

Life-supporting first aid[744]

This should ideally be mastered by all lay persons above about 10–12 years of age, including all health professionals. LSFA includes essentially eight steps (see wallet card at the end of the book): (1) control of external hemorrhage without surgical measures, namely by elevation and pressure (Fig. 34); (2) positioning of the conscious person in shock horizontal with legs elevated (Fig. 36-B); (3) airway control in the unconscious person (Step A) with moderate backward tilt of the head by chin support (mouth open), plus jaw thrust if needed, and immobilization of the neck (Figs. 3–6); (4) manual clearing of foreign matter from mouth and pharynx (Fig. 7); (5) mouth-to-mouth (nose) ventilation (Step B) (Figs. 5 and 6); (6) external cardiac (chest) compressions for pulselessness (Figs. 30–33) (rarely needed and not effective in severe hypovolemia); (7) positioning of an unconscious patient who is breathing adequately in stable side position with the head tilted backward (Fig. 4); and (8) rescue pull (Fig. 36-A).

Advanced trauma life support[22b]

Treatment control of external hemorrhage by *ambulance personnel* includes use of the tourniquet for selected indications, and control of internal hemorrhage below the diaphragm and support of arterial pressure in hypovolemic shock with use of military (medical) anti-shock trousers (MAST), also called pneumatic anti-shock garment (PASG) (Fig. 35)[22b, 397, 455, 902]. These measures are occasionally also indicated in intrahospital emergencies. *Paramedics* may in addition give i.v. fluids and apply other ATLS measures as approved and taught by physicians (Chapter 4).

Emergency care by *physicians* of severely traumatized patients goes beyond the scope of this manual. All physicians are urged to take an advanced trauma life support (ATLS) course, as this provides the basis of trauma stabilization[22b]. *ATLS* includes LSFA (above) with 'primary survey' for Steps A–B–C; all the steps of emergency airway control (Step A) (Chapter 1A), ventilation–oxygenation (Step B) (Chapter 1B), and fluid resuscitation (Chapter 2); immobilization of spine and extremities; clamping of externally bleeding arteries; pericardial drainage for cardiac tamponade; pleural drainage for pneumothorax and hemothorax; 'secondary survey' from head to toes; protection of soft tissue injuries against contamination (wound care); and resuscitative surgical operations for control of internal bleeding via thoracotomy, laparotomy and craniotomy. The three Bs—control of Breathing (airway control) and Bleeding and immobilization of Bones—must have priority over definitive wound repair and major trauma surgery.

External hemorrhage must be controlled immediately since loss of 1 liter of blood or more in an adult (much less in children) can be life threatening. External bleeding from veins and capillaries, as well as most pulsating bleeding from arteries, can be controlled by sealing with *pressure* the torn vessels against tissue underneath, and if possible *elevating* the bleeding site. Compressing arterial pressure points proximal to extremity wounds is less reliable and more difficult to learn. If one cannot keep holding the wound until hospital admission, and a pressure bandage is available, one can replace manual pressure with pressure by bandage (Fig. 34-C, D, E). For the *technique* of controlling external hemorrhage, see the caption to Fig. 34.

Tourniquets should be used only as a last resort and only in cases of extremely traumatized extremities in which major vessels have been injured. Even in traumatic amputations, severed vessels may retract and stop bleeding. When the tourniquet is in place for extended periods, nerves, blood vessels and the entire extremity may be permanently damaged. When applied too loosely, the tourniquet can increase bleeding by impeding venous drainage.

If you decide on using a tourniquet, use a cravat or folded handkerchief, not a rope or wire. Apply a pad over the artery to be compressed (pressure point). Wrap the tourniquet twice around the extremity and tie a half knot. Place a stick, pencil or similar object on top of the half knot and tie the ends of the tourniquet in a square knot above the stick. Twist the stick to tighten the tourniquet until the bleeding stops. Secure it in that position. Write on the patient's forehead 'T' and the time the tourniquet was applied.

Internal hemorrhage below the chest, if suspected, can often be stopped nonsurgically and blood pressure restored with the use of MAST(PASG) (Fig. 35)[397], both in the prehospital setting and inside hospitals. MAST are a pressure suit which surround the legs and abdomen. This pressure suit to some extent controls not only external but also internal hemorrhage below the diaphragm and increases peripheral vascular (aortic) resistance[455]. Whether it can also produce autotransfusion in hypovolemic shock is not certain. It also effectively splints fractures of the pelvis and the lower extremities. Recommended inflation to about 100 mmHg intrasuit pressure can often promptly reverse hypotension in severe traumatic shock, presumably by mobilizing blood volume, compressing bleeding vessels, containing hematomas and perhaps even compressing the abdominal aorta. MAST can cause renal ischemia (if in place longer than 1 hour) and pulmonary congestion, and can augment acidemia after its release. Since abdominal binding restrains the diaphragm, the patient should be given oxygen. If

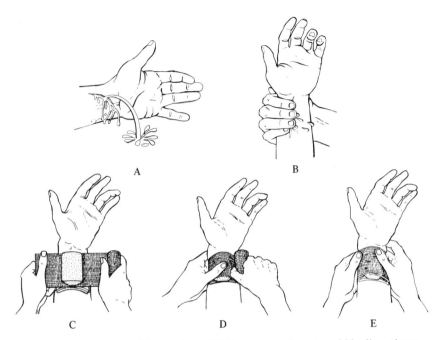

Fig. 34. Control of external hemorrhage. (A) If you recognize external bleeding, elevate the bleeding site and (B) apply direct manual compression with your bare hand, a clean handkerchief or, best, a sterile gauze. (C) If you have a pressure dressing available, apply it without releasing manual pressure. If you use the pictured Laerdal dressing, open the package, hold the bandage with both hands, and place the dressing on the wound with the styrene block directly over the bleeding point. (D) Wrap the bandage over the styrene block several times; do not tighten the bandage more than is necessary to stop the bleeding. (E) Apply the final wrap loosely, press the end gently over the underlying wrap; the bandage is self-adhesive. If professional help is not available, loosen the pressure bandage somewhat after about 30 minutes. If you are the victim and alone, apply the pressure bandage to yourself.

IPPV is needed, it is better performed via endotracheal tube because of a need for high inflation pressures. MAST are relatively contraindicated in cases of head injury, suspected bleeding into the chest, or heart failure with pulmonary edema. For the *technique* of the MAST use, see the caption to Fig. 35. Its exact mechanism of action and indications are still controversial[387, 455, 902].

Deflation of MAST should proceed with the abdominal section, then one leg section, and finally the other leg section, with stabilizing periods of titrated i.v. fluid administration in between. MAST should not be removed until fluid resuscitation is well under way and the team is ready for resuscitative laparotomy, blood pressure support with vasopressor, and sodium bicarbonate to combat washout acidosis. If used for CPR, sponta-

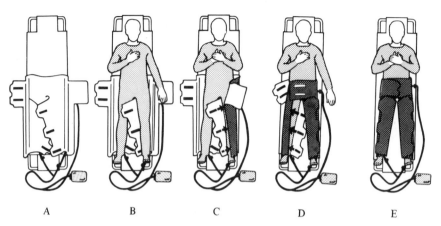

A   B   C   D   E

Fig. 35. Application of military (medical) anti-shock trousers (MAST), also called pneumatic anti-shock garment (PASG)[902]. (From Armstrong Industries, Northbrook, IL; and Caroline N, *Emergency Care in the Streets.* Boston, Little Brown, 1979). (A) Unfold the MAST and lay them flat. If a stretcher is to be used, lay the MAST on it. Attach a foot pump and open the stopcock valves. (B) Put the patient on the MAST face up (supine), so that the top of the garment will be just below the lowest rib. (C) Wrap the left leg of the garment around the patient's left leg and secure it with velcro straps. (D) Wrap the right leg of the garment around the patient's right leg and secure it with velcro straps. (E) Apply the abdominal binder of the garment and secure it with velcro straps. Use the foot pump to inflate the garment until air exhausts through the relief valves and/or the patient's vital signs become stable. Close the stopcock valves. Get the patient to definitive therapy within 1 hour or as soon as possible thereafter, since prolonged MAST inflation causes tissue ischemia. Before releasing MAST, treat shock (in cardiac arrest restore spontaneous circulation). Be prepared for laparotomy or thoracotomy (to clamp the aorta in exsanguinating abdominal hemorrhage). Slowly deflate the abdominal section first, then one leg section and finally the other leg section, with i.v. fluid administration in between. Have vasopressor ready to stabilize blood pressure. Use $NaHCO_3$ i.v. and hyperventilation to combat acidemia.

neous cardiac action should be restarted prior to MAST release. In cases of suspected exsanguinating intra-abdominal hemorrhage, as from ruptured aortic aneurysm, pressure with the fist on the upper abdominal aorta may be life saving when MAST are not available. Some have applied MAST effectively in such cases and left them inflated until the thoracic descending aorta was clamped via thoracotomy[858].

Extrication and Positioning for Shock (Fig. 36)

Circulation support in traumatic-hemorrhagic shock includes extrication of the patient from a wreck without adding injury, and positioning for shock. These measures must be preceded by ascertaining or controlling a patent airway and adequate breathing, and controlling external hemorrhage.

A seriously injured person should not be moved by personnel not trained in field rescue unless it is essential for LSFA, to avoid deterioration of injuries, or to protect against further accidents.

When applying the *rescue pull* (Fig. 36-A), one should move the injured limbs as little as possible and immobilize the patient's head, neck and chest in the aligned position (Fig. 36-A) preferably with helpers. 'Rescue pull' is extrication without equipment. However, ambulance personnel, whenever

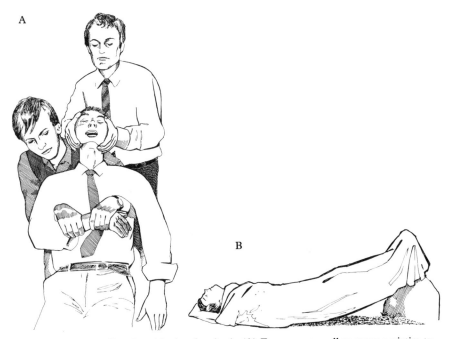

Fig. 36. Rescue pull and positioning for shock. (A) For a rescue pull to move a victim to safety, e.g. from a car wreck, approach him/her from behind, place your arms under the armpits, grasp an unhurt arm, lift gently, and pull the patient along carefully while you move backwards. Avoid aggravating a neck injury by keeping the head, neck and chest aligned, with the head in the mid-position, using your shoulder and chin, or the aid of a by-stander, who should hold the head with both hands. Avoid flexion, lateral rotation and maximal backward tilt of the head. Pull the patient onto a flat surface, preferably a long backboard. Stabilize the head–neck–chest in the aligned supine position by use of a neck collar, sandbags on either side of the head, and taping head and sandbags to the backboard. Support the airway with moderate backward tilt of the head, opening mouth and jaw thrust. Check breathing, stop external bleeding and dress major wounds. If the patient is conscious, reassure him/her. Protect against cold and dampness while waiting for help. (B) Positioning for shock: if the patient is conscious and in 'shock' (restless or stuporous, faint peripheral pulses, cold moist skin, perhaps rapid heart rate), place him/her horizontal, with legs raised. If unresponsive, tilt the head backward and use jaw thrust if necessary. Wrap the patient for warmth, but do not overheat him/her.

possible, should extricate with the help of a short backboard applied before moving the patient, and extricating him/her gently onto a long backboard using established methods of prehospital trauma care[21, 22b, 125a].

Shock is defined as 'a reduction in overall tissue perfusion resulting in vital organ systems malfunction'[163, 799, 948]. The clinical term 'shock' usually implies lower than normal arterial blood pressure. Shock (hypotension) may be due to blood volume loss (the main cause of traumatic shock), cardiac pump failure (cardiogenic shock), vasodilation, blood flow obstruction (pulmonary embolism, cardiac tamponade) or abnormal distribution of microcirculatory blood volumes and tissue blood flows (e.g. septic shock). Trauma and other conditions which lead to external and/or internal blood volume loss produce the clinical picture of overall hypoperfusion—namely, cold moist skin, oliguria, tachycardia (may be absent in infancy, old age or during general anesthesia), faint peripheral pulses, arterial hypotension and CNS excitation followed by depression. The arterial blood pressure may be normal in fit persons until 20–30% of blood volume has been lost because of compensatory vasoconstriction. For blood pressure monitoring, see Chapter 2.

If the patient in shock is conscious, keep him/her horizontal and supine (face-up) and elevate the legs (Fig. 36-B). This may have a slight autotransfusion effect. Keep the patient warm, but avoid overheating. Lightweight thermal blankets are useful. The head-down 'Trendelenburg' position is *not* recommended. If the patient in shock is unconscious and breathing adequately, place him/her in the supported supine aligned position (Fig. 4-A) or move with the head–neck–chest aligned into the stable side position (Fig. 4-B). Do not give the patient anything to drink, as anesthesia may be needed. Even when conscious, the patient may vomit and aspirate.

Prehospital and intrahospital advanced life support for patients with shock (fluid resuscitation and drugs) are covered in Chapter 2.

For *technique* of rescue pull and positioning for shock, see the caption to Fig. 36.

Primary and Secondary Survey of Trauma Cases[22b]

Victims of trauma should be managed with life-supporting first aid (LSFA) and primary survey (started by first responder) going hand in hand; and then with advanced trauma life support (ATLS) and secondary survey (by physician or physician guided paramedic) going hand in hand.

Primary survey. Is the patient conscious? Airway control plus cervical spine immobilization. Is he/she breathing? Ventilate if necessary. Is he/she bleeding externally? Control external hemorrhage. If conscious, does the patient show neurological disability? Undress the patient.

Secondary survey. Examine from head to toe, looking for contusions, wounds, fractures. Examine for intracranial, intrathoracic and intra-abdominal injuries.

Comment: In an unconscious patient, with or without injury, look for a *Medic Alert* bracelet or necklace. An underlying disease (e.g. allergies, diabetes, epilepsy) may call for modification of standard resuscitation procedures.

PHASE II:
ADVANCED LIFE SUPPORT
Restoration of Spontaneous Circulation

After the initiation of basic life support, spontaneous circulation must be restored as promptly as possible, since external CPR produces only borderline blood flow, which may be inadequate to keep the brain and heart viable for longer than a few minutes. Advanced life support (ALS) is meant primarily for restoration of adequate spontaneous circulation, which usually requires intravenous (i.v.) administration of drugs and fluids (Step D) (Figs. 37–41); electrocardiographic diagnosis (Step E) (Figs. 42–46); and fibrillation treatment (Step F) (Figs. 47–50)—in varying sequences depending on circumstances[23c, 720]. ALS also includes open-chest CPR for specific indications (Figs. 51 and 52), the still experimental use of emergency cardiopulmonary bypass (Fig. 53) and advanced trauma life support (ATLS)[22b].

Earliest possible defibrillation with restoration of spontaneous circulation is the key to optimizing chances for good overall and cerebral outcome[3, 217]. Thus, in ventricular fibrillation that occurs while a patient's ECG is being monitored, electric countershock (Step F) should not be delayed by Steps D and E and should precede Steps A–B–C. None of the Steps D, E and F may be required if a spontaneous pulse returns promptly following initiation of artificial ventilation and chest compressions, as is often the case in pulselessness secondary to asphyxia. Needless to say, during attempts at restoring spontaneous circulation, oxygen transport by CPR Steps A–B–C must be maintained with as little interruption as possible.

External CPR Steps A–B–C (basic life support) is meant to be merely a stop-gap measure[429, 709a]—of unpredictable physiologic efficacy for maintaining viability of brain and heart (see Chapter 1C), but at present the only emergency measure available for cardiac arrest outside the hospital—to lead as rapidly as possible to the titrated simultaneous application of Steps A through F (advanced life support).

Chapter 2D
Step D: Drugs and Fluids

Routes for Drugs and Fluids

Peripheral intravenous route (Fig. 37)

A peripheral intravenous (i.v.) route for the administration of drugs and fluids should be established as quickly as possible after the initiation of CPR, but without interrupting CPR, in order to expand the circulating blood volume and provide a route for the administration of drugs. If an i.v. infusion is already running, drugs, fluids and a single bolus of glucose should be given via the existing route. If during CPR there is no infusion in place and if establishment of a percutaneous peripheral venous catheter is not immediately possible, the first i.v. injection of epinephrine (adrenalin) may be made via a temporary stick by small-gauge needle into a large peripheral vein, e.g. the external jugular vein. Sodium bicarbonate, on the other hand, because it requires a large volume for injection, should be withheld until a reliable venous catheter has been inserted. Continuous infusion via metal needles is not recommended, as these are easily dislodged during CPR.

During chest compressions, a member of the team not occupied with ventilation and cardiac compressions should start a peripheral venous infusion, using the largest accessible vein for this purpose. It might be possible to enhance entry of drugs into the heart by use of a large volume of flush solution, elevation of the extremity and/or central venous injection[332, 438]. An antecubital vein is the first choice because it permits insertion of a long central venous catheter; insertion of internal jugular or subclavian central venous catheters would interrupt CPR and infusions into hand and leg veins are more likely to result in thromboses and delayed entry of drugs into the heart. For blood volume replacement, a catheter of 16 gauge or larger is desirable; for drug administration any smaller size is acceptable. A catheter-outside-needle or a catheter-inside-needle may be used, but the former causes less leakage of blood around the catheter and allows a large diameter catheter to be inserted. The *technique* of percutaneous venous puncture and catheterization requires practice (Figs. 37 and 38).

During chest compressions, the *first choice* is a vein you can see, preferably an antecubital vein. Sometimes veins may be palpable but not visible. The external jugular vein is a good *second choice* for puncture as well as insertion of a short catheter-outside-needle; digital compression just above the clavicle distends the external jugular vein and renders it more easily

129

cannulated. The *third choice* is the femoral vein, although invisible; it is located in the inguinal region just medial to the femoral artery, whose pulsations are palpable during cardiac compressions. Finally, the *last choice* for the peripheral venous cannulation is a rapid venous cut-down.

Cut-down is usually more quickly and easily accomplished at the ankle (saphenous vein) than at the wrist or elbow, and can be executed rapidly by making a 1–2 cm transverse incision just anterior to the medial malleolus, then picking up the vein with a hemostat after blunt tissue dissection, inserting a large-bore catheter into the vein, and clamping or ligating the vein distally. To save time, a large blunt metal cannula can be inserted via a small incision in the vein, and a hemostat can be placed over the vein and cannula proximally. No other clamps or sutures are needed initially.

Attempts at cannulating *subclavian* or *internal jugular* veins for central venous catheterization may be problematic during CPR Steps A–B–C, because of the danger of inducing pneumothorax when these measures are attempted in the patient who is being bounced by cardiac compressions; furthermore, such measures may require interruption of CPR at a stage when priority must be given to ventilation, oxygenation, cardiac compressions and defibrillation. However, trained physicians can use these techniques safely and consideration should be given to central venous catheterization if drug effects are not evident from the peripheral venous injection. After spontaneous circulation has been restored, on the other hand, prolonged life-support measures (Phase III) do indicate the use of central venous and arterial catheters in most comatose patients. A pulmonary artery balloon catheter may be inserted in selected cases as well, after the patient is stabilized (see below).

Fig. 37 (opposite). Peripheral venous cannulation for intravenous infusion. (A) Infusion apparatus: 1, Hook for a bottle or bag (preferably) on a pole of adjustable height; 2, air inlet; 3, drip bulb; 4, clamp for controlling flow of fluid; 5, adapter inserted into double three-way stopcock with syringe for drugs or flushing (second stopcock for additional infusion); 6, adapter for insertion into catheter needle. (B) Veins of the arm: 1, cephalic; 2, basilic; 3, antecubital. (C) Veins of the dorsum of the hand: 1, cephalic; 2, basilic. (D) Veins of the dorsum of the foot: 1, great saphenous vein; 2, small saphenous vein; 3, dorsal venous arch. (E) Technique of venipuncture and insertion of catheter-outside-needle: 1, apply venous tourniquet; 2, identify vein; 3, clean site with antiseptic solution; 4, pierce skin with needle and be sure that needle and plastic cannula are through skin (see inset of F); 5, with second (abrupt) definitive but well controlled motion, pierce vein; 6, ascertain blood back-flow; 7, advance catheter over needle, withdraw needle; 8, connect infusion to catheter (see inset of F); 9, tape securely with transparent tape. For catheter-inside-needle (not shown), use similar technique but *never* withdraw catheter from needle, since the sharp needle tip may shear off the end of the catheter, which can disappear into the venous system. (F) Fixation of intravenous catheter needle and tubing to arm, using transparent plastic tape at connector (as 6 of picture A). Note the loop of intravenous tubing and longitudinal tape to prevent inadvertent dislodgment. (Adapted from Dripps RD, Eckenhoff JE and Vandam LD: *Introduction to Anesthesia: The Principles of Safe Practice*, 5th ed. Philadelphia, WB Saunders, 1977.)

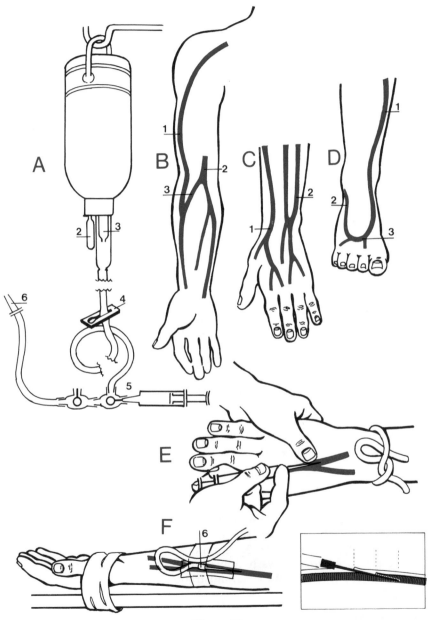

Figure 37

Intrapulmonary route[225, 644, 653, 671]

Intratracheal instillation of selected drugs is recommended in situations where an intravenous route is not readily available. A drug instilled in this fashion is rapidly absorbed across the alveoli, particularly when the drug is injected into the tracheobronchial tree through a suction catheter inserted via the tracheal tube. The effect can be seen almost as rapidly as with i.v. administration. Epinephrine, lidocaine, atropine and other drugs that do not cause tissue damage can safely be given via the tracheal tube, using 1–2 times the intravenous dose diluted in 10 ml of sterile water. Sodium bicarbonate, however, must *not* be given intratracheally, as it may damage the mucosa and alveoli.

Intracardiac route[23b]

The blind intracardiac injection of drugs is *not* recommended during *closed* chest CPR, as it may produce pneumothorax, injury to a coronary artery and prolonged interruption of external cardiac compressions. Inadvertent injection into cardiac muscle rather than a cardiac chamber may, in addition, lead to intractable dysrhythmias. Intracardiac injection of epinephrine should be considered only in the rare instance that a vein is inaccessible and the endotracheal route has not been established, and should be done via a long, thin (e.g. 22 gauge) needle using the paraxyphoid approach (Needle insertion to the left of the xyphoid process and advancement cephalad, posteriorly and laterally is less likely to damage the anterior descending coronary artery.) The position of the needle must be confirmed by free aspiration of blood, since intramyocardial injection can cause irreversible cardiac damage. The parasternal approach is not recommended. During *open* chest CPR, on the other hand, injection into the lumen of the left ventricle is safe and effective if performed under direct vision via thin needle. Epinephrine, antidysrhythmic agents and calcium have been effective in about one-half of the i.v. doses. Sodium bicarbonate must not be given via the intracardiac route.

Intramuscular route[23b, 427]

The intramuscular route has no place in emergency resuscitation because absorption of a given dose from the intramuscular site is unpredictable and thus the onset and duration of drug action cannot be reliably controlled. One may, however, give lidocaine (300 mg) and atropine (2 mg) by intramuscular route for the *prevention* of dysrhythmias, under conditions where peripheral blood flow is adequate and i.v. administration is not possible.

Central venous route (Fig. 38)[836]

During chest compressions, only peripheral i.v. catheters and/or insertion of a long catheter via an antecubital vein into (presumably) a central vein are recommended. Internal jugular and subclavian vein catheterization attempts would hamper CPR. As soon as possible *after* restoration of spontaneous circulation, however, a central venous catheter should be inserted, if possible, to record central venous pressure (CVP) (normal value 3–10 mmHg), to offer an additional route for infusion and to permit sampling of blood for various analyses.

The superior vena cava is the vessel of choice for central venous catheterization. A catheter in the superior vena cava is less dysrhythmogenic than one in the right atrium or pulmonary artery. When mixed venous blood analysis is desired (for instance to follow oxygen values), superior vena cava blood is more representative of pulmonary artery blood than samples from the inferior vena cava or the right atrium.

Many consider the *right internal jugular vein* the preferred approach to superior vena cava catheterization (Fig. 38)[125a, 836]. The *technique* for cannulation through the right internal jugular vein includes turning the patient's head to the left side, palpating the carotid artery with one hand and inserting a catheter needle just lateral to the carotid artery, in a paramedian plane, 45 degrees caudad, piercing the skin at the superior tip of the triangle created by the two portions of the sternocleidomastoid muscle. As with any vascular cannulation, one can either insert a short large-bore metal needle and thread through it a smaller-bore catheter or use a small-bore short catheter-outside-needle first, thread a guide wire through it, then remove the short needle and insert the long CVP catheter over the guide wire. Another option is the catheter-inside-needle method. The catheter-over-wire (after insertion of wire inside needle) is the preferable technique as it causes less leakage around the catheter and carries less risk of trauma. Superior vena cava catheterization via *external* jugular vein is possible with use of a J-wire to get around the vein's angle, but this method is complicated. A peripheral external (short) jugular catheter permits monitoring of relative changes in CVP, as there are no competent valves between external jugular vein and right atrium.

Some prefer *subclavian vein* cannulation (Fig. 38).[125a, 836] The subclavian vein crosses from the axillary vein into the chest, crossing the first rib under the clavicle, anterior to the anterior scalene muscle which separates vein from artery. Insert the needle 1 cm below the junction of the medial and middle thirds of the clavicle, pointing toward the opposite shoulder, in a direction just behind your finger inserted into the suprasternal notch. The apical pleura comes close to the subclavian–jugular junction. Catheterization through the subclavian vein, despite its popularity, remains a definite last choice, for its use is associated with a relatively high incidence of complications, such as pneumothorax and mediastinal infusion.

In all central venous cannulations, strict asepsis is mandatory and one must guard against air embolism whenever the system is open to the atmosphere. The patient's head should be slightly lowered; the conscious patient should be asked to hold his breath, while the unconscious patient should receive positive pressure ventilation; and during unavoidable periods of disconnection, the opening should be occluded by a gloved finger or stopcock. Another complication is bleeding in patients on thrombolytic therapy.

Catheterization of the right internal jugular vein does not require X-ray control since the catheter reliably passes into the superior vena cava. However, when the superior vena cava is catheterized via an arm vein (basilic or cephalic vein) or the subclavian vein, the catheter sometimes passes into the opposite arm or the jugular vein; thus X-ray check of catheter position is desirable. However, central venous catheterization from the right arm (with the patient's head leaned to the right) is a fairly reliable second choice route.

In cardiac arrest, a large volume (e.g. 5 ml/kg) of solution mixed with epinephrine injected rapidly via CVP catheter into or near the right atrium—or injected retrograde via the arterial (aortic) catheter—causes a beneficial effect on the ECG, even before CPR (suggesting retrograde or antegrade coronary flushing)—more rapidly than the same standard dose of epinephrine given via peripheral vein during CPR (Safar P et al, unpublished observations).

Monitoring pulmonary artery catheterization (Fig. 38)[736c, 799, 836, 872]

A pulmonary artery catheter is rarely needed during Phase II of emergency resuscitation; however, it is a useful adjunct for selected cases during long-term life support. The value of pulmonary artery catheterization must in each case be weighed against associated potential complications, which include life-threatening dysrhythmias and distraction of team effort from more important and more simple life support measures. Insertion of a pulmonary artery balloon catheter (Swan–Ganz) is *indicated* to monitor pulmonary artery occlusion (wedge) pressure (PAOP, PAWP) (a reflection of left atrial pressure) in left ventricular failure; to titrate fluid therapy in patients with alveolar-capillary membrane leakage or renal failure; to determine whether increased pulmonary artery pressure is the result of increased pulmonary vascular resistance or of left ventricular failure; and to determine whether increased CVP is due to right or left heart failure. The pulmonary artery catheter also permits monitoring of mixed venous PO_2 (normal value 40–50 mmHg) and oxygen content. A reduction of pulmonary artery PO_2, with arterial PO_2 unchanged, suggests a decrease in arterial oxygen transport (blood flow times oxygen content) below that required for the patient's oxygen consumption. Finally, a pulmonary artery catheter allows monitoring of cardiac output by the thermodilution technique. Normal pulmonary artery pressure is 25/10 mmHg, mean 15 (range 14–17) mmHg. Normal mean pulmonary artery occlusion (wedge) pressure (during occlusion of the peripheral pulmonary artery, reflecting left atrial pressure) is 10 (6–12) mmHg. Pulmonary artery occlusion pressure should not be permitted to exceed plasma colloid osmotic (oncotic) pressure, which is normally 25 mmHg, but can be significantly reduced in severe illness or injury. Monitoring of plasma colloid osmotic pressure (or at least albumin concentration) is desirable in long-term resuscitation[736c, 799, 836].

The *technique* of pulmonary artery catheterization (preferably by balloon-tipped catheter with PA and CV ports, designed for monitoring cardiac output by thermodilution) is an extension of central venous catheterization (above) (Fig. 38). The central venous port is used with guide wire technique to insert a large-bore short introducer sheath into the right internal jugular vein. Through it the pulmonary artery balloon catheter is guided via the right atrium and ventricle into a peripheral pulmonary artery wedge position by continuous monitoring of pressures. The procedure is poten-

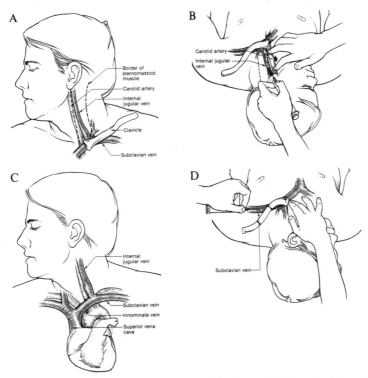

Fig. 38. (A, B) Internal jugular vein cannulation. The internal jugular vein is lateral to, and slightly in front of, the common carotid artery. Puncture is made at the mid-point of the anterior border of the sternocleidomastoid muscle, at 45° to the frontal plane, parallel to the sagittal plane. (C, D) Subclavian vein cannulation. Insert the needle 1 cm below the clavicle, at the junction of its medial and middle thirds, directing it towards the opposite shoulder, with a finger in the suprasternal notch directing the needle behind the fingertip. (From Caroline NL: *Emergency Care in the Streets*, Little Brown, 1987, third edition.)

tially dysrhythmogenic and can cause damage to the heart and vessels. It should not be over-used.

Arterial puncture[736c]

For initial blood gas determinations, arterial puncture is sufficient. Arterial puncture is feasible during cardiac compressions (particularly using the femoral artery) and is essential for proper titration of bicarbonate therapy. It should not, however, interfere with more fundamental therapeutic measures. Emergency hospitals receiving resuscitation cases should have stat blood gas laboratory services available 24 hours a day with results available in minutes.

Arterial puncture is best accomplished using a small, heparin-rinsed syringe with a 25 gauge needle. The radial artery is the site of choice for arterial sampling, since asepsis is more easily assured at that site than in the groin and subsequent bleeding may be more readily controlled. The patency of the ipsilateral ulnar artery should be confirmed before radial artery puncture (Allen's test). The patient is asked to make a tight fist to blanch the hand (or the hand is squeezed). The operator applies occlusive pressure over the radial and ulnar arteries. The patient's opened hand should now be fully blanched. The operator releases pressure on the ulnar artery. If normal color is restored to the hand within a few seconds, ulnar circulation may be considered adequate in the event of radial thrombosis. Blood samples should be drawn bubble-free into the prepared heparin-rinsed syringe. If any delay in processing the sample is anticipated, the syringe should be placed in ice. Potential complications of arterial puncture may be avoided by meticulous care in techniques. Hematoma results from inadequate compression over the puncture site, whereas thrombosis is favored by excessive compression. Excessively frequent punctures at the same site can lead to arterial thrombosis.

Radial artery catheterization[736c]

Peripheral arterial catheterization is indicated for patients requiring long-term life support measures and repeated blood gas determinations over an extended period. The placement of an arterial catheter is not part of the initial stages of resuscitation, but should be performed after restoration of spontaneous circulation in a patient who does not show signs of regaining consciousness. As it can be accomplished during CPR Steps A–B–C, although with difficulty, it can be very useful during prolonged CPR attempts. An indwelling arterial catheter may be desirable in circumstances in which there is a need for frequent and repeated arterial sampling or direct, continuous monitoring of arterial blood pressure. Radial artery catheterization is safe, but only if the catheter is left in place for less than 1–2 days; thereafter the risk of thrombotic occlusion increases significantly. The integrity of the ipsilateral ulnar artery should first be assured. The wrist is splinted on an arm board in supination and dorsiflexion. An 18 gauge needle is used to make a small hole in the anesthetized skin. The 20–22 gauge catheter-outside-needle, held at about a 30° angle to the wrist, is passed through the hole in the skin into the radial artery, puncture of the radial artery being signaled by the appearance of blood in the catheter hub. The needle is advanced another 2–3 mm and then held motionless while the catheter is advanced over the needle into the artery. The needle is withdrawn while holding the catheter securely in place. The catheter is taped in position and attached to the strain gauge via sterile tubing.

Femoral artery catheterization (Fig. 39)[736c]

When long-term arterial catheterization is indicated, we recommend the femoral artery. The puncture site near the inguinal ligament lies between the femoral vein medially and the femoral nerve laterally. The wider the lumen of the artery in relation to the thickness of the catheter, the less likely the occurrence of thrombosis secondary to blood stasis. Therefore the femoral artery is less prone to clotting and thrombosis, even when the catheter is left in place for over a week. It can also be secured in place more easily without having to immobilize the patient's limb. The equipment and techniques used may vary. Some prefer the catheter-outside-needle, others the catheter-inside-needle. One technique found to be satisfactory in our institution is presented here. Under sterile technique, the femoral artery is palpated, a 20 gauge needle is inserted followed by a guide wire and an 18 gauge catheter fed over the wire into the lower abdominal aorta and held firmly in place after the needle is withdrawn over the wire.

In *small children and infants* in whom percutaneous puncture is not successful, a radial or temporal artery catheterization is used via a small skin incision, with catheter insertion through a puncture hole in the artery under direct vision, without ligating the artery.

For *any* arterial catheter, connections to stopcocks for sampling and flushing and to the strain gauge must be nonslipping (locking) to prevent exsanguinating hemorrhage. A continuous flushing device is safer than intermittent flush. Patency can be maintained for weeks by keeping a dilute heparin solution in the catheter (10 mg or 1000 units of heparin in 500 ml isotonic saline) (Fig. 39). Betadine ointment is used to seal the skin puncture site, and sterile gauze is applied over the puncture site and securely taped with adhesive to form a pressure dressing.

When *sampling* arterial or venous blood via catheter for gas and pH determinations, first withdraw slightly more than the dead space volume of fluid and then blood (which may later be reinjected) using a separate syringe. Follow this immediately by sampling into the heparin-rinsed sampling syringe. Sampling must avoid entry of air bubbles into the sampling syringe as well as into the patient's arterial system by handling stopcocks and syringes correctly and skillfully, which includes the use of gravity to control air bubbles. When a continuous flush device is used (a Sorensen device) (Fig. 39), sampling is done via a stopcock on the patient's side of the flush. Although the *complications* of arterial catheterization are potentially greater and more severe than those of arterial puncture, meticulous technique has made safe use of in-dwelling catheters, in the femoral artery for weeks and the radial artery for days, quite routine. Thick catheters in small arteries have resulted occasionally in thromboses. Arterial line flushing with bubbles and thrombi has caused embolization. Both may lead to loss of a limb. Although in exsanguinating hemorrhage and arrest arterial infusion proved very effective[240a, 410, 578], its superiority over venous infusion is controversial[410, 508]. The prevailing opinion at this time is that the arterial route should *not* be used for the administration of drugs and fluids because of the potential for inducing embolic–thrombotic complications.

Note: *Meticulous aseptic, bubble-free, clot-free technique is essential for all vascular cannulations.*

Laboratory Measurement of Blood Gases and pH[36, 787, 808]

Once obtained, whether by direct arterial puncture or via an in-dwelling arterial cannula, bubble-free heparinized arterial blood samples are sent immediately to the laboratory for analysis[786]. Any facility caring for the critically ill and injured should have the capability of providing rapid blood PO_2, PCO_2 and pH determinations on a 24-hour, 7-day basis. Modern laboratory equipment permits these measurements to be made from as little as 0.2 ml of blood within 3–5 minutes. Since it is often desirable to obtain hematocrit and sometimes blood oxygen content values as well, at least 1 ml of arterial blood should be sent to the laboratory.

Instruments used relate change in current to the concentration of ion or gas. *Oxygen electrodes* are based on the 'polarographic' principle developed by Clark. *Carbon dioxide electrodes* are based upon the principles developed by Severinghaus[786] ($CO_2 + H_2O \rightleftharpoons H_2CO_3 \rightleftharpoons H^+ + HCO_3^-$; the resulting H^+ ion concentration is directly proportional to the PCO_2 of the sample). The *pH electrode* has long been in use in industry and medicine. The PO_2, PCO_2 and pH electrodes have been refined and combined by Severinghaus into a *trielectrode* system[786]. These units serve patients better in the hands of specially trained ICU technicians. Unreliable and slow-response blood gas services are a greater hazard to patient care than no blood gas services at all. For determinations of cardiac output, oxygen consumption, shunting and oxygen utilization coefficient[736c], it is necessary to determine, in addition to the PO_2, the actual *oxygen content* of arterial blood (CaO_2) and of mixed venous or central venous blood (CvO_2). Oxygen may be measured by a variety of instruments using chemical, chromatographic and photoelectric techniques.

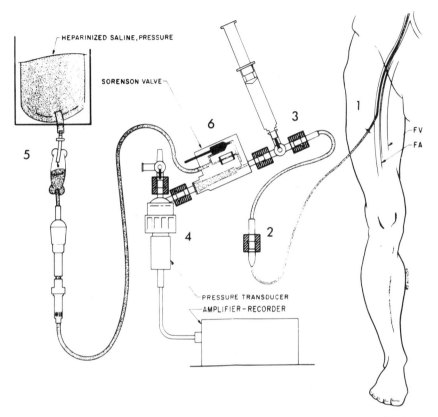

Fig. 39. Arterial catheter system. Femoral artery catheter (1) connected via nonslipping adapters (2) and a three-way stopcock with sampling syringe (3) to a pressure transducer (4). Interposed flushing system (5) with heparin (10 mg or 1000 units/500 ml saline) under pressure and Sorenson valve (6), permitting slow, continuous flush plus intermittent manual flush (see text).

Continuous end-tidal carbon dioxide monitoring (capnography)[454]

In patients with normal lungs, the carbon dioxide concentration or tension of end-tidal gas (PETCO$_2$) equals alveolar carbon dioxide concentration, which equals arterial carbon dioxide concentration. A 1% CO$_2$ equals about 7 torr PCO_2 at sea level. In patients with abnormal lungs, such as when increased alveolar dead space (e.g. emphysema) or hypoperfused lungs (e.g. shock) occur, the end-tidal carbon dioxide tracing will fail to achieve an alveolar plateau and the peak value will be lower than the arterial PCO_2. Continuous monitoring of end-tidal carbon dioxide pressure (PETCO$_2$) curves, using a rapidly responding infrared gas analyzer (capnograph), is a

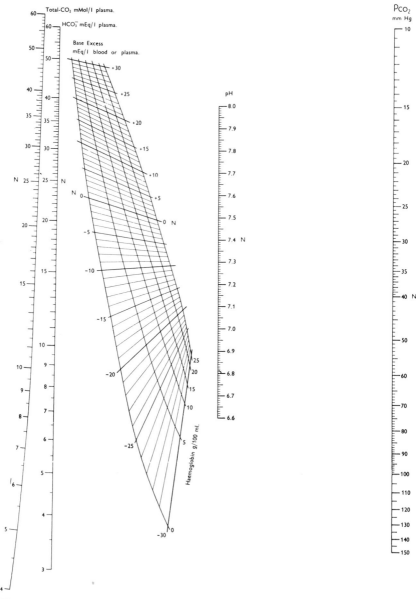

Fig. 40. Blood acid–base alignment nomogram according to Siggaard-Andersen. Measure the blood PCO_2 and pH with appropriate electrodes. Connect the values and read the bicarbonate concentration in milliequivalents per liter (left). Determine the hemoglobin and read the base-excess where the PCO_2–pH–bicarbonate line crosses the base-excess nomogram at the appropriate hemoglobin concentration. N: normal. This nomogram is designed for use with blood at 38°C. (From Siggaard-Andersen: *Scan J Clin Lab Invest* **15:** 211, 1963[808].)

valuable (though not essential) method for critical care, particularly for patients in whom $PaCO_2$ control is important, such as in acute brain failure or cardiac dysrhythmias. Monitoring of $PETCO_2$ permits continuous display, breath by breath, of changes in alveolar carbon dioxide concentration and thereby displays hyperventilation, hypoventilation, apnea and a sudden drop due to increase in dead space caused by reduced lung perfusion, as in pulmonary embolism, severe shock or cardiac arrest. During cardiac arrest and CPR, the better the cardiac output the higher will be the $PETCO_2$ with constant ventilation[946].

Mass spectrometry[454]

Any mixture of gases sampled via a high-vacuum pump into the ionization chamber of a mass spectrometer can be analyzed by being exposed to a beam of electrons. These very expensive systems in use in some anesthesiology and critical care research settings offer little in emergency resuscitation.

Noninvasive (pulse) oximetry[454]

The Waters tissue (ear) oximeter noninvasively measures the hemoglobin oxygen saturation, i.e. the spectral differences between oxyhemoglobin and reduced hemoglobin. In shock, the readings may be low because of low flow from vasoconstriction, increased oxygen extraction and nonarterialization of capillaries and venules. The ear oximeter cannot be used for detecting pulmonary shunting, since a PaO_2 value between 100 and 600 mmHg is not reflected in oxygen saturation decrease. The oximeter is useful as a safety monitor in long-term life support. Currently, pulse oximeters offer beat to beat information about arterial oxygen saturation in the tissue transilluminated (e.g. finger, ear). At the same time they serve as a pulse monitor. These devices, seemingly of great value in the management of the critically ill anesthetized patient[799], should be evaluated in CPR cases.

Transcutaneous PO_2 and PCO_2 analyses[362, 788, 801]

For monitoring arterial PO_2 and PCO_2 continuously and noninvasively through the arterialized (warmed) skin, Huch developed a transcutaneous (tc) PO_2 electrode of the Clark type, which was used first on the scalp of newborns[362], and Severinghaus developed a tcPCO_2 electrode[788]. tcPO_2 depends on PaO_2, arterial oxygen content, and local blood flow. tcPCO_2 is consistently 10–30 torr higher than $PaCO_2$ in dogs, neonates and adults[788]. Relative changes are more meaningful than absolute values. These methods can also be used effectively in adults, not only to follow trends in arterial blood gas changes, but even more importantly to detect decrease in local skin perfusion, which may even precede arterial hypotension, tachycardia and anuria in shock[801]. In the hemodynamically stable patient, tcPO_2 can be used for detecting high alveolar–arterial PO_2 gradients (shunting) in abnormal lungs, which cannot be achieved by ear (skin) oximetry. $tcPO_2$ decrease in low cardiac output states is not an indication of hypoxemia, but with normal PaO_2 monitored simultaneously a $tcPO_2$ below about 40 torr reflects reduced cardiac output and arterial oxygen transport; below 25 torr is life threatening. In shock, $tcPCO_2$ increases while $PaCO_2$ is normal or low. Monitoring of $tcPCO_2$ tracks $PaCO_2$ linearly only as long as there is hemodynamic stability. Thus, $tcPCO_2$ is a trend monitor.

Emergency spirometry (Fig. 41)[736c]

Knowledge of lung volumes is important for long-term respiratory resuscitation of conscious or unconscious patients (Fig. 41). Spirometry is not important in emergency resuscitation. Measurements of vital capacity (VC), total and timed, and increased airway resistance in the conscious patient are useful and readily available. A variety of portable, electronically activated spirometers permit bedside assessment of VC in the form of forced expiratory volume (FEV), total and timed, and maximum mid-expiratory

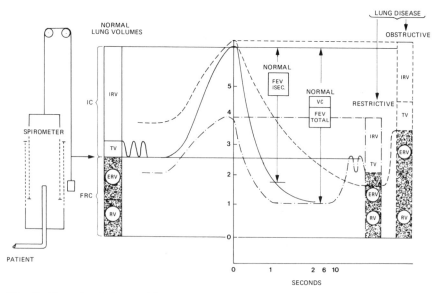

Fig. 41. Normal and abnormal lung volumes and idealized spirometry tracings. Forced expiratory volume (expiratory vital capacity) (FEV) starts at zero seconds. TV, tidal volume; FRC, functional residual capacity; IC, inspiratory capacity; IRV, inspiratory reserve volume; ERV, expiratory reserve volume; RV, residual volume; VC, vital capacity; ——, normal; – – –, primarily obstructive derangement; ....., primarily restrictive derangement.

flow rate (MMFR). Using such a spirometer, the patient is asked to inhale maximally and then exhale as strongly and completely as possible. Leakage can be prevented with a tight-fitting oronasal mask or a mouthpiece with nose clip. Coaching and patient cooperation are required. For use in conscious or unconscious artificially ventilated or spontaneously breathing patients, the ventilation meter (e.g. Wright), a pocket-sized anemometer, can be placed in-line with resuscitation breathing apparatus or be attached to masks or airways for monitoring tidal volume, vital capacity and inspiratory capacity. For monitoring the efficacy of bronchodilators in conscious patients, the peak flowmeter (e.g. Wright) proved practical. For vital capacity measurements, the total volume exhaled (i.e. the vital capacity or total forced expiratory volume, FEV) is compared with the normal (predicted) value of the particular patient (Fig. 41). Total FEV less than 80% of predicted (normal) FEV volume indicates 'restrictive disease'. The normal total vital capacity of a young adult 6 feet (180 cm) tall is 5.0–5.5 liters, which decreases to about 4.5 liters by age 60; it is lower in females and, of course, in shorter people. The volume exhaled in the first second constitutes FEV, which if less than 80% of the total FEV of that patient indicates 'obstructive disease'.

Arterial pressure monitoring

During CPR Steps A–B–C, arterial systolic pressure can be estimated by feeling the carotid or femoral pulse. After restoration of spontaneous circulation, the indirect sphygmomanometric cuff method of Riva-Rocci (1896) should be used. It is based on the principle that pressure transmitted to the major arteries of the upper arm is approximated by the pressure measured in the cuff when flow returns, with a pressure gauge or mercury manometer attached to the cuff. A quick estimate of the systolic arterial pressure can be obtained by feeling the radial artery with one hand, inflating the cuff to about 300 torr and deflating it slowly while detecting the cuff pressure at which the radial pulse returns. Similarly, the manometer will bounce with each pulse at systolic pressure. More accurate is the auscultatory method; a stethoscope over the brachial artery distal to the cuff transmits the Korotkoff sounds, which during cuff deflation appear at systolic and disappear at diastolic pressure. In the unstable resuscitation condition, systolic pressure is more important for the brain, diastolic pressure for the myocardium. When blood pressure sounds cannot be heard, a Doppler flowmeter can pick up flow distal to the cuff. Korotkoff sounds may be faint in hypotension, vasoconstriction, hypothermia and narrow pulse pressure.

Most accurate monitoring of arterial pressure is accomplished directly via radial or femoral artery catheter, stopcock, strain gauge and amplifier to a recorder or oscilloscope screen. Calibrating strain gauges attached to arterial and venous catheters should be with a common zero level, preferably at the level of the right atrium. Central venous pressure (CVP) can also be monitored via a three-way stopcock, which is connected to the venous infusion and to a water (saline) column. The height of the infusion drip chamber, when lowered to see at which point blood returns from the vein, can also be used for estimating CVP. Similarly when an arterial catheter has been inserted primarily for blood sampling and electronic monitoring equipment is not available, long saline filled tubing can be connected from the stopcock to air-filled tubing attached to a mercury or aneroid manometer. The air protects the manometer; the stopcock permits flushing of the arterial catheter. Only mean arterial pressure can be monitored reliably this way. Dilute heparin solution should be used for flushing. For arterial, venous and pulmonary artery catheterization, see above.

Although in skilled hands arterial catheterization can be performed swiftly, it should not distract personnel away from more life supporting measures during CPR.

Drugs

Principal drugs during CPR Steps A–B–C[23b, 373a, 606a, 613a]

Epinephrine (adrenaline) may help restore spontaneous circulation in cardiac arrest of more than about 1–2 minutes duration, irrespective of the electrocardiographic (ECG) pattern, i.e. ventricular fibrillation, ventricular tachycardia, electrical asystole or electromechanical dissociation (EMD) (mechanical asystole with normal or bizarre ECG complexes). In cases of persistent or recurrent ventricular fibrillation or ventricular tachycardia without a pulse—in spite of effective CPR, correctly applied countershock, and normal blood gas and pH values—lidocaine and, if ineffective, bretylium are also indicated during cardiac compressions. Other drugs described below are for the pre- or post-arrest period.

During CPR Steps A–B–C, bolus injections are preferred; during long-term life support, administration of potent cardiovascular drugs by titrated i.v. infusions is preferred, using microdrip sets or infusion pumps. Ideally drugs should be injected piggy back into a running infusion of maintenance fluid to avoid deleterious bolus effects and control volume and doses.

Recommendations call for *epinephrine* first, *lidocaine* as the second agent (for persistent VF), and *sodium bicarbonate* ($NaHCO_3$) as the third agent—only if indicated. This is based in part on the practical fact that the small volume of epinephrine is easily and rapidly administered into a peripheral vein. The longer time taken to infuse the larger volume of bicarbonate, which must be given slowly, should not be permitted to delay the early effect of epinephrine. In cases of asystole or ventricular fibrillation, restoration of spontaneous circulation is usually enhanced by administration of epinephrine i.v. or intratracheally, but is rarely enhanced by sodium bicarbonate ($NaHCO_3$) unless there has been a prolonged arrest time. Occasionally, epinephrine given in asystole or EMD may provoke ventricular fibrillation; this calls for external electric countershock. Controlled hyperventilation with oxygen is more important than bicarbonate to combat the mixed metabolic–respiratory acidemia of cardiac arrest.

In cardiac arrest no drug is effective without IPPV and cardiac (chest) compressions. In *monitored* arrest with ventricular fibrillation or ventricular tachycardia, immediate electric countershock has priority over drugs. In *unwitnessed* arrest and ventricular fibrillation diagnosed by ECG, early countershock usually results in asystole rather than sinus rhythm because of severe acidosis; this calls for prolonged CPR, use of epinephrine and arterial pH control.

Drugs for CPR need reinvestigation. At the present time their use is as much an art as a science. Drug administration must be on a skillfully titrated basis, in concert with CPR Steps A–B–C, electric countershocks and fluid administration—with a feeling of utmost urgency to minimize interruptions of artificial circulation and ventilation and to restore spontaneous circulation as quickly as possible. Epinephrine given during CPR usually results in a hypertensive bout immediately upon resumption of spontaneous heart action, and may be good for recovery of brain perfusion. This must be followed immediately with a titrated infusion of a vasopressor (e.g. dopamine) to prevent rebound hypotension and to control mean arterial pressure (MAP) at normotensive or slightly hypertensive levels throughout post-anoxic coma. Also, recurrent ventricular fibrillation must be guarded against by ECG and MAP by titrated administration of lidocaine. In fact, ventricular fibrillation or tachycardia may be prevented in some patients by prophylactic administration of lidocaine.

Drugs in witnessed cardiac arrest: ventricular tachycardia or ventricular fibrillation

1. If a *defibrillator* is immediately available, apply the quick-look ECG defibrillating paddles, confirm ventricular fibrillation (VF) or ventricular tachycardia (VT) (absence of QRS complexes), and administer within 30 seconds of the patient's collapse three external electric countershocks in rapid sequence, with escalating energy (200–300–360 J). Do not delay countershocks for the administration of drugs or CPR Steps A–B–C. If a defibrillator is not immediately available and the patient is with ECG monitored VF or VT, administer a *chest thump* immediately upon collapse (Chapter 4) and coach him/her to *cough* vigorously every 1–2 seconds to stay conscious (cough producing perfusion of the brain) until the defibrillator arrives.

2. If the three initial countershocks fail to restore a spontaneous pulse immediately, start closed-chest *CPR Steps A–B–C*, check the ECG for persistence of VF or VT, and repeat countershocks every 1–2 minutes.

3. Give *epinephrine* i.v. 0.5–1.0 mg or intratracheally 1 mg in 10 ml water or isotonic saline (in intubated patient without i.v.) (adult doses) as soon as possible after the initiation of CPR. Repeat epinephrine about every 5 minutes during CPR Steps A–B–C. Dilution of epinephrine 0.5–1.0 mg in 5–10 ml or even 25–50 ml of isotonic salt solution is desirable but not essential.

   If countershocks have failed to terminate VF or VT, circulate epinephrine by cardiac compressions for about 1 minute before repeating countershocks with 360 J each.

4. If countershocks fail to terminate VF or VT or if a spontaneous pulse is achieved but then reverts rapidly to VF or VT without pulse, give *lidocaine* 100 mg by *slow* i.v. push, followed by an infusion of lidocaine 1–4 mg/min (adult doses). Then repeat countershocks. If this also fails, try *bretylium* (see below).

5. Give *sodium bicarbonate* (NaHCO$_3$) 1 mEq/kg i.v. slowly into a running i.v. infusion only if initiation of CPR has been delayed (estimated pulselessness without CPR of at least 2–5 minutes) or CPR Steps A–B–C have been prolonged (over about 10 minutes). Do not use NaHCO$_3$ routinely during CPR.

6. During prolonged CPR Steps A–B–C, repeat NaHCO$_3$ 0.5 mEq/kg i.v. about every 10 minutes; or, better, titrate NaHCO$_3$ administration after first dose according to arterial pH and base deficit (see sodium bicarbonate, below).

Drugs in unwitnessed cardiac arrest: asystole or electro-mechanical dissociation

1. Start *CPR Steps A–B–C* as soon as possible.
2. Give *epinephrine* 0.5–1.0 mg i.v. (adult dose), as above. Repeat this or a larger dose (2 mg) i.v. dose every 5 minutes[113a]. If there is no i.v. catheter in place, insert one rapidly or give the epinephrine via needle puncture of a peripheral vein (e.g. external jugular) or via the endotracheal route (1 mg in 10 ml of water or isotonic saline).
3. Give *sodium bicarbonate* ($NaHCO_3$) 1 mEq/kg i.v., slowly into a running infusion, only after estimated arrest time of at least 2–5 minutes or CPR time of at least 10 minutes. Repeat $NaHCO_3$ 0.5 mEq/kg i.v. every 10 minutes of CPR. Once arterial pH values are available, titrated bicarbonate administration should be guided by such measurements and accompanied by moderate hyperventilation. The dose in mEq is equal to body weight (kg) × base deficit/4.
4. Monitor the ECG. Treat VF or VT by *countershocks* (as above).
5. Treat recurrent VF or VT with *lidocaine* i.v. (as above); if ineffective, try *bretylium*. Do not use lidocaine or bretylium in heart block.

Drugs after restoration of spontaneous circulation

1. Maintain arterial normotension with fluid load i.v. (if appropriate) and titrated i.v. infusion of vasopressor (e.g. dopamine or norepinephrine) for hypotension or vasodilator (e.g. trimetaphan) for hypertension.
2. Maintain $PaO_2 > 100$ mmHg, $PaCO_2$ 25–35 mmHg, pHa 7.3–7.5.
3. To prevent re-arrest, control life-threatening tachydysrhythmias (lidocaine–procainamide–bretylium–countershock), bradydysrhythmias (atropine–isoproterenol–pacing), PSVT (verapamil–cardioversion).

Remember: Use antidysrhythmic drugs with caution. They can prevent *and cause* sudden cardiac death[694].

Epinephrine (adrenaline)[169, 652]

This historic cardiovascular stimulant[169] is still unsurpassed by other sympathomimetic amines for use during cardiac arrest and CPR because of its combined strong alpha-receptor and beta-receptor stimulating effects. The alpha-receptor stimulating effect of epinephrine is most important[652]. It increases systemic peripheral vascular resistance (without constricting the coronary and cerebral vessels) and raises systolic and diastolic pressures during cardiac compressions[657], which thereby improves myocardial and cerebral blood flow, which in turn facilitates the return of spontaneous cardiac contractions[109, 534, 588]. The beta-receptor stimulating effect of epinephrine (increased contractile state of the heart) is less important during cardiac compressions, but may become advantageous once spontaneous cardiac contractions resume[477]. The combined alpha and beta effects give a high initial cardiac output and arterial pressure at the beginning of spontaneous reperfusion, which may benefit cerebral and other vital organ system blood flow.

In asystole, epinephrine helps restart spontaneous cardiac action as it elevates perfusion and increases myocardial contractility. In pulselessness with bizarre ECG complexes (electromechanical dissociation), epinephrine often restores a spontaneous pulse. Although epinephrine can produce ventricular fibrillation, particularly in the nonbeating unevenly anoxic (diseased) heart, it also renders the heart in ventricular fibrillation or ventricular tachycardia easier to defibrillate to a pulse-producing rhythm.

During CPR Steps A–B–C, epinephrine hydrochloride 0.5–1.0 mg (adult dose) is given i.v. in a solution of 1 mg/ml or 1 mg/10 ml. The first dose should be given without waiting for ECG diagnosis, and this dose should be repeated every 5 minutes, as the duration of action of epinephrine is short. If the i.v. route is impossible, the intratracheal route should be used (1–2 mg in 10 ml of water or isotonic saline[225, 653, 671]). Although clinical guidelines are not to mix epinephrine and sodium bicarbonate in the same syringe, we found mixtures of epinephrine 1 mg and sodium bicarbonate 1 mEq/kg in a 50 ml bolus by central vein to be effective in dog experiments[745, 911]. We and others[113a] recommend the use during pulselessness of larger doses of epinephrine i.v. (by bolus or infusion) if the recommended doses are ineffective.

After restoration of spontaneous circulation, a continuous i.v. infusion of epinephrine (1 mg in 250 ml) may be used to increase and sustain arterial pressure and cardiac output, starting with 0.01 μg/kg per min and adjusted according to response. Although other sympathomimetic drugs are more commonly used after restoration of spontaneous circulation, in seemingly desperate shock states of anaphylaxis, pump failure or asphyxia (e.g. status asthmaticus), transient use of a titrated i.v. infusion of epinephrine in high concentration was occasionally life-saving. To prevent recurrence of ventricular tachycardia or ventricular fibrillation during administration of a sympathomimetic amine, a simultaneous infusion of lidocaine or bretylium has been suggested.

Sodium bicarbonate[23b, 857]

This is the third drug to be given during CPR Steps A–B–C (after epinephrine and lidocaine), in an initial dose of approximately 1 mEq/kg i.v., but only after prolonged arrest or CPR time. The purpose of administering sodium bicarbonate ($NaHCO_3$) is to neutralize the fixed acids coming from ischemic tissues after circulatory arrest and during the borderline perfusion produced by CPR[857]. Severe acidemia (arterial pH less than 7.2)—actually tissue acidosis—should be reversed because it causes vasodilation, capillary leakage, myocardial depression[147, 481], conduction block[329] and a decrease in fibrillation threshold[271]. Controlled hyperventilation should be the first measure to counteract this tissue acidosis. It is not clear whether the tissue or blood pH or the fixed acids (base deficit) irrespective of pH are in need of control. Acidemia and tissue acidosis reduce the efficacy of epinephrine[360, 409, 617, 652, 893], but epinephrine i.v. in large enough doses is effective without $NaHCO_3$[409, 657]. There are no convincing data showing that $NaHCO_3$ during CPR improves defibrillation success or outcome[409, 546, 654, 888]. More research is needed, with attempts to separate tissue and blood acid–base derangements.

Excessive $NaHCO_3$ (metabolic alkalemia) results in impaired oxygen release from hemoglobin, reduced ionized (effective) to un-ionized calcium ratio, a potassium shift from serum into cells, ventricular tachycardia and fibrillation, and sustained cardiac contraction (stone heart)[450]. $NaHCO_3$ may also be injurious by producing hypernatremia with hyperosmolality[515]. During CPR, less sodium bicarbonate is needed than previously assumed, whereas more is needed after restoration of spontaneous circulation when washout of acids from tissues increases. After cardiac arrest (without CPR) of 2–5 minutes, or after immediately beginning CPR Steps A–B–C of not more than about 10 minutes, acidemia can usually be corrected by moderate hyperventilation alone[86]. During $NaHCO_3$ administration, more than usual hyperventilation is needed to eliminate the carbon dioxide released by $NaHCO_3$. Without hyperventilation, $NaHCO_3$, which raises blood pH, may paradoxically lower brain pH, because carbon dioxide passes through the blood–brain barrier more readily than the charged bicarbonate or hydrogen ions[71, 86], and worsens overall venous acidosis and probably tissue acidosis[947].

In cardiac arrest *during* CPR, the recommended initial 'blindly' administered dose of sodium bicarbonate is 1 mEq/kg i.v. once. $NaHCO_3$ should be given not routinely, but only for suspected arrest times (without CPR) of at least 2–5 minutes or CPR–ABC times of at least 10 minutes. (Bicarbonate is usually available in a solution of 1 mEq/ml in prefilled syringes.) Additional blindly administered doses should not exceed 0.5 mEq/kg for every 10 minutes of CPR. Ideally subsequent administration should be guided by arterial pH measurements, aiming for values near 7.4 (7.3 to 7.5).

Immediately *after* restoration of spontaneous circulation, the release of large amounts of carbonic acid and lactic acid from tissues calls for more controlled *hyperventilation* (IPPV) (titrated according to arterial pH values) and NaHCO$_3$ i.v. (titrated according to calculated base deficit values) (Fig. 40). The optimal approach requires continuous adjustment of ventilation volumes to an arterial PCO_2 of 25–35 mmHg and use of NaHCO$_3$ i.v. solely to correct base deficit (BD) to within about 5 mEq/l, aiming for an arterial pH of 7.3–7.5. BD is negative base excess (BE). The normal blood BD (BE) to aim for is $\pm$ 5 mEq/l. The natural *buffers* that determine BD (BE) in blood are NaHCO$_3$, hemoglobin and proteins.

Base deficit

Base deficit (BD) is *calculated* from arterial pH, PCO_2 and hemoglobin concentration, using the Siggaard-Andersen nomogram (Fig. 40). *Calculation* of the sodium bicarbonate dose required is performed as follows (Astrup):

1. Dose of NaHCO$_3$ in mEq = blood base deficit (mEq/l) × body weight (kg)/4 (i.e. extracellular fluid volume in liters is body weight in kg/4). For example, a 60 kg patient with a BD of 10 mEq/l requires NaHCO$_3$ 150 mEg (10 mEq/l × 60/4).
2. Give the first half of the above dose as a bolus i.v. and titrate the second half, only if needed, to reduce base deficit to 5 mEq/l or less.

Base deficit is *estimated* from arterial pH and PCO_2, while ignoring hemoglobin as a buffer, i.e. simplified teaching by Sladen[815]★:

1. A change in arterial PCO_2 by 10 mmHg up or down changes arterial pH by 0.08.
2. A change in BD (BE) by 10 mEq/l up or down changes arterial pH by 0.15.

★*Example 1*[815]: If during CPR-ABC $PaCO_2$ is 20 mmHg (normal 40 mmHg) and pHa is 7.4 (normal), the respiratory component would account for a pHa of $7.4 + (0.08 \times 2) = 7.56$. The metabolic component (BD) would account for $7.56 - 7.4 = 0.16$. A pH change of 0.15 would be caused by a BD of 10 mEq/l. This would call for a total dose of i.v. NaHCO$_3$ of 70 (kg)/4 × 10 = 17.5 × 10 = 175 mEq (2.5 mEq/kg).
★*Example 2*[815]: If early after restoration of spontaneous circulation following a prolonged cardiac arrest the $PaCO_2$ is 20 mmHg (resulting from controlled hyperventilation) and the pHa is 7.0, the respiratory component would again call for a pHa of 7.56, but the metabolic component has risen to $7.56 - 7.4 = 0.56$. This is caused by a BD of 10 mEq/l for a pHa difference of 0.15, i.e. a total BD of 38 mEq/l. This would call for a total NaHCO$_3$ dose of 70 (kg)/4 × 38 = 17.5 × 38 = 665 mEq (9.5 mEq/kg). One-half should be infused slowly and the other half reconsidered after another blood gas determination.

Tris buffer (THAM)[351b, 646, 888]

This drug has been used in lieu of and in the same dosage (in mEq) as sodium bicarbonate. THAM has the advantage of not being a carbon dioxide donor (and thus not requiring excessive hyperventilation) and entering the intracellular space more readily. However, THAM has the disadvantages of not being available in a readily usable solution and causing apnea, hypoglycemia and venous irritation. A systematic evaluation of THAM and other new hydrogen ion antagonists for CPCR is needed.

Lidocaine (lignocaine, Xylocaine)[123, 485]

All antidysrhythmic drugs are cardiac depressants and not harmless[694]. Lidocaine is the antidysrhythmic agent of choice for the treatment of premature ventricular complexes (PVCs) of the ECG (ventricular ectopy, ventricular extrasystoles) and for preventing progression to ventricular tachycardia (VT) or ventricular fibrillation (VF). In established VF, however, antidysrhythmic drugs should be withheld until several attempts at electric defibrillation have failed, since these drugs depress ventricular ectopy and make initial defibrillation more difficult.

Lidocaine, a local anesthetic of the amide type, was found to *raise* the VF *threshold*[123, 832]. It increases the electric stimulation threshold during diastole and depresses cardiac irritability in cases of frequently recurring VF. Lidocaine raises the VF threshold either by depressing conduction in ischemic areas[441] or by improving conduction in the normal myocardium[263]. It also *raises* the *defibrillation threshold* (increases joules required to defibrillate[40]). In equipotent antidysrhythmic doses, lidocaine produces less myocardial depression than do other antidysrhythmic drugs.

In patients with spontaneous circulation, lidocaine is indicated when there are more than six PVCs per minute, short bursts of two or more PVCs in succession, PVCs of multiple configurations, or PVCs falling on the T wave—also called the R-on-T phenomenon[155]. However, once myocardial infarction is suspected, PVCs of any kind or frequency should be suppressed with lidocaine. Prophylactic use of lidocaine reduces the incidence of primary VF in myocardial infarction[190, 427]. This drug is also the first choice during CPR when VT or VF is resistant to defibrillation.

Lidocaine alone cannot convert VF to a stable rhythm, but might convert VT. In intractable VF lidocaine should be used in conjunction with electric defibrillation attempts, and if ineffective it should be replaced by bretylium (see below).

Side-effects of lidocaine include myocardial depression, which is more likely to be apparent in the presence of cardiogenic shock. In such cases the normal bolus dose may be reduced by half. Doses should also be reduced for patients with right heart failure, since clearance of lidocaine is delayed when there is passive congestion of the liver, and toxic levels of the drug may accumulate rapidly. Lidocaine may cause slurred speech, somnolence and twitching which can be rapidly followed by convulsions, probably at serum levels of over about 10–30 μg/ml. Therefore, resuscitation equipment should be ready. Doses should be reduced in heart failure, shock, patients over 70 years of age, and hepatic disease[146].

Method of administration of lidocaine

1. Give a loading dose of 1 mg/kg by slow i.v. bolus. Follow it immediately by a continuous infusion of 1–4 mg/70 kg per min, preferably via an infusion pump. (Use a solution of 4 mg/ml in 5% dextrose in water.)
2. Give additional boluses of 0.5–1.0 mg/kg every 8–10 minutes, if necessary, to a total of 3 mg/kg.
3. For long-term suppression of ventricular dysrhythmias, after 24 hours at a reduced rate of 1–2 mg/70 kg per min, continue this infusion for several days if necessary. Ideally, monitor serum lidocaine levels and keep them at 1–5 μg/ml to avoid seizures and myocardial depression. Use the same administration mode for prophylaxis against VF in myocardial infarction. Avoid lidocaine in the presence of heart block.

Procaine, procainamide[23b]

Procaine hydrochloride (Novocain) and procainamide hydrochloride (Pronestyl) preceded lidocaine historically for the suppression of PVCs. One of these drugs is indicated when lidocaine is contraindicated. Like lidocaine, these drugs cannot be relied upon to give pharmacologic defibrillation; rather, they are used to enhance the chances of successful electric countershock. In the presence of spontaneous circulation, they are more likely than lidocaine to produce hypotension and reduce conduction, even in normal myocardium. The recommended dose of procainamide is about the same as that of lidocaine, but to a maximum of 1 g. Repeat injections or an infusion of procainamide must be stopped when the dysrhythmia has been controlled, if hypotension occurs, if the QRS of the ECG is widened by 50% or more, or when a cumulative dose of about 1 g of the drug has been reached. Procainamide is eliminated by the kidneys and metabolized by the liver. Quinidine is for long-term use only.

Bretylium[422]

Bretylium (Bretylol), a bromobenzyl quaternary ammonium compound, is an antidysrhythmic agent that *raises* the *VF threshold*, probably through a postganglionic adrenergic blockade (causing hypotension and bradycardia) which, however, is preceded by catecholamine release, causing hypertension and tachycardia. A third phase is blocking re-uptake of catecholamines[422]. In VF it *lowers* the *defibrillation threshold* (decreases joules required); in contrast, the joules required for defibrillation seem to be raised by lidocaine and quinidine[40]. When tried as a first-time antidysrhythmic drug it did not prove superior to lidocaine[600]. Although chemical defibrillation with bretylium tosylate has been reported[115, 766], one must consider this an unreliable rare possibility. It facilitates subsequent electric defibrillation and helps prevent recurrent VT or VF in patients with very sick hearts. Its effects are unpredictable. A variety of side-effects associated with chronic administration, including postural hypotension and nausea, are irrelevant during the emergency use of this drug. It is presently *recommended* as a second line of defense in the control of VT or VF, when countershocks and lidocaine have not been effective, when VF has recurred in spite of lidocaine, or when lidocaine and procainamide have not controlled VT with pulse.

Recommended doses are 5 mg/kg i.v. during CPR in recurrent VF, followed by countershocks. If ineffective in 5–15 minutes, a dose of 10 mg/kg is recommended, which may be repeated until a total of 30 mg/kg has been given[23b]. Continuous infusions of 1–2 mg/70 kg per min have also been used. Bretylium is excreted unchanged through the kidneys.

Cardiovascular stimulants

Vasopressors and cardiac stimulants do not seem to have significant advantages over epinephrine for use *during* CPR Steps A–B–C[109, 169, 588, 604, 651–654, 657, 980]. Sympathomimetic amines with primarily alpha-receptor stimulating properties, such as norepinephrine (Levophed, noradrenaline) and metaraminol (Aramine), and drugs that are pure alpha-receptor stimulants, such as phenylephrine (Neosynephrine) or methoxamine (Vasoxyl, Vasoxine), are also effective in raising diastolic arterial pressure during cardiac compressions and in facilitating restoration of spontaneous circulation in asystole. They do not, however, provide the additional cardiac inotropic (beta-receptor stimulating) effect, which might also be desirable—during CPR Steps A–B–C, as it enhances the vigor of ventricular fibrillation (VF) and thereby seems to enhance the chance for defibrillation, and upon return of spontaneous circulation when it transiently increases stroke volume, heart rate and cardiac output, which is desirable. These drugs have not received the extensive clinical attention that has been accorded to epinephrine. Pure beta-receptor stimulating sympathomimetic amines, such as isoproterenol (Isuprel, isoprenaline), low-dose dopamine, dobutamine and calcium, do *not* aid in the restoration of spontaneous circulation because they lack the ability to increase diastolic arterial pressure and coronary reperfusion during cardiac compressions.

For use *after* CPR Steps A–B–C, for stabilization of cardiovascular parameters, however, vasoactive agents with or without cardiac-stimulating effect are indispensable. One of several individualized approaches is to follow the initial dose of epinephrine given during CPR Steps A–B–C with norepinephrine until the mean arterial pressure (MAP) is stabilized (important for cerebral recovery) and then switch to dopamine or dobutamine for support of cardiac output and normotension (important for overall recovery) and other cardiovascular agents such as antiarrhythmic agents (see above) and vasodilators (see below) (Chapter 3).

All potent vasoactive infusions should be titrated if possible with the aid of direct intra-arterial pressure monitoring, use of microdrips or infusion pumps and (optional) use of pulmonary artery and occlusion pressure (PAP, PAOP) monitoring by balloon catheter[872].

Norepinephrine (noradrenaline)[924]

Norepinephrine (Levophed, noradrenaline), a naturally occurring catecholamine, is primarily an alpha-receptor stimulant and the most potent vasopressor, secondary only to angiotensin II. It also exerts some beta-receptor activity[985]. For use *during* CPR Steps A–B–C, prior to restoration of spontaneous circulation, norepinephrine may be given in the same doses as epinephrine and is effective in helping to restore spontaneous circulation. Experience with norepinephrine during CPR, however, is limited and a controlled comparison with epinephrine in animals is lacking[817].

For use *after* restoration of spontaneous circulation, in the experience of one of us (PS), norepinephrine is less likely than epinephrine (see above), dopamine or dobutamine (see below) to produce recurrent tachydysrhythmias. It compares favorably with dopamine and dobutamine as the first drug for arterial pressure support *after* restoration of spontaneous circulation. Epinephrine for this purpose is usually reserved for this situation when all else fails. Coronary perfusion is increased by raised aortic pressure and coronary vasodilation, but myocardial oxygen consumption may also be increased. Control of normotension, heart rate and cardiac output has been effectively accomplished by the simultaneous titrated i.v. infusion of norepinephrine (alpha-receptor stimulant) plus epinephrine or isoproterenol or dobutamine (primarily as a beta-receptor stimulant) in severe cardiogenic shock[564]. When, in the presence of normovolemia, norepinephrine is cautiously infused merely to maintain normotension, clinical experience indicates that urine flow continues and no evidence of added tissue ischemia is found.

When norepinephrine is given to the point of excessive vasoconstriction, renal and mesenteric blood flow are compromised and a severe metabolic acidosis may develop. The heart rate may slow as a result of a carotid baroreceptor reflex if hypertension occurs. Prolonged administration of norepinephrine in hypovolemia is contraindicated. However, in severe hemorrhage with profound hypotension, if there is delay in replacement of blood volume, particularly in elderly patients, coronary and cerebral perfusion can be protected, and cardiac arrest thereby prevented, by *brief* arterial pressure support with a potent alpha-receptor agonist, such as norepinephrine. This should be accompanied by vigorous volume replacement, titrated at first according to arterial pulse and pressure recovery, and later with use of a pulmonary artery balloon catheter (PAOP) to avoid left heart overloading. In patients with ischemic heart disease, arterial pressure should not be raised above normal for prolonged periods.

In the presence of spontaneous circulation with reduced peripheral resistance and hypotension, norepinephrine is given by titrated i.v. infusion, for example by adding 8 mg of norepinephrine to 500 ml of 5% dextrose in water or isotonic saline (yielding a concentration of 16 μg/ml). One may start with 3 μg (0.2 ml)/70 kg per min. Because the effect of norepinephrine is potent, continuous arterial pressure monitoring is desirable. Infusion should be via a central vein, if possible, since sloughing of superficial tissues may result from extravasation of norepinephrine around superficial venipunctures. If extravasation does occur, phentolamine (10 mg in 10 ml saline solution) should be infiltrated at the site.

Dopamine[282]

This sympathomimetic amine is a biologic precursor of norepinephrine and epinephrine. It exerts dose-dependent cardiac inotropic action (beta-receptor stimulant) in low doses, and vasoconstrictor action (alpha-receptor stimulant) in high doses. Response differs among individuals and with dose and rate of administration[282]. Its vasopressor potency is less than that of norepinephrine.

The principal use of dopamine is in the support of perfusion pressure in cardiogenic or septic shock, using infusion rates of 2–20 μg/kg per min. The infusion rate is increased until arterial pressure and urine flow respond. In CPR cases *after* restoration of spontaneous circulation, dopamine is useful for supporting arterial perfusion pressure once the more potent norepinephrine is no longer required. Some use dopamine as the first choice vasopressor when the epinephrine effect begins to wear off. As when administering any vasopressor, normovolemia or even slight expansion of blood volume should be established. In cardiogenic shock, oliguria may respond to furosemide better when arterial pressure is also supported by dopamine, which is also a diuretic[343]. Dopamine infusion should be discontinued gradually.

Side-effects include tachycardia, increased myocardial oxygen demand, and PVCs, VT and VF (recurrent VF). In conscious patients with prolonged heart failure, carefully titrated cardiac stimulation with dopamine, combined with afterload reduction by nitroprusside, was effective[543].

Dopamine hydrochloride is usually given by titrated i.v. infusion of a solution containing 400 mg of dopamine in 500 ml of 5% dextrose in water or isotonic saline (800 μg/ml). Dopamine by *slow* infusion rate (1–2 μg/kg per min) dilates renal and mesenteric vessels without increasing blood pressure. By *intermediate* infusion rate (2–10 μg/kg per min), it has additional inotropic and vasodilating effects and thus increases cardiac output, but may produce severe tachycardia. *Rapid* infusion of higher concentrations (10–20 μg/kg per min) exert an additional vasoconstrictor effect, and in doses above 20 μg/kg per min the alpha-receptor stimulating effect is predominant and even the renal and mesenteric vessels may be constricted. Cardiac output may decrease and PAOP increase.

Dobutamine[282]

Dobutamine is a new synthetic derivative of isoproterenol with predominantly beta-receptor stimulating (inotropic and vasodilating) effects[251, 904] which proved useful in the treatment of heart failure[282]. Its alpha-receptor (vasoconstrictor) effect, even with large doses, is minimal. It is not surprising, therefore, that it has been found to be inferior to epinephrine and high-dose dopamine for promoting restoration of spontaneous circulation during cardiac arrest[109, 604]. In high doses it can produce ventricular tachycardia. Dobutamine may have certain advantages over isoproterenol, epinephrine and dopamine for increasing cardiac inotropic effects after cardiopulmonary bypass and therefore perhaps also after CPR and restoration of spontaneous circulation[839].

Dobutamine hydrochloride has been used by titrated i.v. infusion of 2.5–10 μg/kg per min (maximum 20 μg/kg per min) in refractory cardiogenic shock. High infusion rates can worsen myocardial ischemia[420]. It has been used in conjunction with reduction of afterload by nitroprusside. Claims of advantages of dobutamine over isoproterenol or low-dose dopamine are not convincing, although less tachycardia may occur with dobutamine.

Amrinone[420]

This is a new nonadrenergic cardiotonic agent with mechanisms of action still unclear. Its cardiovascular effects resemble those of dobutamine, including possible worsening of myocardial ischemia in large doses. It has been used with a 0.75 mg/kg i.v. bolus given slowly over several minutes followed by an infusion of 5–10 μg/kg per min.

Metaraminol[507]

Metaraminol (Aramine) has primarily alpha- and some beta-receptor stimulating action, but is less potent than epinephrine or norepinephrine. It exerts its effect by releasing catecholamine tissue stores and is thus ineffective in situations in which such tissue stores are depleted, such as under the influence of reserpine, guanethidine, chronic heart failure or cardiac arrest. Metaraminol does not usually cause tachycardia and is useful as a mild vasopressor even for prolonged administration. It has been given in individual i.v. boluses of 1–5 mg each and by titrated i.v. infusion of 100 mg in 250 ml (0.4 mg/ml).

Ephedrine[287]

This is the oldest natural sympathomimetic amine. It increases arterial pressure indirectly by causing a release of norepinephrine from tissue stores. In addition, it has a direct cardiac stimulating effect which does not depend on release of norepinephrine. Ephedrine produces not only vasoconstriction and tachycardia, but also CNS arousal. It is widely used in anesthesia for the treatment of hypotension due to spinal or epidural anesthesia, and in obstetrics. It is not recommended for prolonged use or in intermittent doses as its effect fades (tachyphylaxis). It is given in individual i.v. doses of 10–20 mg/70 kg. It is a potent bronchodilator and has been used in the past as an aerosol in asthma.

Isoproterenol[287]

Isoproterenol (Isuprel, isoprenaline) is a synthetic sympathomimetic amine with pure beta-receptor stimulant (cardiac inotropic and vasodilation) action. Because of its lack of peripheral vasoconstricting action, it does not increase arterial pressure and thereby does not enhance selectively cerebral and coronary perfusion during CPR Steps A–B–C. It thus does not by itself enhance restoration of spontaneous circulation[588, 652]; indeed, it dilates peripheral vessels and thereby decreases perfusion pressure. While isoproterenol exerts a potent chronotropic and inotropic effect on the heart, resulting in increased cardiac output, at the same time it increases myocardial oxygen requirements[919]. For these reasons, isoproterenol has no place during cardiac compressions, except in severe atropine-resistant bradycardia and heart block (Stokes–Adams syndrome), pending pacemaker insertion[838]. Even in these cases, however, epinephrine is preferred during CPR Steps A–B–C for restarting the heart.

In myocardial infarction with spontaneous circulation and in cardiogenic shock, isoproterenol may increase myocardial oxygen requirements, leading to extension of the infarction; it is thus less beneficial for decreasing afterload than pure peripheral vasodilators such as nitroglycerin. Isoproterenol may also induce life-threatening tachydysrhythmias. Isoproterenol, when administered for bradycardia in heart block, has been given as a solution of 1 mg in 500 ml (2 μg/ml). Titrated i.v. infusion rates are 0.02–0.2 μg/kg per min. The infusion is adjusted to keep the heart rate at about 60 beats per minute.

In status asthmaticus, isoproterenol has been given for its beta-receptor effect on bronchial smooth muscle (bronchodilator). As a last resort, an i.v. infusion of either isoproterenol[205] or epinephrine[394, 736c], 'pushed' to the point of tachycardia in an attempt to open the intrapulmonary airways, has sometimes helped open the airways and prevent cardiac arrest. This treatment in asthmatic crisis should be considered only after measures with less risk of inducing ventricular fibrillation have failed, i.e. IPPV with oxygen, metaproterenol (a beta-2 receptor stimulant less likely to produce tachyarrhythmias), aminophylline i.v., steroid i.v. and arterial pH normalization[394].

Atropine[287]

This is the classic parasympatholytic drug, which reduces vagal tone, enhances atrioventricular conduction, and—in spite of normally producing tachycardia—reduces the likelihood of ventricular fibrillation triggered by the myocardial hypoperfusion associated with extreme bradycardia. It may increase the heart rate not only in sinus bradycardia but also in high-degree atrioventricular block with bradycardia, but not in complete atrioventricular block, where isoproterenol is indicated. Atropine therefore has essentially no place during cardiac arrest and CPR Steps A–B–C, except possibly in refractory asystole[113]. During spontaneous circulation, however, when the heart rate decreases to less than about 50 beats per minute or when there is bradycardia with PVCs or hypotension, atropine is indicated.

Atropine should be given in doses adequate to increase the heart rate, namely 0.5 mg/70 kg i.v., repeated as needed up to a total dose of about 2 mg, which results in complete vagal blockade[603, 865]. In third-degree atrioventricular block, larger doses may be tried, although a beneficial effect is unlikely. Doses smaller than 0.5 mg/70 kg of atropine may lead to severe bradycardia[180]. This in the sick heart can trigger ventricular fibrillation; the heart rate is slowed, probably via a central vagal stimulus or a peripheral parasympathomimetic action.

In myocardial infarction or ischemia, tachycardia may increase myocardial oxygen demand and the extent of infarct and even lead to ventricular tachycardia or ventricular fibrillation[494, 514]. Thus, atropine should be used with caution in such cases. Atropine may be needed to counteract the bradycardia induced by morphine given for pain in acute myocardial infarction. Atropine is effective by intratracheal instillation.

Calcium[287]

This physiologically important cation is essential for excitation–contraction coupling in muscle. Because calcium increased myocardial contractility[669a], it was tried instead of epinephrine in the early years of CPR, but proved to be less effective in the restoration of spontaneous circulation, since it does not cause peripheral vasoconstriction[652, 657]. Calcium has been recommended for the treatment of electromechanical dissociation, when epinephrine has failed to restart spontaneous cardiac action. Calcium, however, can cause coronary spasm and also increases myocardial irritability. Moreover, excessive doses may cause the heart to stop in contraction, particularly in the fully digitalized patient. The usefulness of calcium in resuscitation is limited, and it may even be contraindicated[187], considering the myocardial and cerebral preservation effects of calcium entry blockers (see below) (Chapter 3). It may be more appropriate to use calcium than sympathomimetic amines in cardiac depression from certain drugs such as barbiturates and other anesthetic agents, but conclusive evidence is lacking. Calcium chloride failed to enhance resuscitability from ventricular fibrillation in dogs[657] and patients[327, 866, 867]. It seemed effective in only 10% of patients with idioventricular rhythm (heart block)[327]. Calcium may enhance digitalis toxicity. It is dangerous in the presence of low potassium. During CPR for pulselessness in heart block, the atropine–isoproterenol (epinephrine)–pacemaker sequence should be tried. For pulselessness with ECG complexes (electromechanical dissociation), an i.v. infusion of epinephrine and perhaps steroid[956]—rather than calcium—should be tried; in calcium entry blocker overdose i.v. calcium is indicated[952].

If, in spite of the foregoing, you decide to try calcium, the preferred salt is calcium chloride (10% solution), given in a dose of 2–4 mg/kg slowly i.v., and repeated if necessary at 10 minute intervals. Since 1 ml of the 10% solution (100 mg of salt) contains 1.36 mEq of ionized calcium, the 5 ml dose contains 6.8 mEq. Other compounds used include calcium gluconate 10%, 10 ml i.v. (4.8 mEq); and calcium gluceptate 10%, 5 ml i.v. (4.5 mEq). Calcium must not be given in the bicarbonate infusion, as the two react to form an insoluble precipitate of calcium carbonate.

Calcium entry blockers[246, 917]

The cerebral resuscitative potentials of calcium entry blockers will be considered in Chapter 3. In the setting of cardiac arrest, calcium entry blockers may have two *beneficial* effects: (1) preservation of the myocardium (protection by pretreatment)[103, 244, 245]; and (2) reduced vulnerability to ventricular fibrillation[665]. In clinical emergency cardiac care, verapamil (the only i.v. calcium entry blocker on the market at this time in the USA) has a clear beneficial effect on paroxysmal supraventricular tachycardias (PSVT), but may also produce hypotension and heart block and worsen congestive heart failure[810].

These agents may also have significant preventative potential[994] and as yet clinically unexplored therapeutic potentials in sudden cardiac death[152]. None, however, has yet been shown to be of benefit in the management of cardiac arrest. Their protective effect on myocardium as well as their vasodilatory effects vary widely from agent to agent[244, 245, 246, 322]. Diltiazem administered as a bolus with reperfusion does not preclude successful resuscitation in dogs, and improves hemodynamics and myocardial oxygen supply/demand relationships, but does not seem to improve outcome[532]. In the ischemic rat heart, reperfusion with lidoflazine seems to enhance functional recovery[636]. Significantly more clinical and laboratory investigation will be needed to clarify the role of calcium entry blockers in attempts to restore spontaneous circulation from cardiac arrest.

Extracellular–intracellular ion concentration gradient (normally 10 000 : 1) and calcium ion fluxes and distributions are crucial for the function of most tissues, particularly muscle cells and neurons[317]. During ischemia and after other types of tissue injury, excessive amounts of free calcium are released from the bound state and enter cells, and accumulate in cytoplasm and mitochondria. During reoxygenation, this is the cause of post-insult vasospasm, and it is suspected to be a trigger for post-insult lipid peroxidation and cell necroses (Chapter 3). Lipid peroxidation, in turn, can worsen hypoperfusion by the formation of vasospastic prostaglandins, platelet-aggregating thromboxane, and membrane-damaging leuko-trienes[246, 806, 918]. There is now substantiated hope that calcium entry blockers will be effective and safe agents for preventing or ameliorating post-insult hypoperfusion and post-insult necrotizing cascades, particularly in the heart and brain[778, 845, 911, 918]. The potential to ameliorate outcome with brain damage after global brain ischemia with calcium entry blocker given early after reperfusion was demonstrated for the first time with lidoflazine in a cardiac arrest dog model[911]; then came nimodipine in a monkey head ischemia model[845]. Except for uncontrolled feasibility trials with verapamil in patients[778], none of the other agents have been tested for cerebral outcome effects. All calcium entry blockers are cerebral vasodilators. Lidoflazine counteracts pathologic vasoconstriction and is less of an active vasodila-tor[916]. Flunarizine[957], lidoflazine[916], nimodipine[17, 845] and diltiazem[917] have been shown to ameliorate postischemic cerebral hypoperfusion.

The use of calcium entry blockers after cardiac arrest is attractive, but confused by the coexistence of multiple beneficial and hazardous cardiovas-cular effects. The *dangerous* effects[103, 917] include: dose-dependent slowing of the conduction system (AV block) with maximal effect being electromecha-nical dissociation and cardiac standstill, particularly with verapamil; vasodilation hypotension (particularly with nimodipine and nifedipine); myocardial negative inotropic effect (perhaps more with verapamil); and tachyarrhythmias in patients with atrial fibrillation (perhaps with lidofla-zine). Diltiazem, which gives side-effects between those of verapamil and nifedipine and apparently also causes hypotension and heart block in large doses, has not yet been studied for use in cardiac arrest.

Verapamil and nifedipine, the only calcium entry blockers on the market in i.v. form at this time, may be tried in patients, even early after cardiac arrest[778], but documentation of their ameliorating effects on cerebral and myocardial ischemia is not yet available. The author's international Brain Resuscitation Clinical Trial study group[3, 404] is conducting in 1984–88 a randomized clinical study of lidoflazine postcardiac arrest. The dose used is 1 mg/kg by continuous, slow, titrated i.v. infusion over more than 10 minutes. In dogs, the post-arrest dose tolerated was lidoflazine 1 mg/kg i.v.[911] Nifedipine[370] or nimodipine[845] were also given to animals, with a moderate hypotensive effect, by titrated infusion. The carefully titrated infusion must be stopped at the first sign of severe hypotension or dysrhythmias. Normotension must be maintained with plasma volume expansion plus small amounts of vasopressor. The calcium entry blocker-induced hypotension is reversible by norepinephrine, dopamine, epinephrine and calcium.

> *Caution*: Ca^{2+} entry blockers can help both prevent and cause life-threatening dysrhythmias and re-arrest early after CPR. If you use Ca^{2+} blocker for heart and brain (see Chapter 3), infuse it slowly, while monitoring pulse and ECG continuously and arterial pressure frequently. Reverse hypotension immediately by stopping Ca^{2+} blocker, giving i.v. fluid load (CVP or PAOP monitoring desirable), and titrate arterial pressure to normotension with dopamine or norepinephrine. If dopamine causes tachydysrhythmias, use norepinephrine. If life-threatening bradycardia occurs, try epinephrine by cautious i.v. infusion. Be prepared with defibrillator and pacemaker. Calcium chloride i.v. may also be useful in reversing hypotension due to calcium entry blockers.

Digitalis[287]

Digitalis preparations increase myocardial contractions, slow the heart rate, reduce AV conduction, and have limited value as inotropic agents in emergency cardiac care[285]. Other drugs are more potent cardiovascular stimulants and have a wider margin of safety and faster action. A variety of digitalis glycosides are the principal agents used for sustained positive inotropic effect (increase in the force of myocardial contraction) for the long-term support of patients in chronic heart failure—principally digoxin. Digitalis is also used to reduce the heart rate in atrial flutter and fibrillation, and in paroxysmal supraventricular tachycardia (PSVT). Digitalis toxicity, combined with potassium depletion (e.g. from diuretics), should also be considered as a possible etiology for intractable dysrhythmias and cardiac arrest in patients undergoing resuscitation. The cardiac symptoms of toxicity are severe bradycardia, ventricular extrasystoles, AV block, atrial fibrillation, and even ventricular tachycardia and fibrillation. The toxic-to-therapeutic dose ratio is narrow. For rapid digitalization, the recommended dose of digoxin is 20 μg/kg i.v., followed by 10 μg/kg 6 hours later, repeated at 12 hours to a total digitalizing dose of 40 μg/kg. For maintenance give 5 μg/kg per day i.v. or p.o. Check digitalis serum levels to keep at 1–2 ng/ml.

Corticosteroids[287]

These drugs may be used for their anti-inflammatory and anti-edema effects in the immediate post-resuscitative period, to ameliorate the reaction of the bronchi to aspiration, which is common in CPR cases. Their ability to reduce postischemic-hypoxic cerebral edema and necrosis has not been documented[398, 741, 956]. Their value in shock and noncardiogenic pulmonary edema is controversial. Suggested beneficial mechanisms by which corticosteroids may act in cardiac arrest include stabilization of lysosomal membranes, prevention of histamine release, vasodilation, and protection of capillary integrity. Postcardiac arrest methylprednisolone exerted some suggestive benefit for brain recovery in an acute rat model[398]. Steroids have not been (but should be) studied in a clinically relevant animal outcome model of cardiac arrest. In a controlled clinical study, early post-CPR steroid medication did not significantly affect survival or cerebral recovery[375b]. Risks associated with prolonged steroid medication, including reduced wound healing, reduced resistance to infection, stress ulcers, osteoporosis and adrenal cortical insufficiency, have not been proved to occur with short-term (3–7 day) use of pharmacologic doses of steroid, or with one massive dose. Large pharmacologic doses of corticosteroids have been recommended for cerebral edema, aspiration or status asthmaticus, i.e. methylprednisolone 1 mg/kg (or dexamethasone 0.2 mg/kg) i.v., repeated every 6 hours up to 48 hours, and then gradually tapered over 1–2 weeks. For septic shock, a single massive dose of methylprednisolone (5–30 mg/kg i.v.) is recommended.

Vasodilators[614]

Vasodilators have no place during CPR-ABC, when efforts must be directed at increasing diastolic arterial pressure. After restoration of spontaneous circulation, however, control of arterial normotension, important for cerebral recovery, and reduction of systemic vascular resistance to reduce myocardial oxygen demand, may require individualized titrated infusions of combinations of vasodilator and vasoconstrictor agents[537, 543]. Vasodilators reduce both arterial pressure (i.e. afterload) and venous return and central venous–right atrial–left atrial pressures (i.e. preload). If diastolic arterial pressure is sustained at the same time (important for coronary perfusion), the heart should benefit. Nitroprusside and nitroglycerin, both direct vasodilators, are popular in cardiac intensive care of conscious patients, but they may not be the agents of choice for the post-CPR state with coma, because they bring about cerebral vasodilation and increased intracranial pressure. The ganglionic blocker trimethaphan (Arfonad) seems a better choice for control of hypertension during coma.

Nitroprusside[614]

This rapidly acting potent peripheral vasodilating agent is very controllable because of its brief effect. It dilates arteries and veins directly. Although nitroprusside has no role during cardiac arrest and cardiac compressions, it has become a valuable adjunct for the reduction of peripheral vascular resistance and venodilation in protracted myocardial failure (to increase cardiac output) and for the control of hypertensive crises[608]. It does not affect cardiac rate and rhythm directly, although it may, through induction of hypotension, lead to reflex tachycardia. In hypertension and in myocardial ischemia with pump failure[211], even minimal reduction in peripheral arterial resistance by nitroprusside can sometimes bring cardiac output toward normal, enhance systolic emptying, relieve pulmonary congestion, decrease myocardial oxygen consumption, and preserve ischemic myocardium. It should be given by infusion pump or microdrip, in a concentration of 50 mg/250–1000 ml, with pressure monitoring by intra-arterial and possibly pulmonary artery catheters (the latter optional). The pulmonary artery wedge pressure should be maintained at or above 15 mmHg. The rapid and short action of nitroprusside calls for a carefully regulated infusion. One may start with 0.1 μg/kg per min. The dose range is 0.5–10 μg/kg per min with an average dose below 3 μg/kg per min. The solution must be wrapped in aluminium foil, since the drug deteriorates with exposure to light. The total dose should not exceed 100 mg/h (single dose, 1.5 mg/kg), lest cyanide intoxication with tissue hypoxia and acidemia develop. The arterial pH should be monitored. Side-effects include hypotension, reflex tachycardia and tachyphylaxis. In the comatose patient, trimethaphan (Arfonad) is less likely to cause cerebral congestion.

Nitroglycerin[373, 523, 614]

This classic direct vasodilator, used for relief of angina pain, is now being used also for the reduction of preload and afterload by peripheral venous and (to a lesser degree) arterial dilation, and for internal phlebotomy—in protracted cardiac failure—as an alternative to nitroprusside. Nitroglycerin also dilates coronary vessels[664] and is beneficial in heart failure due to myocardial infarction[281]. The suggested i.v. solution is 50 mg/250 ml. For the acute relief of angina pain, one nitroglycerin tablet of 0.3–0.4 mg administered sublingually, repeated up to three times at 5 minute intervals, has been recommended. The effect peaks at 5 minutes and lasts 30 minutes. Nitroglycerin tablets have also been administered sublingually in the emergency prehospital situation in the treatment of acute pulmonary edema, a condition in which titrated infusions are not always feasible. Nitroglycerin has no role during cardiac compressions. Again, trimethaphan is preferred immediately post-CPR when the patient is comatose.

Propranolol[23c]

Propranolol (Inderal) is a beta-adrenergic receptor blocking drug that decreases automaticity, conduction and contractility of the heart. It has no place in emergency resuscitation during cardiac compressions because it may make the heart unresuscitable. Its principal use is in the patient with a spontaneous circulation accompanied by recurrent PVCs, or atrial tachy-dysrhythmias, particularly when these dysrhythmias are triggered by pheochromocytoma, thyrotoxicosis, or excessive amounts of beta-receptor stimulating drugs. Ventricular tachycardia and fibrillation may occasionally respond to a beta-blocker[29]. Beta-receptor blockers are hazardous when myocardial contractility is depressed (as is the case after cardiac arrest) and are contraindicated in asthmatics. Propranolol hydrochloride is used in a bolus of up to 1 mg/70 kg i.v. every 5 minutes, to a maximal total dose of 7 mg/70 kg. A test dose of 0.1–0.3 mg/70 kg i.v. has been recommended to avoid dangerous hypotension or bradycardia.

Narcotic analgesics[248]

These agents are not indicated during and immediately following CPR. *Morphine* sulfate is the preferred analgesic for myocardial infarction pain. It is also one of several adjunctive drugs indicated in acute pulmonary edema, which may occur before or after cardiac arrest. Morphine seems to act by dilating capacitance vessels, producing a 'bloodless (pharmacologic) phle-botomy', as well as reducing left ventricular afterload[13, 986]. It may also improve pulmonary edema by relieving anxiety and depressing exaggerated breathing movements. It sometimes has a vagomimetic effect and thus is better avoided in bradycardia or AV block[513]. The drug is best titrated i.v. by repeated individual doses of 2–5 mg/70 kg every 5–30 minutes, until the desired effect is reached. If morphine induces nausea or hypotension, a different analgesic is preferred.

Meperidine (Demerol, pethidine) may also produce hypotension, particu-larly in the presence of hypovolemia and change of posture. Meperidine may slightly depress myocardial contractility[257] (morphine does not), but has an atropine-like effect (morphine is vagomimetic). Meperidine is given by titrated intermittent i.v. doses of 10–20 mg/70 kg every 5–30 minutes. *Fentanyl* (Sublimaze) is shorter acting and less likely to produce hypoten-sion, but more likely to produce breath holding, chest wall spasm and apnea; it is an excellent agent for balanced anesthesia with controlled ventilation, but dangerous in the spontaneously breathing unattended patient. Fentanyl should be used only by personnel experienced with and prepared for tracheal intubation and resuscitation. Because of the ability of fentanyl to produce apnea and asphyxia even with doses which do not induce unresponsiveness, morphine or meperidine is preferred for analgesia in the conscious, non-intubated, patient.

With any narcotic, titrated administration must guard against hypotension and respiratory depression. Narcotics are contraindicated in spontaneously breathing patients with post-anoxic central nervous system depression. In the presence of controlled ventilation, however, any narcotic may be used liberally for analgesia and comfort of the intubated patient. With ventilation and blood pressure controlled, narcotics per se exert no deleterious effects on the brain. In some countries (e.g. Great Britain), *heroin* is available and then becomes the drug of choice for maximal analgesia and euphoria; its dose is 50% that of morphine.

Diuretics[287]

Furosemide (Lasix) (0.5–2 mg/kg i.v.) and ethacrynic acid (Edecrin) (0.5–1 mg/kg i.v.) inhibit the reabsorption of sodium in the loop of Henle. Furosemide has an additional venodilating effect in pulmonary edema[197], and a transient vasoconstrictive effect in chronic heart failure. Diuresis starts within 30 minutes after i.v. administration, peaks at about one-half hour, and lasts for several hours. The diuretic action of these drugs is indicated in pulmonary edema. Furosemide and ethacrynic acid may also reduce intracranial hypertension caused by post-anoxic or post-traumatic cerebral edema, partly because of a reduction in CSF production and increase in CSF clearance; and therefore in the post-arrest period at least one dose is usually indicated, provided normovolemia has been established.

Barbiturates[3, 90, 106, 209, 495, 613]

The barbiturates have been in use throughout the 20th century as sedatives, hypnotics, and anesthetics—primarily because of their CNS depressant effect. Anesthesia is primarily accomplished with larger doses of ultra short-acting agents such as thiopental, particularly as an adjunct of nitrous oxide. There are barbiturates with slow onset and long duration of action (e.g. barbital, phenobarbital); with intermediate speed of onset and duration of action (e.g. secobarbital, pentobarbital); with rapid and short action (e.g. thiopental, thioamylal); and with ultra rapid and ultra short action (e.g. methohexital). These drugs depress, in a dose-dependent fashion, consciousness, breathing, metabolism, and blood pressure. Hypotension is the net result of the direct depression of myocardial contractility and brain stem depression; peripheral vascular tone is first increased, but large doses lead to vasoparalysis.

For barbiturates in brain resuscitation, see Chapter 3. For CPCR cases, after restoration of normotension, the i.v. titration of thiopental (Pentothal) or pentobarbital (Nembutal) is effective in controlling convulsions and restlessness. Safety is provided by controlled ventilation and blood pressure support as needed. A reasonably safe anesthesia induction dose for the normovolemic person with a healthy cardiovascular system is about 3 mg/kg i.v., to be followed by increments of 0.5–1 mg/kg titrated according to response. When thiopental or pentobarbital is used for the prevention or control of seizures, or for specific cerebral resuscitation after ischemic–anoxic insults, or for ICP control, one can usually achieve instantaneous silencing or burst suppression of the EEG with 3–5 mg/kg i.v.. Subsequent doses can be titrated to achieve sustained EEG depression. This usually requires a thiopental or pentobarbital blood level of 3–4 μg/ml. For the emergency treatment of convulsions, barbiturates are being gradually replaced by diazepam, which exerts less cardiovascular depressant effects.

Another resuscitation consideration of barbiturates is the resuscitative treatment of patients poisoned with these drugs—for suicide, accidentally, or by drug abusers. There is no certain 'lethal dose' of barbiturates. As little as 1 g of a barbiturate by mouth has killed fragile elderly persons, who under CNS depression developed upper airway obstruction when the neck was flexed. On the other end of the spectrum, as much as 30 g of a barbiturate taken by mouth has been survived without permanent damage, if the person was found before the onset of apnea and was ventilated and had his blood pressure supported until recovery. The treatment of choice of barbiturate intoxication is general intensive care life support with controlled ventilation, and support of plasma volume and perfusion pressure. This applies to poisoning by any CNS depressant. CNS stimulants without life support have increased mortality; CNS stimulants in addition to life support have not further reduced mortality. In severe acute barbiturate intoxication under controlled ventilation, cardiovascular collapse is the main problem. Hypovolemia must be corrected and a vasopressor used as needed.

Diazepam (Valium)[287]

The benzodiazepines are CNS depressants, causing sedation, hypnosis, anti-convulsant activity and some degree of muscle relaxation—with only large doses causing hypotension or apnea. Diazepam probably works via inhibition of the CNS mediated by gamma-aminobutyric acid (GABA). Its use in resuscitation is mainly for the prevention or control of seizures. It seems to have a wider margin of safety than barbiturates. Diazepam is given by slow i.v. injection in individual doses of about 0.1 mg/kg. Cardiovascular and respiratory depression may occur.

Phenytoin (Diphenylhydantoin, Dilantin)[287]

This is the drug of choice for the long-term treatment of seizure disorders. Phenytoin decreases membrane ion fluxes, similar to local anesthetics, and thereby stabilizes excitable membranes. Although phenytoin is used effectively in titrated fashion for convulsions and cardiac arrhythmias, its i.v. administration in excessive doses can cause cardiac arrhythmias, hypotension and CNS depression. In resuscitation, major generalized convulsions are best controlled initially by thiopental or diazepam i.v. in titrated doses (see above), which is then followed up for long-term suppression of seizures by phenytoin in doses of approximately 5–7 mg/kg per 24 h via i.v. infusion. For i.v. administration of phenytoin boluses the recommendation is not to exceed 1 mg/kg per min. Control of seizures is usually achieved with phenytoin plasma concentrations of 10 μg/ml. Preventive treatment of seizures is often successfully accomplished by phenobarbital or phenytoin or a combination of the two. Due to its membrane stabilizing effect, phenytoin may also have a resuscitation effect post-ischemia on cerebral neurons (see Chapter 3).

Muscle relaxants[209, 247, 287]

Blocking the neuromuscular junctions of patients under resuscitation conditions, with the use of curare or curare-like agents, may be required for rapid tracheal intubation, for the emergency treatment of seizures (in conjunction with a barbiturate or diazepam), or for 'softening' the muscles of patients who are struggling under prolonged controlled ventilation. d-Tubocurarine, gallamine, and pancuronium are relaxants that act by combining with acetylcholine receptors, without activating them (nondepolarizing, competitive relaxants). In contrast, succinylcholine, the most rapidly acting relaxant, and decamethonium (no longer used clinically) exert the same action at the neuromuscular junction as acetylcholine, i.e. by exciting through depolarization of the membrane of the end plate; this causes uncoordinated muscle contractions that are followed by a relaxed refractory period, which is the desired relaxant effect (depolarizing, noncompetitive relaxants). With increased repetitive doses, however, this first depolarizing block is followed by a second competitive-type block.

For emergency endotracheal intubation (see Chapter 1) the most rapidly acting muscle relaxant, succinylcholine, is used in doses of about 1–2 mg/kg i.v. This causes apnea and relaxation of all muscles, including those of pharynx and larynx, within about 1 minute of i.v. injection. This must be accompanied by controlled hyperventilation, preferably with O_2. The required intubation or other procedure must be performed with skillful timing. The fasciculations caused initially by succinylcholine i.v. can be prevented with the preliminary use of a small non-paralyzing dose of tubocurarine i.v. (3 mg/70 kg). Intubation and other uses of muscle relaxants must be by personnel experienced in anesthesia management, including controlled ventilation even without endotracheal tube.

The pharmacologic paralysis induced by these neuromuscular blocking agents can be a life-saving measure. It can also readily kill in the hands of the inexperienced operator. For the long-term suppression of restlessness, coughing on the ventilator, reacting on the endotracheal tube, etc., we favor sedation plus the use of softening doses of a long-acting relaxant given in titrated i.v. doses (e.g., pancuronium, approximately 0.05–0.1 mg/kg). The circulatory side-effects (in the presence of optimal ventilation and oxygenation) are minimal with the use of succinylcholine. d-Tubocurarine tends to cause hypotension, from ganglionic blockade and occasional histamine-like action. Gallamine can cause tachycardia, and pancuronium can cause hypertension and tachycardia which may be avoided by using the newer agents atracurium or vecuronium. The presently favored agent for emergency resuscitation is succinylcholine and for long-term 'softening' (immobilization), to facilitate life support, is pancuronium. Acquisition of knowledge, skills and judgment in the use of these risky agents must be under the direction of an experienced anesthesiologist.

Miscellaneous drugs[144, 287, 373a, 606a, 613a]

The physician should be familiar with the pharmacologic actions of the aforementioned drugs and, in addition, those listed for inclusion in the emergency kit.

Note: Administration of drugs in resuscitation and intensive care must be by *titration*. Titrated drug administration is best by *infusion pumps*, checked for accuracy. This is particularly important for vasoactive drugs. For independent controls of i.v. infusions of multiple drugs and fluids, we recommend a 'piggyback' infusion from each pump separately, into one or more continuously running infusions of drug-free fluid, close to the vein, to minimize dead space delays in drug effects. Using stopcocks between solutions would permit only infusion of one *or* the other drug or fluid into one venous line.

Physician's emergency drug kit

1. Epinephrine (adrenalin)
2. Sodium bicarbonate
3. Vasopressors
    (a) Phenylephrine
    (b) Metaraminol
    (c) Norepinephrine
4. Inotropic agents
    (a) Dopamine
    (b) Dobutamine
    (c) Isoproterenol
    (d) Calcium chloride
5. Calcium entry blockers
    (a) Verapamil or Diltiazem
    (b) Nifedipine or Nimodipine
    (c) Lidoflazine
6. Lidocaine; procainamide; bretylium
7. Propranolol
8. Atropine
9. Nitroprusside for i.v. infusion (shielded)
    Nitroglycerin for i.v. infusion
    Nitroglycerin sublingual tablets
10. Morphine or meperidine (Demerol, pethidine)
11. Furosemide or ethacrynic acid
12. Methylprednisolone or dexamethasone
13. 50% dextrose (for empiric use in coma of unknown etiology)
14. Bronchodilators
    (a) Aminophylline for i.v. infusion
    (b) Metaproterenol for aerosol (a beta-2 receptor stimulator)
15. Diphenhydramine (Benadryl) or pyribenzamine (antihistaminics)
16. Naloxone (Narcan) (narcotic antagonist)
17. Barbiturate, short-acting (pentobarbital) or ultra-short-acting (thiopental)
18. Diazepam (Valium); diphenylhydantoin (phenytoin) (anticonvulsants)
19. Chlorpromazine (thorazine) (vasodilator; for psychiatric emergencies)
20. Muscle relaxants: succinylcholine (Anectine, suxamethonium) and pancuronium (Pavulon) (to be administered only by those trained in anesthesia and experienced in their use, as they produce apnea)
21. Mannitol for i.v. infusion
22. i.v. fluids (see below)—a crystalloid; a colloid

Comment: In using drugs for emergency resuscitation, familiarity with the particular agent, and therefore its skilful use, is more important than small differences in pharmacologic action between similarly acting agents. Not every 'new' drug gives better results.

Fluids

Infusion strategies and hypovolemia[22b, 163, 796, 799, 944]

During emergency resuscitation and post-resuscitative life support, i.v. fluids should be administered with the following objectives in mind:

1. To keep an i.v. route open for drug and fluid administration.
2. To restore normal circulating blood volume immediately after fluid losses, using combinations of electrolytes, colloid and red blood cell containing solutions (see below). Rapid, massive infusion of an isotonic or hypertonic salt or colloid solution can be life-saving, particularly in cases of severe rapid external or internal blood loss.
3. To expand normal circulating blood volume *after* cardiac arrest (e.g. by about 10% of estimated blood volume, 10 ml/kg) in order to reverse the relative loss of blood volume brought about by vasodilation, venous pooling and capillary leakage. During normovolemic cardiac arrest and CPR, however, volume loading can increase right atrial pressure and reduce organ blood flow produced by CPR[199].
4. To help reverse hypotension in acute myocardial infarction with continuous fluid volume loading with CVP and/or PAOP guidance[645].
5. To provide basic hydration and glucose requirements. This may be accomplished by a continuous infusion of 5% dextrose in 0.25–0.5% sodium chloride, 100 ml/kg per 24 hours for each of the first 10 kg of body weight (BW), 50 ml/kg per 24 hours for each of the second 10 kg BW, and 20 ml/kg per 24 hours for each remaining kg over 20 kg. 5% dextrose in water should not be used, as it may augment cerebral edema.
6. To adjust the above therapy for increased or decreased diuresis as soon as possible, keeping urine flow over 0.5 ml/kg per h.
7. To modify i.v. fluids for optimal blood composition in terms of normal electrolyte concentrations, osmolality and colloid osmotic pressure; serum albumin (3–5 g/dl); hematocrit (30–40%); and serum glucose (100–300 mg/dl).
8. To meet special requirements, such as osmotherapy in the early post-arrest period (see Chapter 3) and artificial alimentation (dextrose, amino acids, vitamins) in the late post-arrest period.

In hypovolemic shock without cardiac arrest or in the post-cardiac arrest period, monitoring of arterial pressure, urine flow and pulmonary artery wedge pressure is needed for guiding volume replacement. The heart rate is also an indicator of the adequacy of circulating blood volume, but less reliable. In addition, ECG and arterial blood gases should be monitored when feasible. Overinfusion can be detected from pulmonary rales or rhonchi, a sustained rise in PAOP, or a decrease in arterial PO_2 with unchanged FIO_2 of 50% or 100% (indicating shunting).

For the rapid administration of large amounts of i.v. fluids, a short large-bore cannula and pressure infusion equipment are needed. Doubling the height of the infusion bottle doubles the flow rate, but doubling the internal diameter of the venous cannula increases the flow rate by 16 times. Where glass bottles requiring pressure transfusion by air pressure are still in use, one person must be assigned to guard the pressure infusion continuously to prevent massive venous air embolism. Infusion bags from which embolism risk-free pressure infusion is possible by wrap-around inflatable blood pressure or blood bag cuff are recommended. Long-lasting difficult continuous large vessel hemorrhage (as after major visceral or cardiovascular trauma or liver transplant operations) calls for protracted massive infusions at rates of several liters per minute, which is possible from an emergency cardiopulmonary bypass apparatus or a roller pump infusor-heater with a multi-liter infusion capacity, embolism alarm, and 3–5 mm venous cannula[769]. For the transfusion of banked blood or blood cells, micropore filters are recommended, as well as a blood warmer; massive infusion of cold blood can cause cardiac hypothermic arrest[96]. In exsanguination, arterial pressure infusion can restore perfusion pressure slightly faster and with less volume than venous infusion, but considering the time and risks of vascular cannulation most studies suggest no significant advantage of arterial over venous transfusion[410, 578].

The amount and rate of i.v. infusion depend on the amount and rate of estimated blood volume loss and the type of fluid selected. Circulating blood volume (plasma plus red cell volume) normally accounts for 7–8% of body weight (the figure 10% is used to simplify calculations). In a fit 70 kg person, acute loss of up to about 10% of blood volume (up to 750 ml) is mild hemorrhage and requires merely an electrolyte solution. Loss of about 10–20% of blood volume (750–1500 ml) is moderate hemorrhage, which in most cases results in a picture of shock (pulse > 100, decreased pulse pressure, positive capillary blanch, tachypnea, decreased urine flow, restlessness). Loss of 20–50% of blood volume (1500–2000 ml) is severe hemorrhage, which always results in severe shock, which can progress to secondary cardiac arrest (death) if untreated. Finally, loss of 40–50% of blood volume within 10–20 minutes leads to rapid exsanguination cardiac arrest[22b, 410, 578].

Extracellular fluid volume is normally about 25% of body weight in liters. It includes the intravascular space, i.e. plasma volume (5% of body weight), and the interstitial space (20% of body weight). Electrolyte solutions (isotonic saline, Ringer's solution)[669a] distribute throughout the entire extracellular fluid space—both intravascular and interstitial—and therefore electrolyte solutions should first be given in four times the quantity of blood volume lost. It is apparent that, if moderate to severe blood loss is corrected by electrolyte solutions only, the creation of tissue edema is inevitable. Colloid solutions (blood, plasma, albumin, dextran, gelatin, starch), however, remain longer in the intravascular space (unless there is gross membrane leakage, as after very severe ischemic anoxia) and should therefore be given first in volumes equal to the blood volume lost.

When a *shock state* persists after replacement of estimated blood loss, after cardiac arrest without blood loss, or even following acute myocardial infarction, the hemodynamic state can benefit from incremental blood volume expansion with continuous monitoring of arterial pressure and CVP and/or PAOP. The latter is an important guide for fluid resuscitation in cases of left ventricular failure or shock lung. In the average adult, about 200 ml of electrolyte or colloid solution should be given rapidly i.v. and repeated every 10 minutes until the transiently increased CVP or PAOP does not return to normal, but rather remains higher than 3 mmHg above the previous value[800].

When hemorrhage is being treated concurrently to prevent development of a shock state, moderate deliberate normovolemic *hemodilution* with plasma substitutes is a safe and sound practice in most previously healthy individuals. Hemodilution reduces blood viscosity and thereby improves blood flow and oxygen delivery to tissues, despite the reduced arterial oxygen content, at least down to a hematocrit of about 25%[110, 531, 880]. The previously healthy organism can compensate with increased cardiac output for acute normovolemic anemia to a hematocrit of 25%; it can even survive a reduction in hematocrit to 10%, although with temporary decompensation[880]. The end point of useful hemodilution (uncompensated acute anemia) may, however, be above a 25% hematocrit in patients with cardiopulmonary disease. In any patient, this end-point can be recognized by monitoring several parameters. Blood base deficit will increase due to anaerobiosis and increased lactic acid; furthermore, when the point of excessive hemodilution is reached, mixed venous PO_2 (normal volume 40 mmHg) decreases when oxygen transport does not keep up with oxygen demand. During hemodilution an FIO_2 of 100% is desirable, as an arterial PO_2 of 600 mmHg can add 1.5 ml of oxygen (0.34 ml of oxygen per 100 mmHg PO_2) to 100 ml of blood, which might be significant in severe shock or anemia.

Choice of intravenous fluids[796, 945]

The choice of optimal intravenous fluid for resuscitation remains controversial. Nonetheless, it is clear that replacing all blood loss with blood is neither sound nor necessary[9, 89, 110, 253, 531, 796, 880, 892]. Banked blood can transmit hepatitis and acute immune deficiency syndrome (AIDS), and can cause hemolytic reaction as a result of incompatibility, although modern blood banking techniques minimize these risks. Moreover, typing and cross-matching delays availability of blood. Fresh, type-specific cross-matched whole blood would be ideal, but often is not immediately available and is expensive. Stored, banked blood is also expensive, and entails additional risks, particularly in massive transfusions[96, 361]. These risks include hypothermia (cold blood leading to cardiac arrest), deficiency of clotting factors, high potassium ion concentration, low pH and microemboli. In general, safe blood and blood product services are expensive and may not be available in all regions of the world. Thus, the first line of therapy in blood loss and for blood volume expansion is i.v. infusion of a plasma substitute without red blood cells.

Electrolyte solutions alone, such as isotonic sodium chloride (0.9%) or Ringer's solution[669a], are adequate to maintain blood volume and homeostasis in moderate hemorrhage not exceeding 20% of blood volume. As noted, an electrolyte solution should be given in up to four times the blood volume lost, as it equilibrates thoughout the extracellular (intravascular plus interstitial) space. More must be added to compensate for urine loss. Thus, the plasma volume supporting efficacy in severe blood loss of salt solutions is either brief or depends on the creation of interstitial edema before intravascular volume can be maintained. Although pulmonary edema is rapidly cleared, particularly during IPPV-CPPV, some studies suggest that the use of salt solutions in favor of colloid contributes to pulmonary edema and consolidation after traumatic shock. Lactated Ringer's solution and balanced salt solutions with normal pH (e.g. Normosol) are theoretically more physiologic than 0.9% sodium chloride solution, which is acid. The latter, however, is cheaper and equally effective in treating moderate extracellular fluid loss.

Hypertonic sodium chloride solution (4–6%) attracts interstitial fluid into the intravascular space. It is under investigation for emergency treatment of hypovolemia under field conditions. Small volumes (e.g. 250 ml doses) were effective in animal experiments in preventing cardiac arrest from an otherwise lethal hemorrhage[508a]; the volume effect is brief, unless 4–6% saline is combined with a colloid such as Dextran. This might help in keeping the injured alive until he can receive full fluid resuscitation and be transported to a surgical facility. The possible risks of hypertonic saline (e.g. effects on blood cells and endothelium) remain to be investigated.

In *severe hemorrhage* which is ongoing, whole blood should be used whenever possible—as fresh as possible, warmed, and type O Rhesus negative if there is no time to obtain type-specific blood. When over 30% of blood volume is lost and bleeding controlled, use of electrolyte solutions should be brief as tissue edema is produced if enough is given to maintain plasma volume. Indeed, salt solutions alone under such circumstances may be incapable of maintaining blood volume, cardiac output, arterial pressure and tissue oxygenation, even in 2–4 times replacement volumes; while *colloid plasma substitutes* in 1:1 replacement of volume lost are effective[110, 880, 892]. The choice of a specific colloid solution is controversial. The normal colloid osmotic pressure of 25 mmHg is maintained primarily by a serum albumin concentration of 5 g/dl. A reduction of serum albumin concentration to half normal reduces colloid osmotic pressure by two-thirds, at which level tissue edema tends to develop.

Human serum *albumin* 5% in isotonic saline, or commercial plasma *protein fractions* (e.g. Plasmanate), which contain mainly albumin plus a small amount of globulins, are sterile and safe. They are ideal colloid plasma substitutes. However, they are very expensive and often unnecessary, since serum albumin and globulin levels are fairly rapidly restored from body pools. Therefore, *dextrans, gelatin, starch* solutions, or other adequately tested synthetic colloids are also recommended. These products are inexpensive and suitable for long-term storage, and they support survival as well as albumin and better than salt solutions[796, 880, 945]. Dextran 70, 6% in isotonic saline, has a 30% intravascular retention after 24 hours; Dextran 40, 10% in isotonic saline, has a shorter retention time, but reduces sedimentation rate and may have a more potent antisludging effect[182, 269]. Dextran 40 should, however, be given only after urine flow has been restarted with electrolyte solution, since it tends to plug renal tubules. Hydroxyethyl starch, 6% in isotonic saline, has characteristics similar to Dextran 70. It should be noted that all plasma substitutes and electrolyte and colloid solutions produce hypocoagulability by diluting the clotting factors. Dextrans and starches (particularly Dextran 40), in addition, coat platelets, thus adding further to the anticoagulant effect. This is good for the microcirculation and bad in cases of trauma with incomplete hemostasis. Although synthetic colloids have caused anaphylactic reactions, such reactions are rare and unimportant for emergency resuscitation. For dextrans, haptenes are available for optional prevention of allergic reactions. Synthetic colloids may interfere with typing and cross-matching of blood (therefore, draw blood first), unless a cell washing laboratory technique is used. Hypertonic *glucose* in shock states[525], in the light of negative cerebral data[806], needs re-evaluation.

Plasma pooled from multiple donors may transmit hepatitis. Pasteurized plasma preparations (e.g. 5% plasma protein fraction) are safe, except when occasionally found to contain vasodilator substances. Fresh frozen plasma or cryoprecipitate is indicated in certain hemorrhagic diatheses.

Banked blood or packed red blood cells should be used to sustain the hematocrit at or above 30%. In the absence of hematocrit determinations, whole blood or red cells (if available) should be added to plasma substitutes, when estimated blood loss reaches and exceeds 30% of blood volume, or if the patient was anemic prior to hemorrhage. The preservative-anticoagulant citric acid–phosphate–dextrose (CPD) has replaced citric acid–citrate–dextrose (ACD).

During massive infusions of banked blood or red cells, calcium administration is usually not needed, but blood should be warmed to near body temperature on the way into the patient. Sodium bicarbonate should be given to correct measured base deficit. To prevent coagulation problems, the addition of fresh frozen plasma (250 ml/70 kg for every 1500 ml/70 kg of stored blood infused) has been suggested.

Packed red blood cell solutions, because of their high hematocrit, need dilution with isotonic saline solution added to the bag to enhance flow rate in the infusion for hemorrhage. Undiluted packed red cells are recommended in anemia associated with heart failure or hypertension.

The physician charged with responsibility for resuscitation should be familiar with coagulation problems caused by protracted shock states and massive blood transfusions. He should be conversant with simple clotting tests available for bedside use (e.g. clotting time at 37°C in glass tube, clot retraction, and clot lysis), and with the indications for certain blood components and heparin. Such therapies are beyond the scope of this chapter.

Oxygen-carrying blood substitutes, such as *stroma-free hemoglobin*[20, 52, 192] and *fluorocarbons*[272, 572, 816], have been under laboratory and clinical investigation in recent years. In 1987, neither stroma-free hemoglobin nor Fluosol appears ready for widespread clinical use, as available preparations have not yet been perfected. Improvements may influence the treatment of massive blood loss in the future. Stroma-free hemoglobin is rapidly lost from the circulation and causes pulmonary hypertension and other side-effects attributed to the impurity of the hemoglobin preparation. A polymerized version (Biotest) showed good retention, blood pressure support and oxygen-carrying capability in a hemorrhagic shock monkey model[52]. Stroma-free hemoglobin is more promising than fluorocarbons, which have no advantage over plasma substitutes in subjects breathing air. The fluorocarbon solution Fluosol DA 20%, which has been under clinical trials, requires 100% oxygen breathing and carries less oxygen (8 ml O_2/dl Fluosol at PO_2 600 mmHg) than hemoglobin (20 ml O_2/dl blood at PO_2 100 mmHg with 15 g hemoglobin). Fluosol, however, carries more oxygen than plasma substitutes (0.3 ml O_2/dl per 100 mmHg O_2). The latter, however, promote blood flow better by having lower viscosity. Fluorocarbons may have carcinogenic effects on tissues in which they are stored long-term.

Oral fluid therapy[126]

Emergency resuscitation for hypovolemic shock is required not only in cases of trauma, hemorrhage and burns, but also in cases of severe diarrhea (e.g. cholera). In the out-of-hospital treatment of mass outbreaks of diarrheal disease or of traumatic shock in conscious victims of mass disasters, when i.v. fluid administration is not possible, oral fluids have a place in the treatment of mild to moderate hypovolemic shock. Commercially available oral replacement powders, when diluted as recommended, yield isotonic or one-half isotonic Ringer's solution plus carbohydrates (e.g. 5% dextrose), vitamins, amino acids and flavoring to give them an acceptable taste. The Red Cross recommends adding 1 teaspoon of sodium bicarbonate to each liter of water to be taken by mouth. Fluids should not be given by mouth when the patient is stuporous or comatose—because of the risk of aspiration—or when an operation may be needed.

Conclusion

The most appropriate sequence of choices in treating plasma (blood) volume loss is usually (lactated) Ringer's solution (3–4 × blood volume lost), followed by a colloid plasma substitute (1 × additional blood volume lost), followed by packed red blood cells or whole blood to restore hematocrit to about 30%. Hemorrhagic diatheses are best treated with fresh frozen plasma and fresh whole blood.

Chapter 2E

Step E: Electrocardiographic Diagnosis (Recognition and Treatment of Dysrhythmias)

Techniques of Electrocardiography[23c, 102, 215]

As soon as possible after the start of CPR-ABC, the electrocardiographic (ECG) pattern should be determined, primarily to differentiate between: (1) ventricular fibrillation (or ventricular tachycardia without pulse); (2) electric asystole; and (3) pulselessness (mechanical asystole) with bizarre ECG complexes, also called electromechanical dissociation (Fig. 42). These are the three most common patterns associated with the clinical picture of cardiac arrest (pulselessness of carotid and femoral arteries). Epinephrine is indicated in all three conditions. Sodium bicarbonate is indicated in suspected or proven metabolic acidemia (base deficit) (Fig. 40). In addition, ventricular fibrillation and ventricular tachycardia call for immediate electric countershock, the only reliable means of defibrillation.

The ECG is not an indicator of circulation. Even normal ECG complexes can continue for many minutes in the presence of mechanical asystole, particularly in exsanguination or asphyxial cardiac arrest. Thus, during resuscitation, monitoring of the ECG is important, but only adjunctive to palpation of the carotid, femoral and peripheral pulses; monitoring arterial pressure (by Riva-Rocci cuff technique and, as feasible, via arterial catheter); and examining skin and mucous membranes for color, temperature and capillary refill. In the patient with endotracheal tube in place, an esophageal stethoscope is also recommended, as it is the simplest, cheapest and most reliable device for monitoring breathing and circulation. It permits hearing each heart beat and assessing the strength of cardiac contractions, and also enables clear audition of breath sounds, which gives a clue about tidal volume, bronchospasm and secretions. The esophageal stethoscope is not recommended for use during cardiac compressions. Ideally an endotracheal tube should be inserted first, the gastric tube next, and the esophageal stethoscope last.

The *techniques* for ECG pattern display during emergency resuscitation have been greatly simplified by the fact that modern defibrillator paddles incorporate the ECG pick-up electrodes (Figs. 49 and 50). This permits instantaneous recognition of ventricular tachycardia or ventricular fibrillation and immediate countershock therapy.

178

During CPR, ECG monitoring should be initiated as soon as possible with a method that does not hamper cardiac compressions and artificial ventilation. This is best done by the application of the electrodes to the extremities. For Lead II, one electrode is usually placed on the right arm, another on the left leg, and an indifferent electrode on the left arm.

Long-term ECG monitoring—in emergency cardiac care of patients with spontaneous circulation and during Phase III of CPR—calls for replacement of the extremity electrodes to the chest, so that they do not limit limb motion (e.g. right and left shoulder or upper chest wall, left lower chest wall). They should not interfere with periodic 12-lead ECGs, which might be needed later to diagnose myocardial ischemia. For modified V5 by chest electrode, place the negative electrode just below the left clavicle. For modified lead V1, which is the best lead for distinguishing between right and left ventricular ectopic activity as well as for detecting and recording atrial activity, place the positive electrode over the right fifth intercostal space and the negative electrode over the left shoulder (outer third of the left clavicle); the ground electrode is usually most comfortably attached near the right shoulder (outer right of the right clavicle).

Technique of ECG monitoring during CPR

1. Establish an airway; begin artificial ventilation and external cardiac compressions.
2. Apply quick-look defibrillation paddles to the patient's chest for rapid ECG diagnosis. If ventricular tachycardia or coarse ventricular fibrillation is seen, give immediate countershock. (Cardiac compressions must be interrupted for a few seconds to permit accurate diagnosis.)
3. As soon as possible, apply stick-on electrodes to the patient's extremities. Lead II: right arm (negative); left leg (positive); left arm (ground). Polarity is desirable for exact ECG but not needed for detecting VF or for defibrillating.
4. After restoration of spontaneous circulation, when perfusion is stable, switch from extremity electrodes to stick-on chest electrodes. Modified lead V5: right clavicle (negative); left fifth interspace (cardiac apex) (positive); left clavicle (ground).
5. Modified lead V1 (mcL1): left clavicle (negative); right fourth interspace (positive); right clavicle (ground). Lead V1 is preferred for recognition of PVCs.

The radio-transmission of ECG patterns (ECG telemetry) has been useful for the prevention of cardiac arrest by early recognition of life-threatening dysrhythmias in ambulatory hospitalized patients, and for prehospital emergency cardiac care, when paramedics in the field are under physician direction by radio. The latter, however, does not require ECG telemetry if the paramedics are trained in pattern recognition and the physician giving radio command is experienced in interpreting monitoring sounds and paramedics' verbal reports by radio telephone.

Since most sudden cardiac deaths associated with myocardial ischemia or infarction occur following life-threatening dysrhythmias, ECG monitoring should be used as a *preventive measure* in all patients with suspected myocardial infarction or shock. Cardiac arrest can often be prevented by early detection of premonitory dysrhythmias.

ECG Patterns of Cardiac Arrest (Fig. 42)

Ventricular fibrillation

This is the most common cause of sudden cardiac death. It is an irregular continuous quivering motion of the ventricles of the heart that does not pump blood, i.e. it is synonymous with pulselessness. VF is associated with the characteristic ECG pattern of oscillations without intermittent ventricular complexes. VF may be primary or secondary, and with very rare exceptions does not spontaneously cease in man and large animals. Its mechanisms is still not entirely clear. Primary VF is sudden, without evidence of preceding cardiovascular or pulmonary failure. VF is most often due to spotty areas of hypoperfusion of the myocardium (transient, focal myocardial ischemia, sometimes as a result of vasospasm, sludging or hypotension) in either sick hearts or 'hearts too good to die'[62]. The latter are capable of producing adequate cardiac output once ventricular fibrillation is reversed. Secondary VF may occur spontaneously or be provoked (e.g. by chest compressions) in the weakly beating heart or in EMD or asystole. As to mechanisms, one therapy assumes excitation from many heterotopic foci; another theory assumes a circus movement triggered by one ectopic focus. VF is more likely to occur in large diseased hearts. The only effective treatment of pulselessness due to VF is electric countershocks plus CPR Steps A–B–C.

Electromechanical dissociation and asystole

Electromechanical dissociation (EMD) is pulselessness and cardiac standstill (no blood flow) with the isoelectric ECG intermittently interrupted by normal or abnormal ECG complexes at regular or irregular intervals; this is mechanical but not electric asystole. Protracted EMD can lead to electric asystole or VF. Electric asystole is pulselessness with isoelectric ECG. Primary electric asystole would occur with overdose by myocardial depressant drugs, high-energy electric shock, heart block with severe bradycardia (Stokes–Adams syndrome). The myocardial ischemia from severe bradycardia, EMD or asystole may easily be triggered into VF, particularly under the stimulus of CPR. Increased vagal tone in patients with or without heart disease leads to severe bradycardia, usually to 'vagal escape', but sometimes to cardiac arrest in asystole. Vasovagal syncope in healthy people (e.g. due to emotional insult) can usually be promptly reversed by horizontal positioning with the legs raised. If necessary, oxygen, i.v. fluids and atropine should be used. Pulselessness calls for CPR. Predisposing factors for EMD and asystole include hypercarbia, hypoxemia, hypothermia, hypothyroidism, beta-receptor blocking drugs, reserpine and hyperpotassemia. Asphyxia and exsanguination lead to cardiac arrest in EMD, which over time becomes electric asystole. This is easily resuscitable with CPR. When cardiogenic VF leads over time to electric asystole, or after countershock to EMD or asystole, the prognosis is poor. The pulselessness of EMD may be accompanied by relatively normal or abnormal (agonal, bizarre) ECG patterns, with no characteristic QRS pattern.

When bradycardia due to heart block (usually caused by focal ischemic lesions in the conduction system) lead to syncopy (Stokes–Adams syndrome), it may be due to severe bradycardia, EMD, electric asystole or hypoperfusion-triggered VF.

Treatment of EMD and asystole centers around CPR and abolition of the cause. Attempts at getting the heart restarted include fist pacing (repetitive blows over the pericardium), atropine, isoproterenol, external pacing, transvenous pacing (in heart block without full cardiac arrest); and, in complete pulselessness, myocardial oxygenation with CPR Steps A–B–C and epinephrine, and countershock in the case of secondary VF.

Before accepting a persistent isoelectric ECG asystole, disguised VF should be ruled out by checking the ECG with a second electrode position, 90° to the first one[236].

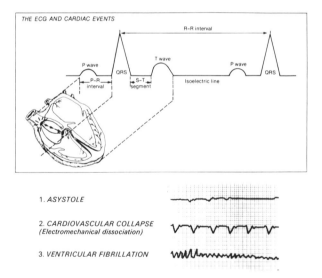

Fig. 42. Electrocardiographic diagnosis of cardiac arrest. Top: relation of normal ECG to cardiac anatomy. The normal ECG consists of the P-wave (depolarization of the atria), the QRS complex (maximum 0.12 seconds) (depolarization of the ventricles), and the T-wave (repolarization). The P–R interval is 0.1–0.2 seconds, and the Q–T interval maximum is 0.4 seconds, related to the heart rate. The S–T segment should be almost isoelectric. Bottom: the three typical ECG patterns associated with pulselessness—1, asystole; 2, electromechanical dissociation (cardiovascular collapse, mechanical without electrical asystole); and 3, ventricular fibrillation. Electromechanical dissociation is not associated with a characteristic QRS pattern. (From Caroline N: *Emergency Care in the Streets*. Boston, Little Brown[125a]; and American Heart Association, Dallas, Texas.)

Life-Threatening Dysrhythmias (Figs. 43–46)[202]

Health professionals providing advanced CPR life support must be able to recognize the following tachy- and bradydysrhythmias (Figs. 42–46)[23b, c]: (1) sinus tachycardia, (2) sinus bradycardia, (3) premature atrial complexes, (4) supraventricular tachycardia (Fig. 43), (5) atrial flutter, (6) atrial fibrillation, (7) junctional (nodal) rhythms (Fig. 44), (8) atrioventricular blocks of all degrees (Fig. 45), (9) premature ventricular complexes, (10) ventricular tachycardia including torsade de pointes, (11) ventricular fibrillation, and (12) cardiac standstill (ventricular asystole) (Fig. 46).

Sinus tachycardia and sinus bradycardia (Fig. 43)

These are easily recognized from a normal ECG, and defined as a heart rate above 100 or below 60 per minute respectively, and a corresponding shortening or lengthening of the distance between P-waves and QRS complexes. For hemodynamic reasons, bradycardia with a heart rate of less than about 40 per minute should be treated with atropine, and a heart rate at rest over 140 per minute should be treated with beta-receptor blocker, if appropriate therapy for the cause of the tachycardia is not effective. Bradycardia is dangerous in the critically ill person when the heart rate is less than 50–60 per minute, irrespective of whether it is sinus bradycardia or bradycardia of ventricular origin. One should always make an attempt to differentiate between these two. Asymptomatic sinus bradycardia is harmless, occurs in healthy persons, and is common in athletes. It can be risky in patients with myocardial disease. Bradycardia of ventricular origin is life-threatening because it is due to a block in the cardiac conduction system. Use lidocaine with caution.

Paroxysmal supraventricular tachycardia (Fig. 43)

PSVT must be differentiated from sinus tachycardia and VT, which may be difficult[482]. Four possibly effective treatments are vagal maneuvers (carotid sinus massage, Valsalva maneuver, face submersion in iced water)[936], drugs (verapamil, digoxin, beta-blocker), overdrive pacing and synchronized d.c. countershock (cardioversion with 75–100 J) under optional sedation (e.g. diazepam). Edrophonium and vasopressors are not recommended. Treatment should be prompt if there is chest pain, hypotension, heart failure or myocardial infarction.

(a) *NORMAL SINUS RHYTHM (NSR)*

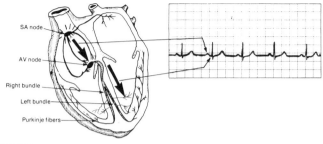

(b) *SINUS TACHYCARDIA*

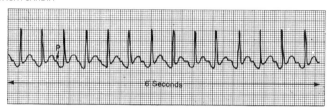

(c) *SINUS BRADYCARDIA*

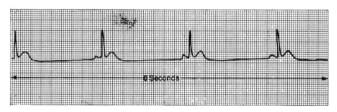

(d) *PREMATURE ATRIAL CONTRACTIONS (PACs)*

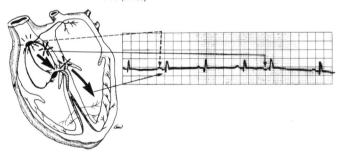

(e) *SUPRAVENTRICULAR TACHYCARDIA*

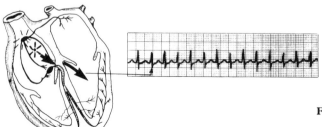

Figure 43.

Fig. 43 (opposite). (a)–(e): ECG patterns of sinus dysrhythmias. (From Caroline N: *Emergency Care in the Streets*. Boston, Little Brown[125a].)

Fig. 43(a). Regular, normal sinus rhythm (NSR). Rate 60–100/min. P waves normal. Pacemaker SA node. P–R interval 0.12–0.2 s. QRS complexes normal. For systematic analysis of the ECG rhythm strip, determine: rhythm (regular or irregular); rate; P waves (before every QRS complex, what is pacemaker site?); P–R interval; QRS complexes (normal or abnormal); S–T segment (isoelectric?); and T waves.

Fig. 43(b). Sinus tachycardia. Rhythm regular. Rate 100–160/min. P waves normal. With very rapid rates, P waves may be buried in the previous T wave. Pacemaker SA node. P–R interval normal. QRS complexes normal. Sinus tachycardia may result from a variety of circumstances, including pain, fever, hypoxemia, shock, and congestive heart failure, as well as from certain drugs (e.g. epinephrine, atropine, isoproterenol). Very rapid heart rates lead in AMI to further ischemia and infarction. Cardiac output may be reduced when heart rate exceeds 120–140/min because of inadequate time for ventricles to fill. Treat underlying cause.

Fig. 43(c). Sinus bradycardia. Rhythm regular or slightly irregular. Rate 35–60/min. P waves normal. Pacemaker SA node. P–R interval normal. QRS complexes normal. In young, healthy individuals, heart rates below 60 per minute may simply reflect good physical conditioning. In AMI, sinus bradycardia implies damage to conduction system, increased vagal tone, or toxic levels of digitalis or other drugs. When heart rate below 50/min, cardiac output, coronary perfusion and electric stability may be reduced and PVCs provoked. *Treatment:* None if blood pressure normal, patient alert, and no PVCs. Treat hypotension and PVCs. PVCs in the context of bradycardia should be treated first with atropine, not lidocaine. Often, merely speeding up the heart rate will abolish PVCs. If atropine ineffective in increasing the heart rate, try isoproterenol infusion, starting at 2 μg/min.

Fig. 43(d). Premature atrial contractions (complexes) (PACs). Rhythm regular. Rate determined by number of PACs. P waves of PACs often different in shape or size. Pacemaker site of the PACs is an ectopic focus in some portion of the atria or AV junction other than the SA node. P–R interval variable. QRS complexes normal. Occasional PACs may occur in normal individuals, but frequent PACs suggest organic heart disease and may lead to atrial tachycardias. No treatment required.

Fig. 43(e). Supraventricular tachycardia (SVT). Rhythm regular. Rate 140–220/min. P waves may be absent or abnormal. Pacemaker site a part of the atria or AV junction other than the SA node. There may be no P–R interval. If a P wave precedes the QRS, the duration of the P–R interval will depend on the distance from the ectopic pacemaker site to the AV junction. QRS complexes usually normal. SVT is sometimes caused by structural damage to the SA or AV node or by digitalis overdose. Paroxysmal atrial tachycardia (PAT) is a relatively benign dysrhythmia, but if it persists for any length of time, PAT may cause congestive heart failure. PAT can be precipitated in susceptible individuals by alcohol, smoking, coffee, hyperventilation and stress. It usually starts abruptly. There is one P wave to every QRS. *Treatment:* 1) Vagal maneuvers (Valsalva maneuver, i.e. straining against a closed glottis; carotid sinus massage; immersion of face in ice water); 2) verapamil 0.1 mg/kg i.v. slowly (do not use if patient on digitalis).

> **Suggested treatment of PSVT**[23b, c]
>
> 1. If the patient is stable, try vagal maneuvers; sedation—verapamil 5 mg i.v., 10 mg i.v. in 15–20 min; cardioversion; digoxin; beta blocker; pacing.
> 2. If the patient is unstable, synchronized cardioversion with 75–100 J, 200 J, 360 J; correct underlying problems; drugs (see 1).
> 3. If cardioversion is successful but PSVT recurs, do not repeat countershock.

Premature atrial complexes (Fig. 43)

Premature atrial complexes are not life-threatening and are usually harmless; they may occur in normal persons. If they are frequent, they may indicate heart or lung disease and may initiate atrial tachycardia. They are important primarily because they need to be distinguished from premature ventricular complexes (PVCs), which are sometimes dangerous. PVCs are followed by a compensatory pause. Therapy for premature atrial complexes consists of sedation, treatment of the underlying problem, if any, and interdiction of coffee and cigarettes.

Atrial fibrillation (Fig. 44)

Atrial fibrillation can also appear occasionally in normal hearts, but is more likely a sign of heart disease. It results in an irregularly irregular ventricular rhythm, which is the hallmark of this dysrhythmia and makes it immediately recognizable even on palpation of the pulse (pulsus irregularis perpetuus). Atrial fibrillation is not life-threatening unless associated with a very rapid ventricular rate. It is usually treated first by a calcium entry blocker (e.g. verapamil), and long-term with digoxin. If unsuccessful, the most effective treatment is synchronized electric (low-energy) d.c. countershock (cardioversion). This should be undertaken with great caution in the digitalized patient. Propranolol may also have a place in the treatment of atrial fibrillation with a rapid ventricular response, especially when the clinical situation permits a more leisurely therapeutic approach. Digoxin remains the most commonly used long-term therapy.

Junctional (nodal) rhythms (Fig. 44)

Junctional (nodal) rhythms may result in a single premature complex or a persistent junctional rhythm. The hallmark is retrograde firing of the atrium which may or may not result in a detectable P-wave. Similarly, there may or may not be a compensating pause depending on whether the sinus node is reset by the premature junctional complex. Junctional escape rhythms typically have a rate of 40–60 per minute, with an inverted P-wave and a short PR interval. Treatment is rarely necessary, but if so atropine is the treatment of choice, followed by isoproterenol if necessary.

Atrioventricular blocks (Fig. 45)

Atrioventricular block (AV block) may be first, second or third degree.

First-degree AV block is merely a delayed passage of the impulse through the AV node, causing a prolonged P–R interval (> 0.2 s). It serves as a warning, but treatment is rarely needed.

Second-degree AV block results in dropped beats and may be one of two types; the Mobitz type I pattern (Wenckebach AV block) and the more dangerous Mobitz type II pattern. Mobitz type I AV block is common in myocardial infarction, usually transient, and if associated with significant bradycardia requires atropine or isoproterenol rather than a pacemaker. In inferior wall myocardial infarction, Mobitz type I AV block may precede Mobitz type II AV block, which occurs in large myocardial infarctions, often as a forerunner to complete AV block. The appearance of Mobitz type II AV block indicates the need for at least a standby pacemaker.

Third-degree (complete) AV block is characterized by an absence of conduction of impulses from the atria to the ventricle, hopefully with a slow idioventricular rate of 30–40 beats per minute, as in Stokes–Adams syndrome. The P-waves are unrelated to the QRS complexes. With a very slow ventricular rate, blood flow may become inadequate to maintain consciousness, and reduced myocardial perfusion can result in congestive heart failure, angina, ventricular tachycardia or ventricular fibrillation. Treatment in the patient who tends to become unconscious or whose heart rate is considered dangerously slow, should consist of external 'fist pacing' (repetitive thumps over the precordium)[720, 998] or use of an external electric pacemaker[999], while an i.v. infusion of isoproterenol is started. With this treatment the patient's heart rate usually can be supported adequately until an i.v. pacemaker is inserted. During CPR Steps A–B–C, when upon restoration of spontaneous circulation there are recurring runs of ventricular tachycardia or even ventricular fibrillation, one should study the ECG in detail to determine whether the tachydysrhythmia is preceded by third-degree (complete) AV block. In this instance lidocaine is contraindicated, and seemingly paradoxic treatment with isoproterenol and pacing may keep the sinus rate high enough to prevent such recurrent ventricular tachydys-rhythmias and cardiac arrest.

In general, atropine is more effective for increasing the heart rate in sinus bradycardia than in ventricular bradycardia (complete heart block), when isoproterenol is more effective. Patients with acute myocardial infarction of the anterior wall (which carries a high mortality) can suddenly develop complete heart block and are usually unresponsive to atropine. In contrast, patients with acute myocardial infarction of the inferior wall (which carries a low mortality) can develop bradycardia due to increased vagal tone with a slow progression to Mobitz II block and finally to third-degree AV block; these sometimes do respond to atropine.

Suggested treatment of bradycardia (< 60 beats per minute)[23b, c]

1. In sinus or junctional (nodal) bradycardia, observe. In symptomatic (hypotension, PVCs, chest pain, dyspnea, stupor, myocardial infarction), use atropine 0.5–1.0 mg i.v. every 5 minutes, to a total of 2 mg.
2. In second-degree AV block type I, use atropine 0.5–1.0 mg i.v.
3. In second-degree AV block type II or third-degree block: if asymptomatic, transvenous electric pacemaker; if symptomatic (above), use atropine 0.5–1.0 mg i.v., external electric pacing for syncope, transient external fist pacing or isoproterenol i.v. infusion (2–20 μg/kg per min), and transvenous electric pacemaker.

ATRIAL FLUTTER

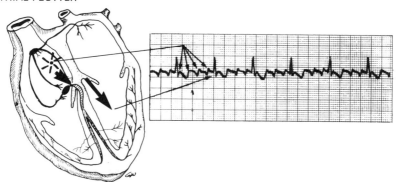

Fig. 44. (a)–(c): ECG patterns of some non-life threatening dysrhythmias. (From Caroline N: *Emergency Care in the Streets*. Boston, Little Brown[125a]).

Fig. 44(a). Atrial flutter. Atrial rhythm regular; ventricular response may be irregular. Atrial rate 240–360/min; ventricular rate 140–160/min. Ventricular rate may be slower if on digitalis. No true P waves. Instead, flutter waves (F waves), often in a jagged, 'sawtooth' pattern. Pacemaker is an ectopic focus in atrium. P–R interval not measurable. QRS complexes usually normal, may follow every second, third, or fourth flutter wave. Caused by underlying disease or damage to heart. If stable, without hypotension, confusion, or coma, then no treatment is indicated. If pulse is in excess of 120–140/min, hypotension, cold skin, confusion, or coma, then use cardioversion. *Note*: Cardioversion may be hazardous in the digitalized patient.

ATRIAL FIBRILLATION

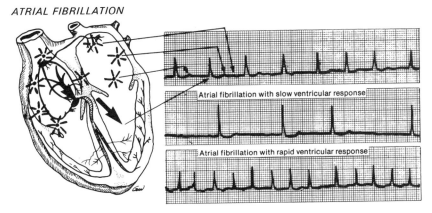

Fig. 44(b). Atrial fibrillation (AF). Rhythm irregularly irregular. Atrial rate 350–600/min, not measurable; ventricular rate 100–160/min if untreated, but slower with digitalis. P waves absent; instead there are fibrillatory waves (f waves), which may be coarse, fine, or resemble a straight line. Multiple ectopic pacemaker sites throughout the atria. P–R interval not measurable. QRS complexes usually normal. Atrial fibrillation is usually associated with underlying heart disease. In AMI, AF may indicate damage to SA node or atria. Cardiac output may decrease. If ventricular response is in excess of 120–140/min, work of heart is increased. *Treatment:* Usually none required immediately. Very rapid AF may require cardioversion or digitalis.

PREMATURE NODAL (JUNCTIONAL) CONTRACTORS (PNCs)

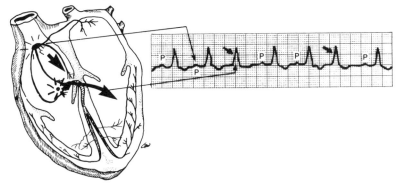

Fig. 44(c). Premature nodal (junctional) contractions (PNCs). Rhythm irregular. The PNC is preceded by a shorter than normal P–R interval. Rate determined by number of PNCs. P waves present or absent in the PNCs; when present, they differ in shape from normal P waves and may occur before, during, or after QRS. An ectopic focus in the AV junction is the pacemaker site for the PNCs. P–R interval less than 0.12 s for the PNC. QRS complexes normal. Occasional PNCs are not significant. When multiple, they indicate irritability of the AV junction. No emergency treatment needed.

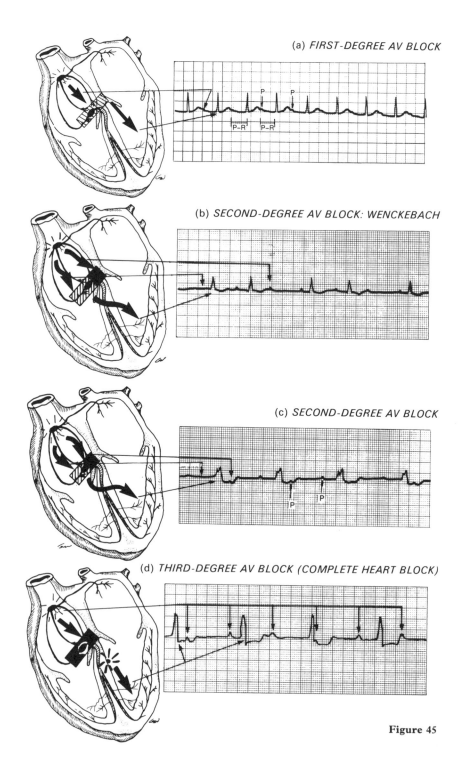

(a) *FIRST-DEGREE AV BLOCK*

(b) *SECOND-DEGREE AV BLOCK: WENCKEBACH*

(c) *SECOND-DEGREE AV BLOCK*

(d) *THIRD-DEGREE AV BLOCK (COMPLETE HEART BLOCK)*

Figure 45

Fig. 45 (opposite).(a)–(f): ECG patterns of potentially life-threatening bradydysrhythmias with atrioventricular (AV) blocks. (From Caroline N: *Emergency Care in the Streets*. Boston, Little Brown[125a].)

Fig. 45(a). First degree AV block. Rhythm regular. Rate normal. P waves normal. Pacemaker site is SA node. P–R interval prolonged beyond 0.2 s. QRS complexes normal. First-degree AV block may be caused by damage to the AV junction, increased vagal tone, or toxicity from digitalis, quinidine, procainamide, etc. May warn of more advanced degrees of block. No emergency treatment required.

Fig. 45(b). Second degree AV block (Wenckebach phenomenon = Mobitz-type I block). Atrial (P wave) rhythm regular; ventricular (QRS) rhythm irregular. P waves more numerous than QRS complexes. Atrial rate normal; ventricular rate normal or slow. P waves normal; a QRS complex is absent after every third, fourth, or fifth P wave. Pacemaker site: SA node. P–R interval progressively widens until atrial impulse blocked and P wave not followed by QRS. QRS complexes normal. Wenckebach block is the less serious type of second-degree block, usually being transient and reversible. However, occasionally Wenckebach block will progress to complete heart block. Monitoring required. No treatment required if heart rate above 50–60/min and cardiac output well maintained. If the heart rate is less than 50–60 min, or if there is hypotension, cold and clammy skin, confusion, or coma, then give atropine 0.5 mg i.v., and repeat at 5-min intervals until the heart rate is 70 or more or until maximum total dose of 2.0 mg.

Fig. 45(c). Second degree AV block (Mobitz-type II block). Atrial (P wave) rhythm regular; ventricular (QRS) rhythm regular or irregular. P waves more numerous than QRS complexes. Atrial rate normal; ventricular rate normal or slow. P waves normal, but not every P wave is followed by a QRS. The ratio of P waves to QRS complexes may be 2:1, 3:1, and so on. Pacemaker site SA node. P–R interval normal or prolonged, but constant. QRS complexes usually normal, each preceded by a P wave; may be widened. Second-degree AV block is serious. It occurs in large anterior wall myocardial infarctions and may progress rapidly to complete AV block (third-degree heart block). Furthermore, if slow ventricular rates are associated with second-degree AV block, cardiac output may be reduced. No treatment necessary if heart rate above 50–60/min and cardiac output well maintained. In slower heart rates, accompanied by signs of inadequate cardiac output, give atropine 0.5 mg i.v., and repeat at 5-min intervals until the heart rate is 70 or more or until maximum total dose of 2.0 mg. Have pacemaker ready. If atropine ineffective, infuse isoproterenol i.v., starting at 2 μg/min.

Fig. 45(d). Third degree AV block (complete heart block). Rhythm regular. Atrial (P wave) rate normal; ventricular (QRS) rate 30–40/min. P waves normal contour; no consistent relationship to QRS complexes. SA node is pacemaker for atria, but impulses from SA node are blocked at AV junction and cannot reach ventricles. Ventricles are driven by a different pacemaker, in the AV junction or below (idioventricular rhythm). The lower the pacemaker lies in the ventricles, the slower the ventricular rate and the more bizarre the QRS complexes. There is no P–R interval since there is no consistent relationship between P waves and QRS complexes. QRS complexes may be normal if ventricular pacemaker lies in AV junction or bundle of His, but usually QRS complexes are wide and bizarre. If heart rate is below 35–50/min, cardiac output may be significantly reduced. In addition, because in third-degree heart block the atria and ventricles are no longer synchronized, the ventricles do not fill completely prior to each contraction, and cardiac output is further reduced. Bradycardia of AV block reduces myocardial perfusion, which can trigger VT or VF. *Emergency treatment*: If complete heart block is associated with signs of inadequate perfusion (e.g. hypotension, syncope, confusion), give atropine 0.5 mg i.v., and repeat at 5-min intervals to maintain pulse above 60, until a maximum total dose of 2.0 mg. If atropine ineffective, infuse isoproterenol, starting at 2 μg/min. No matter how bizarre the QRS complexes, *never give lidocaine to a patient with complete heart block*. Distinguish complete heart block from frequent PVCs! Have pacemaker ready. While waiting for i.v. pacemaker insertion, use fist pacing (repetitive precordial thumping) or external electric pacing or isoproterenol i.v. if heart rate below 30, hypotension, confusion, or syncope. Final treatment: permanent i.v. pacemaker.

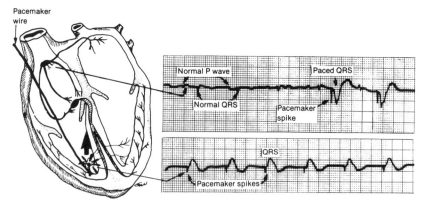

Fig. 45(e). Pacemaker rhythms. Rhythm is regular or irregular. Rate is variable, depending on pacemaker setting. Rate should not be below 60/min if pacemaker functioning properly. P waves normal when present, and may or may not be followed by a QRS. Pacemaker spikes will precede those QRS complexes induced by pacemaker. Pacemaker site is electronic pacemaker and sometimes SA node. P–R interval: May be normal or prolonged when present. QRS complexes following pacemaker spike are wide and bizarre, resembling PVCs. Pacemaker rhythms indicate that patient has an electronic pacemaker in place. Most of the pacemakers used today are demand pacemakers, i.e. they turn on when the patient's heart rate falls below a certain rate (usually about 60/min). Thus, a rhythm strip may show, as above, some normal sinus beats as well as beats originating from the electronic pacemaker. If the pacemaker is not 'kicking in' when the patient's intrinsic heart rate falls below 60–70/min, or if the pacemaker is not sensing the patient's beats but rather is firing right after (or on top of) the normal QRS, the patient must immediately be checked for pacemaker malfunction. In severe bradycardia with syncope, use fist pacing (or external electric pacing)–atropine–isoproterenol–i.v. pacemaker sequence.

(f) *CARDIAC STANDSTILL (ASYSTOLE)*

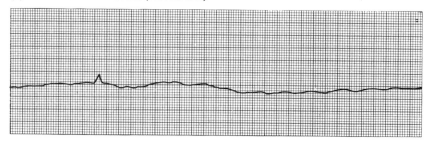

Fig. 45(f). Electric asystole (cardiac standstill). No ECG rhythm, straight line. Rate < 5 ectopic beats/min. QRS complexes absent or very rare and bizarre. Electromechanical dissociation (EMD), i.e. mechanical asystole without electric asystole if untreated leads to electric asystole. So does VF if untreated. *Treatment* consists of CPR with epinephrine and NaHCO$_3$ (see text). If refractory, use fist pacing–external electric pacing–i.v. pacing.

Premature ventricular complexes (PVCs) (Fig. 46)

Premature ventricular complexes (PVCs) are usually bizarre extra ECG complexes triggered by an ectopic focus. PVCs can sometimes be felt as extra pulse beats. Often PVCs do not produce a pulse because of inadequate ventricular filling. The PVC is followed by a compensatory pause, which the patient can sometimes feel as a momentary 'fullness' in the chest. Frequent multifocal PVCs are the most common *precursors* of ventricular tachycardia and ventricular fibrillation (i.e sudden cardiac death), and a PVC falling on a T-wave (R-on-T phenomenon) very often initiates ventricular fibrillation. More than three PVCs in a row are by definition called ventricular tachycardia. If every other beat is preceded by a PVC, it is called 'ventricular bigeminal rhythm'; if it is every third beat, it is called 'trigeminal rhythm'. Single PVCs of similar configuration that do not fall on the T-wave occur in healthy persons and may be harmless; in ischemic hearts, however, they also may represent an increased risk.

Premature ventricular contractions are treated with an i.v. bolus of lidocaine (1 mg/kg), followed by a lidocaine infusion (1–4 mg/min per 70 kg). Later, long-term preventive medication may include procainamide, diphenylhydantoin, propranolol, quinidine, verapamil, or other drugs[263]. In very slow heart rates, such as in heart block (see below), PVCs may represent an 'escape rhythm' and can be prevented by the use of atropine, isoproterenol or pacing. However, atropine and isoproterenol in themselves may result in tachydysrhythmias.

Suggested treatment of ventricular ectopy (PVCs)[23b, c]

1. Search for and treat causes (e.g. digitalis, xanthine, other drugs, bradycardia–heart block, potassium, stress, alcohol).
2. If heart disease is suspected, or if PVCs are frequent, multifocal or R-on-T, administer: lidocaine 1 mg/kg i.v., 0.5 mg/kg every 2–5 minutes, to a maximum 3 mg/kg; procainamide 20 mg/70 kg per min i.v., to a maximum total of 1000 mg/70 kg; bretylium 5–10 mg/kg i.v. over 5–10 minutes; overdrive pacing.
3. When resolved, maintain lidocaine i.v. infusion 2–4 mg/70 kg per min (or use infusion of effective procainamide or bretylium). If infusion over 24 hours is needed, check blood levels (see drugs, above).

Ventricular tachycardia (VT) (Fig. 46)

Ventricular tachycardia (VT) is the most dangerous precursor of ventricular fibrillation (VF). VT is a continuous sequence of PVCs. During VT there may or may not be a palpable pulse, depending in part on the rapidity of the rate. When there is a pulse and the patient is conscious, lidocaine should be

Fig. 46.(a)–(c). ECG patterns of life-threatening tachydysrhythmias (PVCs–VT–VF). (From Caroline N: *Emergency Care in the Streets*, Boston, Little Brown[125a].)

PREMATURE VENTRICULAR CONTRACTIONS (PVCs)

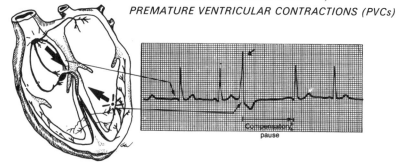

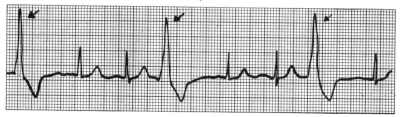

(a/1) *FREQUENT PVCs (MORE THAN SIX PER MINUTE)*

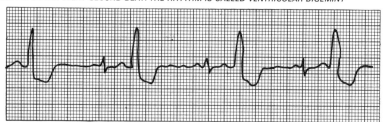

WHEN PVCs OCCUR EVERY SECOND BEAT. THE RHYTHM IS CALLED VENTRICULAR BIGEMINY

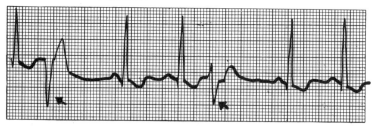

(a/2) *MULTIFOCAL PVCs ARE OF DIFFERENT SIZES AND SHAPES AND INDICATE THAT THERE ARE MULTIPLE ECTOPIC FOCI IN THE VENTRICLE*

(a/3) *BURSTS OF TWO OR MORE PVCs IN A ROW (SALVOS) MAY PROGRESS RAPIDLY TO VENTRICULAR TACHYCARDIA*

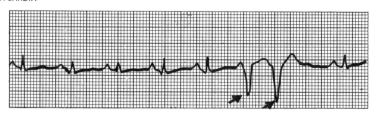

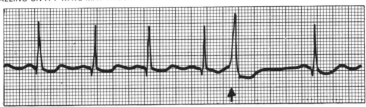

Fig. 46(a) (opposite and above). Premature ventricular contractions (complexes) (PVCs). Rhythm regular. A shorter than normal P–R interval separates the PVC from the preceding normal beat. Most PVCs are followed by a compensatory pause. Rate determined by the number of PCCs. P waves absent before PVCs. The pacemaker site for the PVC is an ectopic focus in one of the ventricles. No P–R interval in the PVC, because it is not preceded by a P wave. QRS complexes of PVCs are distorted, wide (> 0.12 s) and bizarre. The T wave of the PVC is usually oppositely directed (i.e. if the QRS complex is upright, the T wave is inverted). Occasional PVCs may occur in normal persons. However, in the setting of AMI, PVCs indicate increased ventricular irritability and should be treated. Certain types of PVCs are of particular concern because of their tendency to progress to ventricular tachycardia (VT) or fibrillation (VF). Figures 46 a/1, 2, 3, 4 show various dangerous PVC patterns. *Treatment:* In the setting of AMI, probably all PVCs should be treated, but certainly those in categories 1–4 should be treated under any circumstances. Lidocaine 75–100 mg i.v., followed by lidocaine infusion of 2–3 mg/ min per 70 kg. See text.

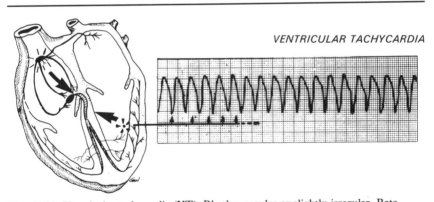

VENTRICULAR TACHYCARDIA

Fig. 46(b). Ventricular tachycardia (VT). Rhythm regular or slightly irregular. Rate 100–250/min. P waves often not seen because they are buried in the QRS complexes; when they are visible, they have no apparent relationship to the QRS complexes. Pacemaker site is an ectopic focus in the ventricle. QRS complexes are distorted, wide (> 0.12 s), bizarre. VT is a very serious and dangerous arrhythmia, which may lead to ventricular fibrillation (VF) and can itself cause marked reduction in cardiac output and even pulselessness. *Treatment:* 1) If the patient is alert and has no signs of inadequate cardiac output (alert without hypotension), give lidocaine 75–100 mg i.v., followed by infusion of lidocaine. If lidocaine is ineffective, try bretylium infusion, 10 mg/kg over 10 min. 2) In a monitored patient who suddenly becomes unconscious and whose rhythm is observed to be VT, a sharp, quick precordial thump may be delivered over the midsternum. If the precordial thump is ineffective and there is continued evidence of inadequate cardiac output (hypotension, coma, or cold and clammy skin), cardioversion (external countershock) is indicated. Cardioversion is more likely to be successful if preceded by a bolus of lidocaine.

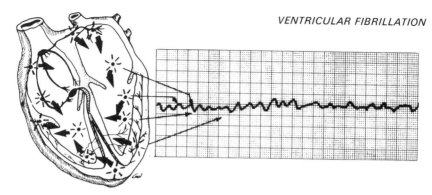

Fig. 46(c). Ventricular fibrillation (VF) = cardiac arrest (pulselessness). Most common cause of sudden cardiac death. Rhythm totally irregular. Rate 150–300 entirely uncoordinated waves per min. P waves not seen. Pacemaker sites are numerous ectopic foci scattered throughout the heart. QRS complexes are absent. In place of QRS complexes there are fibrillatory waves of varying size, shape, and duration. In ventricular fibrillation, the ventricles fire in a totally disorganized fashion, and ventricular muscle simply quivers rather than beating. As a result, there is no cardiac output. Ventricular fibrillation is equivalent to clinical death. When a rhythm resembling VF is seen on the ECG monitor, check the patient rapidly to rule out muscle tremor, loose leads, or patient movement artifact as the source of the oscillating baseline. *Treatment:* 1) If VF occurs in the rescuer's presence (witnessed cardiac arrest) or is identified in a patient who has been in cardiac arrest for less than 1–2 min, an immediate countershock of 200–300 J should be given. If a monitored patient is observed to go into VF and a defibrillator is not immediately available, a sharp, quick precordial thump may be tried. 2) If the patient has been in cardiac arrest for more than 2 min or for an unknown period (unwitnessed cardiac arrest), CPR Steps A–B–C should be initiated and performed for at least 2 min before electric defibrillation is attempted. Usually further measures, such as the administration of epinephrine and sodium bicarbonate, will be required to enable successful defibrillation.

administered intravenously in an attempt to terminate VT; however, VT with unconsciousness or pulselessness must be treated immediately like VF, namely with electric countershock and CPR as needed. Cough[942] or chest thump[541] may be attempted. A defibrillator should be available since these maneuvers can terminate VT or transform it into VF[979].

It is important to differentiate between ventricular and supraventricular tachycardia, since the latter is usually not harmful and the former is life-threatening. If the differentiation is impossible, the hemodynamic effects of the dysrhythmia, as monitored by pulse, arterial pressure and CVP, should guide therapy. Eventually, even atrial tachycardia should be treated, particularly in the elderly with coronary artery disease (Valsalva maneuver, carotid sinus massage, methoxamine, verapamil, digoxin, edrophonium, tensilon, phenylephrine).

Torsade de pointes is VT with changes in amplitude and direction of electric complexes. Torsade de pointes-type VT should be treated with electric pacing, and lidocaine and quinidine are contraindicated[406]. Sometimes magnesium sulfate is effective[906]. This is in contrast to polymorphic VT which may respond to lidocaine.

Suggested treatment of sustained VT with pulse[23b, c]

1. In symptom-free VT with normotension, give oxygen, lidocaine 1 mg/kg i.v., lidocaine 0.5 mg/kg every 5–10 minutes to a maximum 3 mg/kg total, procainamide 20 mg/70 kg per min to a maximum 100 mg/70 kg, and countershock as in (2) below.
2. In cases with hypotension, chest pain, dyspnea, stupor or coma, give oxygen, countershock (cardioversion, synchronized defibrillation) with sedation if conscious (optional), 50 J, 100 J, 200 J, 360 J, i.v. lidocaine, procainamide, bretylium, 360 J, etc.

Ventricular fibrillation (VF) (Fig. 46)[237, 736a]

Ventricular fibrillation (VF) is the most common cause of sudden cardiac death, found in 57–91% of cases[198], with 30% recovery. It is an irregular, continuous, peristaltic, quivering motion of the ventricles of the heart that does not pump blood and is associated with the characteristic ECG pattern of oscillations without intermittent ventricular complexes. Ventricular fibrillation may be primary or secondary (see above). Ventricular fibrillation is most often due to spotty areas of hypoperfusion of the myocardium (transient, focal myocardial ischemia). Coarse (high-amplitude) ventricular fibrillation is easier to terminate with electric shock than fine (low-amplitude) fibrillation[236]. For mechanisms and treatment of VF, see also above and the literature[736a].

Suggested treatment of VT without pulse and VF[23b, c]

In unwitnessed arrest, give CPR until a defibrillator is available.

In witnessed arrest, give precordial thump. If there is then no pulse, give CPR, get a defibrillator with ECG paddles, and if there is VT or VF give countershock with 200 J, 300 J, 360 J. If there is still no pulse, continue CPR, give epinephrine 1 mg i.v. or intratracheal (intubate if possible) and repeat every 5 minutes, followed by 360 J, lidocaine 1 mg/kg i.v., 360 J, bretylium 5 mg/kg i.v., NaHCO$_3$ i.v. 1 mEq/kg (if arrest has continued over 2 minutes or CPR over 10 minutes), 360 J, bretylium 10 mg/kg. i.v., 360 J, and continue. Consider open-chest CPR if possible (physician only).

Electromechanical dissociation (EMD) and asystole (Fig. 46)[113, 236, 589]

EMD is mechanical asystole (pulselessness) with agonal (bizarre, abnormal) or relatively normal ECG patterns. This condition has in the past also been labeled 'cardiovascular collapse'. EMD and resulting asystole are readily reversible by CPR if caused by hypovolemia, hypoxemia–acidemia (asphyxia), anesthetic overdose or vagotonia. 'True EMD' is absent cardiac contractility without apparent cause, perhaps because of impaired calcium shifts in a sick heart. Vigorous CPR and epinephrine can sometimes reverse EMD in spite of its statistically poor prognosis.

Asystole can be mechanical asystole plus electrical asystole (pulselessness with cardiac standstill and isoelectric ECG) or mechanical asystole (pulselessness) with normal or abnormal ECG complexes, i.e. EMD. Asystole may be primary or secondary (see above). Electric asystole in patients with heart disease has been found in 9–27% of prehospital cardiac arrests, with only 10% recovery[113, 202]. Causes of asystole include right coronary artery occlusion, leading to posterior infarct. Before accepting a persistently isoelectric ECG as asystole, 'disguised VF' should be ruled out by checking the ECG with a second electrode postioned 90° to the first one[236, 237].

Suggested treatment of EMD—asystole[23b, c]

1. In syncope (witnessed collapse), place the patient in a horizontal position with the legs up. Give oxygen and atropine (optional) 1 mg i.v. for bradycardia.

2. In pulseless, give CPR Steps A–B–C, epinephrine 1 mg i.v. or i.tr. every 5 minutes, IPPV/O_2, intubation (when possible), $NaHCO_3$ 1 mEq/kg i.v. Recognize and treat hypovolemia, hypoxemia, acidemia, pneumothorax, cardiac tamponade, pulmonary embolism and other causes.

3. In isoelectric ECG, countershock for possible fine VF, atropine 1 mg i.v. (repeat once 5 minutes later), and proceed as in (2) above, followed by pacing (fist–external electric–transvenous).

Note: Dysrhythmias with pulselessness call for immediately resuscitative action. Dysrhythmias with a palpable pulse and consciousness call for thoughtful assessment and *treatment of the whole patient,* not merely the ECG!

Chapter 2F

Step F: Fibrillation Treatment (Defibrillation)

Introduction (Figs. 47–50)

This section of Advanced Life Support (ALS) concerns itself with 'electrical therapy' for life-threatening cardiac dysrhythmias, particularly ventricular tachycardia, ventricular fibrillation, complete heart block (severe bradycardia) and asystole. Electrical therapy includes simple chest thump (for witnessed VT and VF), repetitive chest thumps (fist pacing) (for heart block), cardioversion (synchronized electric countershock) (for atrial fibrillation and VT with pulse), nonsynchronized electric countershocks (for VT without pulse and VF) and pacing (for heart block and asystole).

Rapid electric defibrillation is indicated for the termination of the lethal dysrhythmias of ventricular tachycardia without pulse and ventricular fibrillation[153, 217, 218]. Primary causes of VF include coronary insufficiency, adverse drug reactions, electrocution and cardiac catheterization in an irritable heart. VF may also occur secondarily, during resuscitative efforts for asystole or electromechanical dissociation from asphyxia, drowning, exsanguination and other causes of cardiac arrest[736a].

While appropriate drug therapy can often *prevent* VF, drug treatment cannot by itself be relied upon to *terminate* VF. Lidocaine, bretylium, procainamide and beta-blockers usually cannot in the absence of counter-shock terminate VF, but may instead transform VF into pulselessness with EMD or electric asystole that is subsequently intractable to CPR efforts, including epinephrine.

The most rapid, effective and accepted method for terminating VT and VF is *electric countershock*[39, 61, 167, 226, 232, 235–237, 267a, b, 295, 312, 353, 428, 430, 483–486, 547, 548, 592, 612, 619, 638, 877, 878, 887, 891, 933, 996]. Electric defibrillation has been known since the turn of this century[638], but only after five decades and two world wars did it become part of standard clinical open-chest CPR in the 1940s[61] and closed-chest CPR in 1960. VT can spontaneously revert to sinus rhythm. Spontaneous cessation of VF without countershock is very rare in man and large animals, although common in small animals.

Low-voltage electric shock, which sends less than 2 A through the heart (e.g. electrocution by electric house current), can induce VF. Properly applied *high-voltage* electric shock, which sends more than 2 A through the heart (e.g. shock by lightning) produces, in the normally beating heart, a sustained contraction, and can terminate VF. Such effective therapeutic defibrillating shocks across the chest may be of alternating current (a.c.) with 500 V; or direct current (d.c.) of 100–400 J (i.e. watt-seconds)[353, 428, 430]. Such defibrillating shocks produce simultaneous depolarization of all myocardial fibers, after which spontaneous cardiac contractions may start *if the myocardium is oxygenated and not acidotic*. The amount of current actually passing through the heart cannot be monitored, but delivered energy can and should be monitored.

Energy requirements[167, 178, 235–237, 264, 267a, b, 483, 612, 877, 878]. Defibrillators discharge tension in volts and current in amperes. Volts × amperes gives power in watts. The integrated area under the power curve is energy in watt-seconds or joules (Fig. 47). The amount of current going through the heart

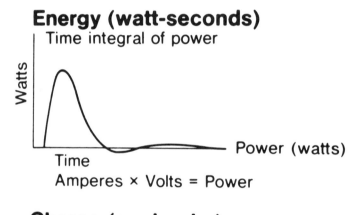

Energy (watt-seconds)
Time integral of power

Watts

Time

Amperes × Volts = Power

Power (watts)

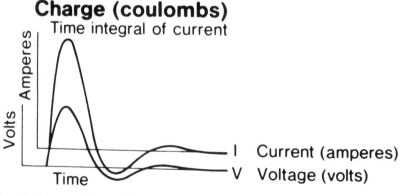

Charge (coulombs)
Time integral of current

Amperes

Volts

Time

I   Current (amperes)

V   Voltage (volts)

Fig. 47. Current, voltage and power waves of a defibrillator discharge delivering a damped half-sinusoidal wave form. (From Ewy GA: *Cardiac Arrest and Resuscitation: Defibrillators and Defibrillation.* Current Problems in Cardiology, vol. 2, no. 2, Chicago, Year Book Medical Publishers, 1978.)

required to defibrillate depends on the resistance between the defibrillator electrodes and the heart (Fig. 48). This in turn depends on many factors[39], including paddle electrode size[891] and the amount of air in the lungs between the electrodes[235]. With constant energy delivered through the defibrillator, defibrillation success is inversely proportional to transthoracic resistance[891]. The larger the electrodes, the lower the resistance. Too large electrodes decrease current density and thereby decrease defibrillation success[891]. Low resistance between electrodes and chest wall, through use of conductive jelly, saline-soaked pads or electrode gel pads, is important. Transthoracic impedance can be reduced by pressing with the electrodes on the chest to lower lung volume and the resistance created by air space in the chest[235]. Transthoracic resistance also decreases with successive countershocks[267b]. Neither adult patients' size[167] nor external energies of about 200–400 J seem to influence defibrillation success rate[938]. The recommended energies presented subsequently are a compromise between the need to consistently deliver above threshold energies and energy-dose related myocardial damage[167, 178, 236, 267b, 486, 612, 877, 938]. The recommendation is to deliver 200–300–360 J externally in cardioversion of VF. Other dysrhythmias require less energy (e.g. 100 J for VT, atrial fibrillation and PSVT; 25–50 J for atrial flutter). For open-chest CPR, 5–50 J should be used[23b].

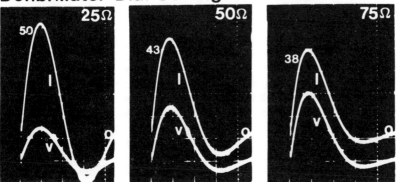

Defibrillator Dial Setting 400 Watt – Seconds

Decreasing delivered peak current with increasing resistance.

Fig. 48. Current (I) and voltage (V) delivered by defibrillators depend on resistance encountered (ohms). Waveforms delivered from a Hewlett Packard model 7802C defibrillator set at 400 J discharged into 25, 50 or 76 ohms resistance. With increasing resistance, voltage increases but current delivered decreases. (From Ewy GA: *Recent Advances in CPR and Defibrillation*. Current Problems in Cardiology, April 1983.)

Techniques for Electric Defibrillation[23b, 61, 638, 996]

ECG diagnosis and electric countershock must go hand in hand. Techniques for electric countershock that minimize chest wall resistance and optimize electric shock wave patterns, durations, delivered voltage in alternating current (a.c.) shock, and delivered energy (watt seconds or joules) of direct current (d.c.) defibrillating shocks now in use have evolved empirically. Direct current countershock rather than a.c. countershock is more effective in enlarged, diseased hearts, as well as in hypothermic patients, and for cardioversion. The short duration of d.c. shocks and the ability for cardioversion of the beating heart to be programmed exactly in relation to the ECG pattern can prevent application of the electric shock on the upstroke of the T-wave of the ECG, which can induce VF. The operator is more endangered by a.c. than by d.c. shock if not protected by insulation. However, even in defibrillation, a.c. countershock has no advantages and some disadvantages over d.c. countershock: a.c. defibrillators depend on wall current and thus are not portable; muscle contractions are strong; the longer impulse required can cause VF in the spontaneously beating heart; and there is an additional hazard to the operator because of nonisolated current flow. Also, the imprecise duration of a.c. countershock may repolarize the myocardium and reinduce VF.

To deliver the required energy to the heart, an *a.c. countershock* (now obsolete) of 500–1000 V (duration 0.1–0.25 s) was applied directly to the outside of the adult's chest. Although lower voltage shocks may sometimes succeed, it was felt that high energy levels should be recommended because failure of the first countershock may delay restarting of spontaneous circulation.

The same applies to the presently used *d.c. countershock*, which has the added advantage of being superior for cardioversion in the beating heart. Direct current countershock is produced by a capacitance discharge-type defibrillator, delivering up to 360 J in old defibrillators (with a setting of 400 J) in about 0.01 second duration. Although subtle histologic changes in the myocardium are related to the amount and duration of current transmitted through the heart, and thereby to the heat produced in the myocardium, external application of such high-energy or high-voltage countershocks does not usually cause enough damage to impair resumption of spontaneous contractions. This risk of producing heat damage may be greater when low voltage or low energy is used frequently, as when the first defibrillation attempt with inadequate energy fails. Also, recovery of the brain is enhanced by immediate restoration of spontaneous circulation. In contrast, direct application of high energy shocks to the heart during open-chest CPR can produce burns on the surface of the heart if used carelessly.

Necrosis of the myocardium (through the epicardium) has been seen in the past, caused by incorrectly applied direct cardiac electrodes during open-chest CPR using high a.c. currents[887]. This was clearly related to current strengths. External countershocks with a.c. current apparently caused no gross damage[353], but a.c. and to a lesser degree d.c. counter-shocks resulted in ECG changes and elevated heart enzyme levels in the serum, suggesting myocardial damage. Animal studies have shown that predominantly subepicardial gross myocardial changes become apparent only several days after multiple d.c. countershocks[933]. In patients with elective cardioversion without cardiac arrest, it seemed that the energies recommended here are safe, and that only cumulative delivered energy doses of over 400 J produce mild myocardial necrosis in patients[232]. Damage is also more likely to come from rapidly repetitive countershocks. In CPR Steps D–E–F, however, the importance of promptly restoring spontaneous circulation far outweighs the slight myocardial damage resulting from electric shocks.

The controversy about the recommended defibrillation energies is still going on. With the same energy, increasing body weight requires higher energies. Immediate countershock is more likely to be effective with low energies than defibrillation attempts after prolonged (unwitnessed) arrests. The proponents of low-energy countershock, who recommend first shocks with 200 J, deal mainly with patients of the former group[167, 612] whereas proponents of a 300–400 J first shock had more often been dealing with the latter group of patients.

The most commonly used initial energy for *external d.c. countershock* is 200 J (3 J/kg) for adults and 2 J/kg for children and infants. Higher energies are rarely necessary, but should be used for repeat countershocks where the initial energy fails. National[23b, c] and international[720] recommendations at present call for an initial two or three shocks of about 3 J/kg in adults (200–400 J) and 2–4 J/kg in children and infants. The ideal amount of energy required in any given case cannot be determined during CPR in advance. While these energy recommendations are for the conventional single-discharge wave form, other wave forms may have different energy requirements. For this the manufacturer's literature should be consulted.

Defibrillators

Defibrillators must be checked frequently to determine the actual energy delivered, since the reading on the dial is not always accurate. A regular maintenance program for defibrillators is essential. Defibrillators should be tested at low and high levels and should be capable of delivering up to 400 J d.c.[592]. There are now improved portable defibrillators and cardio-scopes.

Paddles for *external* electric defibrillation should be large for optimal propagation of current, i.e. 10 cm in diameter for adults, 8 cm for older children, and 4.5 cm for infants. *Paddles* for open-chest *internal* direct electric defibrillation by application on the heart should have diameters of 6 cm for adults, 4 cm for children and 2 cm for infants.

The present recommended technique of *external countershock* is as follows (Fig. 49).

In witnessed arrest, countershock should be applied within 30–60 seconds of the onset of ventricular fibrillation, i.e. before the heart becomes anoxic and acidotic, which would make successful defibrillation and resumption of cardiac contractions impossible. Immediate defibrillation before the start of CPR Steps A–B–C is desirable. If countershock and spontaneous pulse do not occur within 60 seconds of collapse, CPR must be started. If a defibrillator is not immediately available, CPR should be started immediately without waiting for 60 seconds. In *unwitnessed arrest* CPR Steps A–B–C are needed for about 2 minutes (to reoxygenate the myocardium) before an initial attempt to defibrillate has a chance to succeed.

Techniques

An assistant should set up and turn on the defibrillator—presumably a portable battery-powered d.c. defibrillator with 'quick look' paddles. (If using an a.c. defibrillator, the assistant should plug it into the wall outlet.) The helper must be ready to hand the operator the two paddles. Good electric contact between electrodes and skin is essential, but electrode paste should not be used so liberally that it produces a current path between electrodes over the patient's skin. Electrode paste makes the chest slippery for external cardiac compressions, whereas saline-soaked sponges do not. The sponges have the added advantage of being applied more rapidly, thus minimizing interruption of CPR, but again they should not be soaked in such a way that saline oozes between the defibrillator paddles. Just enough electrode paste should be applied to the defibrillator paddles (or saline to the sponges) and to the patient's chest. (Do not use both electrode paste and saline.) The operator should ask the helper to charge the defibrillator, and apply the two standard defibrillator paddles to their appropriate positions: the negative (black) paddle just to the right of the upper half of the sternum below the clavicle and the positive (red) paddle just to the left of the cardiac apex or below the left nipple. Proper polarity facilitates quick lead ECG reading; it has no effect on the success of d.c. defibrillation. The two paddles should be pressed firmly over the sponges to the chest in the appropriate locations. The operator should press hard to force exhalation, as this decreases thoracic impedance. The ECG should be read, as picked up by the defibrillator chest paddles (or ECG electrodes already in place before the arrest), to ascertain VT or VF before triggering the defibrillating shock. When ready, the team should be asked to stand clear of the patient and bed, as the shock will jolt the patient (a convulsive motion caused by skeletal muscle stimulation) and may injure team members. One must know in advance the type of cardioscope-defibrillator in use, as some cardioscopes are protected, but others must be disconnected prior to countershock, lest they be damaged.

The defibrillator should have been preset for 200 J for the *first counter-shock* in an adult (3 J/kg); 2 J/kg for children. If unsuccessful, the second countershock of 300 J (4 J/kg) should be applied as rapidly as recharging permits, and the third and subsequent countershocks with maximal increases to 360 J in the adult (5 J/kg). The countershock is discharged by pushing the appropriate hand switches, preferably one on each paddle to avoid accidental discharge.

The defibrillating shocks are best applied by the individual who directs the CPR team. Immediately after this countershock, the 'quick look' paddles should be left on the chest and the ECG observed, and the carotid or femoral pulse checked, and IPPV and cardiac compressions resumed if no pulse is present. The procedure should be repeated if indicated.

After successful defibrillation (i.e. termination of VT or VF), the ECG may show electric asystole (without spontaneous pulse), abnormal or normal ECG complexes without pulse, or abnormal or normal ECG complexes with pulse. Irrespective of what the ECG monitor shows, cardiac compressions must be continued as long as there is no spontaneous carotid or femoral pulse. If the ECG shows asystole, CPR, epinephrine and bicarbonate must be continued as indicated.

If VT without pulse or VF persists or recurs after the first three electric countershocks of 200–300–360 J (70 kg adult) given in rapid succession, one should repeat CPR Steps A–B–C and countershocks with 360 J in adults (5 J/kg), with CPR between shocks so as not to permit periods of no blood flow (no chest compressions) of more than 10 seconds each. If several maximal energy (360 J) countershocks fail to terminate VF in spite of optimal cardiac compressions and IPPV, and reasonable amounts of epinephrine and bicarbonate have been used, lidocaine 1 mg/kg i.v. should be given. Lidocaine may be repeated and then switched to bretylium if necessary. Efforts to reverse VF with appropriate drug therapy (including bretylium) (see Drugs, above) and repeated high-energy countershocks should be continued until successful, or until irreversible asystole is certain, with signs of myocardial death (intractable electric asystole) of 30 minutes, or more heroic (invasive) measures, such as open-chest CPR or emergency cardiopulmonary bypass are tried.

One should not give up attempts to defibrillate until efforts have been made to improve acid–base status, oxygenation and vasoconstriction by epinephrine. Some patients have recovered consciousness after defibrillation following several hours of VF, during which time external CPR started promptly after collapse[456] must have produced viable cerebral blood flow. Such cases, however, are rare[151, 854].

In *witnessed ECG monitored VF*, a precordial thump should be applied while the defibrillator is charged; an external countershock should then be applied immediately if available, without first giving drugs or starting CPR Steps A–B–C. If unsuccessful, CPR should be started promptly (within 60 seconds of pulselessness) to minimize cerebral and myocardial hypoxia. Drugs should be administered and electric countershocks repeated. The sequence of actions should be adapted to parameters monitored and to the patient's underlying condition. Countershock is more likely to be successful if given 30–120 seconds following the i.v. administration of epinephrine, during CPR. One should, however, never delay the first countershocks to wait for CPR, epinephrine, intubation or bicarbonate. The large volume of bicarbonate takes a long time to be injected, and is rarely needed in witnessed arrest.

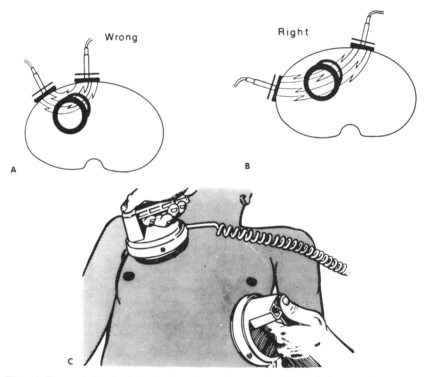

Fig. 49. External electric defibrillation via two bimanually triggered chest paddles applied on conductive jelly or saline-soaked sponge, one paddle just below the right clavicle, the other over the cardiac apex. The paddles incorporate defibrillation outlets and ECG leads. (A) Wrong paddle electrode placement: too close together, current shunted away from the heart. (B) Correct paddle electrode placement: wider spacing, more current through the heart. (From Ewy GA: Defibrillating cardiac arrest victims. *J Cardiovasc Med* 7: 28, 1982.) (C) External placement of 'quick ECG look' defibrillating paddle chest electrodes.

It is desirable to give at least the first three countershocks in rapid succession; if recharging time permits pauses between shocks shorter than 10 seconds each, resuming CPR Steps A–B–C between shocks may not be practical. If recharging takes more than 10 seconds CPR must be applied between shocks. Rapid serial defibrillation attempts are more easily accomplished using the a.c. defibrillator, which does not require recharging. Direct current defibrillators require a few seconds to recharge. Usually, cardiac compressions will have to be interposed between serial countershocks with use of a d.c. defibrillator.

Empirical countershock

In sudden witnessed cardiac arrest (patient unconscious, apneic or gasping, with no pulse in carotid and femoral arteries) with ECG confirmation of VF not available, giving one external d.c. countershock within 30 seconds, even before CPR Steps A–B–C, is acceptable.

This scenario is rare since cardioscope and ECG paddles have become integral components of d.c. defibrillators. Empirical (unmonitored) d.c. countershock for witnessed cardiac arrest is justifiable and safe since the risk of a single shock causing VF or heart damage is very low. Although each shock does cause very slight myocardial damage, myocardial anoxia may be more harmful. Unmonitored countershock in children is not recommended.

Experimental semi-invasive defibrillation techniques using *esophageal-to-chest* surface electrodes reduce the electric resistance between electrodes and therefore the total energy required; this has enabled development of very small portable defibrillators[226].

Technique for external electric defibrillation (Fig. 49)[23b, c]

1. Turn the main power switch *on*. Turn the synchronize switch of the defibrillator *off*.
2. Set the energy to be delivered to the desired reading, i.e. 200 J for adults (approx. 3 J/kg for adults; 2 J/kg for children).
3. Charge the paddles.
4. Lubricate the paddles with electrode paste. If CPR Steps A–B–C are ongoing, interrupt the rescuer's chest compressions as briefly as possible for the countershock, preferably 10 seconds, maximally 20 seconds. Place the paddles on the chest: one paddle just to the right of the upper sternum below the right clavicle, the other paddle just below and to the left of the left nipple.
5. Apply firm pressure with the paddles against the chest to reduce lung volume and electric resistance.
6. Confirm ECG diagnosis of VT or VF if possible.
7. Clear the area.
8. Fire the defibrillator by pushing the appropriate trigger(s). Preferably the defibrillator should have two switches, one on each handle to be pushed simultaneously.
9. Leave the paddles in place 5 seconds to ascertain ECG rhythm from paddle leads; if VT or VF continues, fire a second time with 300 J (4 J/kg) in adults; if VT or VF still continues, fire a third time with 360 J in adults (5 J/kg). (Use 2 J/kg in children for repeat shocks.) If pauses for 'quick look' at the ECG and for recharging the d.c. defibrillator take longer than 10 seconds before the first three shocks, use CPR Steps A–B–C in between.
10. After the first 1–3 shocks check the carotid or femoral pulse. If it is not palpable within 5 seconds, resume CPR Steps A–B–C.
11. If pulseless and VT or VF continues after 1 minute of CPR, repeat single shocks or series of three shocks (as above) using 360 J in adults (5 J/kg in adults; 2 J/kg in children) with CPR Steps A–B–C continued without interruptions of more than 10 seconds every 30–60 seconds; and drugs and fluids given as indicated (Fig. 2).
12. If the ECG shows low amplitude or a flat line, shift quick-look paddle electrodes 90° from the original position, because low-amplitude VF can masquerade as asystole.

Recommendations to *improve defibrillation success*[23b, c, 232, 237]

1. Defibrillation attempts should be as early as possible, even by trained emergency medical technicians.
2. VF may masquerade as asystole (reposition the paddle electrodes).
3. Correct electrode placement is crucial.
4. Transthoracic impedance should be low.
5. Create a good interface between the paddles and the chest wall.
6. Use heavy paddle electrode pressure.
7. Countershock with pressure on the chest with full exhalation.
8. The initial three shocks in adults should be about 200 J–300 J–360 J.
9. The time interval between shocks should be as brief as possible, merely for recharging and reconfirming the persistence of VF or VT on the oscilloscope.
10. In witnessed arrest, defibrillate before CPR if possible, but start CPR within 30–60 seconds. During CPR do not interrupt CPR longer than 10 seconds at a time for shocking and rechecking pulse and ECG.
11. Have a maintenance program for regular checks of defibrillators to *deliver* maximally 360 J.

Synchronized cardioversion[102, 483, 484, 877]

When electric countershock therapy is needed for VT with pulse or for supraventricular dysrhythmias, synchronization of the shock with the ECG complex can minimize the risk of producing VF. One should start with low-energy external shocks (e.g. 0.5–1.0 J/kg) placed in the refractory period of the cardiac cycle—not between R and T waves, so as not to induce VF. Synchronization takes time; therefore, in VT without pulse or with respiratory distress, hypotension or coma, regular unsynchronized cardioversion (defibrillation) is recommended. Modern apparatus for cardioversion detects the R-waves and synchronizes automatically.

Automatic External Electric Defibrillation[176, 193, 219]

Portable defibrillators which read the ECG, recognize VF and discharge countershocks automatically (automatic external defibrillators, AED) are the latest very promising advance in resuscitation technology[176]. The ECG VF pattern is diagnosed over 20–60 seconds and in the case of VF triggers a d.c. countershock. A period of up to 60 seconds to diagnose VF is acceptable. Their use has been shown already to permit defibrillation without delay by emergency medical technicians[176]. Recently their use in the hands of trained laypersons at home has also proved feasible[219]. These new devices (e.g. Laerdal, Physiocontrol) identify VF and deliver automatically external countershocks of 200 J[193]. They perform comparably to manual defibrillators[176]. They may help achieve more widespread early defibrillation in EMS systems which cannot train EMTs in manual defibrillation. The outcome potentials in the hands of laymen have not yet been evaluated, but seem great. In clinical trials, automatic external defibrillators have never shocked a patient inappropriately[176]. The hospital discharge rate was about the same with automatic external defibrillators in the hands of EMTs (28%) as with manual defibrillation (20%). The automatic device permitted shocking slightly faster than the manual device. Training time for use of the manual device is much longer than for use of the automatic device. For crucial immediate termination of VF, we suggest further miniaturization of automatic defibrillators, use by trained laypersons, and trials of VF-threatened patients temporarily using these devices strapped on.

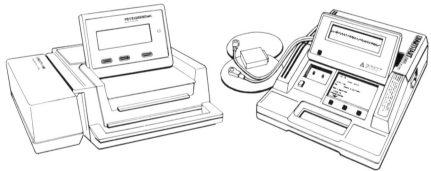

Fig. 50. Automatic external defibrillators. Examples of recently developed semi-automatic external defibrillator of Physio-Control (Lifepack 200) on the left, and of Laerdal (Heartstart 2000) on the right. These units are battery-powered and portable.

Automatic Internal (Implanted) Defibrillation[547, 548]

Automatic implanted defibrillators (AID) have been developed for ambulatory patients at risk of sudden death from VF[547, 548]. The defibrillators monitor the ECG continuously, recognize VF, and defibrillate with 10–20 J from a 250 g implanted biocompatible minidefibrillator, delivering the shock after 20 seconds of VF via two cup electrodes surgically applied over the apex and base of the heart. This result of over two decades of bioengineering efforts by Mirowski and colleagues[547], together with the introduction of a square wave form of countershock[776] which permitted miniaturization of the defibrillator, led to a system and surgical technique with encouraging preliminary clinical results[548]. In one study, 10 out of 23 patients with AID developed VF; all had VF reversed by the AID, and none died during over 1 year follow-up (Fogoros RN, Pittsburgh, 1986, personal communication). The present implantable defibrillators can monitor for 1–3 years and give 100 countershocks. Relative indications for implanting a defibrillator are primarily patients who after myocardial ischemia or infarction have had episodes of syncope, VT or VF, and in whom studies with programmed electric stimulation (dysrhythmia provocation test) including mapping of drug effects found them to be unresponsive to pharmacologic VF prophylaxis[286, 354]. Patients with severe left ventricular failure, and those who have been resuscitated from prehospital VF without evidence of infarction are also at risk of sudden cardiac death[440].

Emergency Cardiac Pacing[23b, c, 102, 995, 999]

For severe bradycardia, EMD or asystole (immediately after onset of syncope), when due to heart block (Stokes–Adams syndrome) with the heart still oxygenated (sudden witnessed arrest), rhythmic (e.g. 70 per minute) low-voltage electric cardiac stimulation can keep the heart beating. *External fist pacing*, i.e. repetitive manual thumping, is always immediately available (Chapters 1C and 4). Even mechanical thumpers are now available[998]. *External electric pacing* introduced in the 1950s[995] was given up because of painful muscle contractions and uncertain effectiveness, but has recently been reintroduced with technical modifications which have succeeded in overcoming these complications[995, 999]. *Transvenous (atrioventricular) pacing*, however, is the method of choice to be eventually established in the presence of spontaneous circulation[283, 890, 995, 997]. *Transthoracic wire pacing* is not recommended. Transthoracic pacemaker insertion takes time and interferes with CPR. Transthoracic intracardiac needle puncture for insertion of a pacing wire is risky.

Indications for pacing include severe sinus or ventricular bradycardia, AV blocks, atrial tachycardia and flutter, recurrent VT, and refractory asystole[283]. The heart must be oxygenated to respond to electric or mechanical stimuli with contractions, and the pink heart without AV block beats without pacing. One should not expect refractory EMD with myocardial hypoxia or acidosis to respond to pacing.

For external electric pacing[995, 999], d.c. shocks of 25–150 V of 2–3 milliseconds duration are applied about 75 times per minute, via two disk skin electrodes. The negative electrode is placed over the cardiac apex (V5 position), and the positive electrode rests over the third intercostal space to the left of the sternum. For internal pacing techniques, see the literature[23b, c, 102].

For temporary *transvenous* pacing, a catheter electrode is inserted percutaneously under ECG guidance into the right atrium or ventricle, via the subclavian, internal jugular, brachial or femoral vein. With insertion of a unipolar electrode (cathode), the indifferent electrode (anode) is placed on the skin. In bipolar electrodes the anode and cathode are in the heart. Unipolar electrodes are safer in terms of preventing inadvertent production of VF. Other possible complications of transvenous pacing include heart perforation, diaphragmatic contractions, and failure of electrode or pacemaker.

Pacing may be temporary (as in CPR cases) or long-term; it may be by fixed-rate (asynchronous, competitive) or by demand (standby) pacemaker[283]. The fixed-rate (nondemand) pacer is suitable only for third-degree AV block. There is a slight risk of an impulse occurring during the vulnerable moment of the spontaneous ECG, leading to VF. For patients with myocardial infarction, a demand pacemaker is recommended. The QRS-inhibited demand pacemaker does not stimulate when the spontaneous heart rate (R-wave) is above a preset level. Whenever the R-wave is not sensed, the pacemaker stimulates. The QRS-triggered demand pacemaker is triggered by the patient's QRS complexes to stimulate the ventricles artificially during refractory periods; without QRS for a preset time interval, the pacemaker stimulates. For patients with intact conduction, there are also AV sequential-demand pacemakers that give an atrial 'kick'. Atrial pacing is used to suppress atrial tachycardia.

Comment on Steps E and F: Dysrhythmias with pulselessness call for immediate resuscitative action. Dysrhythmias with a palpable pulse and consciousness call for thoughtful assessment and *treatment of the whole patient*, not merely the ECG.

Open-Chest Cardiopulmonary Resuscitation (Figs. 51, 52)

Cardiac resuscitation via thoracotomy[82, 851–853] was practiced widely inside hospitals before 1960, when external closed-chest CPR was introduced into clinical medicine[23a, 429, 720]. Open-chest CPR produced high survival rates with good brain function[61, 82, 208, 457, 696, 773, 852].

Open-chest cardiac defibrillation had been worked out in animals at the turn of this century[638], but was used in humans only after Beck's first case of defibrillation in 1947[61]. In 1953, Stephenson published a review of 1200 cases of cardiac arrest treated with open-chest CPR[852]; 28% went home; 14% of the resuscitation attempts were initiated outside the operating room (all inside the hospital), with a 17% survival rate. In autopsies, lacerations of the heart were seen in 10% of cases[6], but massage of up to 2.5 hours could lead to recovery[647, 774]. In 1981, McNulty (Pittsburgh) interviewed physicians who practiced open-chest CPR in the

1950s[185, 208, 380, 457, 647, 720, 852]. This revealed that physicians of various disciplines would perform open-chest CPR, even in emergency rooms and on wards. Restoration of spontaneous circulation with drugs, fluids and countershocks was facilitated by the visual control and touch provided. Most patients either recovered with good brain function (even after 1–2 hours of open-chest CPR), or they died. Infection was reportedly not a problem, even after thoracotomies without sterile techniques. The infection rate in one other study was only two of 43 patients, and the two cases were not lethal[18].

Since the rediscovery of external CPR[429], open-chest CPR has been used almost exclusively in cases of thoracic trauma[48, 49, 368, 516, 518, 556, 846, 847, 852]. In one study, the incidences of wound infection was 8–9% and the incidence of iatrogenic heart damage 0–1.4%; neurologic outcome results were encouraging[49].

Direct cardiac compressions produce better arteriovenous perfusion pressures and overall cerebral and coronary blood flows than do sternal compressions, since the latter increase overall intrathoracic pressure which in turn increases venous pressure simultaneously with arterial pressure. The open-chest technique (Fig. 52) produces higher arteriovenous perfusion pressures and, when cardiac massage is necessary for prolonged periods, also a better chance for sustaining cerebral and myocardial viability and restoring spontaneous circulation[16, 41, 42, 78–83, 118, 185, 650, 837]. In addition, open-chest CPR permits direct palpation and observation of the heart, which helps guide drug and fluid therapy and electric countershock in difficult protracted CPR efforts. Finally, the open chest also permits direct compression of a bleeding site in intrathoracic exsanguination and, in cases of intra-abdominal hemorrhage, allows temporary compression or clamping of the thoracic aorta above the diaphragm.

For most cases of cardiac arrest, closed-chest CPR has replaced open-chest CPR, because the external technique can be started without delay and can be performed by persons not trained in surgical techniques (i.e. outside the hospital). Many physicians fear the possible complications associated with thoracotomy, such as injury to heart and great vessels, and infection. However, in the hands of physicians with the necessary training, experience, skill and supplies, open-chest CPR is safe and hemodynamically superior to the closed-chest technique. To be effective, changing from external CPR to open-chest CPR must be as soon as possible after an adequate but brief trial of external CPR-ALS without restoration of spontaneous circulation[406a, 765b].

Indications for open-chest CPR[22b, 23b, 82]

Open-chest CPR requires a physician trained and experienced (at least in the animal laboratory) in thoracotomy and intratracheal continuous positive pressure ventilation (CPPV). At this time, most consider it appropriate only in the hospital. As re-appraised in recent years after new research, open-chest CPR is indicated—in the hands of trained physicians only—in circumstances for which it may be the only effective method of restoring life:

1. when the chest is already open (in the operating room);
2. in suspected intrathoracic trauma with uncontrollable hemorrhage leading to cardiac arrest, particularly from penetrating wounds of the heart; in crushing injury; in suspected cardiac tamponade; and following cardiothoracic surgery;
3. in suspected intra-abdominal trauma with arterial (aortic) exsanguination and pulselessness—thoracotomy enables CPR, arterial infusion and temporary clamping of the lower thoracic aorta for controlling bleeding in the abdomen, and initiation of cardiopulmonary bypass;
4. in suspected massive pulmonary embolism—here the open-chest technique permits breaking up or removing the emboli and also prompt initiation of cardiopulmonary bypass;
5. in cardiac arrest with hypothermia, where the open-chest CPR technique permits direct rewarming of the heart with warmed saline, which is necessary for defibrillation;
6. when no artificial carotid or femoral pulse is produced by standard external CPR, as is occasionally the case with chest or spine deformities or severe emphysema with barrel chest;
7. after suspected long arrest time, as in unwitnessed arrest, followed by inability of correctly performed external CPR with advanced life support (epinephrine and countershocks) promptly to restore spontaneous circulation within 5–10 minutes.

Indications 1–6 have already been part of national[23b, c] and international[720] recommendations; indication 7 is new; it is based on new thoughts and new research[16, 41, 53, 78–83, 118, 185, 720, 837].

In suspected *cardiac tamponade*, if time permits and the patient is not yet pulseless, rapid drainage of the pericardiac sac by needle puncture (alongside the xiphoid) may postpone or even obviate the need for thoracotomy. If the diagnosis is uncertain, the chest and pericardium should be opened and direct cardiac compressions started.

In cases of suspected exsanguinating *hemorrhage* into the *abdomen* (e.g.

trauma, ruptured aortic aneurysm), immediate application of the MAST can often restore a carotid pulse. Before removal of the MAST for emergency laparotomy, however, and in the case of pulselessness in such patients, emergency thoracotomy should be performed. Carried out on the left side, this procedure permits not only open-chest CPR and aortic infusion but also occlusion of the lower thoracic aorta for temporary hemostasis, to permit removal of the MAST and laparotomy for surgical repair of the aorta[858].

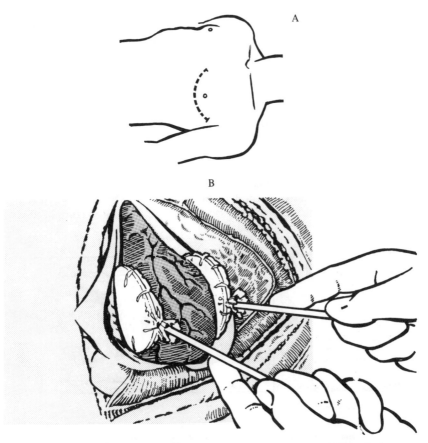

Fig. 51. Open-chest cardiopulmonary resuscitation. (A) Open the chest through the fourth or fifth left intercostal space. Grasp and rhythmically compress the heart as described in the text. (B) Internal direct electric defibrillation. When fibrillation is felt, apply the electrodes and countershock, first with the pericardium closed. (If possible, have electrodes prepared with tied-on saline-soaked gauze.) Apply the internal electrodes as illustrated, wearing rubber gloves, and release the shock (see text). (From Johnson, *Surgery of the Chest*, Chicago, Year Book Medical Publ., 1952.)

Open-chest CPR requires tracheal intubation and continuous positive pressure ventilation (IPPV + PEEP = CPPV) to maintain the lungs expanded while the thorax is open. Concerning hand positions for heart compressions, a recent controlled study in dogs using 60 compressions per minute[53] revealed that perfusion pressures and common carotid blood flows were high when the heart was compressed against the sternum, equally high when heart compressions were with both hands, but relatively lower with use of one hand. If using one hand only, the thumb should be placed posteriorly over the left ventricle, as it can easily perforate the right ventricle (Fig. 52).

As it concerns *personnel*, open-chest CPR is advanced life support by physicians with training and experience in the method, not only surgeons. In the absence of training, external CPR should be used. Dog laboratory practice sessions, used effectively before 1960 for open-chest CPR training[457, 720], are no longer available for all medical students and physicians. Therefore, a realistic open-chest CPR training manikin is needed.

There is considerable evidence to suggest that open-chest CPR may be more efficacious than external CPR and that the risks of thoracotomy are acceptable. Patients who respond to external CPR with advanced life support with resumption of spontaneous normotension within the first 5–10 minutes are unlikely to benefit from open-chest CPR. The benefit to nonresponders, however, may be great, provided open-chest CPR is not started too late for any method to be effective[268]. Open-chest CPR and emergency cardiopulmonary bypass (see below) should be compared with

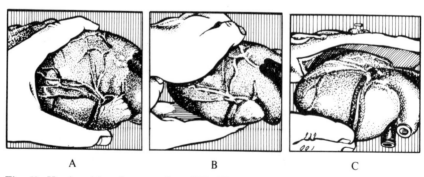

A   B   C

Fig. 52. Hand positions for open-chest CPR. The operator stands on the patient's left side facing cephalad. After thoracotomy, insert the left hand and pump the heart (first without opening the pericardium) either with your thumb posteriorly over the left ventricle and your fingers anteriorly over the right ventricle (A); or with two hands, using palm of your left hand over the right ventricle and fingers 2–5 of your right hand over the left ventricle posteriorly (B); or using fingers 2–5 of your right hand posteriorly over the left ventricle compressing the heart against the sternum upward (C). Methods shown in B and C give better blood flow and are less fatigueing and less traumatic than the method shown in A. (From Barnett WM, et al: *Ann Emerg Med* **13:** 397, 1984[53].)

(prolonged) external CPR attempts in controlled animal outcome experiments, and in a randomized prospective clinical trial, for use in victims of prolonged (unwitnessed) cardiac arrest[82].

Evaluation of open-chest CPR[82]

With the hemodynamic superiority of open-chest CPR over standard external CPR established, the question remains: When does opening the chest offer an advantage? We believe that the indications for open-chest CPR ought to be re-evaluated clinically, and its indications widened, to include cases of prolonged arrest time and failure of external CPR with drugs and countershock to promptly restart spontaneous circulation (indication 7 above). The physiologic superiority of open-chest CPR over all external CPR methods so far studied, in terms of overall blood flow, cerebral blood flow, coronary blood flow, ease of restarting spontaneous circulation, and cerebral outcome, has been convincingly established by clinical observations and experimental work[16, 53, 78–83, 118, 185, 208, 262, 380, 457, 765, 773, 837, 852, 874, 937, 949]. Open-chest CPR (not external CPR methods) can be relied upon to produce perfusion pressures adequate for the required cerebral and coronary blood flows of at least 20% of normal, even after several minutes of no blood flow. There seems to be more blood flow going to the brain than to the face during open-chest CPR,[837] and more to the face than to the brain during external CPR.[78–83] Direct heart compressions squeeze the ventricles only and not the veins, while chest compressions also squeeze the intrathoracic veins and atria. High venous and low perfusion pressures limit the efficacy of external CPR.[502] In patients, during open-chest CPR higher arterial, lower venous and higher perfusion pressures and higher cardiac output were measured as compared with external CPR[185].

Technique for open-chest CPR (Figs. 51, 52)[53, 82, 380, 720, 852]

1. *Thoracotomy.* After initiation of external CPR by a bystander, you, the physician operator, establish tracheal intubation and CPPV (Figs. 21, 25). Ascertain one of the above seven indications; get a knife, preferably sterile, and proceed. *Cut* through skin and muscle directly overlying the fourth or fifth left intercostal space. Pierce the intercostal structures bluntly with the knife handle or bandage scissors and tear open the intercostal space with your fingers. Insert a rib spreader if available (Fig. 51).
2. Immediately *compress the heart*, without at first opening the pericardium. A gloved hand is desirable but use a bare hand if a sterile glove is not available. Standing on the patient's left side, facing cephalad, insert your (left) hand through the thoracotomy incision, place your thumb over the left (thick-walled) ventricle (posteriorly)

and fingers 2–5 over the right (thin-walled) ventricle, anteriorly, in front of the heart. Take care not to pierce the atria or ventricles. When feasible, use one hand behind and one hand in front of the heart to compress it, or place all the fingers of one hand posterior of the heart and compress it against the sternum (Fig. 52). Compress about once per second and adjust the compression force and rate to filling of the heart.

Ask a helper to give i.v. fluid load and epinephrine.

3. First while compressing (and pausing only briefly) try to diagnose VF through the closed pericardium (feel worm-like motions of VF). If you are not certain, open the pericardium, but take care not to interrupt compressions or to injure the heart, vagus nerve or phrenic nerve. In intractable VF or when the first dose of epinephrine has failed to restart cardiac action, open the pericardium to allow direct inspection of the heart and to prevent injury to coronary vessels from multiple needle punctures.

4. *Drug therapy*. When drugs are necessary, have them given i.v. or inject them into the cavity of the left ventricle, *not* into the myocardium. Left ventricular blood must be freely aspirated. Use a 22–25 gauge (thin) needle. Avoid coronary vessels.

(a) Start with epinephrine, 0.5 mg/70 kg.

(b) Atropine and lidocaine may also be given safely via the intracardiac route.

(c) Do *not* give bicarbonate intracardiac—use the i.v. route.

5. *Defibrillation*. Ask a helper to prepare defibrillator and *internal* (presterilized) electrodes. Ideally they should be 6 cm in diameter (4 cm for children; 2 cm for infants).

(a) Use two *paddle electrodes*, with saline-soaked gauze pads attached, with insulated handles.

(b) Place one electrode behind the heart over the left ventricle, the other over the anterior surface of the heart.

(c) *d.c. countershock* is preferred. Have control over the switch that releases the countershock.

(d) Start with 0.5 J/kg (*25 to 50 J* in the average adult). If shock is ineffective at this low energy level, increase the energy level gradually with subsequent shocks. Some recommend to start with 0.25 J/kg (10 J in adults). High-energy shocks applied directly to the heart are more likely than external countershock to produce heart damage, including myocardial burns.

If only external electrodes are available, have a helper countershock externally through the chest wall (with 360 J); remove your hands from the chest and stand back. If only alternating current is available, it is also effective. The a.c. internal defibrillator setting should deliver 110–220 V shocks of 0.1–0.25 seconds duration. If no defibrillator is available, connect two metal spoons—held in rubber-gloved hands—

to a cord with regular male wall plugs, and have a helper briefly push the plug into a wall outlet (110 or 220 V a.c.). This is dangerous and produce myocardial damage.

Do not attempt open-chest CPR without endotracheal tube and controlled ventilation with IPPV plus PEEP (CPPV) (Fig. 21). The self-refilling bag–valve unit should be used with a PEEP valve (Fig. 25). Mouth-to-mouth ventilation during thoracotomy is feasible, but difficult.

Extracorporeal Oxygenation and Circulation (Fig. 53)

Emergency cardiopulmonary bypass[758]

The heart–lung machine was originally developed for the provision of cardiopulmonary bypass (CPB), usually by venoarterial pumping of blood via an oxygenator, to enable open-heart surgery[273]. It was tried for the treatment of cardiogenic shock and given up[47, 677, 864]. It soon became evident during extracorporeal circulation for open-heart surgery[618] that CPB during restarting of perfusion following elective circulatory arrest permits full control over perfusion pressure, flow, temperature and composition of the perfusing fluid. The replacement of the disc and bubble oxygenators of the 1950s and 1960s, which produce blood trauma and limit the safe use of CPB to 1–2 hours, by the less traumatic membrane oxygenators resulted in the safe use of CPB over many hours, even days[984]. The potential of CPB without thoracotomy for emergency resuscitation in addition to or instead of standard external CPR has not been explored for widespread clinical use. We believe that this potential is considerable[758].

Patients dying from massive pulmonary thromboembolism have sometimes been resuscitated from severe shock states, occasionally even from pulselessness, with rapidly begun CPB[517]. These applications were with closed thorax and cannulation by cutdown of femoral artery and vein, in conjunction with CPR for pulselessness, and in preparation for open-heart surgery. Other clinical trials have been for rapid reversal of exposure (hypothermia)-induced cardiac arrest[453, 899]. Bypassing the left ventricle only has been effective, but requires thoracotomy[621, 879]. Limitations for CPB proved to be primarily (a) the time required for inserting a large-bore tube into the venae cavae and cannulating the femoral artery, while the patient is being bounced by external CPR; and (b) the nonavailability of a small portable emergency pump oxygenator primed with plasma substitute. Portable emergency pump oxygenators are now available[462, 517, 637].

The first experimental outcome evaluation of CPB for cardiac arrest was made by Bozhiev in the 1970s[97]. He reported complete recovery of five out of six dogs after 15 minutes of normothermic complete circulatory arrest, using 20 minutes of CPB. Because anesthesia was with barbiturate, the dogs were pre-heparinized and the CPB apparatus was primed with banked blood—clinically unrealistic conditions—the results, although encouraging, were inconclusive. We were encouraged in exploring CPB for CPR by Negovsky's and our observations in the 1960s that in exsanguination brief arterial reinfusion with epinephrine can perfuse the coronaries retrograde and restart cardiac contractions[410, 578]; by our observations in the 1970s that immediate post-CPR arterial hemodilution and heparinization can lead to improved survival and cerebral outcome[733]; and by others' research[640]. We therefore conducted between 1982 and 1987 six dog studies[758]. In *Study 1*, after 20 minutes of normothermic VF cardiac arrest (no flow), CPB of 2 hours (without CPR) enhanced cardiovascular resuscitability over that with external CPR with advanced life support[120]. In *Study II*, asphyxial cardiac arrest of up to 90 minutes of ice water submersion could be reversed to stable spontaneous circulation with CPB for perfusion and rewarming[894]. Studies I and II were short-term and not designed to evaluate cerebral recovery. In *Study III*[637] after 12.5 minutes of normothermic VF cardiac arrest (no flow), CPB oxygenated the myocardium so well that 1–2 countershocks at 1–2 minutes of CPB effectively defibrillated and led to spontaneous normotension in all 10 dogs. After CPB over 2 hours for assisted circulation, seven of 10 survived long-term intensive care and five of the 10 were conscious, but only one neurologically normal. Only 6 of 10 control dogs had spontaneous circulation returned with CPR-ALS and the two long-term survivors remained comatose. The hearts in the CPB group did not show the hemorrhagic contusions seen in the CPR group. In *Study IV*[462] after 4 minutes of VF cardiac arrest (no flow) followed by 30 minutes of CPR Steps A–B–C for BLS (low flow), CPB for restoration of spontaneous circulation and 1 hour assisted circulation gave better long-term recovery than CPR-ALS; survival with complete neurologic recovery was achieved in seven of 10 with CPB versus two of 10 with CPR-ALS. Both groups suffered cardiac trauma from CPR. In *Study V*[29a], VF cardiac arrest of 10 minutes (no flow) plus CPR of 10 minutes (low flow) were followed by CPB, as compared with CPR-ALS; cardiovascular and cerebral recovery was possible with both methods, but more reliably with CPB. CPR-ALS was surprisingly effective because of optimal technique. The controlled reperfusion and assisted circulation possible with CPB, have so far, · *Study VI*[663a], led to good neurologic outcome after up to 15 minutes of normothermic total circulatory arrest, and to restoration of spontaneous circulation after up to 20 minutes of cardiac arrest.

The superiority of CPB over external and probably also over open-chest CPR in promptly restarting perfusion, even after very prolonged cardiac arrest, is apparent. CPB might help enhance conscious survival. It is not yet clear how CPB, which requires several minutes of preparation to be started, would fit into the clinical cardiac arrest–CPR–advanced life support sequence, and whether or not short-term versus long-term (assisted) CPB post-arrest would enhance outcome with better cardiac and cerebral function, as compared to closed-chest or open-chest CPR followed by spontaneous circulation. Since normothermic cardiac arrest of up to 10–20 minutes in man should theoretically be reversible as far as brain recovery potential is concerned, cardiac resuscitability by closed-chest CPR becomes a limiting factor. In this, CPB is competing with open-chest CPR.

Clinical feasibility trials of emergency CPB after prolonged cardiac arrest should be initiated. These should be followed by controlled randomized patient studies. In the laboratory, CPB permits control of reperfusion to test novel brain resuscitation agents, which without CPB might depress spontaneous circulation. In the future some form of closed-chest emergency CPB, with portable apparatus primed with plasma substitute, may become part of the emergency resuscitation armamentarium of physicians inside and outside hospitals.

One possible *technique*, which is probably useful for controlled and assisted circulation and artificial oxygenation, would be similar to the one we have used in studies III–VI above[29a, 462, 517, 637, 785, 663a] (Fig. 53): (1) a rapid

Cardiopulmonary Bypass Circuit Diagram

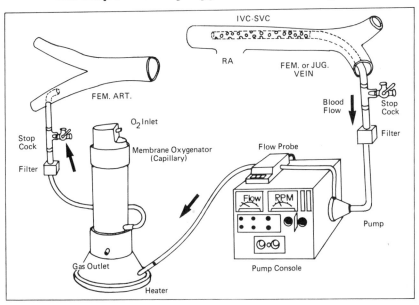

Fig. 53. Portable emergency cardiopulmonary bypass device for resuscitation, with veno-arterial pumping (e.g. Biomedicus centrifugal self-regulating pump) via oxygenator (e.g. Scimed membrane oxygenator) and heat exchanger. Used with priming by plasma substitutes. Vascular access by small femoral cutdown. Multiple-hole large-bore long venae cavae cannula; short large-bore femoral artery cannula. See text[785].

method for inserting a long, large-bore, multiple-hole catheter via the femoral vein into the inferior plus superior venae cavae, and a standard cannula into the femoral artery; (2) draining venous return via a crude filter (there can be intravascular clotting during prolonged cardiac arrest) into a reservoir or a self-regulating pump and fluid administration port; (3) continuing the circuit through a pump (e.g. self-regulating nonocclusive centrifugal Biomedicus pump); (4) a membrane oxygenator; (5) a heat exchanger; (6) a blood filter with bubble trap and injection port; and (7) returning arterial blood into the large-bore femoral artery cannula. Desirable features include a small priming volume of plasma substitute, with still undetermined novel cerebral resuscitation agents added. Heparin (one-half of the fully heparinizing dose in the priming volume and one-half injected into the venae cavae cannulae) should keep the system clot-free. In the future, nonthrombogenic material for the entire circuit will become available, including oxygenators[76a]. This would make artificial circulation by extracorporeal means a futuristic resuscitation approach for medical, surgical and trauma cases. The pumping capacity must allow flows exceeding the patient's normal cardiac output.

Intra-aortic balloon counterpulsation[396]

This method is presently the most popular one for assisted circulation in cardiogenic shock[396, 771, 836]. A special balloon catheter is inserted via the femoral artery into the thoracic aorta. Electrically controlled, heartbeat-synchronized abrupt inflation of the balloon during each diastole and deflation during each systole causes an increase in diastolic ascending aorta pressure (and thus an increase in myocardial blood flow), and a decrease in peripheral resistance (afterload). This method requires a specialized team and expensive apparatus.

Intra-aortic balloon counterpulsation in itself does not seem to improve the low survival rates in cardiogenic shock (10–30%), but helps in supporting life during preparation for a surgically correctable cardiac lesion (e.g. unstable anigna with left coronary artery occlusion), and during weaning of certain patients to stable spontaneous circulation after heart surgery. There has been no controlled study of the possible benefit of this method after cardiac arrest; this is desirable since cardiac output after cardiac arrest can be very low. Other methods for assisted circulation in semi-experimental use include noninvasive external counterpulsation (by pressure suit); and more invasive left heart (without need for oxygenator) and total (with oxygenator) cardiopulmonary bypass pumping (see above).

Extracorporeal membrane oxygenation[984]

When the cardiovascular system functions well, but pulmonary oxygenation failure is resistant to IPPV with high PEEP and supportive measures, extracorporeal membrane oxygenation (ECMO) has been tried[54, 273, 344, 984].

This technique entails prolonged (up to several days) partial bypass pumping of unsaturated venous or arterial blood via an oxygenator, back into a large artery or vein. It requires 24-hour coverage with a highly trained, multidisciplinary critical care team, which must provide bedside vigilance. For this reason, ECMO is appropriate only in large regional centers, i.e. Category I referral hospitals.

A multi-institutional trial of ECMO has given disappointing results[984]. Most of the deaths were from hemorrhage, particularly intracranial hemorrhage in cases of trauma, related to the heparinization required to keep the extracorporeal circuit open. Research on improved technology of ECMO, particularly nonthrombogenic surfaces, and on lung healing may in the future result in a wider and earlier application of ECMO. At this time, increasingly sophisticated respiratory care without ECMO, including IMV with high PEEP, has reduced to a very small figure the number of patients with acute respiratory insufficiency in whom ECMO might be justified. For this reason and because of the uncertain benefits of ECMO, the technique is warranted only in very carefully selected patients—mostly neonates.

According to recommendations of the National Institutes of Health (USA), ECMO[984] is indicated in: (1) patients in whom, despite IPPV with optimized PEEP over 5 cm H_2O and FIO_2 of 100%, PaO_2 has been less than 50 mmHg for more than 2 hours; and (2) patients like those above, but in whom PaO_2 has been less than 50 mmHg for more than 12 hours on FIO_2 of 60% or more and a shunt of over 30% has developed. Also, $PaCO_2$ must be 30–45 mmHg when the indication is considered, the lung failure must be potentially reversible, and the patient must have a reasonable chance for quality survival without severe brain damage. Indications for ECMO must be based on good clinical judgment, and it must not be undertaken until optimized CPPV, diuresis, colloid osmotic pressure normalization, chest physiotherapy, antibiotics, steroids, normothermia, sedation, paralysis, and optimal circulatory, metabolic, acid–base and fluid balance have all been tried. Obviously, these stringent indications will change when the technique becomes safer in the future.

Extracorporeal lung assist[76a, 265, 426, 563, 761, 888a]

A safer and more promising approach to long-term respiratory resuscitation for reversible lung failure seems to be extracorporeal lung assist (ECLA). This concept, introduced by Gattinoni and Kolobow primarily for carbon dioxide removal[265, 426], and by Terasaki and Morioka for oxygenation and carbon dioxide removal[888a], has as its primary objective the avoidance of intratracheal mechanical ventilation. In severe potentially reversible pulmonary shunting (e.g. ARDS, aspiration, overwhelming pneumonitis) or decompensated chronic lung disease, the early application of very low flow partial lung bypass (low-flow veno-arterial or veno-venous pumping via membrane oxygenator), continued for days, has maintained survivable blood gas values in some spontaneously breathing patients with tracheal intubation, and supported them to recovery by 'resting' the lungs to heal.

Contraindications to ECMO or ECLA include: (1) sepsis; (2) irreversible obstructive and destructive lung disease; and (3) irreversible severe central nervous system damage or cardiac function impaired to the extent that a worthwhile existence after recovery from lung failure is impossible.

The *techniques* of ECMO and ECLA are beyond the scope of this chapter. Personnel should study the literature and send a team to an existing program. Among the circuits tried, pumping from the venae cavae (nonocclusive drainage via femoral vein) into the ascending aorta (via the femoral artery) results in better cerebral oxygenation and pulmonary decongestion (required for lung healing) than 5–10% veno-venous pumping for ECLA. For ECMO, bypass flows up to 60–70% of cardiac output were used. Lower flows should be tried early in lethal pulmonary failure. The effects of prophylactic ECMO or ECLA on lung healing should be studied. Full heparinization should increasingly become unnecessary, as long-term chemical bonding of heparin to plastic surfaces is being perfected[76a]. The lungs are ventilated with FIO_2 at 50%, slight PEEP, at a slow rate. Hematologic effects other than heparinization are usually harmless, since the ECMO- and ECLA-induced thrombocytopenia, denaturation of proteins, and hemolysis are mild and reversible.

Concluding Comments on Advanced Life Support

The mechanics of heart and chest compressions in cardiac arrest must be considered a stopgap measure. Optimally performed, standard external CPR, if started immediately upon collapse, can sustain brain viability by providing the critical 20% of normal cerebral blood flow. Even several hours of external CPR have occasionally resulted in cerebral recovery. If not started immediately, CPR times over 20 minutes have rarely resulted in complete cerebral recovery. The longer initiation of external CPR is delayed, i.e. the longer the arrest time without CPR, the less reliable will be the ability of external CPR to reperfuse the brain and reperfuse and restart the heart. Because of the importance of the *time factor* for ultimate intact survival, every effort must be made in cases of cardiac arrest to restart spontaneous circulation immediately, through bystander CPR Steps A–B–C, and after restoration of spontaneous circulation to combat any shock state and thereby minimize the multiple organ systems failure of the post-resuscitation syndrome.

Restoration of spontaneous circulation happens only occasionally with CPR Steps A–B–C alone (as in asphyxial cardiac arrest); it usually requires advanced life support measures, such as i.v. drugs and fluids (Step D), ECG diagnosis (Step E) and fibrillation treatment (Step F). In monitored witnessed arrest, a chest thump and/or electric countershocks (if immediately available) should precede Steps A–B–C, but not delay CPR Steps A–B–C for more than 30–60 seconds. Steps D–E–F should follow as rapidly as possible. Epinephrine i.v. or intratracheal and early defibrillation are still the most important measures. Automatic external defibrillation looks promising. If spontaneous circulation cannot be restored within a few minutes, open-chest CPR for emergency cardiopulmonary bypass may be tried, provided the team is trained and the hospital is appropriately equipped.

Note: Advanced *trauma* life support (ATLS) consists of many resuscitation techniques described above in Chapters 1 and 2, and subsequently in Chapter 3. They are summarized under ATLS in Chapter 4.

PHASE III:

PROLONGED LIFE SUPPORT
Post-Resuscitative
Brain-Oriented Therapy
Cerebral Resuscitation

Chapter 3

Introduction

Phase III of CPCR (Fig. 2), prolonged life support (PLS), is long-term resuscitation; that is, intensive care life support for multiple organ failure. It consists of a combination for which, for memorizing, we have extended the alphabet: Steps *G. gauging* (that is, evaluation and critical care triage); *H, humanizing* the outcome by brain resuscitation measures; and *I, intensive* therapy for general life support[713–715, 720]. These measures require an understanding of the pathophysiologic derangements of the post-resuscitation syndrome (Figs. 54–56) and considerable medical judgment and skills. Steps G, H and I should be taught and applied simultaneously, since long-term life support after emergency resuscitation (Tables 4 and 5) should be brain-oriented (Tables 6 and 7) and applied with reason (Tables 8–10)[721, 722, 739, 747, 758–760]. The latter entails estimation of the severity of the insult (Table 8); evaluation of early predictive criteria, most of which are still under investigation (Table 9); long-term outcome evaluation (Table 10); and criteria and methods for discontinuing resuscitation efforts (Tables 11 and 12). *Copy and use Tables 4–12 as check lists.*

The socioeconomic impact of brain injury secondary to cardiac arrest, stroke, other anoxic states and cerebral trauma is enormous. This impact falls in varying degrees on the sufferer, his family and society. The patient's outcome in terms of survival and overall performance capability (particularly human mentation) depends on the severity and duration of the insult, the speed and quality of emergency resuscitation, and the early start and quality of brain-oriented, post-resuscitative intensive therapy. While such post-resuscitative treatment cannot alter the initial insult, it has been shown to influence *secondary changes* that occur in all vital organ systems after the start of reperfusion and reoxygenation, i.e. 'post-resuscitation disease'[577–580, 749, 759]. Much money and indescribable anguish are drained each year into the long-term nursing care of permanently unconscious 'survivors' of anoxic, traumatic and other cerebral insults[305–308, 634, 635, 929]. Therefore, experimental and clinical searches for brain resuscitation potentials must be accompanied by research into reliable measures to prognosticate outcome with permanent severe brain damage as well as ethical, legal and dignified ways of terminating resuscitation efforts in cases of brain death[300, 305–308].

After several hours of long-term life support, the degree of recovery at each point in time should be noted in terms of 'overall and cerebral performance capability' (Table 10). In case of suspected brain death, orderly brain death determination must be carried out (Table 11). In cases

229

of persistent vegetative state without brain death, 'letting die' is considered ethical and senseless prolongation of the dying process, unethical (Table 12)[24, 168, 635, 929].

Historically, before the 1950s, when modern emergency resuscitation and intensive care were initiated, prevailing perceptions of what resuscitation could accomplish were based on experiences with emergency measures in the absence of post-resuscitative intensive therapy. There was no meaningful support of extracerebral vital organ functions. These perceptions included the observation that normothermic cardiac arrest longer than 4–5 minutes cannot be reversed to normal brain function[154, 342]. *We now know that with advanced brain-oriented post-CPR intensive therapy (special life support throughout unconsciousness), cardiac arrests much longer than 5 minutes can occasionally, although inconsistently, be reversed to complete recovery*[2–4, 106, 759]. Although this challenge for cerebral resuscitation meets complex problems[628] and no breakthrough has yet occurred, systematic research is justified, based on cautious optimism[759, 760].

In the 1950s and 1960s modern long-term resuscitation (intensive therapy) was introduced systematically through the first physician-controlled intensive care units (ICUs) in Europe[150, 352, 364, 436, 590, 594, 595, 849] and America[66, 238, 630, 711, 717, 735]. Most patients admitted to ICUs in the 1950s did not have cardiac arrest, but rather respiratory failure from poisoning, poliomyelitis, trauma or major operations. In the 1960s, increasing attention was paid to life support for victims of cerebral trauma[448, 493]. For victims of stroke (focal brain ischemia, cerebral hemorrhage), research has been carried out since the turn of the century, but resuscitation and life support, although available, have generally not been used and evaluated. The advent of external CPR in 1960 brought an increasing number of comatose CPR survivors into ICUs.

In spite of ICU support, many immediate survivors of CPR attempts developed secondary brain death or cardiac failure within days, and 10–40% of long-term survivors remained with permanent brain damage[2–4, 153, 216, 465, 466, 831]. The concept of 'hearts too good to die', introduced by Beck in the 1950s[62], justified a concerted attack on sudden cardiac death through worldwide programs for training and delivery of CPR basic and advanced life support[23, 720]. The concept of 'brains too good to die' after cardiac arrest, introduced by Safar around 1970[392, 722, 737], was based on the reversibility of (treatable) secondary pathologic changes[27, 357–359, 473, 474, 580, 733, 825]. This initiated research into 'brain resuscitation' after cardiac arrest[733, 734], which extended CPR to CPCR[720]. Indeed, one of the first post-cardiac arrest animal studies showed the possibility of successfully combating secondary changes after reperfusion and thereby improving outcome[733]. The first extensive long-term animal outcome studies revealed the profound effect that extracerebral complications and the prevention of reversal with prolonged post-arrest life support might have on cerebral outcome[92, 745].

Negovsky had coined the term 'post-resuscitation disease'[580] (we prefer the term 'post-resuscitation syndrome') for multiple organ failure after clinical death and emergency resuscitation[749, 759]. This syndrome proved to affect primarily the brain, but also to some extent the extracerebral organs, even when blood pressure, blood gases and blood composition were controlled by prolonged intensive care[760]. Thus, brain-oriented intensive care life support[722, 737, 743] is based on general intensive therapy for conscious patients with multiple organ systems failure[736b, 799].

Concerning clinical death, we are engaged in pursuing three goals simultaneously: (1) determine biologic limits; (2) develop therapeutic potentials; and (3) develop predictive measurements. As of 1987, this rapidly changing field of cerebral resuscitation research has seen hope and some progress, but still awaits a breakthrough.

In sudden total circulatory arrest, brain tissue oxygen stores are exhausted in 10 seconds[683, 806] and brain glucose and ATP in 5 minutes[535, 806]. Under ideal experimental conditions, however, some cerebral neurons seem to tolerate complete normothermic ischemia of up to 20 minutes[28], and perhaps even 60 minutes[357, 358]. However, no specific therapy has yet been identified by which such long periods of cardiac arrest can be reproducibly reversed to complete recovery in animals or humans.

At least six post-cardiac arrest treatments currently in various stages of exploration have been shown, in long-term animal outcome models of global brain ischemia or cardiac arrest, to ameliorate post-ischemic brain damage (compared with 'usual' post-arrest care), but not with certainty or reproducibility. These treatments, which are discussed later in this chapter, are[759]:

1. general brain-oriented life support by protocol (recommended for general clinical use);
2. intracarotid hypertensive hemodilution (still experimental);
3. barbiturates (which have undergone controlled clinical trial and have adjunctive value, but are not recommended for routine clinical use);
4. calcium-entry blockers (promising; now undergoing controlled clinical trials);
5. free radical scavengers (still experimental);
6. etiology-specific multifaceted treatment protocols (still to be worked out in the laboratory).

Although the results derived from semi-empirical studies of brain resuscitation potentials after global ischemic anoxia have not yet yielded the hoped-for breakthrough, we have shown that monkeys, dogs and patients can occasionally recover with normal neurologic function after up to 17 minutes of global head ischemia and up to 12 minutes of cardiac arrest[2-4, 106, 277–280, 720, 733, 760, 911]. The importance of brain resuscitation research crosses over many clinical areas. If novel treatment protocols under investigation proved effective in preventing or ameliorating secondary brain damage after cardiac arrest, they would, perhaps in modified form, also prove effective after conditions that more often injure young people (i.e. severe shock, polytrauma, cerebral trauma, and cerebral hemorrhage)[45]. The protocols also might be effective in victims of stroke[349] and encephalitis[511, 737, 738, 834]. Relevance of CPCR research results for transplantation medicine is considerable: (1) increasing the availability of donors with brain death (and in the future perhaps also those with cerebral death); (2) prolonging survival time of harvested organs (preischemic protective therapy) to make transplantation surgery elective and thereby less expensive; (3) helping prevent early rejection of organs due to reoxygenation injury (postischemic resuscitative therapy); (4) helping develop methods to determine viability of organs; (5) improving the management of donors for multiple organ harvesting; (6) developing a bridge from emergency resuscitation attempts to heart transplantations, through prolonged cardiopulmonary bypass and other measures.

Post-Resuscitation Syndrome (Figs. 54, 55, 56)

After cardiac arrest of several minutes' duration and subsequent restoration of spontaneous normotension, followed by unconsciousness of at least several hours, the patient usually suffers from multiple organ failure, which may last several days. Negovsky was the first, in the 1950s, to describe this 'post-resuscitation disease' in cardiac arrest animal models; cardiovascular-pulmonary, hepatic, renal, hematologic, metabolic and endocrine derangements occurred without post-arrest control of normotension, blood gases and other vital parameters[580]. We have found this post-resuscitation syndrome (PRS) to include protracted tissue acidosis and reduced cardiac output[393] which probably result from a combination of microcirculatory obstruction and cardiac failure, even in the presence of controlled normotension and blood gases[121, 134, 748, 821]. With controlled ventilation, we found no pulmonary failure. Clinically, the situation may be complicated by aspiration syndrome, flail chest from sternal compressions, acute pulmonary edema from left heart failure, or progressive pulmonary consolidation—adult respiratory distress syndrome (ARDS), shock lung—from protracted hypoperfusion, trauma or sepsis. Special post-arrest life support challenges are posed by near-drowning, septic shock, blood loss, acute intracranial mass lesion, spinal cord injury, intoxication and anesthesia accidents (Chapter 4).

Total circulatory arrest without reperfusion leads to uniform tissue *autolysis*, which probably starts in the brain after only 1–2 hours of no blood flow[389]. When *reperfusion* is delayed after 5 minutes or more of cardiac arrest, it provokes multifocal reperfusion failure, which is proved to occur in the brain[27, 388] and suspected in other organs, and which represents the main component of the post-resuscitation syndrome (Fig. 54). Complex secondary changes may develop[582, 584, 736a, 759, 760]; some of these are documented, but others as well as their interactions are still only hypotheses. The end results are known as typical histopathologic damage patterns throughout the brain[108, 277, 296a, 540, 558–560, 581, 641, 910, 911].

We *hypothesize*[737, 759, 760] that cerebral recovery from cardiac arrest is hampered by the interaction of the following three secondary derangements: (1) cerebral reperfusion failure, from multifocal initial no reflow to global hypoperfusion, which may last 1–3 days (Fig. 55)[27, 64, 474, 580, 825]; (2) cerebral reoxygenation injury (cell necrotizing cascades resembling oxygen poisoning), perhaps triggered by free radical reactions and calcium shifts, leading to lipid peroxidation (Fig. 56)[32, 230, 759, 770, 806, 807, 958, 959]—proved in some extracerebral organs[104], but merely suspected for brain ischemia; and (3) cerebral intoxication due to ischemic damage of extracerebral organs, such as leaking gastrointestinal tract and hepatic failure (hypothesis only)[580]. The fourth factor, which may tie these together, is blood, made toxic and more viscous by stasis, interacting with tissue[320, 321, 421]. We hypothesize that after clarification of these factors, combinations of etiology-specific therapies directed at these derangements can improve functional and morphologic recovery of all organ systems better than any single therapy. We believe that complete recovery after more than 5 minutes of cardiac arrest has been rare because of the multifactorial pathogenesis of the post-resuscitation syndrome. The secondary pathophysiologic changes that accompany attempts to reoxygenate tissues seem to be similar in brain[759] and heart[76b]. The limit for tolerable complete arrest of perfusion for both organs seems to be between 10 and 20 minutes at 37°C. These phenomena are under intensive investigation by us and others.

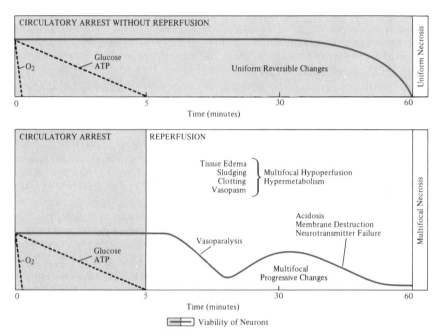

Fig. 54. Diagram of hypothetical events in the brain following total circulatory arrest (no blood flow). Vertical axes: viability of brain tissue, from pre-ischemic normal (left) to post-ischemic brain death (right). Top: *without* reperfusion, brain damage becomes clearly irreversible (necrosis) after only 30–60 minutes of no flow (complete ischemia). Bottom: *With* reperfusion after no flow for at least 5 minutes, secondary changes are provoked, which, added to the initial insult, result in multifocal necroses. Brain resuscitation research seeks to ameliorate these secondary changes and thereby help recovery of neurons (from Safar P; *Hospital Practice* **16:** 67, 1981).

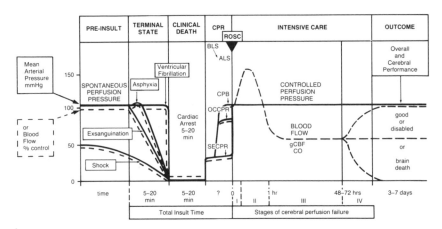

Fig. 55. Diagrammatic presentation of mean arterial (perfusion) pressure (MAP), cardiac output (CO), and global cerebral blood flow (gCBF)—during (a) dying (terminal state) and clinical death (cardiac arrest) [left]; (b) artificial circulation by standard external cardiopulmonary resuscitation (SECPR), open-chest CPR (OCCPR), or cardiopulmonary bypass (CPB) [center]; (c) restoration of spontaneous circulation (ROSC) [center]; and (d) post-arrest controlled normotension and ventilation until long-term outcome [right]. Four stages of cerebral perfusion failure post-arrest: stage I, multifocal no-reflow; stage II, global hyperemia; stage III, protracted global and multifocal hypoperfusion: and stage IV, outcome with improvement, continued hypoperfusion, or progression to zero flow (brain death). Summary of data from animal experiments[27,82,429,474,580,758,759,825]. Adapted from Safar P: *Circulation* **74:**138 (suppl. IV), 1986[759].

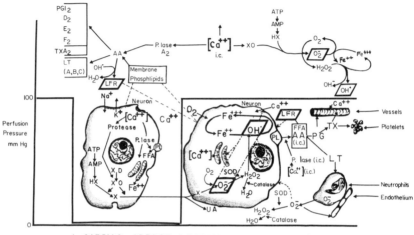

|←CARDIAC ARREST →|←REPERFUSION + REOXYGENATION →|

Fig. 56. Reoxygenation injury in brain (suspected) and extracerebral organs (proven) after cardiac arrest[39,72,113-116,121,145]. Diagrammatic summary of hypothesized cell-necrotizing cascades during temporary circulatory arrest (left) and reoxygenation (right). Under normal homeostatic conditions, intracellular (i.c.) free calcium (Ca^{2+}), is strictly maintained at approximately 100 nM. The regulation of $[Ca^{2+}]i$ is achieved by the plasma membrane Ca/Mg ATPase (Ca^{2+} gate), and the ATP-dependent uptake of Ca^{2+} into the endoplasmic reticulum (ER) and mitochondria. The release of bound Ca^{2+} from the ER store is believed to be triggered by inositol-1,4,5 triphosphate (IP_3) and/or by free arachidonic acid (AA). Release of Ca^{2+} bound in mitochondria is not thought to occur until the ER stores are depleted. The initial response of many different cell types to stimulation—i.e., ligand–receptor interaction, whether this be hormone-receptor binding, chemotactic peptide binding to polymorphonuclear leukocytes, or presynaptic or postsynaptic neurotransmitter binding, is an increase in $[Ca^{2+}]i$ due to release of intracellular ER-bound Ca^{2+}, an influx of extracellular Ca^{2+}, or both. Changes in many intracellular enzyme activities, including phospholipases and protein kinases, the polymerization of g-actin to f-actin, and that of tubulin to microtubules, all occur at different 'set points' of $[Ca^{2+}]i$. Therefore, much of the control of intracellular processes is related to the level of $[Ca^{2+}]i$. During anoxia (left), in all cells (including neurons) the level of ATP decreases rapidly to near zero. This causes an increase in free calcium $[Ca^{2+}]i$, even without an increase in IP_3. The addition of 2-deoxyglucose to cells, which acts as an ATP sink, causes a rapid increase in $[Ca^{2+}]i$. Increases in $[Ca^{2+}]i$ activate phospholipase A_2 (P.lase), which breaks down membrane phospholipids (PL) into free fatty acids (FFA), particularly AA. The AA causes increased activity of the cyclooxygenase pathway to produce prostaglandins (PG), including thromboxane (TX) A_2, the lipoxygenase pathway to produce leukotrienes (LT), or both. Furthermore, during anoxia, the hydrolysis of ATP via AMP leads to an accumulation of hypoxanthine (HX). Increased $[Ca^{2+}]i$ enhances the conversion of xanthine dehydrogenase (XD) to xanthine oxidase (XO), priming the neuron for the production of the oxygen free radical O_2^- intracellularly, once O_2 is reintroduced. During reoxygenation (right), significantly increased levels of at least three free-radical species (in oblique boxes) that break down membranes and collagen and worsen microcirculatory failure may be formed: O_2^-, OH·, and free lipid radicals (FLR). O_2^- may be formed from two sources: (1) the previously described XO system and (2) activation of neutrophils in the microvasculature due to increased LT production by the neurons or simply by decreased blood flow and increased margination and diapedesis of neutrophils from the microvasculature. Increased O_2^- production leads to increased H_2O_2 production as a result of the intracellular action of SOD. H_2O_2 is controlled by intracellular catalase. Increased O_2^- further leads to increased OH·, due to the Fenton reaction ($Fe^{2+} + H_2O_2 \rightarrow Fe^{3+} + OH + OH·$), with iron liberated from ferritin, and the Haber–Weiss reaction ($O_2^- + H_2O_2 \rightarrow OH^- + OH·$). Each or all of these oxidants can result in lipid peroxidation and the production of LFRs. All free radicals can cause leaky membranes and cell death. Furthermore, reoxygenation restores ATP via oxidative phosphorylation, which may result in massive uptake of $[Ca^{2+}]i$ into mitochondria. Loading of mitochondria with bound Ca^{2+} results in the self-destruction of mitochondria. Thus, increased $[Ca^{2+}]i$ as a result of anoxia and reoxygenation, by itself, and by triggering free radical reactions, may well be the principal cause of neuronal necrosis during reoxygenation. Figure prepared by Safar P, Basford R, and Ernster L. Adapted from Safar P: *Circulation* **74:** 138 (suppl IV), 1986[759].

Stabilization of Extracerebral Organ Function
(Tables 4, 5)[780, 799]

After cardiac arrest and restoration of spontaneous circulation and after terminal states without cardiac arrest requiring resuscitation, the patient's cardiovascular-pulmonary and other extracerebral organ systems functions should be monitored and optimized. First an i.v. line should be established (Fig. 37), and later consideration given to central venous, pulmonary artery (Fig. 38) and arterial catheters (Fig. 40) (Chapter 2).

During transportation of the resuscitated patient, either from the scene to the hospital or within the hospital to the ICU or to a diagnostic facility, life support must be continued without interruption, with support of ventilation and oxygenation (best by intracheal IPPV-CPPV with self-refilling bag–valve–mask–oxygen); and monitoring of ECG, carotid or femoral pulse, heart and breath sounds (esophageal stethoscope), and arterial pressure (cuff technique until arterial catheterization is possible). Transportation should be accompanied by a portable ECG monitor-defibrillator, portable oxygen cylinder, and portable suction, as well as appropriate resuscitative drugs, all on the patient's transportation carriage.

Derangements of the organ systems to be prevented or ameliorated are the result of a combination of the patient's baseline characteristics, the underlying disease, the insult that led to the terminal state, the promptness and adequacy of emergency resuscitation, and the reversibility of primarily cardiovascular-pulmonary malfunction after emergency resuscitation. After emergency resuscitation, as long as the patient is unconscious or shows an unstable cardiovascular-pulmonary system, life-support measures should be continued (Tables 4–6), modified according to the specific case.

If the patient regains consciousness promptly (within about 6 hours), cerebral function will most likely return to pre-arrest levels without special cerebral resuscitative measures. Early mental stimulation and neurologic activity might enhance return of normal cerebral function and emotional stability. Extracerebral organs may still need support (Tables 4 and 5).

If after cardiac arrest and CPR the patient regains consciousness within a few hours and has been weaned to spontaneous breathing (with normal blood gas values on air or low-flow oxygen), and has normotension without drug support and adequate urine output, probably little further life support is needed. Nevertheless, the patient should remain in an ICU setting until the cause of the arrest and full recovery have been ascertained. During this period the patient should continue to be continuously observed and noninvasively monitored, with an attendant at the bedside at all times. The patient should receive: (1) ECG monitoring and supplemental oxygen (by nasal prongs or open face mask with humidification); (2) an i.v. infusion of 5% dextrose in water; and (3) general physical examination, including chest radiogram, 12-lead ECG, arterial blood gas values on air and 100% oxygen, serum electrolytes, glucose and cardiac isoenzymes, and a detailed neurologic examination. If the arrest was due to VF, a prophylactic infusion of lidocaine to prevent re-arrest is indicated; for transient bradycardia, atropine is indicated; and for persistent severe bradycardia with heart block, continuous i.v. pacing is indicated. For pain, a narcotic should be given by i.v. titration. If dysrhythmias continue, advanced life support equipment, including a defibrillator, should remain near the bedside.

If after restoration of spontaneous circulation prompt weaning to spontaneous breathing and stable spontaneous circulation without drug support proves impossible, the patient should be monitored and treated long-term for cardiovascular-pulmonary and other extracerebral organ system derangements. If he/she is unconscious, these measures should be adapted to enhance cerebral recovery (Table 6).

Pulmonary support (Table 4, Chapters 1A, 1B)[533, 736c, 799, 815, 821, 827]

Pulmonary support begins with continuous observation of breathing movements and chest auscultation and percussion. Rule out unilateral breath sounds resulting from accidental bronchial intubation, pneumothorax and interstitial emphysema at the neck from lung rupture. Rule out bronchospasm, pulmonary edema and bronchial secretions. Examine suctioned pulmonary secretions for aspiration (pH, appearance, Gram stain, culture and antibiotic sensitivity). On chest films, check for tube and catheter positions, rib fractures, and pleural fluid and air (with appropriate positioning).

The comatose patient should have a cuffed endotracheal tube in place. Tracheal intubation in the stuporous or comatose not relaxed patient who has an obstructed airway, seizures or vomit in the airway, and whose traumatized or anoxic brain is vulnerable, needs an expert who can use a relaxant (e.g. succinylcholine) safely (Chapter 1A). Once the patient is intubated, ventilation should be stabilized, if necessary with partial curarization (e.g. by pancuronium). Start with continuous mechanical ventilation or, in its absence, uninterrupted manual ventilation by bag–valve unit (Fig. 21). The mechanical ventilator should be volume-set or volume readable. Start with tidal volumes of about 15 ml/kg, a ventilatory frequency of about 12 per minute, an inspiratory/expiratory ratio of about 1:2 and an inspired oxygen concentration (FIO_2) of about 50% (in suspected pulmonary edema or consolidation, an FIO_2 of 90–100%). If available, use a heated humidifier that delivers gas at the patient's airway at 36°C (96.8°F). Use controlled ventilation with assist (high-sensitivity) or intermittent mandatory ventilation (IMV) standby. Use IMV later for weaning. A positive end-expiratory pressure (PEEP) of 5 cmH$_2$O used prophylactically helps prevent collapse of alveoli. A PEEP greater than 5 cmH$_2$O should be used only if the ventilation volumes just specified do not yield an arterial PO_2 of at least 90 mmHg with an FIO_2 of 50%. Unnecessary high PEEP can hurt the postischemic brain. The effect of incremental increases of PEEP can be monitored by arterial blood gas, arterial pressure and airway pressure changes and, if available, by cardiac output and shunt determinations, which require mixed venous (central venous) oxygen content determinations. If increased PEEP reduces shunt and cardiac output, the latter should be supported by i.v. fluids and vasoactive (cardiac) drugs as indicated. Optimal PEEP and FIO_2 may be adjusted by monitoring and optimizing effective compliance (lowest peak airway pressure at constant lung volume ventilation), PaO_2 and venous oxygen values (oxygen supply/demand)[736c].

If the patient is conscious or unconscious, but returns with spontaneous breathing without straining or bucking, IMV with continued PEEP is useful in weaning gradually to spontaneous breathing. Reduce the controlled ventilation rate of IMV gradually to zero, i.e. spontaneous breathing, while checking arterial blood gases. Finally, if shunting continues, maintain spontaneous breathing with continuous positive airway pressure (SB-CPAP) (Chapter 1B) (Fig. 22). SB-CPAP should be continued and switched to atmospheric airway pressure only when the patient can maintain an arterial PaO_2 of about 100 mmHg without PEEP with an FIO_2 of 50% and a normal arterial PCO_2 and pH. Another mode suitable for difficult weaning to spontaneous breathing is high-frequency positive pressure jet ventilation (HFPPJV) (Chapter 1B).

For ascertaining a safe airway in the unconscious patient, an orotracheal or nasotracheal tube with a large soft cuff is appropriate. Tracheobronchial secretions and pulmonary edema fluid should be suctioned, after FIO_2 90–100% is given. Suctioning should be brief to prevent deoxygenation, and the ventilator and bag–valve unit should be ready. Ideally, the tracheal tube cuff should be inflated to the point of abolishing leakage and then slightly more, not exceeding an intracuff pressure (equals tracheal wall pressure with use of large soft cuffs) of 25 mmHg (Chapter 1A).

Arterial blood gases and acid–base status (Fig. 40)[736c, 815]

This should be monitored by intermittent arterial puncture via small-bore needle into heparinized syringe, or by indwelling catheter in the radial or femoral artery (Chapter 2). Ideally, blood gas values should be obtained with an FIO_2 considered clinically adequate at the time, and then after at least 5 minutes of FIO_2 90–100%. The arterial PCO_2 should be maintained at 25–35 mmHg during unconsciousness and anywhere between 20 and 45 mmHg during spontaneous breathing. Arterial PCO_2 is controlled by adjusting ventilation volumes, first frequency and then tidal volume. Arterial pH will vary with arterial PCO_2 and fixed acids, as reflected by calculated base excess and by blood bicarbonate. If the arterial PCO_2 is less than 30 mmHg and the arterial pH is greater than 7.5, measures should be taken to correct this respiratory alkalosis, because it can result in reduced serum potassium and dysrhythmias. If arterial PCO_2 is above 45 mmHg, controlled ventilation or IMV should be continued to maintain arterial PCO_2 below 40 mmHg. Respiratory acidemia should be treated by ventilation; metabolic acidemia by improving perfusion and transiently giving sodium bicarbonate ($NaHCO_3$) i.v.; respiratory alkalemia by reducing ventilation volumes; and metabolic alkalemia (sometimes seen with excessive gastric suctioning, or loop diuretic) by potassium chloride i.v., since it is often associated with hypokalemia (shift of potassium from extracellular into intracellular space and urinary excretion of potassium to retain hydrogen ions). Potassium chloride administration may start with 10 mEq/h and may be continued with about 200 mEq/24 hours. If metabolic alkalemia continues after correction of serum potassium, hydrochloric acid 0.1 N (100 mEq H^+/1000 ml) may be given via a central vein (do not exceed 100 ml/h). An alternative would be infusion of acetazolamide (Diamox) 250–500 mg, a carbonic anhydrase inhibitor.

Cardiovascular support (Table 4, Chapters 1C, 2)[800, 821, 827, 945, 948]

Cardiovascular support also begins with observation. Carotid, femoral and peripheral pulses and the skin should be felt; the heart and lungs auscultated; and the veins and color of mucous membranes and skin inspected. A bladder catheter and a central venous catheter should be inserted. If the patient remains unconscious or if there is suspicion of cardiac failure (and if these techniques are established in the hospital), a radial or femoral artery catheter as well as a pulmonary artery balloon catheter should be inserted. The ECG should be monitored continuously (lead 2), and a 12-lead ECG should be determined intermittently. Secondary cardiac arrhythmias are common[298]. Serum electrolytes, protein, albumin (or colloid osmotic pressure) and cardiac enzymes should be determined.

The central venous catheter provides right-heart filling pressure (CVP), and the pulmonary artery catheter in the occluded (wedge) position provides left-heart filling pressure (PAOP). The pulmonary artery balloon (flow-directed) catheter should ideally have a CV channel and a thermistor probe. The latter permits measurement of cardiac output by the thermodilution method; with use of a bedside computer, cardiac output measurements can be repeated frequently. Repeated measurement of cardiac output, pulmonary artery pressure (PAP), pulmonary artery occlusion pressure (PAOP), systemic blood pressure, heart rate, and arterial and pulmonary artery (mixed venous) oxygen content ($Ca\text{-}\bar{v}O_2$) will permit calculation of systemic and pulmonary vascular resistances (SVR, PVR), arterial oxygen transport (CaO_2), oxygen consumption (VO_2), and other variables, all used to guide fluid and drug therapy in support of the cardiovascular-pulmonary systems.

Titration of cardiovascular-pulmonary variables with fluids and drugs may be crucial in the early post-resuscitative period for supporting cerebral recovery and preventing multi-organ systems failure. During coma, normotension must be maintained, usually with a combination of sympathomimetic amines by titrated infusion, balancing alpha- and beta-agonist effects (dopamine, dobutamine, norepinephrine, epinephrine). These should be infused by calibrated pump rather than by drip. Intravenous volume load should be adjusted to keep central venous pressure (CVP) and PAOP between 5 and 15 mmHg, thereby enabling the patient to be weaned from a vasopressor. Pulmonary edema is detected by serial determinations of arterial PO_2 during 100% O_2 administration (PA-aO_2 on FIO_2 100%), auscultation and chest films; and is prevented by keeping the PAOP below 15–20 mmHg and plasma colloid osmotic pressure (COP) near 25 mmHg. Alveolar edema occurs when COP is less than 5 mmHg above PAOP. When

Table 4. Cardiovascular-pulmonary support guidelines* (P. Safar, RRC, 1987).

Immediate measures
Prevent hypoperfusion: restore blood volume-pump-pressure
Insert bladder and CVP catheter; arterial catheter (optional)
Maintain and optimize arterial pressure, CVP, urine flow (UF) (maintain UF over 0.5 ml/kg
  per h)
Monitor ECG, prevent/control dysrhythmias (antidysrhythmic drugs, pacing, cardioversion)
Monitor and normalize (optimize) body temperature
Use intratracheal IPPV + PEEP (5 cmH$_2$O prophylactic PEEP) until stable
  Optimize PEEP (effective compliance, changes in PA (or CV) O$_2$
  Wean from IPPV via IMV to spontaneous breathing
  Tracheal tube and cuff care; extubate
Maintain and optimize arterial PO_2, PCO_2, pH, BE
  Start with FIO_2 90–100%; 50% as soon as possible
Insert pulmonary artery balloon catheter if cardiac failure or pulmonary edema is suspected
  (for PAOP)
Maintain and optimize pulmonary arterial pressure; CVP and PAOP 5–15 mmHg
Keep COP-PAOP over 5 mmHg
Monitor cardiac output (thermodilution) (optional)

Urgent measures
Chest X-ray; sputum examination
Aseptic airway and catheter care
Drain stomach; drain pus; drain hematomas
Control fluid intake and output; monitor body weight
Monitor and optimize blood: hematocrit, glucose, cell count, clotting variables
Maintain and optimize plasma COP and serum and urine osmolality, electrolytes, proteins

Additional measures
Diuresis; dialysis if needed
Albumin 5% i.v. test with 200 ml, effect on PaO_2, CVP, PAOP
Alimentation i.v. or GI: 2000–4000 cal/24 h per 70 kg (i.e. dextrose 10–20%, amino acids,
  vitamins, essential fatty acids, etc.)
Steroid (?); Dextran 40 (?); heparin (?)
Correct the underlying problem that led to shock, terminal state or cardiac arrest

* For conscious or unconscious critically ill or injured patients with spontaneous circulation, and after emergency resuscitation from severe shock, preterminal state, or cardiac arrest. For abbreviations, see glossary.

pulmonary edema is evident with normal PAOP and COP, it is of the noncardiogenic variety, usually due to membrane failure (e.g. secondary to aspiration, sepsis or traumatic shock).

Prevention and treatment of pulmonary edema includes: (1) alveolar recruitment by IPPV plus PEEP with high FIO_2; (2) diuretic, digitalis and restriction of fluids for cardiogenic pulmonary edema; (3) albumin for low COP; and (4) steroid for membrane failure. Restlessness may be blocked with morphine, after hypoxemia has been excluded as its cause.

Cardiogenic shock is present when there is a persistently low arterial pressure, a very low cardiac index, a PAOP over 20 mmHg, and lactic acidemia. In this case, titrated infusion of cardiovascular drugs and fluids is tried first, and assisted circulation by intra-aortic balloon counterpulsation might be considered next. If there is second- or third-degree heart block, a transvenous pacemaker should be inserted and used with a demand pacing unit, which triggers only when the R–R interval of the spontaneous ECG exceeds a preset value.

Other organ system support (Table 5)[799]

This is less urgent than cardiovascular-pulmonary support, although hematologic-coagulation assessment and therapy should receive more and earlier attention than is the custom.

Gastrointestinal system support starts with prophylaxis by gastric tube suction, prophylactic antacid and maintenance of cardiac output. Liver function should be monitored as well. Hematologic and visceral derangements after cardiac arrest and CPR are under investigation[580, 760]. Preventive measures that might help overall recovery (e.g. plasmapheresis, detoxification) have been suggested[580], but their efficacy post-CPR has not yet been established. If derangements become evident, standard therapies for renal failure and hepatic failure are indicated.

Renal system support[736b, 799] starts with carefully adjusted i.v. fluid administration, according to fluid output (i.e. gastric suction, vomit, diarrhea, urine flow, fluid loss through skin and lungs); serum electrolytes (particularly potassium), blood urea nitrogen (BUN), creatinine, protein, albumin and osmolality; and urine electrolytes, nitrogen, creatinine and osmolality. Pre-renal failure is usually caused by hypovolemic hypotension and reduced cardiac output. Post-renal failure (mechanical blockage of urine flow) is bypassed by bladder catheter. Oliguric renal failure exists when urine flow is less than 400 ml/24 h per 70 kg. In acute renal failure (with pre-renal causes excluded), the index of urine sodium divided by urine/plasma creatinine is greater than 1. In polyuric renal failure, i.v. potassium should be avoided, electrolytes titrated, essential amino acids administered, loop diuretic given, and dialysis used early (peritoneal dialysis; veno-venous femoral catheter hemodialysis).

Table 5. Multiple organ systems support guidelines: summary of prolonged life support, CPCR Phase III (P. Safar, RRC, 1987).

Cardiovascular-Pulmonary Support (Table 4) (for conscious or unconscious patients)
Most important variables to be monitored and controlled:
  MAP, CVP, UF, ECG, temperature, PAOP
  Arterial PO_2, PCO_2, pH, BE

Standard Brain Support (Table 6) (for unconscious patients)
Most important variables to be monitored and *controlled* during critical post-insult phase:
  Normotension, hyperoxia, hypocapnia, moderate hemodilution, moderate hyperglycemia
  Normal blood electrolytes, osmolality, fluid balance, ICP (in selected cases); seizure
    prevention/control

Special brain resuscitation potentials (Table 7) (for unconscious patients)
For general cases (outside controlled randomized clinical trials), select patients and special
treatments carefully, weighing potential risks *vs.* benefits for each case

Renal support
Monitor fluid intake (i.v., p.o.); fluid output (GI suction, diarrhea, vomit, UF, skin, lungs);
  serum electrolytes, BUN, creatinine, protein, albumin, osmolality; urine electrolytes, N_2,
  creatinine, osmolality
Correct hypovolemia, hypotension, low cardiac output (most common cause of acute renal
  failure)
Oliguric renal failure = < 400 ml/24 h per 70 kg
Nonoliguric renal failure with rising BUN and creatinine
Prerenal failure = urine Na < 10 mEq/l, urine osmolality high
Adjust i.v. fluids, give i.v. alimentation, consider insulin for hyperglycemia, loop diuretic,
  inotropic drugs, mannitol, hemofiltration (for water), peritoneal dialysis, hemodialysis

Hepatic/gastrointestinal support
Detect liver failure (alkaline phosphatase, SGOT/SGPT, bilirubin, albumin, prothrombin
  time [PT])
Insert gastric tube
Prevent GI hemorrhage (maintain gastric pH > 3.5 with antacids, cimetidine 300 mg/6 h i.v.)

Bleeding/clotting
PT, partial thromboplastin time (PTT), platelet count, thrombin time (TT), fibrinogen, fibrin
  split products (DIC?)
Consider heparin, protamin, EACA, vitamin K, fresh frozen plasma, fresh blood, blood
  components
Simple bedside monitoring available: clotting time (CT)–clot retraction–clot lysis; activated
  clotting time (ACT); thromboelastogram; bleeding time

Infection control
Obtain infectious disease consult
Sputum smear gram stain
Culture blood, sputum, urine
Treat/eliminate focus, use specific antibiotics

For abbreviations and normal values, see Glossary.

Standard Brain-Oriented Intensive Therapy (Table 6)

The objectives of 'post-resuscitative brain-oriented intensive therapy' are:

1. to optimize respiratory, cardiovascular, metabolic, renal and hepatic-gastrointestinal function for survival of the entire organism;
2. to apply these measures in a way that will benefit the recovery of cerebral neurons in particular (standard, noncontroversial measures of brain-oriented life support);
3. to investigate in patients the benefits and risks of additional measures for resuscitation of the central nervous system (CNS), most of which are still experimental and controversial.

The guidelines listed in Tables 4 and 5 are for care of the conscious or unconscious patient; those in Table 6 are for the unconscious patient. These guidelines are by no means absolute; they serve merely as checklists for patient care, which should be adapted according to the patient's underlying disease and the available resources and intensive therapy services.

There are several accepted measures, based on experimental evidence or extensive clinical experience, which are useful after a severe ischemic-anoxic insult for supporting recovery of cerebral neurons. These measures are for: (1) extracranial homeostasis, i.e. to control extracerebral organ systems function in ways that would benefit the brain (Table 6-A); and (2) intracranial homeostasis, particularly control of intracranial pressure (ICP) (Table 6-B).

Extracranial homeostasis measures (Table 6-A)[3, 404, 743, 759]

The comatose patient must have his/her arterial blood pressure controlled by i.v. fluids and vasoactive agents (e.g. dopamine or norepinephrine vs. trimethaphan). After cardiac arrest, immediately upon restoration of spontaneous circulation, a brief period of moderate hypertension (which usually occurs as the result of epinephrine given during CPR) may help overcome the multifocal no-reflow phenomenon (initial sludging and stasis in the cerebral microcirculation)[27, 122, 357–359, 580, 733, 742]. Thereafter any degree of hypotension (systolic pressure below about 100 mmHg or higher in hypertension) as well as severe hypertension (systolic pressure over about 170 mmHg or MAP over 150 mmHg) should be avoided. After cardiac arrest, normotension or mild sustained hypertension may be beneficial (MAP 100–120 mmHg). After head trauma the hypertensive bout should be avoided and normotension (MAP 90–100 mmHg) or mild hypotension (MAP 70–90 mmHg) maintained. In suspected or monitored ICP rise, however, arterial pressure must be raised and/or ICP lowered to maintain cerebral perfusion pressure (MAP-ICP) at 50–100 (maximally 150) mmHg.

Endotracheal intubation and mechanically controlled ventilation, if necessary, with partial neuromuscular blockade by a curare-like agent such as pancuronium (Pavulon), allow for immobilization, which facilitates control of arterial pressure and blood gases and may thereby reduce the severity of brain injury. Avoidance of complete curarization and use of controlled moderate hyperventilation are recommended to retain the ability to recognize awakening, seizures or focal neurologic signs.

It was found in animals that routine use of post-CPR controlled ventilation and immobilization beyond 6 hours, if not needed for blood gas control, did not influence cerebral outcome[277]. Prolonged moderate hyperventilation (arterial PCO_2 25–35 mmHg) after cerebral trauma seems to enhance survival, but may have little effect on outcome with disability[293, 682]. Hyperventilation (better by mechanical ventilation than by the patient himself) counteracts cerebral acidosis; decreases ICP and increases intracranial compliance by decreasing intracranial blood volume; and improves intracerebral blood flow distribution from reactive areas to those with lost autoregulation. The arterial PO_2 should be maintained over 100 mmHg with the highest inhaled oxygen concentration considered safe (50% long-term) and avoidance of mean airway pressure higher than necessary (minimal PEEP). Such levels can be safely achieved without pulmonary oxygen toxicity by applying, at least for the first 6–12 hours, FIO_2 levels of 50–90%[900]. This recommendation is based on the hypothesis that increased blood PO_2 is more likely to create the necessary PO_2 gradient through tissue edema into neurons. In the conscious patient, arterial PO_2 should not be permitted to drop below 60 mmHg (the 'knee' of the oxyhemoglobin dissociation curve).

The arterial pH should be maintained at 7.3–7.6. Arterial pH is less important for guiding brain homeostasis than is the pH of the CSF[293]. Carbon dioxide equilibrates promptly between brain and blood; the charged ions of hydrogen and bicarbonate equilibrate only slowly. Lumbar CSF composition equilibrates with cerebral CSF only over hours. If ventricular or lumbar CSF is accessible, life support might be adjusted to keep CSF pH near the normal value of 7.3. This may require considerable controlled hyperventilation, which will raise arterial pH above normal. Avoidance of fully paralyzing doses of the relaxant enables recognition of awakening and of focal lesions.

Noxious afferent stimuli should be avoided, as they can cause dramatic increases in MAP and ICP. Prevention or treatment of restlessness, straining, 'bucking' on the tracheal tube, shivering, exhaustive spontaneous hyperventilation and seizures may require a CNS depressant, such as i.v. thiopental (Pentothal) or pentobarbital (Nembutal) in conventional anesthetic doses that do not depress the cardiovascular system, diazepam (Valium) and/or diphenylhydantoin (Dilantin, phenytoin). 'Therapeutic coma' with these agents requires intratracheal controlled ventilation and hemodynamic monitoring. Management problems increase as coma is extended beyond 6–12 hours. Severe generalized convulsions should be controlled with relaxant plus CNS (EEG) depressant agents.

The effect on outcome of the early use of a corticosteroid following cardiac arrest has not been clarified[375a, 741]. Since adjunctive benefits cannot be ruled out[418, 741] and short-term use of steroids is safe, they are included in the protocol for optional use. Maintenance of optimal hematocrit (about 30%), electrolytes, plasma colloid osmotic pressure, serum osmolality, blood glucose, hydration and alimentation must be ensured. Normothermia should be maintained; hyperthermia must be avoided. When the hyperthermic patient is being cooled to normothermia, a barbiturate, a narcotic or chlorpromazine in cautious i.v. doses (to avoid hypotension) may be useful. The evolution (continuance, progression or resolution) of post-cardiac arrest cytotoxic (intracellular) and vasogenic (extracellular) cerebral edema is unclear.

In summary, with the standard treatment protocol suggested in Table 6, hypoperfusion and cerebral edema are counteracted by a combination of arterial normotension, moderate hyperventilation, mild hyperoxia, loop diuretic, normothermia or mild hypothermia, ICP normalization, and normalization of blood glucose and serum osmolality, which can be abnormally high in severe hyperglycemia, in uremia and by excessive use of sodium bicarbonate. Standard brain-oriented intensive care (even without CNS depressants) seems to ameliorate post-ischemic brain damage, compared with 'usual care', in both animals[92, 743, 745] and patients[2-4, 106].

Intracranial homeostasis and pressure control
(Table 6-B, Chapter 4)[448, 493, 539, 574, 790, 826, 926]

Intracranial homeostasis measures start with the ruling out of an intracranial mass lesion that would require immediate operation, such as epidural, subdural, subarachnoid (CSF) or intracerebral hemorrhage. Unwitnessed asphyxia or cardiac arrest is sometimes the result of cranial trauma. Even in the patient under the influence of a relaxant or an anesthetic, a mass lesion can be suspected from the history and from unilateral mydriasis or other focal signs, and proved by computed tomographic (CT) scanning, magnetic resonance imaging (MRI) or cerebral angiography[300, 886].

Monitoring of intracranial pressure (ICP) has become increasingly common for guiding interventions to control ICP after head injury. After moderate global ischemic-anoxic insults (cardiac arrest), cerebral edema is rarely severe enough to increase ICP[90, 474, 581, 825]. However, if there is initial neurologic improvement followed by secondary deterioration (usually on the second or third day), ICP may rise and should be monitored, where facilities for safe, atraumatic, aseptic ICP monitoring are well established. The hollow skull screw[926] is favored in medical coma, and the ventricular catheter[493] is favored after head trauma. Both methods carry a slight risk of infection. In recent trials, new epidural pressure probes appear promising. ICP monitoring is indicated in coma after head injury or encephalitis more often than after cardiac arrest[574].

Table 6. Standard brain-oriented life support guidelines for coma* (P. Safar, RRC, 1987).

A. *Extracranial homeostasis*
For cardiovascular-pulmonary support, see also Table 4.
1. Control MAP and normalize blood volume with i.v. vasopressor/vasodilator and fluids. Post-anoxia plasma volume expansion (e.g. Ringer's solution or Dextran 40, 10 ml/kg) optional.
(a) Induce brief mild hypertension (MAP 120–140 mmHg) for 1–5 min, desirable with restoration of spontaneous circulation (often automatic owing to epinephrine during CPR). Hypertension contraindicated after cerebral trauma.
(b) Maintain normotension (MAP 90 mmHg; systolic AP 120–130 mmHg, or normal for patient) throughout coma; accept spontaneous slight hypertension (MAP 100–120 mmHg) after cardiac arrest; accept spontaneous slight hypotension (MAP 60–90 mmHg) after cerebral trauma. If ICP monitored, keep CPP (MAP-ICP) over 50 mmHg.
(c) Insert bladder, CVP, arterial catheters; pulmonary arterial balloon catheter optional.
(d) Position head up 10–30°, turn entire patient side/side every 2 hours without causing straining.
2. Immobilize with softening (not fully paralyzing) doses of relaxant (e.g. pancuronium i.v.) if necessary, to facilitate controlled ventilation. Maintain controlled ventilation for at least 2 hours post-arrest, longer if necessary.
3. Control (essential) or prevent (optional) restlessness, straining, seizures:
(a) Thiopental or pentobarbital 5 mg/kg per h (aim for plasma level 2–4 mg/dl), total 30 mg/kg (more for recurrent seizures); or
(b) Diphenylhydantoin (Dilantin, phenytoin) 7 mg/kg i.v. bolus + 7 mg/kg/24 h maintenance; or
(c) Diazepam (Valium) 5 mg/70 kg i.v. titrated as needed. For pain (when awake) narcotic by i.v. titration.
4. Maintain arterial PCO_2 at 25–35 mmHg during controlled ventilation: 20–40 mmHg during spontaneous breathing.

5. Maintain arterial pH at 7.3–7.6 (with ventilation and $NaHCO_3$ i.v. as needed).
6. Maintain arterial PO_2 over 100 mmHg, with FIO_2 90–100%; after 1–6 hours FIO_2 50%. Minimal PEEP during coma.
7. Give corticosteroid (optional):
(a) methylprednisolone 1 mg/kg i.v. followed by 0.5 mg/kg per 6 h i.v., or
(b) dexamethasone 0.2 mg/kg i.v. followed by 0.1 mg/kg per 6 h i.v.
(c) *Stop* or taper corticosteroid at 48–72 h. (Optional 1 early larger steroid dose.)
8. Blood variables—control:
(a) Hematocrit 30–35%; electrolytes normal.
(b) Plasma COP over 15 mmHg, serum albumin over 3 g/dl.
(c) Serum osmolality 280–330 mOsm/l.
(d) Glucose 100–300 mg/dl.
9. Maintain normothermia; avoid hyperthermia.
10. Give fluids i.v.—no dextrose in water alone:
(a) Use dextrose 5–10% in 0.25–0.5% NaCl i.v., 30–50 ml/kg per 24 h (100 ml/kg per 24 h in infants); add potassium as needed.
(b) Give alimentation; dextrose 20%, amino acids, electrolytes, vitamins. (Start at 24–48 hours, i.v.—GI).

B. *Intracranial homeostasis*
1. Rule out mass lesion; history, clinical picture; X-ray film; CT scan or cerebral angiogram in selected cases. MRI. Prevent straining during examination with use of partial paralysis (pancuronium).
2. Monitor ICP (only if safe technique established); optional after CPR; recommended after cerebral trauma and in encephalitis:
(a) Hollow skull screw preferred in nontraumatic coma.
(b) Ventricular catheter preferred in traumatic coma.
Control ICP at or below 15 mmHg by:
(i) Further controlled hyperventilation ($PaCO_2$ to 20 mmHg) with relaxation and sedation (no coughing!)

Table 6 *(cont.)*

(ii) Ventricular CSF drainage.
(iii) Mannitol 0.5 g/kg i.v. plus 0.3 g/
kg per h, i.v., short-term; or
mannitol 1 g/kg once i.v.,
empirical, without ICP
monitoring, immediately following
restoration of spontaneous
circulation after cardiac arrest, and
at neurologic deterioration
(optional).
(iv) Loop diuretic i.v. (e.g. furosemide,
0.5–1.0 mg/kg i.v.).
(v) Thiopental or pentobarbital 2–5
mg/kg i.v.; repeat as needed.
(vi) Corticosteroid (above).
(vii) Hypothermia, 30–32°C, short-
term (with controlled ventilation,
relaxant, anesthetic, vasodilator);
short-term hypothermia optional;
long-term hypothermia not
recommended.
3. Monitor (optional).
(a) Regular EEG.
(b) Computerized EEG (cerebral function
monitor).

(c) Evoked potentials (experimental).
(d) Treat EEG seizures (A2, A3 above).
4. Monitor neurologic recovery and
prognosis.
(a) Determine CSF CPK-BB at 48–72
hours.
(b) Monitor depth of coma by Glasgow
Coma Score or Pittsburgh–Glasgow
Coma Score (Table 9).
(c) Monitor cerebral blood flow and
metabolism (experimental).
5. Determine and manage outcome.
(a) Determine periodically cerebral and
overall performance categories 1–5
(Table 10).
(b) Determine accurately and certify brain
death (CPC 5) (Table 11), starting 6
hours after cardiac arrest. If brain death
is certified, remove donor organs with
permission and discontinue IPPV.
(c) Determine persistent vegetative state
(CPC 4). If unresponsive 1–2 weeks
after cardiac arrest (1 year post-cerebral
trauma) consider 'letting die' (Table
12).

For abbreviations, see Glossary.
* For unconscious, critically ill or injured patients; for use after global ischemic-anoxic insult,
modify guidelines for other causes of coma.

Monitored increases in ICP above the 'normal' level of about 15 mmHg (zeroed at the level of the midcranium) can be expected or unpredictable. They are used to guide titrated stepwise measures for ICP reduction (Table 6-B): further hyperventilation; ventricular CSF drainage; an osmotic diuretic such as mannitol; a loop diuretic such as furosemide; an i.v. anesthetic such as thiopental; a steroid; and hypothermia.

Although short-term (12–48 hours) low-dose osmotherapy with mannitol should be considered early[376, 418, 448], intracranial hypertension is increasingly being controlled with additional anesthetic doses of i.v. thiopental or pentobarbital. This is particularly the case when the need for treatment extends for more than 24 hours or when large doses of osmotic agents are required for ICP control. In the last circumstance, rebound edema and severe disturbance of blood volume, fluid and electrolyte balance may be major complications of osmotherapy and may thus limit its usefulness.

It should be noted that although these ICP-controlling measures were developed from experience with patients after brain surgery or head injury, they are also appropriate for selected patients in coma with encephalitis, with severe stroke, or after cardiac arrest. Furthermore, ICP monitoring assists in detecting circumstances that may inadvertently increase ICP (e.g. tracheal suctioning or change of body position).

Other advanced measures[306] for promoting intracranial homeostasis, most of which are still experimental, include: (1) regular and computation EEG analysis and recording of evoked EEG potentials (technically difficult in the ICU setting[639a, 780a]); (2) measurements of cerebral blood flow and metabolism, which would require sampling of cerebral venous (superior jugular bulb) blood or a highly complex, expensive CT technique[975]; (3) measurement of cerebral electric impedance (shift of ECF into cells increases impedance); and (4) analysis of CSF for pH (normal value 7.3), lactate (normal value 1.5–2 μmol/ml, i.e. 14–18 mg/dl), and the cerebral intracellular enzyme creatine phosphokinase (CPK–BB) (normal value below 20 units/ml)[213, 567, 910a–c, 911]. Evaluating insult and outcome as well as neurologic signs early after the insult, which might permit prediction of outcome (described below), should be part of standard management of the comatose patient after emergency resuscitation.

Special Brain Resuscitation Potentials (Table 7)[759]

The clinical, socioeconomic and scientific importance of searching for increasingly effective post-cardiac arrest measures to prevent or reverse post-ischemic-anoxic encephalopathy is obvious. Most of the special brain resuscitation measures to be discussed here are new or under reinvestigation and are still controversial[759]. None should be used routinely after cardiac arrest. Confusion and controversy have arisen because of conclusions drawn from comparisons of experimental results with different animal models, treatment modalities and post-insult management. One must keep in mind the differences between the kinds of injury produced in the brain by ischemia, anoxia, hypoglycemia, anemia, trauma, hemorrhage, metabolic or toxic abnormalities and inflammation, or by different combinations of these processes. With ischemic insults, there are also important distinctions between *global* ischemia, as in shock states or cardiac arrest, and the focal ischemia of cerebral infarction or embolism. There are also differences between *incomplete* ischemia, as in shock, and total cessation of blood flow, as in cardiac arrest. Finally, in considering therapeutic measures, one must differentiate between *protection* (measures instituted before and during an insult) and *resuscitation* (measures taken *after* an insult).

Some of the measures that appear most promising for saving neurons, if applied during or after CPR, are controversial because their possible benefit is accompanied by known risks. These treatments include anesthetics such as barbiturates, anticonvulsants, prolonged immobilization, osmotherapy and hypothermia. Other procedures, such as moderate hemodilution and administration of certain calcium-entry blockers, are associated with low risk. Expensive or risky innovative therapies should be tested in controlled patient trials before they are used routinely in patients. Controlled randomized patient trials take years to complete and are expensive[3, 404]. It therefore seems reasonable for inexpensive, probably harmless novel therapies that have been effective in animal outcome models to be used in general clinical practice without prior controlled clinical trials.

Only special cardiac arrest *animal models*, with post-insult intensive care and evaluation of long-term outcome[745], should be relied upon to determine protective clinical benefit of brain resuscitation potentials[338, 406a, 463, 605, 745, 750, 759, 760]. At this time (1987), only six brain resuscitation measures used immediately following restoration of normal perfusion pressure after prolonged total circulatory arrest have been found by us and others in such animal experiments to ameliorate post-ischemic brain damage (Table 7): (1) general brain-oriented intensive therapy by protocol (recommended for routine clinical use); (2) promotion of reperfusion with intracarotid hemodilution, transient hypertension and other measures (promising but still experimental); (3) barbiturates (adjunctive value only); (4) calcium-entry blockers (under controlled clinical trial); (5) free radical scavengers (experimental); (6) etiology-specific combinations (future). Clinical benefits were more than statistically significant.

(1) General brain-oriented intensive therapy by protocol[734a, 759]

This control of extracerebral organ systems (standard therapy protocol), described above (Table 6), has extended the maximal period of reversible normothermic cardiac arrest beyond the 5 minute limit encountered so far with 'usual care', in both animals[92, 745] and patients[2-4, 106] (Table 6). These standard treatment protocols attempt to: (1) overcome reperfusion failure; (2) optimize blood gas values and blood composition; and (3) support multiple-organ systems with intensive care.

(2) Promotion of reperfusion[733, 758] (Fig. 55)

The first phase of post-arrest reperfusion failure, namely multifocal no-reflow in the brain (and possibly also in other vital organs)[27, 64, 241, 580, 583, 825], can be counteracted to some extent by reperfusing with induced transient, moderate hypertension (by fluid load and vasopressor) and moderate normovolemic hemodilution (e.g. to hematocrit 25–30%). The delayed protracted cerebral hypoperfusion (Fig. 55)[825] may be counteracted by the same plus additional treatments. Multifocal CBF measurements over time are needed to clarify recommendations for reperfusion therapies[759, 975].

For *hypertension* therapy, the optimal reperfusion pressure pattern has not yet been determined. At present, immediate post-ischemic transient moderate hypertension (e.g. after defibrillation) or artificial (e.g. by cardiopulmonary bypass) raising of MAP to about 130–140 mmHg for 5–15 minutes by i.v. fluids and/or vasopressor[122, 241, 358, 733, 972] is recommended. Repeated or prolonged severe hypertension can worsen brain damage probably by inducing vasogenic edema[91, 418].

For *hemodilution* therapy, combinations of electrolyte and colloid solutions have been used. Normovolemic hemodilution to hematocrit 25–30% looks promising for cerebral infarction[870] and experimental contusion[386]. In exsanguination cardiac arrest, brief retrograde intra-aortic infusion of plasma substitute helped restore spontaneous cardiac action[410, 411, 578]. In the first outcome study in dogs of brain resuscitation after cardiac arrest (12 minutes VF cardiac arrest) the combined use of intracarotid hemodilution (flush) with Dextran 40, transient moderate hypertension with norepinephrine, and heparinization ameliorated brain damage[549, 733]. In a subsequent study of head ischemia in monkeys, i.v. hemodilution alone did not ameliorate brain damage[742]. Intracarotid (rather than i.v.) hypertensive hemodilution with a plasma substitute should be re-examined, first in animals. In dogs with VF cardiac arrest, we have found this treatment delivered by cardiopulmonary bypass (CPB) (venae cavae to femoral artery pumping via oxygenator) to be superior to CPR advanced life support (ALS) for restoration of spontaneous circulation[758]; it thereby enhanced conscious survival[462, 637]. Normovolemic or hypervolemic hemodilution[531, 880, 881] is effective in focal ischemia[275, 276, 870]. Acellular oxygen-carrying blood substitutes should be evaluated post-arrest[192, 816].

Heparinization looks promising[868] and should be reinvestigated. Heparinization i.v. after global head ischemia in monkeys did not improve outcome[742]. If very prolonged stasis during clinical cardiac arrest results in intravascular clotting[358, 894], or the post-resuscitation syndrome provokes clotting[580, 749], heparin or *streptokinase* should be studied as a component of the initial 'flush' perfusion fluid[469].

Adding a *calcium-entry blocker* to the initial perfusion fluid, which might help protect neurons against necrotizing processes[958], is now under investigation[663a]. Free radical scavengers looks promising[913]. A combination of a *free radical scavenger* such as superoxide dismutase (SOD), an *iron chelator* such as deferoxamine[133, 230, 959], a xanthinoxidase inhibitor (lodoxamide) and a calcium entry blocker (lidoflazine) in the initial perfusion fluid might theoretically enhance cerebral tissue recovery, by helping prevent the necrotizing chemical cascades started with reperfusion; this matter is presently under investigation[663a].

Osmotherapy (e.g. mannitol i.v.)[376, 448, 539, 971] can also be considered a potentially reperfusion-promoting measure, since it reduces cerebral edema after head injury or neurosurgery. The value of this treatment for the promotion of reperfusion and other objectives after cardiac arrest is unclear and is in need of reinvestigation. The role and progression of cytotoxic (intracellular)[915] and delayed vasogenic (extracellular) cerebral edema during and after cardiac arrest remain to be clarified[418].

Hypothermia is listed here because perfusion and metabolism should be matched. Hypothermia reduces cerebral metabolism and blood flow[75], and is the most potent protective (pretreatment) measure for cerebral ischemia[666, 680, 681, 973, 991]. A temperature of 30°C during total circulatory arrest of up to about 30 minutes, and of 20°C during ischemia up to 60 minutes, can protect against post-ischemic brain damage. Barbiturates reduce cerebral metabolism to a minimum of 50% of normal by reducing neuronal activity. Phenytoin[14, 175] and local anesthetics[35, 348], in addition, can reduce energy requirement for ion fluxes across membranes[35]; however, only hypothermia can stop all metabolic activity[35]. Hypothermia has also been shown to stabilize enzyme systems and membranes. Hypothermia induced *after* cardiac arrest is of debatable value, since curiously its use has not yet been studied in a clinically relevant reproducible animal outcome model. Hypothermia induced in adults after brain insults reduces the rate of brain metabolism, the magnitude of cerebral edema, and the size of experimental infarcts[680, 681]. Hypothermia has not gained acceptance for use after cardiac arrest because it entails difficult management problems, especially if prolonged to 12–24 hours; it is also associated with a variety of injurious side-effects, such as increased incidence of dysrhythmias and shock, elevated blood viscosity with reduced blood flow, and increased susceptibility to infection and stress ulceration. Hypothermia does not improve reperfusion and may even hamper it by increasing blood viscosity[842]. Protective external head and brain cooling during prolonged CPR is feasible[100], but its effect on outcome has not been demonstrated.

In patients with a previously healthy cardiovascular system (e.g. children after drowning) short-term moderate hypothermia is justified[158]. One feasible technique is the reduction of body temperature to 30–32°C for 3–6 hours, as early as possible after the insult, followed by gradual rewarming to normothermia. To use hypothermia safely, the patient's defense reaction to cooling must be blocked, so that poikilothermia will be induced. Therefore, cooling must be accompanied by relaxation (using a neuromuscular blocking agent), controlled ventilation and drugs to block (prevent) hypothermia-induced shivering, hypermetabolism, vasoconstriction and dysrhythmias. All this can be accomplished by a slow intravenous infusion of chlorpromazine (Thorazine) 5–10 mg, repeated with titration as necessary (avoiding hypotension) or by anesthetics such as thiopental or pentobarbital[442].

(3) Barbiturates[3, 90, 278, 740, 759, 982, 983]

Although barbiturates are clearly not a breakthrough therapy for cardiac arrest (see below), these agents *do* exert potentially beneficial adjunctive effects on the injured brain. Barbiturates are known to reduce cerebral metabolic rate[940]; enhance restoration of cerebral energy state[593]; decrease formation of cerebral edema[819], free fatty acids[795] and cyclic adenosine monophosphate (AMP)[470, 503]; suppress seizure activity[895]; block noxious stimuli[495]; shift metabolism to synthesizing pathways[319]; reduce intracranial blood volume and ICP[511, 790]; improve cerebral differential perfusion in relation to metabolism[239, 425]; scavenge free radicals (thiopental)[188, 820]; and rest the brain by silencing EEG activity (with thiopental or pentobarbital plasma levels of about 3–5 mg/dl)[511, 674]. Whereas *during* complete global ischemia there is no activity and metabolism to be suppressed, *after* reperfusion the multifocal (incomplete) ischemia of the cerebral post-resuscitation syndrome might benefit from the activity- and metabolism-depressant effects of barbiturates.

Large and moderate doses of thiopental and pentobarbital, given before or after experimental permanent *focal* (i.e. incomplete) ischemia (ischemic stroke), have been shown to reduce the size of the infarct[536, 818]. There have been beneficial results when barbiturates were given to animals *before complete global* ischemia[284, 782] (protection)—although not duplicated by another group[840]—or during or after *incomplete global* ischemia (hypoxia)[464, 982]. In patients, thiopental pretreatment has been shown to protect open-heart surgery patients against neuropsychiatric deficits from the incomplete multifocal cerebral ischemia of emboli[597]. The value of anesthetic doses of thiopental or pentobarbital to reduce ICP has been demonstrated[790]; but the prophylactic use of a barbiturate after head injury was not effective[931]. Barbiturates seem to increase tolerance of temporary carotid occlusion[953].

Barbiturate loading *after complete global* brain ischemia was studied for the first time in rhesus monkeys with a long-term intensive care outcome model of global head ischemia, with a positive therapeutic effect[90]. The main *rationale* was that postischemic encephalopathy entails secondary multifocal incomplete ischemia which might benefit from reduction in cerebral metabolism. The beneficial results could not be repeated later in the same laboratory with a more consistently controlled reperfusion pressure and long-term life support protocol in pigtail monkeys[278]. In another laboratory, barbiturate loading in cats after VF resulted in lower mortality from seizures, but not in improved neurologic deficit of the survivors[895]. Others' results were variable[464, 824, 982].

After promising pilot studies in patients[106], the first multi-institutional international randomized clinical study of CPCR after cardiac arrest, in 1979–1984, tested the efficacy of thiopental loading after cardiac arrest[2-4]. Starting 10–50 minutes after restoration of normotension, thiopental 30 mg/kg i.v. was given slowly. There was no statistically significant difference between the thiopental and standard therapy groups in the proportion of patients who achieved good outcome (cerebral performance categories (CPC) 1, normal; and 2, moderate disability) rather than poor outcome (CPC 3, severe disability; 4, coma; and 5, brain death) (Table 10). A subgroup of patients with cardiac arrest times (without CPR) of 5 minutes or longer showed a trend toward benefit from thiopental. The treatment proved feasible and safe, even in patients with myocardial infarction. Hypotension might offset a beneficial effect.

The clinician must bear in mind that the vasodilating and cardiac depressant effects of large doses of thiopental or pentobarbital are considerable, particularly in the patient with heart disease or hypovolemia. The risk : benefit ratios of loading doses versus conventional (safe) doses have not been determined. Conventional anesthetic doses of thiopental or pentobarbital (2–5 mg/kg i.v.), repeated as needed, may not depress the circulation and may require only occasionally small amounts of vasopressor and plasma volume expansion. They may be clinically indicated in post-CPR states to sedate, suppress seizures, facilitate controlled ventilation, reduce 'brain stress' and normalize monitored rise in ICP. Even this less controversial treatment should be used only by physicians skilled in the administration of anesthetics, and only in patients who are comatose after a severe global or focal ischemic-anoxic or other brain insult.

We do *not* at this time (1987) recommend the routine use of barbiturates after cardiac arrest. Selective use of anesthetic doses of a barbiturate in patients early after cardiac arrest is justified, particularly for seizure prophylaxis, seizure control, sedation and ICP control. Seizure prophylaxis, of course, may be accomplished also by other agents, such as diazepam or phenytoin. Barbiturate anesthesia for protection against anticipated (incomplete) brain ischemia during neurosurgical[826, 953] and cardiothoracic surgical[597] cases is indicated. After head injury or encephalitis, administration of prophylactic barbiturate without ICP monitoring is controversial[306, 539, 953]. In shock states with coma, cardiovascular stabilization has therapeutic priority, since barbiturate may precipitate cardiac arrest in hypovolemia. Furthermore, because barbiturates suppress neurologic function and the usual clinical signs are depressed, careful diagnostic evaluation is necessary before CNS depressants are used.

Phenytoin (Dilantin) looks promising for brain resuscitation[14, 175] and also has ion-flux and membrane stabilizing properties. *Halothane*, which reduces cerebral metabolism and increases blood flow and intracranial pressure, worsens focal ischemia[818]. *Isoflurane* shows potential for cerebral protection and resuscitation[932].

(4) Calcium entry blockers (Fig. 56)[759]

Calcium blockers are known to exert both beneficial and deleterious cardiovascular effects (Chapter 2)[103, 244, 245, 916, 917]. The mechanisms of calcium channel blocking effects are not the same among the most investigated agents: verapamil, nifedipine, nimodipine, diltiazem, flunarizine and lidoflazine. The general cardiovascular and cerebral vasodilating effects of these calcium-entry blockers have been documented, but not compared[17, 400, 576, 661, 843–845, 911–913, 957, 958]. There is suggestive evidence that lidoflazine is less likely than nifedipine or nimodipine to produce hypotension, and is less likely than verapamil to produce heart block; lidoflazine might play a role in VT and VF of patients with myocardial ischemia and atrial fibrillation. Flameng used lidoflazine 1 mg/kg i.v. in more than 1000 patients for myocardial protection before cardiopulmonary bypass for heart surgery, without any serious side-effects (unpublished data). In dogs and patients, lidoflazine given before circulatory arrest in cardiopulmonary bypass exerted significant myocardial protection against ischemia[244, 245]. Calcium entry blockers reverse cerebral vasospasm[17, 400, 843, 957]. They are suspected to (but have not yet been proved to) reduce the intraneuronal liberation and accumulation of free Ca^{2+} and blockage of mitochondria (Fig. 56), which seems to occur during ischemia and reperfusion[95, 145, 358, 576, 770, 806, 807, 917, 958, 959]. Controlled data on the effect of calcium entry blocker therapy after cerebral trauma are lacking; for intracranial hemorrhage, the data look promising[17, 917]; and before or after focal ischemia (cerebral infarct), results are inconclusive[661].

Improved neurologic *outcome* after calcium entry blocker therapy following complete *global* cerebral ischemia in animals has been demonstrated in four studies:

1. Lidoflazine[916] 1 mg/kg i.v. immediately after cardiac arrest in dogs improved early (12-hour) neurologic recovery[968].
2. Lidoflazine 1 mg/kg i.v. over 10 minutes, after 10 minutes of VF cardiac arrest in dogs, immediately after restoration of spontaneous circulation, and repeated at 8 and 16 hours, ameliorated brain damage significantly at 96

hours[911]. In this first positive long-term outcome study of a calcium entry blocker after cardiac arrest, five of 11 treated dogs recovered completely (Overall Performance Category 1), whereas none of 11 control dogs did. Also, in the lidoflazine group, early post-arrest cardiac output was better, dysrhythmias were less severe, and norepinephrine requirement for early post-arrest control of normotension was not higher than in the control group. After asphyxial cardiac arrest (a more severe brain insult) the same dose of lidoflazine had no effect on outcome[912a].

3. Nimodipine infused i.v. before, during and after ascending aorta occlusion in dogs improved early (24-hour) neurologic recovery[843], but when given only after the same insult, it had minimal beneficial effects[844].

4. Nimodipine 10 μg/kg i.v. bolus plus 1 μg/kg per minute over 10 hours[845], using the Pittsburgh monkey model of global head ischemia by neck tourniquet with long-term intensive care[581], ameliorated neurologic deficit in one-half of the treatment series[845]. This achieved encouraging results, similar to those of Vaagenes et al, after cardiac arrest with lidoflazine[911].

Global cerebral blood flow changes per se, above a certain minimum of local CBF required for tissue viability (probably 20% normal), cannot be expected to influence outcome. This indeed seems to be the case. Nimodipine, which somewhat ameliorated global cerebral hypoperfusion post-ischemia[843], and lidoflazine, which does not seem to have this effect[246a], both seem to ameliorate brain damage[845, 911]. Also, these two different calcium entry blockers gave the same improvement in outcome, whether myocardial ischemia was included in the insult[911] or not[845]. Thus, the effect seems to be directly on brain tissue.

Verapamil 0.1 mg/kg i.v. after VF cardiac arrest, in a pilot study of five dogs, did not improve outcome[912b]. In patients, an uncontrolled feasibility trial of verapamil caused hypotension, but gave encouraging outcome results[778]. Flunarizine improved post-cardiac arrest cerebral blood flow[957] but caused hypotension and pulmonary edema (Mullie; Michenfelder; personal communication). The effects on long-term post-cardiac arrest neurologic outcome of diltiazem and nifedipine have not yet been investigated. The evidence presented above caused us to initiate a new randomized study (1984–1988) of the effects of a calcium entry blocker (lidoflazine) in patients after cardiac arrest, using established methodology[4].

(5) Free Radical Scavengers[186, 759] (Fig. 56)

The rationale for studying free radical scavengers as potential brain resuscitation agents after cardiac arrest is that reperfusion injury may start with free iron-triggered[32, 43, 230] oxygen (O_2^-) and hydroxyl ($OH\cdot$) radicals which, concomitant with calcium loading of mitochondria, create cascades of chemical reactions leading to membrane damage and cell necrosis[345, 346, 521] (Fig. 56). In vitro evidence and suggestive observations in extracerebral organs[116] support the combined roles of $Fe^{3+} \rightarrow Fe^{2+}$[32, 230, 959], the 'oxygen paradox' (O_2^- and OH· accumulation)[32, 186, 188, 230, 258, 346, 521, 759], and the 'calcium paradox'[76b, 246, 521, 759 770, 917, 958, 990] in lipid peroxidation. The calcium-triggered formation of arachidonic acid during reperfusion in turn leads to prostaglandins, thromboxane and leukotrienes, which might worsen the microcirculatory states and make reperfusion failure and reperfusion injury feed on each other.

Free radical scavengers have not yet been tested satisfactorily in outcome animal models, with the exception of a small study of 7-minute asphyxial cardiac arrest in dogs, in which a free radical scavenger solution (a mixture of mannitol, dextran 40, l-methionine, tromethamine (THAM) and magnesium sulfate) seemed to improve outcome over standard care[913]. The same combination therapy after 10 minutes of VF cardiac arrest did not ameliorate brain damage. Another free radical scavenger combination produced no effect[775a]. Studies are now underway by us and others on single and combination therapies, including some of the following known free radical scavengers[663a]: superoxide dismutase (SOD), thiopental, vitamin E, vitamin C, catalase, glutathione, l-methionine, chlorpromazine, promethazine and others. Xanthinoxidase inhibitors (al'opurinol, lodoxamide) are also under investigation. Since free radicals cannot be captured as markers in such studies, the results of treatment trials in reliable animal models may have to be used to answer the question of whether free radicals play a significant role in cell-necrotizing processes after cardiac arrest.

(6) Etiology-specific combination therapies[279, 759, 760]

We predict that a calcium entry blocker, a barbiturate, or any other single agent alone will not produce the maximal protective or resuscitative effect. This will more likely come from etiology-specific therapies which combine agents aimed at one or more derangements of the post-resuscitation syndrome (PRS)[749]. Multifactorial problems require multifaceted approaches. In our laboratory, two animal studies using multifaceted therapy protocols with brain resuscitation potential gave statistically significant improvement in outcome: (1) in dogs, the combination of intracarotid hemodilution, hypertension and heparinization[733]; (2) in monkeys, the combination of immediate post-arrest hypertension, i.v. hemodilution, barbiturate, steroid and hypothermia[279]. In the latter study amelioration was not dramatic, perhaps because negative side-effects of one treatment (e.g. hypothermia) can offset the beneficial effects of another.

Treatable extracerebral organ dysfunction might worsen brain damage[580, 749]. With combined therapies, we have occasionally seen complete recovery in animals after up to 18 minutes of head ischemia[90, 279, 743], but after only up to 12 minutes of total body circulatory arrest[733, 911]. Negovsky's results in animals without post-arrest intensive care and our results with maintained normotension and intensive care[121, 393, 911] have shown a prolonged post-CPR decrease of cardiac output and increase of systemic vascular resistance, which parallel the changes in cerebral blood flow[358, 825]. Thus, in 1985 we have embarked on a systematic study of the post-resuscitation syndrome in animal models[749, 760].

Miscellaneous brain resuscitation measures[759, 760]

Other treatments that on the basis of past studies and clinical impressions might be beneficial in saving neurons post-arrest, and deserve investigation for use immediately post-arrest, include: (1) Hypertonic glucose–insulin–adenosine triphosphatase (ATP)–$MgCl_2$[163, 432, 525, 829]; (2) CSF pH normalization[663]; (3) various anesthetics, sedatives, free radical scavengers and calcium blockers that do not depress the blood pressure[759]; (4) any safe combination therapy that minimizes brain metabolism, improves capillary

Table 7. Special brain resuscitation potentials* (P. Safar, RRC, 1987).

Treatment	Ready for clinical trials after cardiac arrest	Cardiac arrest		Brain infarct		Cerebral trauma acute ICP rise cerebral edema	
		Animal	Man	Animal	Man	Animal	Man
Moderate, brief, induced hypertension	Yes	+		(+)	(+)		
Hemodilution (i.v.)	Yes	(+)		+	(+)	(+)	
Intracarotid hypertensive hemodilution ('flush')		+					
Heparinization	?	0		−	−	−	−
Cardiopulmonary bypass	Yes	+		−	−	−	−
Barbiturate high dose	†	(+)	0(†)	+		(+)	(+)
Barbiturate anesthetic dose		(+)		+		+	+
Phenytoin (Dilantin)	Yes	(+)					
Immobilization and IPPV during coma		(+)	(+)	(+)		+	+
Osmotherapy	Yes			(+)		+	+
Hypothermia		(+)		+		(+)	(+)
Calcium entry blocker	Ongoing†	+	†	(+)			(+)
Free radical scavenger		(+)					

* See text and references to Chapter 3.
† = International collaborative randomized clinical study (Resuscitation Research Center, University of Pittsburgh) 1979–1989[3].
Key: + = Reduces brain damage; (+) = possibly reduces brain damage; − = may be harmful; 0 = studies showed no effect; blanks = not studied for effect on outcome.

blood flow, reduces brain edema, normalizes brain pH, or stabilizes membranes[759]; (5) control of reperfusion pressure, flow, blood composition, and temperature by emergency cardiopulmonary bypass[97, 120, 462, 637, 758, 894]; and (6) understanding and ameliorating the complex hematologic-rheologic changes which interact with endothelium[320, 321, 421]. Other specific treatments to consider for animal model studies include allopurinol[173], DMSO[11], naloxone[355], phenoxybenzamine[431], heparin[320, 868], streptokinase[469], indomethacin[320], prostacyclin I_2[320] and leukopheresis[320, 421, 439].

Volatile anesthetics such as halothane (which, like barbiturates, reduce metabolism) may be harmful to the damaged brain, because they increase cerebral blood flow and ICP and depress blood flow autoregulation within the brain[503, 818]. Isoflurane might protect[932]. 'Therapeutic anesthesia' is not a new idea[363, 442]. The issues of when to rest the injured brain and when to stimulate it need investigation. The number of brain resuscitation potentials worth investigating in animal models is vast[759, 760].

To *conclude*[760c], animals and patients have occasionally completely recovered neurologically after more than 10 minutes of complete normothermic global brain ischemia or cardiac arrest. The limit of resuscitability from normothermic circulatory arrest seems to be the same for heart and brain, namely between 10 and 20 minutes, both in animals[760a] and patients[760b]. This justifies cautious optimism about cerebral resuscitation potentials. Semi-empirical studies in animals have not yet yielded the hoped-for breakthrough, because of the many poorly understood pre-arrest and post-arrest factors that influence outcome, particularly the increasingly recognized complexity of the post-resuscitation syndrome. A systematic collaborative search for novel CPCR methods is warranted, to extend the reversible duration of clinical death to a maximum[760c]. This should be accompanied by studies which determine the biologic limits to the reversibility of clinical death, and by a search for reliable measurements early post-arrest which could be used to predict outcome with permanent brain damage. In the meantime, clinicians should participate in randomized clinical trials of risky or expensive treatments, and select for non-research clinical use inexpensive, simple to use, and risk-free treatment potentials that improved outcome in clinically relevant animal models.

Evaluating Insult, Progress and Outcome (Tables 8–10)

In every emergency and critical care setting—be it department, hospital, community or region—attempts should be made to quantitate the clinical material in terms of types and severity of insult at the time the patient enters the EMS system (Table 8), the appropriateness of measures used and their influence on the progress of the disease (Table 9), and the *outcome* in terms of mortality and permanent disability (performance capability) (Tables 10 and 11). The purpose of evaluation is not only for research, but also for gauging the quality of services, guiding service priorities for the future, and—in the individual case—helping predict outcome and thereby determine the appropriate level of care (Table 12).

The simple methods summarized here for estimating or quantitating a cardiac arrest insult (Table 7), post-CPR progress of recovery (Table 9), and outcome (Table 10) have withstood the tests of time and controlled clinical trials[2–4, 214, 306, 377, 404, 736b, 885]. We recommend their widespread use to enable comparision of data between different patient populations. This chapter concerns primarily cardiac arrest. For cases of trauma (see Chapter 4), trauma scores permit quantitation of severity of insult[22b, 138].

Evaluating insult (Table 8)

The severity and duration of the ischemic-anoxic (cardiac arrest) insult influence the outcome of cerebral and overall function, as do the adequacy of

Table 8. Estimation of global ischemic-anoxic insult.

1. *Hypoxia time prior to arrest* Time of severe hypotension, severe hypoxemia, or severe anemia	.... min
2. *Arrest time* Time without spontaneous or artificial pulse in large arteries. Must *not* include CPR time. No blood flow	.... min
3. *CPR time* Equals time of CPR-ABC, i.e. borderline perfusion by cardiac compression during cardiac arrest. Low blood flow	.... min
4. *Hypoxia time after arrest* Time of severe hypotension, severe hypoxemia, or severe anemia following restoration of spontaneous circulation	.... min
5. *Total insult time★* Sum of 1, 2, 3 and 4	.... min

★ Repeated arrests and repeated restoration of spontaneous circulation within one resuscitation effort should be stated as the sum of all times without circulation (total arrest time) and the sum of all times of hypotension, hypoxemia and anemia (one total hypoxia time), whether this occurred before or after the first or subsequent arrest.

Source: Based on data form of Brain Resuscitation Clinical Trial (Safar P, Abramson N et al, 1979–1989).

resuscitation, the underlying disease and the secondary complications. The severity of traumatic brain insult is in itself almost impossible to quantitate (Chapter 4). However, the severity of a global ischemic-anoxic insult, like cardiac arrest, can be estimated immediately retrospectively by interviewing

Table 9. Glasgow–Pittsburgh coma scoring method (1984) (Teasdale G, et al; Safar P, Smyder J, Reimmuth O, Abramson N, et al: Brain Resuscitation Clinical Trial II, 1984–1989).

Glasgow coma score (GCS) (at time of examination)	Pittsburgh brain stem score (PBSS) (at time of examination)

Glasgow coma score (GCS) (at time of examination)

If patient is under the influence of anesthetics, sedatives or neuromuscular blockers, give best estimate of each item.

Write number in box to indicate status at time of this exam.

(A) *Eye opening*

Spontaneous	= 4
To speech	= 3
To pain	= 2
None	= 1

(B) *Best motor response*
(extremities of best side)

Obeys	= 6
Localizes	= 5
Withdraws	= 4
Abnormal flexion	= 3
Extends	= 2
None	= 1

(C) *Best verbal response*
(If patient intubated, give best estimate.)

Oriented	= 5
Confused conversation	= 4
Inappropriate words	= 3
Incomprehensible sounds	= 2
None	= 1

Total GCS
(Best   GCS = 15)
(Worst GCS = 3)

Pittsburgh brain stem score (PBSS) (at time of examination)

Add to GCS (A, B, C)

Lash reflex present (either side)	yes = 2 no = 1	☐
Corneal reflex present (either side)	yes = 2 no = 1	☐
Doll's eye or iced water calorics reflex present (either side)	yes = 5 no = 1	☐
Right pupil: reacts to light	yes = 2 no = 1	☐
Left pupil: reacts to light	yes = 2 no = 1	☐
Gag or cough reflex present	yes = 2 no = 1	☐

Total PBSS
(Best   PBSS = 15)
(Worst PBSS = 6)   ☐

Patient condition at time of examination:
Check (√) all that apply.

☐ Anesthesia/heavy sedation

☐ Paralysis (partial or complete neuromuscular blockade)

☐ Intubation

☐ None of the above

Note: The primary purpose of this scoring system is to identify a hierarchical *level* of function from brain stem to cerebrum, not to indicate laterality of disease.

bystanders, relatives, ambulance personnel and other health care personnel (Table 8). We recommend estimating 'arrest time' (without CPR), 'CPR time', 'hypoxia times before and after the arrest and CPR', and 'total insult time' (Table 8).

Evaluating progress and coma (Table 9)

The degree of unresponsiveness (depth of coma) and its change over time (progress) can and should be followed, at least as long as the patient is in the ICU after a cerebral insult. This may be accomplished by standard neurologic evaluation[629] and by using the following two coma scales:

1. *The Glasgow Coma Scale* (Table 9)[885] has become popular for quantitating the depth of CNS depression in cases of head injury. It uses a score of total 15 points, the best score of 15 being composed of 4 points for consciousness (eye opening), plus 6 points for best motor response, plus 5 points for best orientation (verbal response). The worst score, for coma with brain death, is 3 points—one point for each of the three categories. This scale has been tested and used primarily to evaluate patients with cerebral trauma.

2. *The Glasgow–Pittsburgh Coma Scale* (Table 9)[214, 743] was designed to evaluate comatose patients after any type of insult—trauma, cardiac arrest and others. When we applied the Glasgow Scale to cases of medical coma, we found a need to score or at least record in addition brain stem reflexes and breathing. We thus have retained the Glasgow score of 15 points (best) and first added $4 \times 5 = 20$ points (5 each for pupils, brain stem reflexes, absence of seizures and breathing)[743]. This 35-point scale was used in the first phase of our randomized clinical trial of CPCR for cardiac arrest[2–4, 404] and correlated well with outcome[214]. Since there were no problems with seizures and apnea on controlled ventilation, we simplified it for the second phase of our study (1984–) to the scale shown in Table 9, which is now in use. The Pittsburgh brain stem score (PBSS) is added to the Glasgow Scale; breathing pattern is commented on separately. The prognostic correlations with outcome of brain stem reflexes have been determined by others[465, 466]

Any coma score will be lower (worse) if the patient is under the influence of a CNS depressant or a neuromuscular blocker. Thus, it is preferable that the depth of coma following CPR be scored before their administration. It should then be repeated at 6–24 hour intervals, until recovery of consciousness.

Scoring technique with Glasgow–Pittsburgh coma scale (Table 9) primarily for patients who do not respond to verbal command

I. Glasgow coma scale (GCS)[885]

(A) *Eye opening.* Watch for spontaneous eye opening (without stimulation). Spontaneous eye opening does not necessarily imply awareness. If there is no spontaneous eye opening, speak loudly to the patient (e.g. "open your eyes"). If there is no response, apply pain by forcefully pressing on fingertips (pressure on the face can cause grimacing and eye closure).

(B) *Best motor response.* First stimulate the patient with a verbal command. If there is no response, apply a painful stimulus; first use forceful pressure on the fingertips to induce any response, then pressure on the supraorbital notch to test for localization. 'Obeys' is judged from the response to instructions such as to lift the arm or protrude the tongue. Asking the patient to squeeze the examiner's fingers is not a reliable test, since reflex grasping may occur in unconscious patients. If there is no response to command, apply a painful stimulus. The significance of the response to pain is not always easy to interpret unless stimulation is applied in a standardized way and is maintained until the maximal response is obtained. Initially, apply pressure to the fingernail bed with a pencil; this may result in either flexion or extension at the elbow. If you see flexion, stimulate the head, neck and trunk, to test for localization. A 'localizing' response means that a stimulus applied at more than one site causes a limb to move to attempt to remove the stimulus. A flexion response may vary from rapid withdrawal, associated with abduction of the shoulder ('withdraws' = score 4), to a slower, stereotyped assumption of the hemiplegic or decorticate posture with adduction of the shoulder ('abnormal flexion' = score 3). Extensor posturing is obviously abnormal and is usually associated with adduction, internal rotation of the shoulder, and pronation of the forearm ('extends' = score 2). Test each side separately, and record best side as indicated on the form.

(C) *Best verbal response.* The stimulus is conversational questioning. 'Oriented' means that the patient knows who and where he/she is and the date. If conversational exchange is possible, but the patient lacks the above orientation, it is termed 'confused'. 'Inappropriate words' refers to intelligible articulations used in an exclamatory or random way; no sustained conversational exchange is possible. 'Incomprehensible sounds' refers to moaning and groaning but no recognizable words.

II. Pittsburgh brain stem score (PBSS)[2-4, 214, 404, 743]

(A) *Eyelash reflex.* Test by stroking the eyelashes and observing contraction of the lower lid.

(B) *Corneal reflex.* Test by touching the rim of the cornea with a moistened cotton swab and observing closure of the eyelids.

(C) *Doll's eye reflex.* (Do *not* use in suspected head–neck injury!) Test by turning the head abruptly from side to side. A positive response (i.e. reflex present) is contraverse conjugate eye deviation (e.g. if the head is rotated to the right, the eyes deviate to the left).

(D) *Iced water calorics* (After checking that the tympanic membrane is undamaged and removing impacted cerumen). Elevate the head 30° above horizontal. Irrigate the external auditory canal with up to 120 ml of iced water, slowly introduced through a small catheter. Absence of reflex is indicated by a lack of deviation of eyes.

(E) *Carinal reflex.* Test by inserting a suction catheter through the tracheal or tracheostomy tube, deep enough to touch the bifurcation of the trachea. Watch for coughing motions. In the unlikely event that the patient has absent reflexes but is still without tracheal tube, check for a gag reflex instead of a carinal reflex by stimulating the posterior pharyngeal wall with a tongue blade or laryngoscope. Watch for gagging motions.

Note: If the patient is paralyzed, anesthetized, intubated or on controlled ventilation, the coma score will be affected. Presence of any of these conditions at the time of examination must be indicated on the form. Examination in the absence of any or all of these factors gives a more accurate neurologic assessment.

Predicting outcome

In assessment of depth of coma, rapid recovery of eye and upper airway reflexes should be considered good prognostic signs. Poor (but not hopeless) prognostic signs, on the other hand, include absence of the oculocephalic (doll's eye) or oculovestibular (caloric) reflex at 6–12 hours post-arrest, continuing unconsciousness and nonreactivity of the pupils, and progressive deterioration of reflexes after initial partial recovery[466]. Pupil size, eye and lid movements, EEG activity[313–315, 381, 382, 639a, 981] (difficult to determine reliably in the ICU setting) and return time of spontaneous breathing are less reliable as prognosticating indicators[88, 466, 479]. Important for prognosticating outcome with brain damage are the time lapses over hours or days for the recovery of coordinated breathing movements, cranial nerve reflexes, flexor positioning, defensive motor and verbal responses and recovery of purposeful responses to verbal stimuli[381]. Electrocortical activity recovers first intermittently, then continuously, and may or may not normalize[381]. Early post-arrest recovery patterns of evoked potentials[133] and EEG spectra[135] are being explored for their prognosticating values.

It is possible that CPCR causes some conditions that were previously not survived now to be survived with permanent coma. Certifying brain death is not a problem, since it equals death[65, 305–307, 634]. Survival in a persistent vegetative state is more difficult to prevent[305, 929]. In comatose patients, outcome predictions can be uncertain. The longest reported unresponsiveness followed by complete recovery has been 2 weeks after cardiac arrest[2–4, 106, 466] and about 1 year after head injury[307, 639]. Neurologic assessment and EEG changes may be misleading and complicated by therapy[151, 307, 382, 466, 639]. Cerebrospinal fluid (CSF) enzyme activity measurements look promising as predictive 'chemical brain biopsy'[213, 567, 910]. Severe damage to brain cell membranes results in leakage of large molecular cytosolic enzymes into the CSF. The level of various cytosolic enzymes, particularly brain-specific creatine phosphokinase (CPK-BB), rises in the CSF (not in the blood), peaking at about 48 hours after cardiac arrest. Studies showed an excellent correlation between 48–72 hours post-insult CSF CPK-BB peaks, the severity of the insult, and the resulting neurologic and histologic damage, both in animals and in patients[213, 478, 567, 910a, b, c]. After cardiac arrest, CSF CPK-BB levels above 80 unit/l support prognosis of PVS, and levels above 20 unit/l are abnormal (normal CFS CPK-BB = < 5 unit/l)[910]. After focal brain lesions, high CSF CPK-BB levels early post-insult may be seen even when good outcome follows.

Evaluating outcome (Table 10)

After emergency resuscitation, the outcome should be evaluated in terms of quality of life, as evident from patient performance capability. The Glasgow outcome categories 1 (best) through 5 (worst)[377] have provided a simple

Table 10. Progress and outcome evaluation: Glasgow–Pittsburgh outcome categories 1–5 (Jennett B, et al; Safar P, Abramson N, et al: Brain Resuscitation Clinical Trial I and II, 1979–1989).

Cerebral performance category (CPC)

Evaluate *only* cerebral performance capabilities.

Check (√) one

Overall performance category (OPC)

Reflects cerebral *plus* noncerebral status. Evaluate *actual* overall performance.

Check (√) one

CPC 1. Good cerebral performance
Conscious, alert, normal cerebral function. May have minor psychological or neurologic deficits which do not significantly compromise cerebral or physical function. ☐

OPC 1. Good overall performance
Conscious, alert, capable of normal life. Good cerebral performance (CPC 1) plus slight or no functional disability from noncerebral organ system dysfunction. ☐

CPC 2. Moderate cerebral disability
Conscious, alert, sufficient cerebral function for activities of daily life (e.g. dress, travel by public transportation, food preparation). May have hemiplegia, seizures, ataxia, dysarthria, dysphasia or permanent memory or mental changes. ☐

OPC 2. Moderate overall disability
Conscious, alert. Moderate cerebral disability alone (CPC 2) *or* moderate disability from noncerebral organ system dysfunction alone, *or both*. Performs independent activities of daily life (dress, travel, food preparation) *or* able to work in part-time sheltered environment. Disabled for competitive work. ☐

CPC 3. Severe cerebral disability
Conscious, has at least limited cognition. Dependent on others for daily support (i.e. institutionalized or at home with exceptional family effort), because of impaired brain function. Includes wide range of cerebral abnormalities, from ambulatory patients who have severe memory disturbance or dementia precluding independent existence, to paralyzed patients who can only communicate with their eyes (e.g. the locked-in syndrome). ☐

OPC 3. Severe overall disability
Conscious. Severe cerebral disability alone (CPC 3) *or* severe disability from noncerebral organ system dysfunction *or both*. Dependent on others for daily support. ☐

OPC 4. Coma/vegetative state
Definition same as CPC 4. ☐

OPC 5. Death (without beating heart)
Apnea, areflexia, 'coma', no pulses (see text). ☐

CPC 4. Coma/vegetative state
Not conscious, unaware of surroundings, *no cognition*. No verbal and/or psychological interaction with environment. May *appear* awake because of spontaneous eye opening or sleep–wake cycle. Includes all degrees of unresponsiveness which are neither CPC 3 (conscious) nor CPC 5 (coma which satisfies brain death criteria). ☐

OPC A. Anesthesia (CNS depressant)
Uncertain as to above categories because anesthetic, other CNS depressant drug or relaxant effects. ☐

Time achieved: ☐ ☐
Hour   Minute

CPC 5. Brain death (with beating heart) or death (without beating heart)
Apnea, areflexia, 'coma', EEG silence ☐

Compared with baseline status *before* the insult, the patient's *intellectual* function *now* is (check [√] one in each column):

CPC A. Anesthesia (CNS) depressants
Uncertain as to above categories because of anesthetic, other CNS depressant drug or relaxant effects. ☐

Time achieved: ☐ ☐
Hour   Minute

	Patient opinion	Family opinion	Examiner opinion
Unchanged (1)	☐	☐	☐
Worsened (2)	☐	☐	☐
Unsure (3)	☐	☐	☐
Other or unable to determine (4)	☐	☐	☐

Explain: _____
_____

mechanism for classifying patient outcome in terms of performance capability after head injury. The Glasgow–Pittsburgh cerebral performance categories (CPC) and overall performance categories (OPC) separate the cerebral from the extracerebral disabilities. The CPC-OPC evaluation was designed for post-cardiac arrest states[2-4, 720], where it proved important to evaluate the effect of new treatments on cerebral recovery versus mortality and morbidity due to the underlying disease (most commonly cardiovascular failure). Overall and cerebral performance should be assessed upon discharge from the ICU and periodically thereafter up to at least 6 months in cases of ischemia; longer in cases of head injury. Of particular interest for brain resuscitation studies is the *best* cerebral performance category that the patient achieves at any time post-resuscitation. Although the separate evaluation of CPC and OPC was designed for cases of medical coma[2-4, 404, 720], it should also be preferable over OPC alone in patients with head injury, who may have suffered polytrauma.

Briefly, the cerebral (CPC) and overall performance categories (OPC) are as follows (Table 10): *Category 1*, conscious and normal, without disability. *Category 2*, conscious with moderate disability. *Category 3*, conscious with severe disability. *Category 4*, coma or vegetative state, without brain death. *Category 5*, brain death or death. For example, a conscious, mentally active, bedridden post-CPR patient with severe heart disease would have a CPC 1 and OPC 3. Differences between CPC and OPC are for categories 1, 2 and 3; OPC 4 and 5 are determined by the cerebral status, thus identical to CPC 4 and 5. Overall performance category (OPC) 5—death—may be due to primary extracerebral organ failure or to primary brain death (CPC 5), with the heart still beating or stopped.

Starting and Terminating Emergency Resuscitation

When not to undertake emergency resuscitation

Resuscitation should not be undertaken when the patient is in the terminal stages of an incurable disease, when the physician's orders include 'do not resuscitate' or 'no CPR', or when there is another acceptable reason to withhold CPR[305, 929]. Among such acceptable reasons are situations in which there is no reasonable chance to restore human mentation (e.g. when clinical death has progressed to the point of rigor mortis, evidence of tissue decomposition, or extreme dependent lividity), and, of course, gross traumatic destruction of the brain.

Uncertainty regarding the possibility of brain death (Table 11) should *not* deter resuscitative efforts, since brain death cannot be determined immediately, and newer techniques for post-arrest treatment show promise of mitigating the damaging effects of ischemia-anoxia on the brain.

When to terminate emergency resuscitation

In acute respiratory or circulatory distress, the medical professional or trained lay person on the spot must start resuscitation immediately. There is no time for contemplation or consultation[713]. *After* the start of emergency resuscitation, however, when it becomes known that the patient is in the terminal stage of an incurable disease or that he is almost certainly incapable of regaining cerebral function (e.g. after 30 minutes to 1 hour of proven pulselessness at normothermia without CPR), all the resuscitation efforts may be discontinued[713]. Whenever possible, the decision to terminate resuscitation should be made by the physician, on the basis of his own and his colleagues' experience and knowledge. Common sense must play a large role in determining when to stop resuscitation in any given case.

In multicasualty incidents or mass disasters, of course, sorting of patients according to appropriate treatment priorities (resuscitation triage) will often justify withholding or discontinuing emergency resuscitation efforts in seemingly hopeless cases without availability of consultants or laboratory tests.

Cardiac death (irreversible cardiac arrest)

In all salvageable patients, CPR efforts should be continued until spontaneous circulation is restored or signs of cardiac death (irreversible cardiac arrest) are present. Cardiac death is evident when there has been intractable electric asystole (a flat line on the ECG) for at least 30 minutes, despite optimal CPR and drug therapy. Pulselessness in the presence of ECG complexes (mechanical asystole without electrical asystole) is *not* proof of irreversibility[713]. As long as ECG activity continues, even in the form of ventricular fibrillation (VF) or agonal QRS complexes, one must assume that there is still a chance of restarting spontaneous circulation. Near-normal or abnormal ECG activity may continue for many minutes after cardiac arrest without resuscitation and for hours during CPR. During closed-chest CPR without ECG monitoring, irreversibility cannot be proved, since VF may be present, and VF is always potentially reversible. There have been occasional cases of VF with CPR of several hours' duration, followed by successful defibrillation and recovery of conscious-ness. The previously healthy heart experiencing clinical death without pretreatment can be made to beat again effectively after up to about 20 minutes of normothermic and 90 minutes of hypothermic complete global myocardial ischemia—particularly with controlled reperfusion by emergency cardiopulmonary bypass[120, 713, 894]. The use of such high technology for artificial circulation in resuscitation in the future might bridge the gap from irreversible heart failure to the emergency implantation of an artificial or natural (donor) heart.

Apparent brain death during emergency resuscitation

It is impossible to judge the salvageability of the brain during emergency resuscitation. Therefore, terminating emergency CPR efforts in the presence of apparent brain death is justified only when there is also cardiac death[713, 720].

During CPR Steps A–B–C, before restoration of spontaneous circulation, patients may regain pupillary constriction and spontaneous respiratory movements, but almost never awareness. During CPR, electroencephalographic (EEG) activity cannot be monitored reliably because of movement artifacts; EEG activity would be of poor prognosticating value, because it does not correlate with the degree and speed of neurologic recovery.

After restoration of spontaneous circulation, reactive pupils, increased responsiveness, spontaneous movements and resumption of spontaneous breathing efforts are strong indicators that there is some cerebral oxygenation. On the other hand, dilated, fixed pupils and absence of spontaneous breathing efforts for at least 1–2 hours after the restoration of spontaneous circulation are usually, but not always, followed by brain death or recovery with severe brain damage. Dilated, fixed pupils, however, can also occur in the absence of cerebral death, as the result of brain contusion, skull fracture, intracranial hemorrhage, catecholamines given for resuscitation, or over-dose of a hypnotic or anesthetic.

When brain death persists after restoration of spontaneous circulation, it is frequently associated with pressor-resistant hypotension and cardiac arrest, secondary to medullary herniation from cerebral edema. If circulation continues, however, with or without vasopressors, brain death should not be certified until life support has been optimized and the patient's condition has stabilized for at least 24 hours. Most patients who develop the criteria of brain death do so on the second day post-arrest, after various degrees of initial neurologic improvement.

As a rough guide, most patients who begin to wake up within 10 minutes of restoration of spontaneous circulation will recover with normal brain function. On the other hand, most patients who show no purposeful response to painful stimuli (e.g. forceful pressure on the angles of the mandible), with no oculocephalic (doll's eye) reflex or oculovestibular (caloric) reflex by 6–12 hours after restoration of normotension, and who receive standard post-resuscitative care, will suffer some degree of permanent brain damage[465]. Such damage may range from minor psychologic-behavioral changes to the persistent vegetative state. Note that these tests of function may not be feasible under conditions in which the use of anesthetics and other central nervous system depressants or relaxants is required to stabilize the patient.

Even after recovery from anesthetics or relaxants, a persistent vegetative state (with active EEG and reflexes) cannot be diagnosed with certainty until 1–2 weeks of unconsciousness has elapsed after the CPR effort. This is particularly true when treatment has included new brain resuscitation methods, because these newer techniques have occasionally achieved complete recovery even after 10–20 minutes of circulatory arrest in normothermia (or up to 40 minutes in hypothermia) and 1–2 weeks of unresponsiveness following CPR[151, 647, 804, 854].

In summary, in potentially salvageable patients, termination of emergency resuscitation efforts is justified when there is solid evidence of irreversible cardiac arrest; however, it is *not* justified solely on the basis of neurologic signs suggesting cerebral or brain death, since these signs are not reliable prognostic indicators during and immediately after CPR.

Terminating Long-Term Resuscitation (Tables 11, 12)

Brain death determination and certification (Table 11)

Modern resuscitation has changed the definition of death (Fig. 1)[65, 519, 553, 713, 736a, 848, 941]. *Clinical death* is apnea (no spontaneous breathing movements) plus total circulatory (cardiac) arrest, with all cerebral activity suspended but not irreversibly. Clinical death is the early period of death during which initiation of resuscitation, provided therapy is optimal, might be followed by restoration of all vital organ systems function, including normal brain function.

Cerebral death (cortical death) is irreversible destruction (necrosis) of the cerebrum, particularly the neocortex and other supratentorial structures—not the medulla. It is the EEG and morphologic picture associated with deep vegetative state (apallic syndrome), i.e. coma with spontaneous breathing present but a silent or diffusely grossly abnormal electrocorticogram.

Brain death (total brain death) is cerebral death plus necrosis of the entire brain, including cerebellum, midbrain and brain stem[65, 307, 519, 553, 634, 687, 713, 736a, 941]. Cerebral death and brain death often become apparent following restoration of circulation by CPR, with or without initial transient improvement of neurologic status. When brain death develops after cardiac arrest, it is usually after initial neurologic improvement, which reverts to brain death within the first week. Most medical and legal authorities now define 'death' in terms of brain death, even though the heart may continue to beat as artificial ventilation is maintained[634]. With permission, organs may be removed from the brain-dead (i.e. dead) heart-beating donor for transplantation[305, 307].

Biologic death (panorganic death) inevitably follows clinical death when there is no invervention with CPR or when resuscitation efforts are abandoned (Fig. 1)[736a]. Biologic death is an autolytic process in all tissues, starting with cerebral neurons, which become necrotic after about 1 hour without circulation, followed by heart, kidneys, lungs and liver, which become necrotic after about 2 hours without circulation, and the skin, which may not become necrotic for many hours or days.

'Social death' is persistent vegetative state (PVS), the apallic syndrome. It represents irreversible severe brain damage in a patient who remains unconscious and unresponsive but has some EEG activity, some reflexes, and is capable of breathing spontaneously. This is to be distinguished from *cerebral death*, in which the cortical EEG is silent and the brain stem (partially) also continues to produce spontaneous breathing; and from *brain death*, in which all cranial nerve reflexes and spontaneous breathing efforts are also absent. In the vegetative state, there can be wake–sleep cycles.

Terminating 'life support' in brain death. Brain death is the permanent loss of all integrated neuronal functioning, including cerebrum, brain stem, pons, midbrain and cerebellum[65, 305, 634, 720]. Brain death following cardiac arrest and CPR is usually the result of cerebral ischemic encephalopathy, hypoperfusion, necrosis, edema and consequent brain herniation, sometimes occurring after a brief period of neurologic improvement. Brain death is more likely to ensue after severe, prolonged insults or inadequate resuscitation. Destruction of the medullary centers results in intractable arterial hypotension and secondary cardiac arrest in spite of use of vasopressors and artificial ventilation. Secondary cardiac arrest usually occurs within 72 hours after the onset of the clinical picture of brain death, although in rare instances hearts of artificially ventilated patients with brain death have been kept beating for up to 1 month, with circulation supported by fluids and drugs. Nonetheless, once at least two licensed physicians have determined and certified total brain death, most ethical and legal views permit cessation of all treatment, including artificial ventilation and airway control (Table 11)[65, 305, 307, 634, 720, 929].

Specific criteria for determining brain death have been proposed by many groups. Such criteria should be established at the community, state or national level, but should be consistent with internationally accepted guidelines and practices. Although there is agreement on concepts, guidelines differ concerning which tests are required. All require detailed neurologic examination. The criteria in various states may or may not demand repeat evaluation after 2, 3, 6 or 12 hours. Although most guidelines require EEG determination, in hospitals where reliable EEG tracings cannot be obtained, it is acceptable to determine brain death without proof of EEG silence if all other criteria are present. In ICUs, EEG tracings without artifacts are often impossible to obtain.

Brain death criteria in use at the University of Pittsburgh since 1968, as developed and modified by Grenvik[305, 307], include (Table 11): (1) complete absence of cerebral and brain stem activity on two clinical examinations performed at least 2 hours apart, in the absence of CNS depressants, relaxants or hypothermia; and (2) one isoelectric EEG recording with auditory stimulation for at least 30 minutes. Part of the EEG record must be with an amplification of 2 $\mu V/mm$. The EEG is usually obtained during the interval between the first and second clinical examination. Succinylcholine may be used to abolish muscle artifacts that interfere with the EEG tracing, but its effect must be absent (tested by nerve-muscle stimulator) before the subsequent clinical examination. There should be no spontaneous breathing activity within 3 minutes of apnea, with arterial PCO_2 permitted to rise to 50 mmHg. Oxygen 100% should be given to prevent hypoxemia during the test, and blood gas analysis should be used for confirmation when available. Cranial nerve reflexes and responses, including pupillary reflexes, must be absent. The heart rate must not increase following atropine.

In short, all evidence of brain stem activity must be absent. Spinal cord activity (e.g. reflex spasms), however, may be present, since spinal cord neurons may remain viable after brain death. Two physicians must sign the certification document (Table 11).

Table 11. Brain death determination and certification (1984) (Grenvik A, et al, Presbyterian University Hospital of Pittsburgh, USA).

Note: The patient must be observed in the hospital during treatment of potentially correctable abnormalities (e.g. hypovolemic shock). Two clinical examinations must then be performed; the second no sooner than 2 hours after the first.

Date and time of 1st exam _____   2nd exam _____

A.   Coma of established cause and absence of induced hypothermia and central nervous system depressant drugs. A blood ethanol level and/or other appropriate toxicology studies should be performed if indicated. Body temperature should be recorded.

	1st exam	2nd exam
1. Body temperature	_____	_____
2. Blood ethanol	_____	_____
3. Toxicology studies	_____	_____

B.   No spontaneous muscular movements and no evidence of decerebrate or decorticate posturing or shivering (in the absence of muscle relaxant). Spinal reflexes (stimuli causing movements) may be present.

C.   Cranial nerve reflexes and responses:
1. Pupils light-fixed _____
2. Absent corneal reflexes _____
3. Unresponsiveness to intensely painful stimuli, e.g. supraorbital pressure _____
4. Absent response to upper and lower airway stimulation (e.g. pharyngeal and endotracheal suctioning) _____
5. Absent ocular response to head turning (no eye movement) _____
6. Absent ocular response to irrigation of the ears with 50 ml of ice water (no eye movement) _____

D. Absence of spontaneous breathing movements for 3 minutes and $PaCO_2$ above 60 mmHg at end of test (in absence of muscle relaxant). If a history suggestive of dependence on a hypoxic stimulus for ventilation (e.g. emphysema) is present, the PaO_2 at end of test must be less than 50 mmHg.
   1. $PaCO_2$ at end of apnea test _____
   2. PaO_2 at end of apnea test _____

E. An isoelectric electroencephalogram recorded in part at full gain (see text). _____

F. Failure to increase heart rate by more than 5 per minute following 1 mg atropine intravenously:
   1. Heart rate before atropine _____
   2. Heart rate after atropine _____

G. Comments: _____

CERTIFICATION
Having considered the above findings, we hereby certify the death of:

_____

Date _____   Time _____

Physician's Signature   Names Printed

                               Dr. _____

                               Dr. _____

(*This document should be signed by two physicians.*)

These criteria are only guidelines. When EEG or blood gas monitoring is not available, carotid angiography and demonstration of the absence of intracranial perfusion is an acceptable alternative way to prove brain death. When no laboratory determinations are available, clinical signs alone must suffice.

Brain death determination and certification should be done after stabilization of the patient in the ICU and after sufficient time has been allowed for the course of CNS deterioration to be assessed in an orderly fashion. Family consent is not required for certification of brain death, but the family should be kept fully informed of the patient's condition and be counseled and emotionally supported.

Once total brain death has been certified, procedures to be fulfilled will depend on the local, regional and national criteria. In the USA, once brain death has been certified organs may be removed for transplantation, with signed consent from the family, while the donor's heart is beating. After organ removal, all treatments including artificial ventilation are discontinued, and circulatory arrest is permitted to occur[305, 307, 634, 929].

Critical care triage (Table 12)

In the context of resuscitation, 'triage' refers to the process of sorting critically ill patients in terms of expected outcome and possible treatment regimens, i.e. 'appropriate' levels of care. At Pittsburgh's Presbyterian-University Hospital, critical care triage, as pioneered by Grenvik et al, is facilitated by the custom that two physicians classify and periodically reclassify each ICU patient into one of four categories (Table 12)[305, 307, 720, 929]: (1) total support (all ICU patients fall into this category at the time of ICU admission); (2) full support, short of CPR; (3) 'letting die' (extraordinary measures are withdrawn); (4) brain death certification (all measures are withdrawn).

Letting die in persistent vegetative state (Table 12)

'Letting die' should be carried out according to medical, legal and ethical customs of the community[168, 305, 527, 635, 713, 831]. These determine the degree of care appropriate in hopeless, moribund patients.

The most common indications for 'letting die' are irreversible coma with spontaneous breathing, due to cerebral (cortical) death (EEG silence, no apnea); and persistent vegetative state (no EEG silence, no apnea). The latter differs from brain death in many ways, since the patient may have an active EEG, cranial nerve reflexes and spontaneous breathing; he is simply 'disconnected' from his surroundings.

The socioeconomic tragedy of severely brain-damaged survivors is obvious, for such cases may impose an unbearable financial and emotional burden on the family. The decision to discontinue extraordinary means of life support is a medical one. It should be made by an experienced physician who is thoroughly familiar with the case, in consultation with experienced specialists (e.g. anesthesiologist, critical care physician, neurologist), and should consider the patient's previously expressed wishes, the family's attitude, prognostic signs and measurements (see previous section), and the best quality of life expected. Although relatives should not be asked to make this decision, their agreement with the physician's decision should be sought[929].

The criteria for brain death certification are objective and reliable (Table 11). On the other hand, in a given patient, completely reliable proof of the irreversibility of the vegetative state (apallic syndrome) (irreversible coma without brain death), or of permanent severe neurologic deficit with consciousness, is usually not possible. Thus, the hopelessness of the situation must often be determined from a combination of published

Table 12. Critical care triage: selecting appropriate levels of care*.

1. *Total support*
   For critically ill or injured patients in whom survival without persistent severe brain failure is expected. Vital organ systems, although usually affected, are not irreversibly damaged. Everything possible is done to reduce mortality and morbidity.

2. *All but CPR*
   For patients with continuing brain function or hope for brain recovery, who have irreversible cardiopulmonary or other multiple organ failure, or are in the terminal stages of incurable disease, e.g. advanced carcinomatosis. Everything possible is done for comfort. Prolongation of life is not carried beyond cardiac arrest. When this occurs, CPR is not provided and the patient is permitted to die.

3. *No extraordinary measures, letting die*
   For patients in whom some forms of treatment seem meaningless, serving only to prolong death rather than life. Examples are patients with minimal brain function in whom there is no hope for improvement and thus no prospect for future human mentation. Extraordinary measures are not initiated for such patients or are discontinued if such discontinuation is not expected to result in immediate demise. Such extraordinary measures may include admission to the ICU; CPR; dysrhythmia control; tracheal intubation; mechanical ventilation; use of artificial organs; transplantation; blood transfusion; invasive monitoring; i.v. infusion of potent vasoactive drugs; and total parenteral nutrition. In some circumstances, the responsible physician may consider it medically sound and ethical also to withdraw gastric tube feeding, i.v. fluids, and antibiotics. The conscious moribund hopeless patient is made comfortable and pain free.

4. *Brain death determination and certification; termination of all life support*
   For patients with irreversible cessation of all brain function. Once brain death has been demonstrated by established criteria, the patient is declared dead and all therapy is stopped. If organ donation is being considered, cardiopulmonary support is continued until the required organs have been removed.

* Adapted from Grenvik et al[305], Presbyterian-University Hospital of Pittsburgh, USA.

predictive criteria (none of which are 100% reliable), clinical judgment and laboratory data; the latter may include CSF CPK-BB elevation at 48–72 hours[213, 567, 910], persistently low cerebral blood flow and metabolism[111, 789], and brain shrinkage on CT or NMR imaging[992].

Although brain death certification calls for withdrawal of *all* life support measures, 'letting die' (passive euthanasia) calls for discontinuance of *extraordinary measures only* (Table 12). Extraordinary measures may be defined differently in different countries, depending on priorities and available resources, which are finite everywhere. In most industrialized countries, extraordinary measures include mechanical ventilation, blood administration, dysrhythmia control and life-supporting drugs; they may or may not include i.v. fluids and alimentation. Airway care is usually considered 'ordinary' care. In irreversible vegetative state, antibiotics and artificial feeding and hydration (intravenously or by gastric tube) may justifiably be withheld[24, 929]. In the terminal state of a hopeless case, honoring the patient's wishes (as previously expressed if presently unconscious), a dignified departure from life, for the patient (if aware) and his surroundings (family, friends), is part of the art of medicine and should receive priority over prolonging the dying process[929].

Once irreversibility of coma is determined by a combination of clinical judgment, the patient's history and laboratory data, letting the patient die of natural causes, in a dignified setting, is ethical and feasible. Prolonged expensive intensive care in the clearly hopeless case is inappropriate, undignified, socioeconomically counterproductive and unethical[46, 929]. The brain is the target organ of resuscitation. Resuscitation must reach beyond technological advances and concern itself also with the quality of life (see Chapter 7).

Chapter 4

Special Considerations

Introduction

This chapter concerns itself with several considerations and conditions for which the resuscitation methods described in Chapters 1, 2 and 3 are appropriate, but which may require some special emphases or modifications. First, we shall discuss 4 special technical considerations of resuscitation: (1) pediatric resuscitation; (2) neonatal resuscitation; (3) witnessed arrest; and (4) complications and pitfalls of CPR. Second, we shall summarize a few important practical points concerning 8 common special dying mechanisms (Fig. 1)[736a]: (1) sudden cardiac death, myocardial ischemia and infarction; (2) alveolar anoxia; (3) asphyxia; (4) exsanguination cardiac arrest; (5) hypoglycemia; (6) hypothermia; (7) hyperthermia; and (8) electrolyte and acid–base derangements. Third, we shall comment on 9 selected special emergency conditions in which one or more of the above dying mechanisms may be encountered[736a]: (1) electric shock; (2) drowning; (3) acute pulmonary edema; (4) pulmonary embolism; (5) status asthmaticus; (6) carbon monoxide poisoning; (7) anesthesia-related cardiac arrest; (8) drugs and poisons; (9) anaphylaxis. This section has been adapted from previous publications[736a]. Fourth, we shall summarize 11 topics of trauma requiring resuscitation, adapted from the advanced trauma life support (ATLS) material of the American College of Surgeons[22b]: (1) introduction and patient assessment (including trauma scale); (2) severe polytrauma; (3) circulatory shock; (4) burns; (5) radiation injuries; (6) cerebral trauma; (7) spinal cord trauma; (8) thoracic trauma (including tension pneumothorax and cardiac tamponade); (9) abdominal trauma (including peritoneal lavage); (10) extremity trauma; (11) anesthesia in disasters.

Special Technical Considerations

Pediatric cardiopulmonary resuscitation (Fig. 57)[23b, 784a, 985a]

For purposes of resuscitation, an *infant* is defined as younger than 1 year and a *child* as 1–8 years old. Children more than eight years old may be treated with the techniques described for adult resuscitation. The major differences in CPR for the child compared with the adult are: (1) the etiology of cardiopulmonary arrest, which in children is predominantly asphyxia rather than primarily ventricular fibrillation; (2) differences in the size of victims;

and (3) the availability of specialized physicians and nurses for the care of neonates, infants and children.

In terms of teaching and organization, it is worthwhile to coordinate teaching of pediatric resuscitation with that of adult resuscitation. Trainees should learn adult resuscitation techniques before embarking on training programs for resuscitation of infants and children. Neonatal resuscitation, however, should be taught in separate courses because of its importance and unique features (see neonatal resuscitation, below).

The sequence of steps of CPR and general resuscitation principles are the same for infants, children and adults. However, priorities and techniques differ somewhat for different age groups.

Cardiac arrest in children and infants is usually the result of suffocation by foreign body obstruction, near-drowning, trauma, burns, smoke inhalation, poisoning, upper airway infection or sudden infant death syndrome. Primary ventricular fibrillation or asystole is rare and in newborns almost unheard of. Thus, prevention of accidents is most important in this age group. Once an emergency occurs, however, Steps A and B of CPR are most important to prevent cardiac arrest. With prolonged hypoxemia usually preceding cardiac arrest in children, outcome results of CPR attempts, once pulselessness has occurred, have been poor[490]. Thus, prompt application of Steps A and B before the onset of pulselessness is crucial. Parents, child care personnel and teachers should be taught prevention of accidents and pediatric CPR. Young children should not be left unsupervised. In automobiles, all age groups should use seat belts. In developed countries, almost half of all deaths in children and infants are the results of accidents, with almost one-half of these motor vehicle accidents.

Basic life support without equipment differs somewhat from that in adults. If the child is unconscious, the same sequence of steps as in adults is recommended. Head-tilt by chin support is favored. Extreme backward tilt of the head might occlude the small infant's upper air passage. Often moderate head-tilt alone is all that is needed to open the airway. If not, gentle jaw thrust plus opening of the mouth should be added. The infant's mouth should not be closed, as nasal obstruction is common. If the child is struggling to breathe, but is conscious, he/she should be rapidly transported to an advanced life support facility.

Although air is easily blown into the infant's stomach, maintaining manual pressure on the epigastrium is not favored, as this can provoke regurgitation. Only if abdominal distension makes ventilation impossible should one press over the epigastrium for gastric decompression, and then only after the child has been turned on his/her side. Pressure over the epigastrium should be accompanied by gentle clearing of the pharynx by finger or suction. Gastric distension can be minimized by gentle slow inflations[528, 529].

In the case of acute airway obstruction, when there has been a history of fever and barking cough, one should suspect *croup or epiglottis*. The usual measures for managing foreign body obstruction are contraindicated in such cases, and the patient should instead be rushed to the hospital, where emergency tracheal intubation may be required. Oxygen should be given en route, if available. Pre-hospital attempts at tracheal intubation in such cases should only be by a highly experienced operator and as a last resort.

When circumstances suggest that obstruction has been caused by a *foreign body*[324] and the child is conscious, he/she should be encouraged to take a deep breath and to cough up the foreign body. If cough is ineffective, or if the child becomes cyanotic or unconscious, a (still controversial)[23b] combination of gentle finger sweeps of the pharynx (Fig. 7) and back blows and abdominal thrusts (Figs. 8–10) should be used. Some discourage blind finger sweeps in infants and children, fearing to push the foreign body deeper[23b]. The authors find gentle finger sweep more likely to be effective in children than in adults, as insertion of the hooked finger along the inside of the cheek can reach to the larynx entrance to dislodge the foreign body. Jaw thrust plus inflation attempts can sometimes transform complete into partial obstruction. Chest thrusts are preferred over abdominal thrusts by the authors, for simplicity of teaching (chest thrusts are the same as chest compressions for CPR). Abdominal thrusts are *not* recommended in infants, because of the danger of causing internal injuries[889], but are permissible in children[23b].

Chapters 1 and 2 include some reference to children and infants. The most important changes in adult CPR that one must consider in resuscitating children and infants, for basic and advanced life support[985a] are evident from Fig. 57 and the following instructions. Prolonged life support for infants and small children calls for special expertise in pediatric intensive care[44, 350, 395]. Further details may be obtained from the literature[23b, 72, 137, 324, 490, 601].

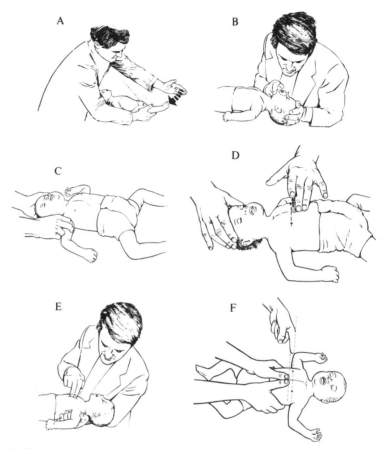

Fig. 57. Resuscitation of the newborn or infant. (A) If unconscious, stimulate sole of foot for arousal. (B) If not breathing or breathing inadequately, perform mouth-to-mouth-plus-nose ventilation, with moderate backward tilt of the head by chin support. (In newborn, ventilate with puffs from your cheeks rather than from your lungs.) In newborn resuscitation, use bag–valve–mask–oxygen unit if available. (C) After two inflations, feel brachial artery pulse. If no pulse (or if in newborn heart rate below 60 per minute), start external chest (cardiac) compressions. (D) For external chest compressions, locate lower half of sternum by drawing an imaginary line between nipples, which divides the sternum in half; and compress the sternum with two or three fingers, one finger's width below that line. (E) Compress sternum 0.5–1 inch (1.3–2.5 cm) at the rate of about 120 per minute (2 compressions per second). Compression–relaxation ratio should be 50:50. After every fifth sternal compression, pause briefly and give one lung inflation; continue with compressions at 5:1 ratio. During CPR, support the chest with one hand (or ask an assistant to support the chest) to maintain the head tilted backward; this may make it unnecessary to switch one hand to the forehead for ventilations. (F) An alternative method for chest compressions in small infants is to encircle the chest with both hands, with the fingers at the back and thumbs pressing over the sternum one fingerbreadth below the midsternum, as described above.

Technique for resuscitation of infants and children: Steps A–B–C without equipment (Fig. 57)[23b]

Differences from adult methods are in italic.
1. Determine unresponsiveness (gently shake and shout). If the patient is unconscious, place him/her on firm flat surface, supine (face up), and horizontal, with the legs elevated (if hypovolemic). Call for help.
2. Open the airway by head-tilt with chin support. Place one hand on the forehead, the other supporting the chin and mouth slightly open. If necessary, add jaw thrust; in cases of trauma, use moderate head-tilt plus jaw thrust and open mouth (Fig. 6).
3. Determine breathlessness (apnea). Look for chest movements, listen for exhaled air, and feel for air flow.
4. If the patient is not breathing, begin artificial ventilation. In infants and small children, use *mouth-to-mouth plus nose*. Encircle the mouth *and* nose with your mouth. In larger children, use mouth-to-mouth *or* mouth-to-nose. Pinch the nose with your hand on the forehead.

Start rescue breathing with *two slow inflations* (1–2 seconds each), and remove your mouth and let him/her completely exhale passively.

Adjust the inflation force and volume to make the chest rise. Moderately slow inflations help avoid gastric distension. Inflate in infants once every *3 seconds (20 per minute)*. Inflate in children once every *4 seconds (15 per minute)*.

You may use cricoid pressure, if you are a health professional trained in its use, to limit gastric insufflation.
5. If the chest does not rise, the airway is obstructed; readjust head-tilt and chin support, and add jaw thrust (Fig. 6). Try again to ventilate. If the chest still does not rise, or at any time when foreign matter is visible at the mouth, use finger sweeps of the mouth and throat (Fig. 7).
6. Determine pulselessness—feel a large artery (5–10 seconds). In children over 1 year feel the *carotid or femoral* artery; under 1 year the *brachial or femoral* artery, since the infant's short chubby neck make carotid palpation difficult.

Palpate the carotid artery with two fingers of one hand, at your side of the larynx, while maintaining head-tilt with the other hand on the forehead. Press gently, do not occlude.

Feel the femoral artery in the groin just below the inguinal ligament, approximately midway between the symphysis pubis and the anterior superior iliac spine. Feel the *brachial artery* on the inside of the upper arm between the elbow and shoulder.

Precordial pulses are unreliable. Also look for abdominal (aortic) pulsations.
7. If there is no pulse, start external chest compressions to provide

artificial circulation. Activate the EMS system (ask a helper to call the emergency phone number). Do not leave the victim.

In infants, perform chest (heart) compressions in the horizontal supine positon on a hard surface (e.g. the *palm of one hand*). Maintain *head-tilt* as necessary by *lifting the shoulders. Compress the lower half of the sternum, one finger breadth below where the line connecting both nipples* crosses the sternum at the midline. Use *2–3 fingers,* pressing *0.5–1.0 inch* (1.3–2.5 cm), at *120 per minute* (approx. 2 compressions per second). Keep your fingers on the sternum during relaxation. Use a compression/inflation ratio of *5 : 1* for both *one and two operators;* add a pause after every 5th sternal compression for one ventilation (total 1–2 seconds per inflation). After 1 minute of CPR, check the pulse, and check it again after several minutes.

In children, perform chest (heart) compressions, also over the lower half of the sternum. Locate the lower margin of the *rib cage* on one side with your middle finger and follow to the base of the sternum. Place your index finger next and cephalad to the middle finger, and place the *heel of your other hand* next to the index finger on the *lower half of the sternum.* Compress the sternum with the heel of one hand *1–1.5 inches* (2.5–3.5 cm) at a rate of *80–100 per minute.* Keep your fingers off the ribs. Keep your hand on the sternum during relaxation. Use a 50:50 ratio for compression and relaxation.

In children over 8 years, use the adult methods.

Removal of foreign body without equipment in infants and children (Fig. 8–10)[23b]

In infants, if you suspect foreign body airway obstruction place him/her prone (face down), *straddled over your arm,* with the head down, supported with your hand on the jaw. Rest your forearm on your thigh. With the heel of your other hand give four *backblows* between the shoulder blades. Sandwich the infant between your two arms and hands and turn him/her around face up (Fig. 10). Apply *four chest thrusts* in rapid succession, like external chest compressions for CPR. Do *not* use *abdominal thrusts* in infants.

If the infant is unconscious, try to *ventilate.* Apply gentle *finger sweep* (Fig. 7). Repeat *backblows* and *chest thrusts.* Repeat ventilation attempts, finger sweeps (follow the inside of the cheek with your index finger to hook the foreign body out of the throat), back blows, and chest thrusts; and repeat until you can ventilate or help arrives.

In children the technique is the same, but use the side position for *backblows.* (The American Heart Association and the Resuscitation

Council (UK) no longer teach back blows; the International Red Cross does.) In children you may use chest thrusts[311] or *abdominal thrusts*[23b, 334-336]—with the victim standing or sitting if conscious; or with victim lying if unconscious—as for adults (Figs. 8–10).

If the child is relaxed, use the tongue jaw lift maneuver (Fig. 7) which may release an obstruction, and if you see the foreign body, remove it with your hooked finger or use finger tweezers (Fig. 7).

Note: The best and ultimate method for foreign body obstruction is extraction under direct vision with the use of a laryngoscope (or flashlight and tongue blade) and forceps, suction or finger.

Step F: defibrillation in infants and children[23b, 316]

1. Use external defibrillator chest electrodes (with built-in ECG electrodes) of 4.5 cm diameter for infants and small children, and 8 cm diameter for older children.
2. Treat ventricular fibrillation (and ventricular tachycardia with unconsciousness) by external countershock with *2 J/kg*. Use techniques and sequences as in adults.
3. If the above fails, repeat the shock with *4 J/kg*; and repeat again. After three serial shocks, before increasing the dose further, improve oxygenation, give epinephrine and correct arterial PO_2, PCO_2, pH and hypothermia.
4. If countershocks again fail, use lidocaine followed by bretylium if necessary, as in adults (in pediatric doses).

For ECG synchronized cardioversion use one-tenth to one-half energy (0.1–1.0 J/kg).

Step D: Drugs for resuscitation of infants and children[23b]

Use the same drugs for adults, for the same indications, but in slightly different doses (Chapter 3)[23b, 985a].

Drug	*Dose*
Epinephrine (adrenaline)	For CPR: 0.01 mg/kg (0.1 ml/kg of 1 : 10 000) i.v. (if not i.v. consider intratracheal or bone marrow instillation, using the same dose). For spontaneous circulation support: 0.1–2.0

	μg/kg per min i.v. titrated to direct arterial pressure measurement.
Sodium bicarbonate	1 mEq/kg i.v. (plus hyperventilation!) (solution 1 mEq/ml in children, 0.5 mEq/ml in infants). As soon as possible, titrate against arterial base deficit (BD) (0.3 mEq/kg × BD × kg) as determined by an arterial blood gas (Fig. 40).
Atropine sulfate	0.02 mg/kg (maximal 1 mg total). Doses may be repeated three times.
Calcium chloride 10%	20 mg/kg i.v. (0.2 ml/kg solution). Calcium should not be given routinely during CPR, only if there is hypocalcemia, hyperkalemia, hypermagnesemia; or anesthetic or calcium entry blocker-induced hypotension.
Dopamine	2–20 μg/kg per min titrated to direct arterial pressure (AP) measurement.
Lidocaine (Xylocaine, lignocaine)	Bolus 1 mg/kg i.v. Infusion 20–50 μg/kg per min i.v.
Dobutamine	5–15 μg/kg per min titrated to AP.
Isoproterenol	0.1–1.0 μg/kg per min i.v., titrated to heart rate and AP.
Norepinephrine (Levophed)	Start 0.1 μg/kg per min titrated to AP. 1 mg/500 ml—infants 2 mg/500 ml—children
Naloxone (Narcan)	0.01 mg/kg i.v. May be repeated as needed.

Respiratory stimulants (coramine, cardiazol, picrotoxin, etc.) are *not* indicated for resuscitation!

Neonatal resuscitation (Table 13)[23b, 229, 302, 375, 896]

by Peter Safar and Ian Holzman

When cardiac arrest in the newborn occurs outside the hospital, in the absence of health care personnel, the basic life support measures summarized above for infants and children are the only ones available for treating the newborn infant in distress. Wherever possible, deliveries should be conducted in a hospital with complete obstetric and newborn resuscitation services. If conducted outside the hospital, the presence of personnel experienced in newborn resuscitation techniques, including the use of equipment, is essential.

The importance of neonatal resuscitation is evident from the fact that any degree of asphyxia in the first few minutes of life can cripple a child for life. Airway obstruction by mucus, blood, meconium or the tongue; brain damage during traumatic birth; drugs given to the mother; and blood loss from cord compression or hemorrhage can all result in asphyxia and shock in the newborn infant and cause lasting brain damage.

Evaluation of the neonate with the *Apgar score* has been adopted worldwide and is recommended as a simple, uniform way of assessing the infant's condition[30]. This is best done at 1 and 5 minutes after full delivery. However, *resuscitation should never wait for determination of the Apgar score.* The scoring system uses five objective signs which are evaluated and scored with 0, 1 or 2—making the best score 10, and the worst score 0 (Table 13).

Normal *deliveries*, and particularly complicated deliveries, should be managed in a way that permits immediate treatment, in the event of asphyxia, hypothermia, shock, acidemia or hypoglycemia[302, 374, 375, 419].

Immediately after delivery of the infant's head, gently clear the nose and pharynx with suction. A hand-operated bulb aspirator is preferred unless meconium is present. If a mechanical device is used, the vacuum should not exceed 30 cmH$_2$O. The catheter used for suction may also be used to check for nasal-choanal patency, but the operator should be aware of the risk of inducing bradycardia with deep suctioning in the first few minutes after delivery[160].

If the infant is breathing and pink upon full delivery, quickly dry the skin and place on his/her side, with the head tilted backward, against the mother's body or in a heated isolette to prevent heat loss. If in need of

Table 13. Apgar scoring system for evaluating newborn infants (e.g. at 1 and 5 minutes after full delivery).

	Score*		
Clinical sign	*0 points*	*1 point*	*2 points*
A: Appearance (color)	blue, pale	body pink, extremities blue	completely pink
P: Pulse	absent	less than 100	over 100
G: Grimace (reflex irritability)	no response	grimaces	cries
A: Activity (muscle tone)	limp	some flexion of extremities	active motion
R: Respiratory effort	absent	slow, irregular	good, strong cry
Total score	worst: 0		best: 10

* Score 10 = optimal condition.
Score 6 or less = depression; resuscitative measures required.

resuscitation, keep the baby supine (horizontal, face-up) with the head held in a moderate backward tilt. Add jaw thrust or a pharyngeal tube if necessary. If the breathing is shallow or cyanosis is present, use *exhaled air ventilation* (mouth-to-mouth plus nose with gentle puffing). This may require skillfully adjusted assisted breathing superimposed on the patient's own respirations (when the patient breathes in, you breathe out). Cyanosis as a sign of hypoxemia is more reliable in infants than in adults, because of the infant's higher hemoglobin content. Significant polycythemia in small-for-gestational-age infants, infants of diabetic mothers and twin-to-twin transfusions can lead to cutaneous sludging and the appearance of cyanosis.

For neonatal *respiratory resuscitation* in the hospital, a bag–mask–oxygen unit is recommended—using either a valveless to-and-fro unit (which requires an anesthesiologist's skills) or the infant version of a self-refilling bag–valve–mask unit with oxygen reservoir (e.g. Laerdal or Ambu infant unit). The bag–mask unit should have a pressure-limiting pop-off valve, preset at 30–35 cmH$_2$O with a 60 cmH$_2$O override, since high pressure may be necessary for initial lung inflation. In the absence of a pop-off valve, an airway pressure gauge should be attached to the bag–valve–mask unit and observed carefully in order to avoid pressure over 20 cmH$_2$O. The unit should have a low dead space, an effectively sealing infant mask, and an oxygen reservoir permitting delivery of 50–100% oxygen to the infant. Manually triggered oxygen-powered ventilation devices are not recommended.

When ventilation by mask fails, *intubate the trachea* using a 3.0–3.5 mm ID tube in a term neonate (Table 2, Figs. 14–16). For intubation there are special anatomic considerations[212] (Chapter 1A). Initiate ventilation by bag–valve–tracheal tube or, in its absence, mouth-to-tracheal tube. Oxygen enrichment of your exhaled air can be accomplished by filling your own mouth with oxygen via a nasal or oral cannula.

If thick *meconium* is present during delivery, it is essential to clear the oro- and nasopharynx prior to the onset of breathing. This can be accomplished by suction when the head is delivered but prior to delivery of the thorax, to prevent aspiration. After delivery, a depressed infant will require suction of the oropharynx and visual inspection of the vocal cords for the presence of meconium. If meconium is suspected to be below the cords, the trachea should be intubated and suction applied to the tube with your mouth (via a DeLee suction trap if available) to remove meconium. If thick meconium occludes the tube, it may be necessary to remove the tube and reintubate. The overall goal is to remove as much meconium as is feasible within a relatively short time (less than 1 minute) prior to initiating positive pressure ventilation which would force particulate meconium into distal airways[130].

Endotracheal intubation and ventilation with oxygen by mouth-to-tube or bag–valve–tube are indicated if, in spite of assisted ventilation by bag–mask–oxygen, oronasal suctioning, warming and external stimuli, breathing remains depressed or the heart rate drops *below 100* beats per minute. With severe asphyxia (Apgar score < 2) it is often necessary to intubate during the first minute of life[68, 229]. Drugs are only rarely necessary for resuscitating infants. Usually ventilation-oxygenation restores a normal heart rate of over 100 per minute. Also, failure to achieve adequate oxygenation and heart rate may indicate the presence of a pneumothorax, pulmonary hypoplasia or a congenital anomaly such as diaphragmatic hernia.

Prolonged respiratory distress calls for continuous positive pressure breathing, which is being increasingly recommended as a prophylactic measure in severely premature or asphyxiated infants, to prevent the development of respiratory distress syndrome (Fig. 22). Spontaneous breathing with positive airway pressure is possible via mask or nasal prongs, whereas IPPV with PEEP requires an endotracheal tube. Both are specialized measures to be carried out wherever possible in neonatal intensive care units[302].

If respiratory resuscitation fails to restore adequate *circulation*, external cardiac compressions for assisted circulation should be considered whenever the heart rate is *below 60–80* beats per minute. In circulatory distress, a catheter should be inserted into the umbilical vein for drug and fluid administration. Insert it approximately 3–4 cm, which should place it into the portal sinus. Free aspiration of blood must be confirmed prior to injecting drugs. Care should be taken to avoid infusing hypertonic solutions. Blood gas monitoring and pressure monitoring can be accomplished by inserting a size 3.5–5 French catheter via one of the two thick-walled umbilical arteries. The distance can be determined by a standard graph[210, 414].

If there is *hypotension*, as measured by umbilical artery transducer or infant-cuff technique, in spite of adequate oxygenation, infuse a 15 ml/kg dose of 5% albumin, lactated Ringer's solution or blood. In addition, give dextrose 10 or 25% in water (an initial dose of 0.5 g/kg), since hypoglycemia is common in neonates. Fluid overload must be avoided, as there is little room for error in treating the neonate. Attention to temperature control is essential throughout the resuscitation. The use of radiant heat is mandatory and polyethylene wrapping may be efficacious as well.

Determine arterial PO_2, pH, PCO_2 and hemoglobin, and calculate the base deficit[374]. Correct the base deficit slowly with sodium bicarbonate. The overall dose in mEq needed is equal to the arterial base deficit in mEq/l × body weight (kg) × 0.3 (Fig. 40). Correct, at most, one-half of this base deficit initially, and only if it remains greater than 10 mEq/l when adequate oxygenation and perfusion have been obtained. In many cases, lactic acid is metabolized within 1–2 hours and no $NaHCO_3$ is needed. Rapid bicarbonate administration may lead to cerebral acidosis from increased carbon dioxide and to intracranial hemorrhage from hypernatremia. If the baby is intubated during bicarbonate administration, hyperventilate.

If there is *cardiac arrest*, severe asphyxia (as suggested by prenatal fetal heart rate monitoring or pH determination from scalp blood samples) or shock, and if blood gas analyses are not available, *slowly* inject sodium bicarbonate 1–2 mEq/kg diluted 1:1 with sterile water (0.5 mEq/ml solution) into the umbilical vein. For shock add i.v. dextrose 10% in Ringer's solution. Bicarbonate 1 mEq/kg may be repeated every 10 minutes of arrest, but is preferably titrated to arterial base deficit and pH. In cardiac arrest, epinephrine is also indicated in 1:10 000 dilution (1 mg/10 ml), 0.1 ml/kg (0.01 mg/kg) i.v. The dose is 0.1 ml/kg of 1:10 000 and can be given via the endotracheal tube if no other access is available.

Cardiac resuscitation is not always justified in clinically dead newborn infants. Obviously, where there is only transient pulselessness following a complicated delivery, a brief period of closed-chest CPR may quickly restart the asphyxiated asystolic heart and is therefore justified. After CPR for prolonged pulselessness, however, irreversible brain damage (cerebral palsy) is almost certain to follow, since cardiac arrest in the newborn infant occurs secondary to asphyxia or shock, which are usually associated with prolonged intrauterine hypoxia. Obviously, in infants and children beyond the first few hours of life (provided there are no defects incompatible with ultimate survival), sudden pulselessness should be treated with all-out CPR. There are several different ways of performing CPR in infants[23b, 896] (see above section on infants) (Fig. 57).

In the newborn, respiratory resuscitation, fluid and acid–base control, temperature control, and treatment of hypoglycemia must be carried out vigorously; however, prolonged cardiac resuscitation efforts are unwise because they may result in the survival of a severely brain-damaged child. It is useful to be aware of the time from the onset of resuscitation to the beginning of respiration (first gasp) since more than 20 minutes of adequate resuscitation without the onset of gasping often indicates severe cerebral damage[181].

Equipment available in the *delivery room* should include: radiant warmers; ECG with neonatal electrodes; adjustable suction with vacuum manometer; suction catheters size 5, 6 and 8 French gauge; an oxygen source; bag–valve–mask unit with mask sizes 0 and 1 and with oxygen reservoir; oropharyngeal tubes sizes 0, 00 and 000; tracheal tubes 2.5–3.5 mm diameter with stylet; laryngoscope with straight blades sizes 0 and 1; umbilical artery and venous catheterization tray with catheters 2.5 and 5 French gauge; three-way stopcocks; drugs as above; intravenous fluids; and an 18 gauge catheter-inside-needle to evacuate a pneumothorax.

Monitoring resuscitation and intensive care of the fetus and neonate in hospitals are highly specialized subjects and therefore beyond the scope of this book. We would like to stress, however, that resuscitation services for newborn infants should integrate basic life support, advanced life support and post-resuscitative intensive therapy as part of *community-wide* emergency medical services[784a]. All general advanced life support facilities should be staffed and equipped to provide basic and advanced life support, not only for adults but also for children, infants and neonates (Chapter 6).

Resuscitation from cardiac arrest in infants and children is required less often than in adults. Inhospital pediatric resuscitation carries an excellent prognosis, even though pre-hospital prognosis has been disappointing[218]. Conversely, inadequate resuscitation of a child is more likely to result in lifelong brain-damaged survival.

It is highly recommended that all hospitals with obstetric services be equipped and staffed for advanced maternal–fetal monitoring, neonatal resuscitation, and for transfer of the infant with life support to a neonatal intensive care unit. Ideally, neonatal intensive care services should be established on a regional basis, as should obstetric units for identified high-risk pregnancies.

Within hospitals with obstetric services, newborn resuscitation should be organized and quality controlled by an interdisciplinary committee. For neonatal resuscitation at least two persons are required, one to ventilate and intubate and the other to monitor, insert catheters and inject medications. Performing cardiac compressions, if necessary, requires a third person.

Witnessed arrest (cough CPR and precordial thump) (Fig. 58)[23a]

There are a number of special considerations and controversies that apply to the management of witnessed sudden cardiac arrest, among them: (1) use of the C–A–B sequence in place of the usual A–B–C sequence (Chapter 1C); (2) empirical electric countershock ('blind defibrillation') in the absence of an ECG tracing (Chapter 2F); (3) cough-CPR; and (4) precordial thump. Of these four techniques, the authors endorse (2), (3) and (4).

Empirical countershock[295]

We recommend[23b, 720] in sudden witnessed cardiac arrest without ECG monitoring, but when a d.c. defibrillator is available, empirical application of one external countershock of about 200 J (3 J/kg), and continued CPR. This situation has become very rare, since most portable defibrillators include ECG monitors with ECG electrodes incorporated in the defibrillating paddles. Treatment of witnessed, monitored sudden ventricular fibrillation or ventricular tachycardia by immediate external electric countershock, without preliminary CPR Steps A–B–C, has become routine in cardiac care units. This method is effective as long as the heart remains oxygenated, i.e. for about 30–60 seconds after the onset of pulselessness. Therefore, each patient at risk of cardiac arrest should have a defibrillator in immediate readiness. New devices for immediate automatic defibrillation are available (see Step F).

Cough CPR[170]

When sudden ventricular fibrillation (VF) without gasping or coughing induces cardiac arrest instantaneously, the victim becomes unconscious within 10–15 seconds. Spontaneous vigorous gasping or, even better, repeated vigorous coordinated coughing can produce limited blood flow due to intrathoracic pressure fluctuations. Each gasp preceding a cough (Mueller maneuver) produces a thoracic 'diastole'; each subsequent glottic closure and pressure build-up during cough (Valsalva maneuver) produces a thoracic 'systole'. In the cardiac catheterization laboratory, patients who have been coached to cough have kept themselves conscious by coughing for up to 90 seconds during VF, after which they were defibrillated[170]. Cough-CPR has been investigated in animals and patients[80, 585, 675]. It is still not known how long, following sudden onset of VF, active coughing can maintain sufficient oxygen transport to the brain to keep the patient conscious. Animal studies, however, suggest that coughing during cardiac arrest is a short-lived phenomenon.

The authors recommend the following. (1) Health care personnel should be taught how to coach repeated coughing when an ECG monitored patient suddenly develops VF; this should be considered an emergency standby measure while a precordial thump is given (see below) and a defibrillator is obtained. (2) Selected patients at risk of sudden cardiac death could be taught, "if you feel that your heart has stopped, call for help and cough forcefully once every second, with deep breaths in between coughs; this might keep you conscious until help arrives". Although the efficacy of this recommendation has not yet been examined, cough-CPR is at present the only possible self-help measure available for sudden cardiac death. (High-risk patients should be considered for automatic implantable defibrillators or home defibrillators.) When considering trials of cough-CPR one must keep in mind potential harm from coughing in the absence of cardiac arrest, such as the possiblity of inducing hypoxemia, bradycardia or VF in patients with severe heart disease; and the possibility of syncope from a sustained Valsalva maneuver.

Precordial thumping (Fig. 58)[620]

There is no evidence that the electric current produced in the heart by precordial thump is strong enough to reproducibly terminate VF. There is, on the other hand, some experimental and anecdotal clinical evidence that one precordial thump can convert ventricular tachycardia (VT) (unpredictably)[620] and occasionally even VF back to sinus rhythm[119]. The thump can also, however, unexpectedly induce VF[656]. In severe bradycardia or asystole from heart block (Stokes–Adams syndrome), repeated precordial thumping, if started within about 30 seconds of syncope, can often induce spontaneous cardiac contractions and serve as an external mechanical method for cardiac pacing ('fist pacing'). Standard external cardiac compressions (CPR), however, can accomplish the same, and in addition circulate blood, which thumps cannot do. Thumping may be less painful than sternal compressions. In severe bradycardia, precordial thumping or external cardiac compressions do not have to be synchronized with spontaneous cardiac contractions. Because a thump can be delivered by anyone immediately, it is recommended for use by any rescuer as the first step, in witnessed cardiac arrest: (1) without ECG monitored when a defibrillator is not immediately available; and (2) with ECG monitored in VT without pulse or VF. Precordial thumping can neither defibrillate nor stimulate cardiac contractions when the heart is anoxic; thus thumping is not a substitute for CPR.

For precordial thumping, the recommended *sequence of techniques* is as follows[23b, 720]. In witnessed cardiac arrest *without ECG monitoring*, use standard CPR, i.e. head tilt–ventilation–palpation for pulse–external cardiac compressions. If the victim becomes unconscious and continues to breathe adequately while you find the carotid pulse absent, go straight to

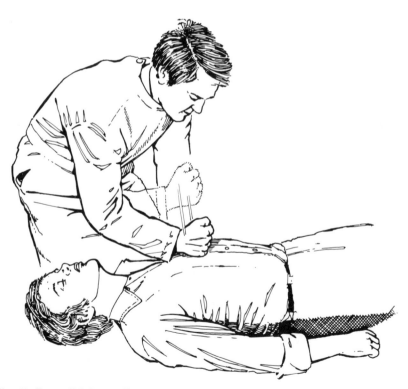

Fig. 58. Precordial thump. From a height of 8–12 inches above the chest, deliver a sharp quick single blow over the midportion of the sternum, using the fleshy bottom portion of your fist. For indications for precordial thump, see text.

Step C (external cardiac compressions), since he/she is already providing Steps A and B. The unconscious patient is, however, unlikely to maintain the airway or adequate tidal volume. Patency of the airway and adequacy of breathing must be continuously reassessed and Steps A and B instituted immediately when needed. If the patient has a very slow heart rate (less than 40 beats per minute), or is known to have heart block, and develops syncope, use the less painful repetitive thumping (fist pacing) when he/she is conscious; use external cardiac compressions when he/she is unconscious. Apply repeated thumping at a rate of about 60 per minute. If the necessary apparatus is available, use external mechanical[998] or electric[995] pacing. Ask an assistant to give atropine or isoproterenol i.v., and initiate insertion of an intravenous pacemaker once the diagnosis of heart block has been established.

In witnessed cardiac arrest *with ECG monitoring*, treat VT or VF with immediate electric countershock, without first starting CPR Steps A–B–C. As soon as VT or VF is suspected, feel for the carotid or femoral pulse. If it is absent, apply three sequential countershocks. Immediately recheck the pulse. If the patient remains pulseless, tilt the head backward, give four quick lung inflations, check the pulse again, begin external cardiac compressions, and continue with standard CPR. Repeat countershocks as needed (Chapter 2F). If you see VT on the ECG tracing and find the patient pulseless, and a defibrillator is not immediately available, apply one precordial thump. If VT or VF is successfully converted to sinus rhythm, check the pulse and beware of recurrence of VT/VF. If this does not terminate VT or VF, continue CPR and use the defibrillator when it arrives. If you see sudden severe bradycardia or asystole on the ECG tracing, give repetitive precordial thumps (about 60 per minute) while the patient is conscious and switch to standard CPR when he/she becomes unconscious. In *unwitnessed* cardiac arrest and in witnessed arrest in infants and small children, precordial thumping is *not* recommended.

Complications and pitfalls of CPR[23b, 37]

CPR can cause complications, even if performed correctly. Some are minor compared with the certain death if CPR is not started; others leave residual problems. The following are only a few examples.

Backward tilt of the head and positive pressure *inflation attempts* to ventilate the lungs rarely by themselves produce serious complications, even in patients who do not need them, provided they are performed correctly. If the airway is inadequate or inflations are too forceful, however, gastric insufflation may occur and provoke regurgitation and inhalation of gastric contents.

In the aged with atherosclerosis, maximal backward tilt of the head, particularly when the head is turned to the side, can cause circulatory impairment of the vertebrobasilar artery system, resulting in brain stem ischemia. In accident victims, maximal backward tilt of the head, turning the head to the side, and flexion of the head may all aggravate a cervical spinal cord injury and cause paralysis; thus, in these patients, maintenance of the neutral position with in-line traction or only moderate backward tilt of the head, as part of a triple airway maneuver, is recommended.

External cardiac compressions may result in costochondral separations or multiple rib fractures, especially in elderly patients, even if sternal compressions are performed correctly. This is not necessarily a serious complication. Should a flail chest result, prolonged controlled ventilation may be necessary after resuscitation. Pressure applied too high may cause sternal fracture. Pressure applied too low may rupture the liver or cause regurgitation. Pressure applied laterally may fracture ribs, leading to pneumo- or hemothorax or lung contusion. Bone marrow emboli are possible, but are not necessarily obstacles to recovery. Every patient after an episode of external cardiac compressions should have a chest X-ray as soon as practically possible[87, 570]. Sternal compressions cause (unavoidable?) hemorrhagic contusions and necroses of the heart[462, 637]. Gastro-esophageal laceration can also occur[522].

The previously recommended initial *stepwise inflation* of the lungs without waiting for full exhalation has not been proved to help reinflating alveoli. As it can also increase pharyngeal pressure to such an extent that the stomach becomes distended, it is no longer recommended[23b, 529]. Lung rupture with tension pneumothorax is possible when excessive volumes are blown into the lungs of infants or when the patient's lungs are diseased, e.g. in emphysema.

Endotracheal intubation attempts, if prolonged, may produce asphyxia and cardiac arrest. Although needed and safe in cardiac arrest, endotracheal intubation attempts in the patient with spontaneous breathing and retained reflexes can aggravate life-threatening dysrhythmias and increase intracranial pressure, even without producing hypoxemia. Thus, endotracheal intubation should be done with a clear understanding of the risks, benefits and alternatives.

Central venous catheter insertion via the *subclavian route* interrupts cardiac compressions and may cause pneumothorax, hemothorax and mediastinal infusion. Thus, this procedure should only be performed by properly trained health care providers.

The American Heart Association enumerates these *salient points*[23a, b]:

1. Do not interrupt CPR for more than 7 seconds, except for tracheal intubation, moving the victim over stairways or telephoning for help as a lone rescuer. These maneuvers should not exceed 60 seconds each.
2. Do not, under most circumstances, move the patient until stabilized; restoring spontaneous circulation at the scene has resulted in higher survival rates than transporting the patient with CPR and restarting spontaneous circulation in the emergency department. Stabilization includes ventilation,

oxygenation, venous lifeline, ECG monitoring, restarting spontaneous circulation, communication for consultation and arrangement for hospital admission.

There are exceptions to the requirement for stabilization at the scene, where ambulance personnel are not trained or equipped to use the invasive treatment required for life-threatening conditions, such as airway closure by laryngeal edema, tension pneumothorax, pericardial tamponade, intractable heart block requiring pacemaker insertion, hypothermic cardiac arrest requiring warm infusions or thoracotomy, and internal hemorrhage requiring resuscitative surgery. Under such circumstances rapid transportation without prior stabilization, and with life support measures as feasible en route, is necessary.

3. To avoid injury to the liver, do not maintain pressure on the abdomen to decompress the stomach while CPR is being performed.

4. Pay attention to the details of techniques. The objective is to minimize the risk of iatrogenic complications.

Special Dying Mechanisms

Sudden cardiac death, myocardial ischemia and infarction[23c]

In the USA, one-fifth of those who die from coronary heart disease are under 65 years old[23c]. Coronary artery disease is the most frequent cause of 'sudden cardiac death', which is defined as 'unexpected cardiac arrest without pre-arrest symptoms or with symptoms of less than 1 hour's duration'. Two-thirds of these sudden cardiac deaths occur outside hospitals. Although three-fourths of these victims have advanced coronary artery disease at autopsy, in more than 50% myocardial infarction is not evident as a precipitating factor; it is likely that this group suffers primary ventricular fibrillation (VF), perhaps triggered by temporary focal myocardial ischemia in 'hearts too good to die'[7, 62]. Cases of sudden cardiac death with or without myocardial infarction (the latter usually being diagnosed after hospital admission) have up to a 40% chance to awaken and be discharged from hospital, if CPR basic life support (BLS) by bystanders is started within 4 minutes and advanced life support (ALS) by ambulance personnel restarts spontaneous circulation within 8 minutes of collapse[216a, 440, 492, 938]. For the USA it has been estimated that such ideal (but feasible) implementation of CPR could save 100 000–200 000 lives each year. In spite of an overall decrease in cardiovascular disease mortality of about 20% and cerebrovascular disease mortality of about 40% over the past 2 years, the mortality of the 1.5 million myocardial infarctions each year still is about 20–30%. Also, 4.5 million Americans are at increased risk of sudden cardiac death due to having had a previous myocardial infarction.

Overall *risk factors* for coronary artery disease include: smoking, hypertension, low density lipoprotein cholesterol, diabetes, lack of exercise, obesity, stress, male sex, age and family history[23b, 485]. Education on prevention, warning signs, CPR-BLS and emergency telephone number (911 in the USA) should start in schools but continue for all age groups, as control of the above factors even later in life reduces the risk[23b, 485]. Additional pathogenetic factors under study include the roles of coronary spasm, the sympathetic nervous system, and platelets[23b].

Sudden ventricular fibrillation is often preceded by recognizable *warning signs* (chest–arm–shoulder pain, nausea, sweat, shortness of breath); and by premature ventricular complexes (PVCs) or ventricular tachycardia (VT), which the patient can 'feel' or suspect only occasionally. These tachydysrhythmias are sometimes triggered by bradycardia, particularly in acute myocardial infarction. Therefore, in uncomplicated acute myocardial infarction, suspected or proven, the measures listed below are crucial for the prevention of sudden cardiac death[23b, 153, 492, 610].

In acute myocardial infarction with *hypotension* (systolic arterial pressure below 90 mmHg), i.e. *cardiogenic shock*[38a, 250, 564, 799, 948], one should normalize the heart rate, control dysrhythmias and use invasive arterial and pulmonary artery pressure monitoring for titration of hemodynamic life support including pHa, PCO_2[951] and pulmonary artery occlusion (wedge) pressure (PAOP)[872] (Chapter 2D). With mean PAOP below 12 mmHg, one should use 100–200 ml i.v. rapidly administered fluid challenges and aim for a mean PAOP of 15–22 mmHg and for optimal cardiac output. For severe myocardial failure, increased filling pressures may be required. Among vasoactive agents, dopamine is popular because it increases cardiac contractility without producing much vasoconstriction at infusion rates of 1–10 μg/kg per min; however, dopamine may worsen tachycardia. Dobutamine is chosen for primarily beta-adrenergic activity, and norepinephrine, with primarily alpha-adrenergic activity, may be preferable for arterial pressure support. Simultaneous balanced titration of both has been effective.

In cases of profound hypotension, in additon to cardiac stimulants and vasoconstrictors, assisted circulation by *intra-aortic balloon pumping*[396], systole-synchronized high airway pressure jet ventilation[417, 626, 627] or cardiopulmonary bypass[47, 758] may be tried (Chapter 2). Intra-aortic balloon pumping reduces peripheral resistance during systole and increases diastolic coronary blood flow. In cardiogenic shock an intermittent increase in intrathoracic pressure by IPPV or CPPV is not only well tolerated, but improves ventricular transmural pressures and cardiac output[303, 627]. The mortality in cardiogenic shock is still over 80%. Therefore, intra-aortic balloon pumping[396], an expensive, specialized measure requiring an experienced intensive care team, is indicated where available, as it can occasionally turn the tide. Methods of assisted circulation should in general be reserved for those patients in whom operative repair (e.g. coronary angioplasty, coronary revascularization, valve replacement or heart transplant) is feasible. The use of assisted circulation as adjunct for medical treatment only helps rarely.

In acute myocardial infarction with *hypertension* (systolic blood pressure above 130 mmHg), attempts to normalize the blood pressure should be with i.v. beta-adrenergic blockade sublingual or i.v. nitroglycerin, i.v. furosemide or ethacrynic acid, and titrated i.v. infusion of nitroprusside with arterial pressure monitoring (Chapter 2D). Calcium entry blockers may also be useful for acute control of ischemia accompanied by hypertension.

In *acute* myocardial infarction with acute *pulmonary edema*, one should give 100% oxygen first by mask, preferably with spontaneous continuous positive pressure breathing (SB-CPAP) (Chapter 1B); place the patient into a full upright sitting position with the legs in a dependent position; normalize arterial pressure using direct pressure measurement (see above), and give morphine i.v. in titrated doses of 0.03 mg/kg each, to relieve anxiety and tachypnea and to produce 'bloodless phlebotomy'. Vasodilation by a calcium entry blocker (e.g. nifedipine) has also been effective. These drugs should be used with caution, so as not to induce severe hypotension. If morphine fails, actual phlebotomy of 500 ml of blood may provide dramatic improvement. One should monitor and normalize PAOP if possible. Arterial hypotension must be guarded against. If all of the above fails and arterial PO_2 cannot be maintained above about 80 mmHg with oxygen by mask, or if foam fills the tracheobronchial tree, the trachea should be intubated (smoothly!) and ventilation controlled with IPPV plus PEEP (i.e. CPPV) (Chapter 1B). If necessary, one should use heavy sedation and muscle relaxation.

Survivors of sudden cardiac death and CPR, patients with episodes of life-threatening dysrhythmias (with or without syncope), those who had suffered myocardial infarction with shock, pulmonary edema or severe dysrhythmia, and those with unstable angina are all at an increased risk of sudden cardiac death[566]. Prevention of such a lethal event is often possible with programmed electric stimulation studies with mapping of responses to various antiarrhythmic drugs[354], and long-term prevention of VT and VF by optimal drug therapy, physical measures or an automatic implanted pacemaker or defibrillator (Chapter 2F). Not every person who has frequent PVCs, however, is at increased risk of sudden cardiac death, as some healthy subjects can be prone to PVCs[695].

Prevention of sudden cardiac death in suspected acute myocardial ischemia

1. Administer *oxygen* at the earliest possible moment to any adult with chest pain.
2. Establish a keep-open *i.v. line* with 5% dextrose in water.
3. Begin ECG *monitoring*.
4. *Relieve chest pain*
(a) Nitroglycerin 0.4 mg sublingual every 5 min, max. 3 times.

(b) Morphine in small, titrated doses of 2–5 mg i.v. each, without producing hypotension.

(c) 50% oxygen/50% nitrous oxide self-administered by patient.

5. For *PVC-VT prophylaxis*, give a lidocaine infusion 1–4 mg/70 kg per min.

6. For *PVC-VT treatment*, give lidocaine bolus 1 mg/kg i.v. if:

(a) there are more than six PVCs per min,

(b) there are multifocal PVCs,

(c) there are two or more PVCs in a row,

(d) PVCs fall on a T-wave (R-on-T).

7. For severe bradycardia (and PVCs with a heart rate of less than 60 per minute), the *first* drug to use is atropine 0.5 mg i.v., every 5 minutes, up to four doses, followed by cautiously administered isoproterenol as needed, to be followed perhaps by a temporary pacemaker in second and third degree heart block.

8. If VT occurs without loss of pulse or consciousness, give lidocaine bolus, 1 mg/kg i.v. If lidocaine fails, give procainamide. If procainamide also fails, give bretylium. If bretylium also fails, use electric cardioversion.

9. Severe sinus tachycardia compromising cardiac output for which no cause can be found (e.g. hypoxemia, hypovolemia) may be suppressed with propranolol; PSVT with vagal maneuvers, verapamil and cardioversion. Avoid worsening cardiac failure with drug therapy.

10. Atrial fibrillation with a rapid ventricular rate should be controlled acutely with verapamil and chronically with digitalis if the patient is conscious, and with electrical cardioversion if the patient is unconscious or hemodynamically unstable.

11. One may try to reduce infarct size with cautiously titrated use of nitroglycerin and/or a beta-receptor blocker by i.v. titration[692]. Intracoronary thrombolytic therapy[405], emergency coronary artery angioplasty, and emergency coronary artery bypass operation are controversial.

Alveolar anoxia[736a, 873]

True alveolar anoxia is relatively rare. Examples are patients who have inhaled oxygen-free gas (e.g. laboratory, industrial, mining or anesthetic accidents), or who have suffered rapid decompression (in high-altitude flying). A sudden switch from breathing air or oxygen to breathing oxygen-free inert gas causes cerebral failure, followed rapidly by cessation of breathing movements and circulation. There is continued removal of carbon dioxide and other metabolites from anoxic tissue until oxygen lack stops the heart. The resulting neuronal failure may therefore be associated with less acidosis than in asphyxia. A sudden change to breathing oxygen-free gas results in spontaneous hyperventilation, and within 1 minute in hypotension, bradycardia and pupillary dilatation. Within 3–7 minutes, cardiac arrest develops in asystole. Clinical death after about 5 minutes is easily reversed with CPR. Rapid decompression causes cerebral brain failure almost as rapidly as in neck-cuff occlusion, which produces unconsciousness within 10 seconds[683].

Less fulminating alveolar hypoxia is common, in exposure to *high altitude* or inhalation of *gas mixtures* with decreased oxygen concentration. Alveolar hypoxia kills by the same mechanism as hypoxemia from pulmonary disease. At an arterial PO_2 of 30 mmHg, cerebral vessels are maximally dilated and a further decrease in PaO_2 will lead to cerebral anaerobiosis. Cardiac arrest may occur at a PaO_2 of 15–25 mmHg. In 'acclimated' chronic obstructive lung disease, pulse and some cortical function can continue with PaO_2 values to as low as 20 mmHg. Obviously, such severe degrees of hypoxemia cannot be tolerated long by the heart and brain. 'Resuscitation' from high-altitude pulmonary and/or cerebral edema consists of rapid descent and increased FIO_2 if possible[716].

Asphyxia[435, 651, 736a, 745, 873]

Hypoxemia denotes reduced arterial PO_2; *hypercarbia* (hypercapnia), increased arterial PCO_2; and *asphyxia* a combination of both. Hypoventilation is a reduction in alveolar ventilation (minute volume minus deadspace minute ventilation). This results, in the air-breathing animal or person, in a progressive increase in arterial PCO_2 and in an inversely related decrease of arterial PO_2. The extremes of hypoventilation are complete airway obstruction and apnea (no breathing movements), and these comprise the two principal causes of asphyxia.

By far the most common cause of rapid dying from obstructive asphyxia is *coma*, irrespective of the cause. Coma may result in: (1) upper airway soft-tissue obstruction from malpositioning (flexion) of the head; or (2) airway obstruction by foreign matter (e.g. vomitus) (Chapter 1). Other causes of upper airway obstruction include trauma with soft-tissue obstruction or inhalation of blood, inflammatory swelling of tissues (e.g. cellulitis of the floor of the mouth, croup, epiglottis) and food bolus obstruction. Laryngospasm may result in hypoxia-induced apnea, but usually the larynx relaxes before cardiac arrest.

Foreign matter may trigger reflex laryngospasm. If started prior to cardiac arrest, skilfully applied positive pressure artificial ventilation can usually revive the patient even if the foreign matter is not removed.

Moderate *partial airway obstruction* as in bronchospasm (asthmatic crisis) first stimulates increased respiratory efforts. When the patient becomes exhausted or the obstruction worsens, asphyxia develops, with rapidly progressive hypoxemia and hypercarbia leading to secondary apnea and cardiac arrest.

Complete airway obstruction results in increased breathing efforts (exaggerated intrathoracic pressure fluctuations causing intercostal and suprasternal retractions) and sympathetic discharge (arterial hypertension and tachycardia). This leads to unconsciousness within about 2 minutes, when the PaO_2 reaches about 30 mmHg (arterial oxygen saturation 50%). Apnea occurs at 2–6 minutes, and pulselessness (asystole in diastole) at 5–10 minutes. Hypoxia and acidosis (from accumulation of carbon dioxide and fixed acids) in blood and tissues combine as a cause of circulatory failure. Pulselessness occurs when the PaO_2 is about 10 mmHg and pHa 6.5–6.8[435].

When IPPV is started before the critical MAP of about 40–50 mmHg is reached, resuscitation is prompt. When CPR is started within 2–5 minutes of cardiac arrest, recovery with an intact CNS is common. After up to 20 minutes of pulselessness from asphyxia in animals, restoration of spontaneous circulation by CPR is still possible, although the severe acidemia requires both administration of large amounts of epinephrine and correction of low pH using sodium bicarbonate.

In dogs, asphyxia-induced normothermic cardiac arrest of 5 minutes or less could be reversed to complete cerebral recovery; when it was 7 minutes or longer, it invariably resulted in permanent brain damage even with special brain resuscitation measures. In some human cases of slow asphyxiation, as little as 1–2 minutes of arrest or even no circulatory arrest at all has resulted in permanent neurologic deficit, particularly when pre-existing illness or injury caused a prolonged decrease in PaO_2 and cardiac output (arterial oxygen transport) prior to airway obstruction. Probably the brain acidosis during asphyxiation leads to more brain damage than the same period of VF-induced cardiac arrest.

Sudden apnea in an air-breathing patient or animal results in a similar course toward asphyxial cardiac arrest, but events proceed at a somewhat slower pace than in complete airway obstruction, because in apnea struggling entails lower oxygen consumption during the dying process[745]. Sudden apnea may occur as a result of high-energy electric shock; intravenous injection of a paralyzing dose of muscle relaxant (as used during anesthesia); sudden severe increase in intracranial pressure with brain herniation; and large doses of anesthetics, narcotics, or hypnotics.

Hypercarbia without hypoxemia can be produced by inhalation of an oxygen-enriched atmosphere prior to hypoventilation or apnea. The rate of $PaCO_2$ rise in apnea is about 5 mmHg/min. Preventilation and complete denitrogenation with 100% oxygen can initially produce a PaO_2 of over 600 mmHg and subsequently during apnea, sustain the PaO_2 above 75 mmHg for over 30 minutes, provided the oxygen-filled alveoli and airways remain connected to an oxygen reservoir without other gases (apneic diffusion oxygenation)[207, 259, 351a, 417]. Apneic diffusion oxygenation is a principle applied in prophylactic oxygen inhalation for patients whose respiratory movements or airway patency are at risk (e.g. convulsive states).

Exsanguination cardiac arrest[22b, 410, 411, 578–580, 736a, 881, 897, 902]

Exsanguination usually leads to an agonal state (no pulse, gasping) and, after loss of more than 50% of blood volume, to clinical death in asystole[410, 578]. Resuscitative efforts may subsequently elicit ventricular fibrillation (VF).

Resuscitation from exsanguination to pulselessness consists of the *simultaneous* application of the following[410, 578, 881]:

1. *Ventilation* (with oxygen if available) plus external cardiac compressions.
2. *Control of hemorrhage* by external compression of the bleeding sites, tourniquet, shock trousers (MAST suit, see Chapter 1C), laparotomy or thoracotomy.
3. *Massive i.v. infusions* through large-bore cannulas (e.g. 8.5 Fr sheath introducer placed by Seldinger technique), of the most immediately available plasma substitute—sodium chloride, lactated Ringer's solution, dextran, hydroxyethyl starch, polygelatin or albumin. Plasma substitutes should be infused in quantities up to a volume equal to estimated loss, until spontaneous cardiac action has restarted; then the flow rate can be reduced. Banked or fresh whole blood or packed red cells (group O rhesus negative or typed and cross-matched) are optional. Blood should preferably be given via a blood warmer and micropore filter. Immediate massive infusion of plasma substitutes is more effective than delayed infusion of blood!
4. *Epinephrine* (1 mg) and *sodium bicarbonate* (1 mEq/kg) should be administered i.v. without mixing them (3, above).
5. *ECG monitoring*; if VF or VT occurs, defibrillation.

In experimental animals with asystole from exsanguination, spontaneous cardiac activity is usually restored during external cardiac compressions when about 50% of shed blood volume has been replaced. The other 50%, plus an additional 10–20% of estimated leakage, should be restored more slowly, while monitoring arterial pressure and blood gases, central venous pressure and ideally pulmonary artery pressure, to avoid overloading. When exsanguination cardiac arrest is reversed with electrolyte solutions only, colloid should be added within 1–2 hours, since salt solutions do not remain in the intravascular compartment[880].

Hemoglobin is usually not needed to restart the circulation, provided that the hemorrhage is controlled[410]. Rapid exsanguination leaves 40–50% of total red cell mass in the body. Continued blood loss, accompanied by further washout of hemoglobin with plasma substitutes, however, may reduce hematocrit below 20%. If this is the case, typed and cross-matched blood, immediately available, should be used in conjunction with plasma substitutes. After restoration of spontaneous circulation and control of hemorrhage, a hematocrit of 25–35% should be restored and clotting factors replaced as needed.

Intra-abdominal hemorrhage should be treated, to prevent cardiac arrest, with application of a pressure suit (MAST suit)[397]. The suit should stay inflated at 100 mmHg until the team is ready for laparotomy and massive infusion. In case of cardiac arrest, left thoracotomy and clamping of the lower thoracic aorta can stop the hemorrhage before deflation of the pressure suit[858].

In experimental conditions with use of warm oxygenated, heparinized blood with epinephrine[578], exsanguination cardiac arrest can be reversed somewhat more rapidly and with less volume by using the *intra-arterial* route of infusion. Intra-arterial infusion can restart the heart even without cardiac compressions, due to retrograde perfusion of the coronary arteries. This can be done in the hospital using emergency cardiopulmonary bypass with femoral arteriovenous access (Chapter 2C). When clinically available plasma substitute or cold banked blood was used via the arterial route in animals, the heart did not restart without cardiac compressions; while massive venous infusion of plasma substitutes at room temperature plus CPR were effective in restarting the heart, as the infused fluids are oxygenated and diluted in passage through the lungs[410, 411]. Hazards of intra-arterial infusion include delay in artery cannulation, retrograde air or thromboembolism, and post-cannulation thrombosis with ischemia of the extremity[508].

Hypoglycemia[736a, 742]

The CNS depends on glucose and oxygen for energy metabolism. Fat and proteins are unable to substitute for glucose. Whereas oxygen deprivation is the principal cause of sudden cardiac death, glucose deprivation is rare and kills more slowly—probably because the favored nutrients for heart and lung are fatty acids and amino acids rather than glucose. Hypoglycemia, however, results in brain failure, even without cardiac arrest.

Hypoglycemia occurs in patients with overdose of insulin, islet cell tumor of the pancreas, alcohol intoxication and salicylate overdose. The symptomatology and outcome depend on the degree and speed of reduction in blood glucose, the underlying disease, and other factors. A decrease of blood glucose levels to about 30–50 mg/dl results in hunger, yawning, irritability, sweating, hyperventilation, tachycardia and arterial hypertension (release of epinephrine). A rapid reduction in blood glucose to 30 mg/dl or less produces exhaustion of glucose and glycogen stores, which results in coma, convulsions, wide pupils, pale skin, hypoventilation, bradycardia and hypotension (insulin shock)—and cardiac arrest in asystole, if the blood glucose drops further and remains below 30 mg/dl over 1–2 hours. Beyond that time and degree of hypoglycemia, CNS recovery may be with neurologic deficit. Neurohistologically, the damage caused by hypoglycemia is similar to that caused by ischemic anoxia[108, 807].

Since hypoglycemia could be a factor in any case of convulsions and cardiac arrest, and since glucose transport and brain glucose stores are reduced in ischemic anoxia, administration of 30–50% glucose during resuscitation—irrespective of the underlying problem—is a reasonable recommendation. *Hyperglycemia* at the time of cardiac arrest (compared with normoglycemia) worsens brain damage, as it increases cerebral lactacidosis[480, 662, 805]. Hyperglycemia for resuscitation from cardiac arrest might be more beneficial than detrimental. Hyperglycemia for treatment of shock proved beneficial[525, 863]. A combination of hypertonic glucose, potassium and insulin i.v. has been recommended for critically ill patients with myocardial infarction[829]. Hypoglycemia before, during or after ischemic anoxia may be harmful. The optimal blood glucose levels for resuscitation have not been worked out.

Hypothermia[15, 19, 75, 158, 453, 680, 736a, 764, 830, 850, 894, 899, 962, 974, 987, 991, 993]

Man is homeothermic through a delicate mechanism that maintains core body temperature near 37°C (98.6°F). The hypothalamic temperature-regulating center controls the required balance of heat production (primarily from muscular work and hepatic metabolism) and heat retention or elimination (primarily through cutaneous vasoconstriction and vasodilatation, sweating and pulmonary ventilation).

By reducing the consumption of oxygen by body tissues, hypothermia protects vital organs during apnea and circulatory arrest (Chapter 3). However, hypothermia can itself cause cardiac arrest in man when the heart temperature reaches about 22–28°C (72–84°F). Healthy, unmedicated humans exposed to low environmental temperatures without protection fight the cold with cutaneous vasoconstriction, shivering and catecholamine release, which result in a transient increase in oxygen consumption, heart rate, arterial pressure and cardiac irritability. The latter can cause cardiac arrest in cardiac disease patients during cold exposure, even before core temperature decreases. With persisting exposure, the defense mechanism finally becomes depressed and the core body temperature decreases. When core temperature falls to 30–35°C (86–96°F), a further decrease in temperature will usually be unopposed by shivering and vasoconstriction. CNS depressant and vasodilating drugs (including alcohol) and muscle relaxants (used in anesthesia) foster a more rapid downward drift in core temperature in a cold environment. The decline in body temperature is accompanied by a decline in total and cerebral oxygen consumption, cardiac output, cerebral blood flow, microcirculation (hence, increased blood sludging and viscosity), arterial pressure, heart rate, respiratory minute volume, and electrical activity of the brain. While hypothermia endangers heart action, it protects the brain, through reduction in brain metabolism and acidosis and preservation of cerebral enzyme and membrane functions.

Oxygen consumption falls to about 50% of normal at a core temperature of 30°C (86°F) and 15% of normal at 20°C (68°F), at which point the EEG is isoelectric. Core temperatures below about 22–28°C (70–82°F) stop the human heart in asystole or VF. Restoration of spontaneous circulation, including defibrillation, may be difficult unless the heart temperature is rapidly increased during cardiac compressions; this may require thoracotomy and direct rewarming of the heart, or extracorporeal circulation with a heat exchanger. During rewarming, VF may occur, triggered by shivering with increased oxygen consumption, uncontrolled acidemia, mechanical stimulation of the heart by CPR, or other factors. To prevent this, rewarming under spontaneous circulation should be slow, with control of shivering by drugs and blood gas and pH normalization. Rewarming methods during resuscitation include—in order of increasing effectiveness—surface warming, warming of inhaled gas, warm i.v. fluids, warm gastric or peritoneal lavage, and veno-arterial pumping via oxygenator and heat exchanger (emergency cardiopulmonary bypass)[758].

One must appreciate the basic pathophysiologic differences in the following hypothermic states encountered in clinical medicine:

1. Induced hypothermia in *surgical* patients for elective cardiac arrest or temporary vessel occlusion for surgical operations, preceded by normal circulation and oxygenation, permits complete cerebral recovery after circulatory arrest of up to about 30 minutes at 30°C, 60 minutes at 20°C or 90 minutes at 15°C, but requires extracorporeal cooling and warming by cardiopulmonary bypass.

2. Accidental hypothermia from *exposure*, without submersion, without asphyxia, results in cardiac arrest at 25–28°C, and in further cooling; there are anecdotal reports of complete recovery when bodies with a 10–15°C core temperature were rewarmed and ventilated after apparent clinical death of several hours. In the presence of a spontaneous (possibly very slow) pulse, slow rewarming should be accompanied by gentle artificial ventilation, but *no* chest (heart) compressions, as the latter can induce VF. If pulseless, the patient should be transported—with ongoing external CPR and slow rewarming (which is controversial)—to a facility where controlled external and pulmonary warming, thoracotomy for intrathoracic warming, and extracorporeal circulation are available to raise the core temperature to the 28–30°C required for defibrillation and restoration of spontaneous normotension. Warming from 30°C to 36°C should be slow.

3. Cold water *drowning* results in cooling during asphyxiation[15, 894]. Cardiac arrest can occur without water in the lungs (due to laryngospasm or air lock), with fresh water in the lungs (which may be absorbed), or with seawater in the lungs (which causes severe lung damage) (see Drowning, below). Cardiac arrest in cold water drowning is less easily reversible than exposure hypothermia, because of tissue acidosis and anoxia at the time of hypothermic cardiac arrest.

In maritime disasters in icy waters, many victims with life vests may be immersed without submersion of the face, without drowning. In regular clothes, they can cool within 2–5 minutes to apnea and cardiac arrest.

Hyperthermia[768, 793]

Emergencies arising from increased body temperature vary from benign electrolyte imbalance to rapidly lethal derangements of multiple organ systems. These reflect both normal (but exaggerated) and defective responses to increased temperature. Each year in the USA, 4000–9000 persons die from hyperthermia-related crises, such as heat stroke and febrile convulsions.

Heat cramps are usually most marked in the muscles of the legs and abdomen. They are relatively benign sequelae of electrolyte loss through sweating.

Heat exhaustion is a form of hypovolemic shock caused by the body's exaggerated response to high environmental temperatures; massive fluid loss through sweating leads to peripheral vasomotor collapse. The patient has a pale, *cold*, clammy *skin*, wide pupils, arterial hypotension, tachycardia, and an increased core temperature. Nausea and vomiting frequently accompany this syndrome and further exacerbate hypovolemia. Emergency treatment is aimed at restoring vascular volume, providing a cool environment, positioning the patient supine with legs raised, and infusing isotonic saline or Ringer's solution.

Heat stroke (heat pyrexia) represents a failure of heat regulation through sweating. The pathogenesis of heat stroke is usually a combination of external heat, severe exercise, dehydration and (viral) infection. The patient has a flushed, *hot*, dry *skin*. Cardiac output, arterial pressure, heart rate, minute volume of breathing and core temperature are all increased. Blood glucose levels may be very low. The cerebral cortex can suffer irreversible heat damage, especially at temperatures of about 40°C (106°F) or above. The insult to the brain depends on the duration and degree of hyperthermia above 40°C as well as on the adequacy of PaO_2 and cardiac output (arterial oxygen transport) and blood glucose. Treatment consists of rapid cooling; ventilation with oxygen; intensive therapy for shock, respiratory failure and brain failure; and CPR when appropriate, which can restore spontaneous circulation[768]. Cooling should be cautiously carried to the point of normothermia—using external means, cold i.v. and rectal fluids, and perhaps extracorporeal circulation with heat exchanger. A core temperature of about 42°C or higher results in an irreversible shock state resembling the clinical picture of a combination of hypovolemic, cardiogenic and septic shock, in spite of correction of blood glucose, temperature and other monitored variables.

Malignant hyperpyrexia during anesthesia[209, 542] is a very rare, sudden, unexpected and fulminating increase in metabolism and body temperature that occurs during induction or maintenance of anesthesia with a variety of agents, principally succinylcholine and halothane. It happens in apparently healthy individuals because of a familial error in skeletal muscle metabolism. Susceptible patients may have high serum creatine phosphokinase (CPK) levels and muscle biopsies which demonstrate abnormal contracture with halothane and caffeine. They should be given dantrolene prophylactically before anesthesia. Local anesthesia is favored. Regional procaine or tetracaine rather than lidocaine should be used although this is controversial. Immediate recognition should usually result in complete recovery if standard resuscitation principles are followed, plus rapid cooling, hyperventilation, pHa normalization and i.v. dantrolene. The latter seems to normalize calcium flux in excitation–contraction coupling.

Electrolyte and acid–base derangements[736c]

Electrolyte disturbances can be the primary cause of cardiac arrest. A normal serum sodium level is required to maintain cardiac excitability and contractility. Disturbances of the calcium/potassium ratio can cause asystole or VF. Calcium increases myocardial contractility and, if present in excessive concentration, stops the heart in systole. Potassium, on the other hand, depresses myocardial contractility and stops the heart in diastole or VF. Not only the absolute values of each electrolyte but also their ratios are important. Hyperpotassemia, occurring in patients with extensive burns (worsened by succinylcholine), may precipitate cardiac arrest. Magnesium, which may be absorbed in high concentration during aspiration of sea water, can stop the heart in diastole. An abnormal increase in sodium and other osmotically active substances such as glucose and urea can result in hyperosomolality.

Severe acid–base disturbances, as reflected in grossly abnormal arterial pH values (which often do not reflect the acid–base milieu in tissues), can also cause cardiac arrest. Well compensated arterial pH abnormalities usually lie between 7.2 and 7.6. In humans, such arterial pH extremes as under 6.9 or over 7.8 can result rapidly in shock states or cardiac arrest. Extreme acidemia can result in circulatory collapse and cardiac standstill, extreme alkalemia in VT and VF.

One must keep in mind the possibility of paradoxic phenomena, such as the following:

1. Cerebral acidosis due to $NaHCO_3$[646, 807, 947, 948a]. During dying and its reversal, alkalemia may at times coexist with tissue acidosis. For example, giving $NaHCO_3$ i.v. raises arterial pH, but a shift to the left of the oxygen–hemoglobin dissociation curve may reduce oxygen release at the tissue level. This adds to the shock-induced tissue acidity for which bicarbonate was administered. Moreover, brain tissue acidosis is worsened by the carbon dioxide released from $NaHCO_3$. Without hyperventilation, carbon dioxide diffuses readily into the brain, while the blood–brain barrier remains relatively impermeable to hydrogen and bicarbonate ions.

2. Cerebral alkalosis due to passive hyperventilation (IPPV)[685, 726]. In patients with high carbon dioxide and bicarbonate (e.g emphysema), rapid lowering of $PaCO_2$ by artificial hyperventilation may lead to coma due to cerebral vasospasm caused by high CSF pH, when carbon dioxide

molecules but not bicarbonate ions diffuse out of the brain.
3. Lungs vs. brain. Increased hydrogen ion concentration from low oxygen and/or high carbon dioxide in the extracellular fluid causes vasodilatation in the brain and vasoconstriction in the lungs.
4. Direct vs. indirect carbon dioxide effects. Hypercarbia in the healthy person causes little circulatory disturbance, because it releases norepinephrine from nerve endings, causing vasoconstriction and cardiac stimulation, which are offset by the direct carbon dioxide effects of vasodilatation and myocardial depression.

Special Emergencies

Electric shock[23b, 159, 353, 647, 736a, 882]

In electric shock several special considerations apply. Household a.c. current (110 V in the USA, 220 V in Europe) may cause ventricular fibrillation (VF). High-voltage current passing through the heart causes a contraction only as long as the current flows, and passing through the brain can cause apnea (reversible by Steps A and B alone). Apnea leads to secondary asphyxial cardiac arrest (in electromechanical dissociation asystole), which might be reversed by CPR without the need for defibrillation. In addition, electric shock can cause tissue burns.

The likelihood of electric current producing VF depends on the intensity of the current, its frequency of oscillations, its path (whether or not the heart is included), and the duration of contact. Direct current is more injurious than alternating current of the same voltage, as d.c. produces electrolytic tissue damage and burns. Chances of recovery are best when neither brain nor heart lies directly in the path of the current.

Lightning[159, 647, 882] may produce millions of volts. Many persons struck by lightning are merely stunned and may transiently have difficulty moving, hearing or feeling. Some suffer burns, primarily at the entry and exit points of the often erratic paths travelled by lightning current. If the current passes through brain and heart, the victim suddenly loses consciousness (electronarcosis) and becomes apneic (probably because of instantaneous cessation of brain metabolism). At the same time, the heart is thrown into a sustained contraction. Soon after termination of the lightning shock, the contracted heart relaxes and resumes spontaneous contractions with sinus rhythm, while the respiratory center remains paralyzed. Then, owing to the apnea, the heart asphyxiates to secondary asystole, unless artificial ventilation is started before the onset of cardiac arrest. Usually, the brain arrest is reversible. Very high voltage, however, can burn and destroy brain tissue. On the other hand, some victims of lightning stroke have survived more than 10 minutes of clinical death treated by CPR and prolonged IPPV, with complete CNS recovery[647].

Household voltage. When 100–120 V a.c. (50–60 cycles per second) traverse the human heart from hand to foot, VF usually results. In hospitalized patients even very low currents have killed via improperly grounded apparatus connected to patients with catheter or wire leads going into the heart. In patients with heart disease, low-voltage currents may cause arrhythmias without cardiac arrest, which in turn can subsequently trigger VF.

Household voltage seems to produce little long-term deleterious effect on the myocardium if exposure is only momentary. Noxious effects depend on resistances which determine the amperage going through the heart. The resistance of an adult person's thorax is about 70–100 ohms and varies with the type of skin contact. Dry skin offers resistance of several thousand ohms. Inside the body, bone tissue and air-filled lungs offer high resistance, but the extracellular fluid is an excellent conductor.

At 100 V, a 60-cycle a.c. current in humans applied from hand to foot, of less than 0.01 A will cause merely a 'funny' sensation; with 0.01 A, the person will experience tetanic muscle contraction; between 0.1 and 1 A, the likelihood of inducing VF and sudden death is greatest; and with more than 1 A the myocardium contracts, and if it was in VF may be defibrillated (the original a.c. external defibrillator, which discharged 500 V at 5 A, probably got 1.5–2 A through the heart) (Chapter 2F). High-voltage line accidents result in either VF or the pattern described above for lightning, depending on the amount of current traversing the heart and brain.

Treatment of victims of electric shock

1. Make sure the victim is no longer in contact with the current source! Guard against getting shocked yourself.
(a) If possible, shut off the current source.
(b) Otherwise, dislodge the victim from contact with the current source using a stick, rope or other nonconductive implement.
2. Administer CPR-ABC and DEF (defibrillation) as needed.
3. Special considerations:
(a) Tetanic muscle spasms may cause fractures to long bones and damage to the spine. Handle the patient accordingly.
(b) The magnitude and severity of internal tissue damage cannot be gauged from external burns. Thus, even patients who wake up quickly after electrocution must be hospitalized.

If cardiac arrest develops on the *pole top*, one should deliver a precordial thump and initiate mouth-to-mouth breathing as feasible, while lowering the victim as rapidly as possible to the ground. CPR is not effective when the victim is in the upright position, for it does not permit adequate venous return. Thus, the victim should be placed supine with all possible speed.

Drowning[15, 158, 551, 648, 649, 736a, 764, 873, 894]

Submersion accidents kill more than 100 000 people per year worldwide. One must differentiate between near-drowning (which implies that the victim was removed from the water with a pulse present) and drowning (where the victim was removed pulseless, in clinical death). In either case, the victim may or may not survive, depending on resuscitation and numerous other factors. Victims removed from the water with a pulse, and before anoxic relaxation of the larynx and agonal gasps occur, are easily resuscitated with IPPV/exhaled air or air, since the lungs are normal[648a]. If water or vomitus is inhaled, the picture becomes more complicated[648, 649, 873, 920].

Inhaled *fresh water*[648c] rapidly passes into the circulation, so that a subject removed prior to circulatory arrest may have dry lungs. The results of fresh water aspiration are not only hypoxemia, hypercarbia and acidemia, but also hypervolemia, hemodilution (with reduced serum electrolyte concentrations), hemolysis and hyperpotassemia (from acidemia and hemolysis). Dogs with fresh water flooding of the lungs developed VF within less than 3 minutes. At the moment of VF, the dogs had inhaled and absorbed about 40 ml/kg of water (50% of blood volume). With CPR, IPPV/100% oxygen, epinephrine and electric countershock, most dogs could be fully resuscitated. It appears that VF is primarily the result of anoxia and hypervolemia, not of the moderate hyperpotassemia and hemolysis to which it was attributed in the past. Chlorinated water (customary swimming pool concentration) causes about the same pattern of dying as does fresh water[551].

Inhaled *sea water*[648b] (which is hypertonic, 3–5% salt) leads in dogs to transudation of fluid from the circulation into the alveoli, resulting in hypovolemia (about 30% decrease in blood volume) and hemoconcentration with absorption (and increases in the serum) of sodium, magnesium, potassium and chloride. Sea water damages the capillary-alveolar membrane, resulting in plasma protein loss into the alveoli and fulminating pulmonary edema with hypoxemia, which is proportional to the quantity of sea water inhaled. Hypoxemia, bradycardia and oligemic hypotension lead to asystole. If resuscitation is started before the onset of pulselessness, prolonged IPPV with 100% oxygen and plasma volume normalization should result in survival. About twice as much inhaled sea water as fresh water is needed to cause cardiac arrest. Sea water is worse for the lungs; fresh water is worse for the heart; both damage the brain through asphyxiation.

In human victims of near-drowning with evidence of fresh or sea water inhalation who are rescued *before* cardiac arrest, electrolyte disturbances are minimal or absent 30 minutes to 1 hour after removal from the water.

Apparently, the organism can rapidly correct the electrolyte changes and clear the free plasma hemoglobin[550]. The main limiting factor in human near-drowning is severe and prolonged hypoxemia from the damage any type of water causes in the lungs. The pulmonary lesion, however, is usually reversible with modern respiratory care. The brain can survive often very low PaO_2 values, provided there is good cardiac output and arterial pressure. As little as 2 ml/kg of any type of water inhaled can produce hypoxemia, bronchospasm and pulmonary vasospasm. Larger amounts of fresh or brackish water inhaled cause primarily alveolar atelectasis from loss of surfactant, whereas sea water produces pulmonary edema in addition. Additional regurgitation and aspiration of gastric contents, which is not uncommon, complicates the pulmonary pathologic changes.

The main limiting factor during resuscitation attempts in human drowning cases—i.e. victims rescued *after* the onset of cardiac arrest—is brain damage. Prevention of brain damage calls for immediate special post-resuscitative therapy (Chapter 3).

Absence of early awakening is no reason to give up, particularly if drowning occurred in *cold water*, which protects the brain. This is illustrated by the survival with normal CNS of a 5-year-old boy after a documented 40 minutes of submersion in ice-cold fresh water; his heart was restarted by external CPR and rewarming, his pulmonary edema was controlled by respiratory care, and he regained consciousness within about 2 days[804]. In dogs the restoration of adequate spontaneous circulation was possible after up to 90 minutes of iced water submersion[894]. At least 25 case reports have been published on victims of cold water drowning, with submersion times of 7–30 minutes, who survived with good brain function[158a]. This is most likely due to protective brain temperatures (30°C/86°F or less) reached at the time heart action ceases due to asphyxia[15, 894].

In victims of near-drowning (with pulse)[551] or drowning (without pulse)[649], who may or may not have water in their lungs (depending upon reflex laryngospasm), reoxygenation should not be delayed by attempts to drain fluid from the lungs. A good swimmer can start mouth-to-mouth or mouth-to-nose resuscitation while treading water. Otherwise, one can start mouth-to-mouth ventilation while standing in shallow water, placing the victim's head and chest over one's knee. Sternal compressions are not possible until the victim is removed from the water. In general, the principles of CPCR (Chapters 1–3) should be followed. Water and vomitus may drain by gravity before and during resuscitative efforts. One should intermittently clear the pharynx. If the abdomen is distended after the victim has been removed from the water, he/she may be turned briefly on the side and the upper abdomen compressed to expel water and gas. Some recommend later turning him/her quickly into the prone position and lift with hands under the stomach to force water out ('breaking' the victim). Abdominal thrusts[336] should not be routine, as they may delay reoxygenation and do not seem to enhance recovery of the lungs[955]. One should switch ventilation from exhaled air to 100% oxygen as soon as possible because pulmonary changes occur with even small amounts of inhaled water. Hospital admission is mandatory, even if the victim recovers consciousness at the scene or during transportation. Late pulmonary edema is not unusual. Victims of sea water submersion should have early intratracheal IPPV with 100% O_2 and plasma substitute infusion i.v. After submersion to pulseless-ness, CPCR (advanced and prolonged life support with cerebral resuscitation) started early and continued throughout coma (including barbiturate, steroid, mannitol, hypothermia and ICP normalization) has occasionally resulted in recovery[158].

If neck injury is suspected following diving into shallow water, one should try to float the victim onto a backboard before removal from the water. If mouth-to-mouth ventilation is needed, one should use jaw thrust with moderate backward tilt of the head, asking a helper to hold the head–neck–chest aligned, to avoid aggravating a possible spinal cord injury. One should not flex the neck.

Rescue swimming should be attempted only by strong swimmers. Others should quickly find a floating device. Teaching rapid rescue from water is as important as teaching resuscitation. 'Reach' with a pole. 'Row' a boat or surfboard. 'Throw' a life preserver, and 'Go' (swim) toward a drowning person only as a last resort.

Scuba divers may drown secondarily to complications from increased pressure, which may cause coma and loss of reflexes. These hyperbaric injuries can be due to the following[161]:

1. *Nitrogen narcosis.* This may occur below 200 feet depth when breathing air.
2. *Decompression sickness ('the bends').* Nitrogen bubbles released into all tissues, including the brain, during rapid ascent after nitrogen loading at a depth of over 30 feet. Decompression sickness can be avoided by slow ascent according to decompression tables.
3. *Cerebral air embolism.* Systemic arterial air embolism, fortunately rare, is the most threatening potentially lethal complication, because it cannot always be avoided, even with sound diving practices. This accident can be caused by rapid ascent of just a few feet, resulting in expansion of trapped gas in the lungs (trapped because of breath holding, emphysema, asthma or other causes) and alveolar rupture. This may lead to entry of air into the pulmonary veins, causing cerebral and/or coronary air embolism and sudden death.

Acute pulmonary edema[673, 736a–c]

Acute pulmonary edema kills by hypoxemia. Thus, the first priority of treatment is to improve oxygenation. Immediate increase in arterial PO_2 is usually possible with 100% oxygen administered by some form of continuous positive airway pressure. The simplest positive-pressure treatment is spontaneous breathing (SB) with continuous positive airway pressure (CPAP) by mask or mouthpiece (Chapter 1B, Fig. 22). Unnecessary tracheal intubation, a potentially dysrhythmia-inducing procedure, should be avoided in cardiogenic pulmonary edema. However, if the patient is stuporous or comatose or cannot cough up the edema fluid, or if PaO_2 cannot be kept above 60 mmHg with spontaneous breathing of 100% oxygen by CPAP, or if CO_2 rises, tracheal intubation and controlled mechanical ventilation with IPPV plus PEEP and 100% oxygen—facilitated if necessary by relaxants—are indicated. In pulmonary edema, increasing airway pressure raises the PaO_2 not by increasing the alveolar capillary pressure gradient (since the capillaries are exposed to the same positive pressure), but by increasing FRC, i.e. fluid-filled alveoli are 'recruited' and edema fluid may be thinned out, thereby facilitating oxygen diffusion into blood. In addition, reopening alveoli may facilitate the healing process in the lung.

Acute pulmonary edema, particularly of the cardiogenic type, benefits from a reduction in venous return. This is best accomplished by the measure which also increases PaO_2, namely an increase in airway pressure. The resultant increase in intrathoracic pressure is transmitted to the venae cavae, thereby reducing overall venous return. Morphine, titrated i.v. to the point of relieving dyspnea, tachypnea and anxiety (but not to the point of hypotension), may cause vasodilation (particularly of capacitance vessels) and reduce venous return, gasping and negative intrathoracic pressure. If there is suspicion of left heart failure, the patient should be rapidly digitalized. The choice of further therapy depends on the mechanism and cause of pulmonary edema. It may include use of a vasodilator more potent than morphine (e.g. trimethaphan [Arfonad], nitroglycerin, chlorpromazine, nitroprusside); phlebotomy; postural adjustment (sitting position); rapid diuresis with i.v. furosemide to reduce blood volume; possible peritoneal or hemodialysis (in the presence of uremia); bronchodilation with aminophylline (which also increases sodium and water excretion, promotes systemic and pulmonary vasodilation, and enhances cardiac contractility); arrhythmia control; and normalization of pHa, $PaCO_2$, base deficit and oncotic pressure. The use of rotating tourniquets, although traditionally advocated in pulmonary edema, is of no clinically proved benefit and indeed may produce deleterious degrees of tissue acidosis and increased afterload. Finally, the underlying cause of the pulmonary edema should be sought and treated.

Therapy of acute pulmonary edema should be guided by careful monitoring of vital signs and arterial blood gas values on known increased FIO_2. Furthermore, periodic measurements of pulmonary artery wedge pressure as well as on-line determinations of cardiac output are of great help in the management of pulmonary edema. Cardiogenic pulmonary edema may require increased inotropic support. Continuous or intermittent monitoring of mixed venous oxygen saturation may also be useful in assessing the adequacy of arterial oxygen transport.

Pulmonary embolism[736a–c, 767]

Massive pulmonary embolism may produce circulatory shock (low arterial pressure, low cardiac output) as a result of blood flow obstruction. Potentially lethal obstruction may be caused by embolized thrombi, gas, fat, tissue or amniotic fluid. Some of these agents may cause sudden massive main pulmonary artery obstruction; others may produce showers of small obstructive matter, clogging peripheral pulmonary vessels. The majority of pulmonary emboli are thrombi which arise from major veins in the legs or pelvis.

Acute pulmonary thromboembolism may be the most common cause of death in hospitals, particularly among old and chronically ill patients. There are humoral and nervous factors which may affect pulmonary vessels and bronchi remote from the embolic obstruction. The overriding factor determining the degree of shock and the likelihood of sudden death is the proportion of the total cross-sectional area of the pulmonary arterial tree blocked by thrombus. In patients with previously healthy lungs and heart, more than about 50% of the vascular tree must be obstructed to produce shock. Sudden cardiac arrest from pulmonary thromboembolism is usually caused by a large thrombus blocking the pulmonary artery bifurcation. Under such circumstances, CPR may be of limited utility. In patients with cardiopulmonary disease, a smaller proportion of the pulmonary vasculature suddenly blocked may cause shock or cardiac arrest. Sudden death may be the result of vasovagal shock, right ventricular failure or severe hypoxemia in addition to obstructive shock.

In shock or cardiac arrest from pulmonary thromboembolism, there is no pulmonary infarction, and thus no hemoptysis. Pulmonary infarction is more likely to occur when a pulmonary end artery becomes blocked in a patient with left heart failure and pulmonary congestion. About 50% obstruction of the pulmonary vascular bed results in arterial hypotension, tachycardia, venous hypertension, diffuse pulmonary artery spasm and bronchospasm. Chest roentgenography may reveal reduced pulmonary vascularity. A normal lung scan and normal PaO_2 virtually rule out significant embolization. If the lung scan is positive and time permits, a pulmonary angiogram confirms the diagnosis. Pulmonary embolism increases not only the physiologic deadspace but also right-to-left shunting, the cause of hypoxemia. Although the exact mechanism is not clearly understood, it is related at least in part to complex ventilation–perfusion disturbances (patchy bronchoconstriction and pulmonary edema in hyperemic vascular beds).

Management is aimed at prevention of recurrent embolization and support of vital functions during the days that Nature requires to achieve thrombolysis and recanalization of obstructed vessels. Embolectomy has been associated with very poor results. Heparinization primarily prevents secondary thrombus formation. In shock, management should include IPPV/100% oxygen with PEEP, maintenance of arterial perfusion pressure by vasopressor, use of bronchodilator and pulmonary vasodilators (the best pulmonary vasodilator is 100% oxygen), and more definitive measures. These include intravenous infusion of a thrombolytic agent (such as urokinase or streptokinase) and emergency cardiopulmonary bypass (closed chest) with venoarterial pumping via membrane oxygenator to ameliorate right heart overload, improve arterial flow (provide assisted circulation) and facilitate pulmonary embolectomy (which is controversial) (Chapter 2C).

Status asthmaticus[205, 394, 736a–c, 799]

The *diagnosis of status asthmaticus* is made if two doses of epinephrine given subcutaneously (at least 20 minutes apart), each 0.01 mg/kg (0.5 mg in an adult), do not improve the obstruction. *Therapy for status asthmaticus* requires the use of sophisticated measures by an experienced team. Priorities for therapy are: (1) oxygenation with IPPB by mask, or IPPV (FIO_2 at 0.5–1.0) via tracheal tube if indicated (with 'titrated' expiratory retardation); (2) bronchodilation and pHa normalization; and (3) steroid i.v., hydration and additional measures.

The bronchodilator effect of catecholamines is decreased by acidosis; pHa normalization restores this effect and may thereby obviate the need for tracheal intubation and mechanical ventilation. Normalization of pHa is possible with adequate hydration and then bicarbonate (1–2 mEq/kg, followed by titrated doses according to base deficit)[394]. The advantages of THAM for pHa control over $NaHCO_3$ should be re-explored[351b]. Bronchodilator titration is best accomplished with the combined effects of aminophylline i.v. (e.g. 4 mg/kg per 6 h) and metaproterenol by aerosol. Long-term administration of aminophylline i.v. should ideally be titrated by plasma levels (aiming for 10–20 μg/dl). In intractable bronchospasm, intravenous titration of epinephrine or isoproterenol[205] by infusion, and as a last resort general anesthesia with halothane, may be used (see appropriate drugs, Chapter 2D). In all cases of status asthmaticus, ECG and blood pressure and gas monitoring are mandatory, as the combination of hypoxemia, acidemia and bronchodilator can cause life-threatening dysrhythmias, hypotension, tachycardia and cardiac arrest.

Hydrocortisone 5 mg/kg (or dexamethasone 0.2 mg/kg, or methylprednisolone 1 mg/kg) should be given i.v. immediately, even though the effect of steroid begins only after about 1 hour and peaks at 1–3 hours. Some would use two to three times these doses. Steroid doses should be repeated every 6 hours so long as there is severe wheezing. A broad-spectrum antibiotic should be started and readjusted according to sputum smear and culture results. Circulatory support is essential because hypovolemia (plasma loss) and reduction in cardiac output from increased intrathoracic pressure are common. Thus hydration is essential, e.g. with 5% dextrose in 0.25% NaCl (plus potassium, 2 mEq/dl), over 24 hours—100 ml/kg for the first 10 kg body weight, 50 ml/kg for the second 10 kg, and 20 ml/kg for each kilogram over 20. Additionally about 50 ml/kg should be given for rehydration over 24 hours. Colloid may also be indicated. Sedation, muscle relaxation, tracheal intubation and controlled ventilation are indicated when the patient cannot clear secretions spontaneously or becomes comatose.

Carbon monoxide poisoning[249, 575, 577, 736a]

Carbon monoxide (CO), an inert odorless gas, is probably not a cellular poison per se; by virtue of its affinity for hemoglobin, however, it produces acute normovolemic 'anemic' hypoxia. Hemoglobin binds carbon monoxide about 200–300 times more readily than it binds oxygen; the carboxyhemoglobin produced is subsequently not available for oxygen transport. In carbon monoxide poisoning there is normal arterial PO_2 with low available oxygen content. Carbon monoxide poisoning may occur with exposure to products of combustion in closed spaces, automobile exhaust, or carbon monoxide-containing gases used in industry.

As little as 0.2% CO inhaled, will form carboxyhemoglobin at a rate of 1% per minute. If the patient is doing heavy work, this rate will be 2.4% per minute, and within about 45 minutes carbon monoxide will saturate 76% of the hemoglobin—a lethal concentration. Conscious dogs inhaling 1% CO reach 80% CO hemoglobin saturation almost instantaneously, and death is sudden[577, 578]. There is no increase in respiratory drive, since the peripheral chemoreceptors are sensitive to a decrease in arterial PO_2, not oxygen content. The sequence of events is loss of consciousness, rapidly followed by hypotension, convulsions, apnea and cardiac arrest in asystole. If, prior to cardiac arrest, IPPV with 100% oxygen is begun, the animal survives and resumes spontaneous breathing but may have permanent cerebral damage. Dogs inhaling lower concentrations develop cardiac arrest in hours. Resuscitation of cardiac function and spontaneous breathing is easily achieved, but the animals die in coma within days. Irreversible cerebral damage apparently occurs before cardiac arrest. Hypotension seems to be a more crucial parameter in determining the outcome of the brain than the percentage of carboxyhemoglobin and duration of exposure.

The organism tolerates normovolemic hemodilution better than the same degree of reduction of available hemoglobin by blockage with carbon monoxide. This may be because carbon monoxide, with hematocrit unchanged, does not increase tissue blood flow because it shifts the oxyhemoglobin dissociation curve to the left and because certain respiratory enzymes have greater affinity for carbon monoxide than for oxygen. The question of whether carbon monoxide also damages the brain directly has not been resolved. Neurohistologically, there are not only the well described areas of necrosis in the globus pallidus but also nonspecific changes as in ischemic-anoxic encephalopathy of other types.

Humans breathing low concentrations of carbon monoxide develop a sequence of headache, vertigo, yawning, dimmed vision, tachycardia and vomiting. Higher concentrations or longer exposure result in coma, twitching, collapse, pupillary dilatation, Cheyne–Stokes respirations, apnea and cardiac arrest (asystole). The skin is warm; and a cherry-red tint, while allegedly pathognomonic of carbon monoxide poisoning, is only rarely seen. The *treatment* includes IPPV/100% oxygen and CPR when indicated. Inhalation of carbon dioxide has not proved valuable; hyperbaric oxygenation has, but is rarely available early enough to influence the outcome. Early hypothermia or other measures to ameliorate postanoxic brain damage should be considered (Chapter 3) but, as above, need to be instituted rapidly in order to be efficacious.

Anesthesia-related cardiac arrest[70, 209, 402, 542, 623, 920]

The common causes of cardiac arrest associated with anesthesia management seem to be, in this order of incidence: (1) airway obstruction–hypoventilation–apnea; (2) regurgitation and aspiration; (3) relative overdose of myocardial depressant anesthetics (general as well as local anesthetics) or para-anesthetic agents; (4) uncontrolled or unreplaced blood loss; and (5) uncontrolled hypotension from total sympathetic block secondary to spinal or epidural anesthesia[402, 623]. Cardiac arrest occurs more usually in the very old or the very young; in patients with pre-anesthetic physical status (PS) 3–5 (American Society of Anesthesiologists) (PS 1 = normal; 2 = mild derangement without disability; 3 = moderate derangement with general disability; 4 = life-threatening condition; 5 = moribund); in patients with heart disease; and during induction or emergence. Prevention requires skill, knowledge, judgment, constant vigilance, and continuous monitoring of ventilation, oxygenation and pulse. Lasting morbidity has been caused by many types of anesthetic mishap, particularly those that resulted in permanent brain damage after asphyxiation and procrastination with resuscitation. The prompt action that can prevent post-CPR brain damage requires knowledge and experience with most of the resuscitative measures described in this book, their appropriate selection for the given emergency, and their quick, effective application. Brain protection against periods of circulatory arrest is definitely provided by hypothermia and is probably provided by barbiturate anesthesia, induced before the occurrence of profound hypotension, cardiac arrest or embolization. Even a barbiturate given early during the start of resuscitation from an anesthesia related cardiac arrest may have a mild brain damage-ameliorating effect (Chapter 3). Prevention of anesthesia-related deaths requires skilled vigilant personnel who use their senses, not necessarily expensive monitoring devices.

Drugs and poisons[31, 287, 461, 891a]

Sudden death from poisons, taken by mistake or for suicide, or given for murder, is as old as mankind. Some poisons we have adapted for therapeutic use. Often, poisons kill by nonspecific means, i.e. by inducing coma, hypotension, pulmonary edema or bronchospasm, all of which are often reversible by standard resuscitation and life support measures. A comprehensive discussion of toxicology is beyond the scope of this book. All acute care physicians (in emergency room, anesthesiology, ICU) are strongly encouraged to develop familiarity with the very broad spectrum of drug intoxications/poisoning that they may encounter.

One third of sudden deaths in previously healthy adults seem to be the direct result of *alcohol* intoxication, which usually kills through asphyxia (coma resulting in upper airway soft-tissue obstruction, regurgitation and aspiration). Arterial hypotension from vasodilation and myocardial depression, as well as accidental hypothermia, are additional factors leading to morbidity and mortality in the alcohol-intoxicated patient. *Cocaine* overdose is also an increasingly frequent event in the USA[287, 461].

Barbiturates and many other anesthetics, when given in doses much larger than those causing coma and vasodilatation, may also depress myocardial contractility and produce cardiac arrest, particularly in the presence of hypovolemia or cardiac disease. Other *hypnotics* such as glutethamide (Doriden) cause, in addition, capillary and pulmonary membrane damage, arterial hypotension, and pupillary dilatation. These toxic manifestations do not obviate complete CNS recovery if support of arterial oxygenation and circulation is started early. *Narcotics* (e.g. heroin), injected intravascularly, may cause fulminating pulmonary edema through mechanisms that are not well understood. Talcs and other adulterants contaminating illicitly used narcotics may produce pneumonitis and vascular damage. Cardiac arrest in narcotic overdose is usually secondary to airway obstruction and apnea, as with other depressants. Fentanyl (more so than morphine or meperidine) tends to cause involuntary apnea (breath holding—unless the patient is coached to breathe) with spasm of respiratory muscles, coma, and apneic asphyxia. Other CNS depressants may endanger life also by causing postural hypotension. *Phenothiazines* and other mood modifying agents can cause excitation, sympathetic discharge, and life-threatening dysrhythmias. *Local anesthetics* first produce convulsions followed by apnea and cardiovascular collapse if oxygen is not immediately administered. *Anticholinesterases* (e.g. neostigmine without atropine, nerve gases, some insecticides, poisonous mushrooms) may kill through the muscarinic actions of acetylcholine (salivation, vomiting, defecation, bronchospasm, bronchorrhea, obstructive asphyxia, hypotension, bradycardia and asystole) or its nicotinic actions on ganglia and skeletal muscles (first stimulation then depression) resulting in synaptic block, paralysis and apnea. Atropine reverses the muscarinic effects, while IPPV supports life until the nicotinic effects subside. *Salicylates* stimulate spontaneous hyperventilation (hypocarbia, respiratory alkalemia), which is followed by metabolic acidemia, circulatory collapse, coma, convulsions and asphyxial death, unless artificial ventilation, intravenous bicarbonate and other life support measures interrupt the sequence. *Arsenic*, a cellular poison, causes death by unknown mechanisms. The terminal event appears related to defibrillation-resistant VT and VF. *Cyanide*, the most rapidly lethal poison, inhibits the cytochrome oxidase system for cellular oxygen utilization, producing cellular anoxia. Cyanide poisoning can result almost simultaneously in cerebral silence, apnea and asystole, without hypoxemia or hypercarbia (unless dying is slow). Reversibility of coma and cardiac arrest from cyanide poisoning have not been studied. Specific antidotes to cyanide are amyl nitrite or sodium nitrite, which produce ferric iron, displacing cyanide from cytochrome oxidase; and sodium thiosulfate, which converts cyanide to nontoxic thiocyanide.

Anaphylaxis[287, 736a, 780, 799]

Anaphylaxis may be viewed as a manifestation of the immune system gone berserk in which antibodies (IgE), elaborated in response to a previous exposure to an antigen—usually a foreign protein—reappear in full force upon re-exposure to the antigen and trigger a potentially lethal process. The antigens most often incriminated include insect poisons, vaccine proteins, antitoxin sera (especially those derived from heterologous sources) and drugs (e.g. penicillin). Any antigen or haptene may elicit an anaphylactic response in the specifically sensitized individual.

In anaphylactic shock, the antigen–antibody complex absorbs into cells (primarily mast cells) that liberate histamine and probably also serotonin, slow-reacting substance (SRS), acetylcholine, kinins and other vasoactive materials. These are smooth muscle and membrane poisons, and their most significant target organs are the airway, lungs and vascular bed. Development of pharyngeal and laryngeal edema, bronchospasm, and edema of the bronchial mucosa is virtually instantaneous and leads rapidly to asphyxia. The peripheral vascular bed reacts with vasodilatation, capillary leakage and shock. The chemical mediators of anaphylaxis may also exert direct effects on the myocardium.

Management should include i.v. or intratracheal epinephrine 0.2–0.5 mg/70 kg, IPPV/ oxygen, CPR and i.v. colloid plasma substitute as needed to restore plasma volume and reverse hemoconcentration. Laryngeal edema may call for tracheal intubation or cricothyrotomy. When the antigen has been introduced by injection in an extremity (as in insect stings or injection of medication), a tourniquet may be applied proximal to the injection site to delay absorption of the antigen. A corticosteroid is also indicated, although its effects will be delayed and it should be continued for at least 24 hours. Antihistamines are unlikely to be of value in full blown anaphylaxis, since they cannot reverse the action of histamine already liberated and are entirely ineffective against the many other chemical mediators (serotonin, kinins) involved in anaphylaxis.

Advanced Trauma Life Support[22a, b, 164a, 799, 902, 966a]

Introduction and patient assessment

Trauma is the leading cause of death in those under 40 in many industrialized countries; and malnutrition, infectious diseases and trauma the leading causes of death before old age in the 'third world'. In the USA there are about 10 million disabling injuries per year, and accidents cause 150 000 deaths per year. Although trauma was already recognized as a major public health problem in the 1950s[783], serious medical efforts to combat the problem on a large scale did not start until the 1960s in Europe and the 1970s in the USA. Not every trauma victim 'dead on admission to hospital' is a hopeless case[164, 794, 897, 902].

Instantaneous death is often the result of exsanguination from a large vessel or irreparable destruction of the brain. Cases of rapid exsanguination are salvageable only in cities with a few minutes of transport to a trauma center. Many subacute and late deaths due to (1) airway obstruction, (2) severe blood loss (intrathoracic, intra-abdominal, into tissues around multiple fractures), and/or (3) head injury (with or without epidural or subdural hematomas) are preventable by basic and advanced trauma life support measures (BTLS, ATLS) within the first 'golden hour' after injury—at the scene, during transport and in the hospital. Late deaths (days to weeks) are usually the result of sepsis and/or multiple organ failure due to the inadequately controlled initial sequence of trauma–hypovolemia–infection–sepsis.

The most important initial action by bystanders must be life supporting first aid (*LSFA*), which is *BTLS* (Chapter 1, Table 1) (Fig. 60). Efforts toward implementing early *ATLS* include the two training 'packages' from which this section of the book has been adapted—the US Department of Transportation's course for ambulance paramedics[125] and the American College of Surgeons (ACS) ATLS course for physicians[22]. The decision on which invasive measures of ATLS the trained nonphysician should be permitted to apply outside or inside hospitals varies between countries and communities.

We recommend not separating advanced cardiac from advanced trauma life support, but rather teaching resuscitation medicine for both medical and surgical conditions. Therefore, the reader will find most of the knowledge items of the ATLS course distributed throughout the chapters of this book. Here, for quick reference, we refer to the key topics of the ACS ATLS course and where to find them[22]: initial assessment (primary and secondary survey) (Table 1, Chapter 1C); upper airway management and oxygenation (Chapters 1A and 1B, Figs. 6, 11–19, 23–28); treatment of shock including pressure suit (MAST, PASG) (Chapter 1C, Fig. 35) and i.v. infusions (Chapter 2D, Figs. 37–40); chest trauma management (see below in Chapter 4, and Chapter 1A, Fig. 19 and 20, Chapter 1B and Fig. 21 and 51); abdominal trauma, including peritoneal lavage (see below in Chapter 4); head trauma (see below in Chapter 4, and Chapter 3, Tables 4–7); spinal cord trauma (see below in Chapter 4); burns (see below in Chapter 4); trauma to extremities (see below in Chapter 4). For general wound care, pediatric trauma and special organ injuries, see introductory trauma teaching texts[22, 799, 902]. For disaster preparedness, see Chapter 6.

After stabilization at the scene, the decision as to when to transport to which hospital is a matter of judgment based on experience. There is evidence that patients with severe life-threatening trauma (particularly of head, chest, abdomen, pelvis or femur, or with polytrauma) should have the airway and ventilation controlled at the scene and then be rushed to the closest major trauma center, with ongoing life support. Prolonged efforts at stabilization in the field, as recommended for cardiac emergencies, are *not* recommended for cases of trauma, as internal hemorrhage may continue to exsanguination. The decision on whether a trauma victim should be transferred to a special trauma center can be aided by quick assessment in the field, by: (1) primary survey; (2) secondary survey; (3) assessing the loss of consciousness by coma scale (Table 9); and (4) determining a trauma scale (see below).

After initial assessment, the paramedic or physician at the scene should speak directly to the physician in the trauma center which is to receive the patient. A record with patient data, injury mechanism, general history if available, vital signs and emergency management and stabilization should accompany the patient if possible. Transfer from scene to trauma center or from primary hospital to trauma center should be with life support, controlled by a traumatology experienced physician, or by paramedics under physician guidance or using standing orders.

Immediately following an injury, uninjured laymen or 'first responders' (e.g. police, fire fighters, life guards) should apply life supporting first aid (LSFA) (Fig. 60)[81, 107, 234, 443, 444, 744]. Making an injured person accessible for resuscitation may require simple rescue pull (Fig. 36) or elaborate rescue procedures to be carried out by rescue personnel who must also be skilled in LSFA. Immediately upon arrival of health professionals such as emergency medical technicians (EMTs), ambulance paramedics, emergency care physicians or nurses, they should begin at the scene with more advanced resuscitation and stabilization accompanied by primary and secondary surveys (the latter preferably by a physician).

Trauma scale

One of several popular *trauma scales* (scoring systems) is that proposed by Champion[138]:

	Trauma score*	Points/score
Respiratory rate	36 per minute or greater	2
	25–35 per minute	3
	10–24 per minute	4
	0–9 per minute	1
	none	0
Respiratory expansion	normal	1
	shallow	0
Systolic blood pressure	90 or greater	4
	70–89	3
	50–69	2
	0–49	1
	no pulse	0
Capillary refill	normal	2
(fingernail bed)	delayed	1
	none	0

* A trauma score of 12 or less calls for transfer to a trauma center.

The *primary survey* is initial assessment accompanied by management of 'A–E': *A*irway, *B*reathing, *C*irculation (hemorrhage control), *D*isability (neurologic status) and *E*xposure (completely undress the patient). Airway control must be while holding head–neck–chest aligned so as not to aggravate a cervical spine injury. The triple airway maneuver (moderate backward tilt of the head, plus jaw-thrust, plus open mouth) may be necessary. For other measures, see Chapter 1A. Assume cervical spine injury in any patient with injury above the clavicle. For breathing support, see Chapter 1B. For circulation support, one should start with recognizing shock (pulse, skin color, capillary refill, blood pressure). If the radial pulse is faint or absent and the femoral or carotid pulse palpable, the systolic blood pressure will probably be 60–70 mmHg. External bleeding should be controlled by pressure, pneumatic splints (or leg portion of pressure suit), or (rarely needed) a tourniquet. Internal bleeding in the chest or abdomen or around major fractures or penetrating injuries requires surgical control in a mobile or stationary operating room setting; transport to such a facility should not be delayed. For major external or internal bleeding below the diaphragm, with signs of shock, many emergency physicians favor early application (in the field or during transportation) of the pressure suit (MAST, PASG) (Fig. 35). During transportation, large-bore i.v. infusions should be started with balanced salt solution. Most traumatic shock is due to hypovolemia. Blood should be drawn for crossmatching later. Balanced salt solution i.v. may be followed by a colloid solution and then by blood or red blood cells to keep the hematocrit above about 20% (Chapter 2D). Traumatic-hypovolemic shock is not to be treated with drugs. A vasopressor is only transiently justified to sustain a pulse in threatening exsanguination cardiac arrest, while replacing the lost blood volume. Airway control in maxillofacial trauma may be difficult and must be improvised (Chapter 1A). Patients with maxillofacial trauma and head trauma are cervical spinal cord injury suspects. The absence of neurologic deficit does not rule out cervical spine injury. It should be presumed until ruled out by roentgenographic examination. One should insert a gastric tube into the severely traumatized, stuporous or comatose patient, unless a basal skull fracture is suspected; a urinary catheter should be inserted unless urethral transsection is suspected. ECG monitoring is indicated. The patient should be completely undressed to facilitate thorough examination.

Neurologic evaluation may follow the AVPU principle[22]: A—Alert, V—response to Vocal stimuli, P—response to Painful stimuli, U—Unresponsive. This is later followed by formal coma scoring (Table 9). Resuscitation must accompany primary survey and rapid transportation to a trauma hospital or to an advanced mobile ICU operating room facility in the field.

The *secondary survey* should be conducted by the physician, if one is available. It starts with detailed examination of the head (eyes, pupils, fundi, lens, penetrating injuries, face, skull) and continues with examination of face, cervical spine and neck, with continuous support of head–neck–chest aligned. A sports helmet should be removed with great care if cervical injury is suspected and in the absence of other vital priorities may be left in place until a roentgenogram is taken. Then follow examination of chest, abdomen, rectum (sphincter tone, blood), extremities (wounds, fractures) and the neurologic picture. For chest, abdominal, head and extremity injuries, see the discussion below.

Neurologic examination during the secondary survey includes repeated determinations of the level of consciousness, pupils, and (in the conscious victim) motor and sensory function or (in unresponsive patients) coma scoring (Table 9). Until ruled out, any severe injury calls for immobilization on a long spine board, with cervical collar, sand bags and tape to prevent head–neck motion, throughout transport to an advanced facility. Most important is suspicion of intracranial hemorrhage and drainage of epidural or subdural hematoma by the closest competent surgeon, within 1 hour of injury if possible! In suspected intracranial hemorrhage, rapid transfer to an appropriate facility is essential. The secondary survey ends with appropriate X-rays, laboratory tests and special studies. Definitive surgical care is beyond the scope of this book; it is covered by other texts[22, 163, 164, 799, 902].

Primary and secondary surveys include external hemorrhage control and general principles of wound care. The latter include prevention of contamination by sterile dressings in the field; thorough cleaning, removal of devitalized tissue and foreign bodies in the ATLS facility or hospital; and tetanus prophylaxis[22b]. Most patients will have had two or more prior injections of tetanus toxoid. They should be given 0.5 ml of 'absorbed toxoid' for both tetanus-prone and non-tetanus-prone wounds. No passive immunization is needed. Patients without previous toxoid but with non-tetanus-prone wounds should receive 0.5 ml of toxoid, but in the case of tetanus-prone wounds 0.5 ml of toxoid, plus human tetanus immune globulin (250 units), plus antibiotics should be given. Tetanus antitoxin horse serum should not be used. It is assumed that increasingly more people will have had four injections of diphtheria–pertussis–tetanus immunization in early childhood, a fifth dose at 4–6 years of age and a booster every 10 years; a previously nonimmunized adult will have had three injections of toxoid and a booster every 10 years.

Management in the hospital includes obtaining AMPLE history[22b]: A—allergies, M—medications, P—past illnesses, L—last meal, and E—events preceding the injury. There should be frequent re-evaluation, determining the mechanism of injury, record keeping, and legal considerations.

This section of the book is meant to highlight a few knowledge items. For skill acquisition of ATLS measures, we recommend first scanning Chapters 1–3 and this section of Chapter 4, and then taking an ATLS course which includes skill practice stations. A simplified ATLS course without animal laboratory practice, although a compromise, is better than no ATLS course, as it is suitable for introducing the majority of physician nonsurgeons and medical students into everyday emergency care. This would provide some effectiveness in the case of a disaster.

Severe polytrauma[163, 164a, 799, 902]

The fate of the victim of severe multiple injuries is usually determined by: the location and extent of brain tissue destruction; the degree and rate of initial hemorrhage; and whether or not there is exsanguination cardiac arrest before help arrives. Ameliorating factors include: early hemostasis and fluid resuscitation; initial airway and breathing control; ATLS within the first hour; and the speed with which resuscitative surgery is carried out for intracranial, intrathoracic or intra-abdominal trauma. Early fluid resuscitation, immobilization and wound care can prevent late deaths after polytrauma due to fat embolism, thromboembolism, sepsis and multiple organ failure. The latter include acute tubular necrosis of the kidney (ATN) and adult respiratory distress syndrome (ARDS), also called 'shock lung' in the absence of chest injury[557, 622, 725]. It is not hypovolemia alone but probably a combination of tissue trauma, hypovolemia and sepsis which causes so-called 'irreversible shock'[163, 796–800]. All the subsequent subheadings represent conditions which contribute to the mortality of polytrauma. The interaction of multiple organ derangements includes: brain trauma–ischemia–increased intracranial pressure (ICP), which can cause neurogenic pulmonary edema; cardiovascular failure causing low perfusion pressure, which can reduce the chance of recovery after cerebral trauma; hypoxemia after chest injury or airway problems, which can add to brain failure; abdominal trauma with peritoneal spillage of intestinal contents, which can add sepsis and mediator effects contributing to hypovolemic shock; and gastrointestinal–hepatic tissue injury, which can cause overall microcirculatory disturbances, including ATN and ARDS. For effective treatment of polytrauma, a general trauma surgeon should remain the coordinating primary physician of multidisciplinary team action, and the most experienced and skilled anesthesiologist of the team should guide or help with resuscitation.

Circulatory shock[163, 270, 796–800, 902, 943–945, 948]

Shock is the 'clinical picture of overall tissue perfusion inadequate to meet tissue needs'[736a]. Shock, if not reversed in time, may lead to lethal multiple organ failure due to hypoperfusion. In slow dying from shock, vital organs may become irreversibly damaged before circulation ceases entirely.

Shock states may be classified as follows[948]:

1. oligemia (decrease in circulating blood volume, e.g. from external or internal loss of blood);
2. cardiac pump failure (cardiogenic shock);
3. total blood flow obstruction (e.g. pulmonary embolism, cardiac tamponade);
4. altered blood flow distribution (e.g. septicemia, intoxication, sympathetic paralysis)[802].

Traumatic shock may consist of a sequence of three insults: (1) tissue injury, (2) hypovolemic shock, and (3) sepsis. With prompt treatment of (1), one can often prevent (2) and (3).

In shock states, there is usually time for compensatory mechanisms to come into play. These may give short-term protection through cerebral and coronary vasodilatation and systemic vasoconstriction. In spite of these mechanisms, however, the brain may suffer permanent damage during shock if MAP drops below about 30–40 mmHg for prolonged periods, particularly if accompanied by low arterial PO_2. Shock states predispose the sick heart to VF or asystole, which can be triggered by minor interventions, such as transportation or airway suctioning (hypoxemia).

In *hypovolemic (traumatic) shock*, highest priority must be given to the venous access routes for fluid resuscitation. One should seek insertion of several largest possible cannulae, percutaneously, in this order of preference: arm vein; external jugular vein; subclavian vein; right internal jugular vein to superior vena cava; femoral vein. A plastic introducer cannula, 8 French, inserted over a guide wire (Seldinger technique), serves multiple purposes. In some cases, venous cutdown is required, preferably of an arm vein (or saphenous vein at the ankle, but only in the absence of severe trauma below the diaphragm). Ideally, each trauma hospital should have available in the emergency room and operating room, rapid infusion devices with blood warmers. Those with roller pumps are particularly effective, permitting infusion of 1–10 liters per minute[462, 796].

Adequate concurrent treatment of acute hemorrhage with plasma substitutes (Ringer's solution, dextrans, hydroxyethyl starch, polygelatin, albumin) is essential in the absence of immediate blood transfusions and leads to acute *normovolemic hemodilution*[531, 880]. We have demonstrated four sequential phases of response during hemodilution without hypovolemic shock[110, 880, 881]:

1. complete compensation of arterial oxygen transport through increase in cardiac output until the hemoglobin values had decreased to approximately 5.5 g/dl (about 20% hematocrit);
2. partial compensation when the hemoglobin levels fell to between 5.5 and 4 g/dl (about 15% hematocrit);
3. reversible decompensation when the hemoglobin had fallen to about 3–4 g/dl (about 10–15% hematocrit); at this point, cardiac output declined, heart failure started, and blood lactate increased; animals could survive without requiring blood transfusion;
4. irreversible decompensation when the hemoglobin dropped below approximately 3 g/dl (10% hematocrit) breathing air or below about 2 g/dl (6% hematocrit) breathing 100% oxygen. A dramatic decrease in cardiac output, oxygen consumption and venous oxygen values was followed by cardiac arrest in asystole.

Patients with oligemia or cardiopulmonary disease may decompensate earlier. Monitoring may include central or mixed venous PO_2 and base deficit. When mixed venous PO_2 reaches about 30–35 mmHg, metabolism in vital organs can be assumed to become anaerobic, and there is consequently a need for increasing the arterial oxygen-carrying capacity by infusion of blood or red blood cells. In most patients treated for blood loss with normovolemic (or hypervolemic) hemodilution, it is wise not to let the hematocrit fall below 30%. The widely accepted sequence of action is: Ringer's solution or isotonic NaCl–colloid plasma substitute–red cells or whole blood.

Hypertonic salt solution (4–7%) in small amounts (200 ml) can attract interstitial fluid and help maintain arterial pressure while waiting for ATLS[508a]. It thus seems valuable in field and transport.

Stroma-free hemoglobin, an acellular oxygen-carrying blood substitute, appears promising[20, 52, 192] but has not yet been perfected for general clinical use.

Fluorocarbons require 100% O_2 breathing to offer advantage over plasma substitutes[572, 816]. Hypertonic glucose may be beneficial[163, 432, 525, 768, 829] or create deleterious cerebral acidosis[663, 806]. These and other agents need critical evaluation in animal outcome models of cardiac arrest[745] and shock[52, 163].

For fluid resuscitation in hypovolemic shock see Chapter 2D; for management of multiple organ failure see Chapter 3.

Burns[22a, b, 33, 164a, 575, 755d, 799, 902]

In the USA about 12 000 persons burn to death every year. Most burn injuries are due to flame; some are due to scalds, electric current, chemicals or radiation (see disasters, Chapter 6). Most dangerous are upper and lower airway burns due to heat, ash, gases and other combustion products. They call for continuous respiratory observation and perhaps tracheal intubation. While controlling Steps A–B–C, one should obtain a brief history and assess the extent and steps of the burn injury, assess associated injuries and weigh the patient for subsequent fluid therapy. Blood carbon monoxide levels should be obtained. Airway control should be aggressive, and include tracheal intubation and mechanical ventilation if indicated. Pulmonary care should be guided by frequent arterial PO_2 measurements on constant FIO_2 to detect early shunting.

The extent of surface burns should be assessed by the rule of 9's (anatomical regions, each representing 9% of total body surface area): each arm counts as 9%; each leg, 18%; the front trunk, 18%; the back trunk, 18%; and the head, 9% (in a child, 18%).

One should determine the depth of the burn wounds[902]: first degree (erythema), second degree (red or mottled skin with swelling and blisters), and third degree (full thickness burn with leathery appearance, dry or moist, coagulation necrosis). Water loss through skin areas with third degree burns may be over 10 times the normal water loss through skin, which for the entire body is about 1000 ml/70 kg per day. Besides fluid loss, major burns result in heat loss (several thousand kilocalories per day deficit), paralleled by greatly increased oxygen consumption. Increased capillary permeability occurs first in the burn area, but in extensive surface burns can become systemic. Thus, the greatest danger in burn injury is *hypovolemic shock*, which if not promptly corrected can lead to ATN and multiple organ failure. In contrast to mechanical trauma, whole blood is not lost in large quantities. Thus, a combination of balanced salt solution (e.g. lactated Ringer's) and colloid solution (e.g. plasma protein fraction or albumin) is needed. A negative nitrogen balance calls for early oral or parenteral hyperalimentation. Pulmonary edema may develop as the result of pulmonary burns, overinfusion and overall increased capillary permeability.

The overall severity of a burn injury is best assessed by considering as *critical* (for admission to a burn center)[902]: any degree burn involving over 25% body surface area; third degree burns over more than 10% of the body surface area; all burns of the face, eyes, ears, hands, feet or perineum; suspected pulmonary burns of any extent; associated major other injuries; lesser burns in patients with pre-existing major disease; burns of over 20% of body surface area in the young or the old; and high-voltage electric burns.

Early i.v. fluid resuscitation is recommended for any degree burn greater than 20% of body surface area, titrated according to hourly urinary output (bladder catheter) and measurements of body weight. Fluid therapy must be individualized. Urine flow should be kept at about 1 ml/kg per hour for children and 0.5 ml/kg per hour for adults. Usually, electrolyte solution 2–4 ml/kg × percent body surface burn per 24 hours is required (the Baxter formula).

The Brooke US Army Hospital guidelines call for more electrolytes than colloid solution during the initial 24 hours, and colloid during the second 24 hours. The guidelines include for the first 24 hours: lactated Ringer's solution 1.5 ml/kg × percent body surface area burn (50% maximal), plus a colloid (albumin, plasmanate, fresh frozen plasma, dextran 10, polygelatin, or hydroxyethyl starch) 0.5 ml/kg × percent body surface burn, including 2000 ml of water. More should be given in the first 8 hours and the rest in the subsequent 16 hours. The guidelines call for the second 24 hours to give electrolyte solution 0.75 ml/kg × percent body surface burn, plus the same amount of colloid and water as in the first 24 hours. Several other fluid resuscitation formulas are also acceptable. Hypertonic salt solutions for initial burn shock therapy are controversial. If they are used, serum sodium should be kept at less than 158 mEq/l. Most burn centers follow isotonic salt solutions with a colloid solution. Maintaining urine flow may require pushing fluids i.v. Serum albumin should be maintained above 2.5 g/dl.

Other considerations for the acute management of burn victims include:

1. Early life support to follow the principles of this chapter (above).
2. Cold water application for minor burns, but not for extensive burns. Application of sterile moist dressings in the field (optional). Preserving second degree burn blisters intact and applying topical antibiotic ointment. Cautious titrated use of narcotic analgesics i.v.
3. Cleansing of all burn wounds with mild antiseptic solution. Early conservative debridement. For severely burnt patients, application of topical antimicrobial agents, e.g. silver sulfadiazine, or (for better eschar penetration) mafenide acetate.
4. Definitive burn wound care, prevention and treatment of sepsis (the major cause of late deaths), and reconstructive plastic surgery are beyond the scope of this book. Neomycin dressings are used by some after grafting.

5. Laboratory blood tests to include hematology, clotting data, and arterial blood gas values. Chest roentgenograms. Maintaining a flow sheet.
6. Maintaining circulation of burned swollen extremities by escharotomy and perhaps even fasciotomy. Topical enzymes (e.g. Travase) may be substituted for escharotomy.

Radiation injuries

Human error, technologic failure, terrorism or war can result in radiation injuries, ranging from a subtle leak of radioactive material to the explosion of a nuclear weapon. The latter causes instantaneous death or injuries through blast and thermal burns, to be followed by the effects of acute radiation. Emergency treatment is hampered by the need to resuscitate while providing protective clothing to victims for isolation and to rescuers for reverse isolation, and by the need for early decontamination.

The medical literature concerning the harmful biological effects of radiation is quite extensive. The effects on human beings of whole-body irradiation begin with the acute radiation syndrome or radiation sickness, mentioned above. Exposure to radiation is difficult to quantitate in real terms. Therefore, symptomatology as described above will suggest the extent and severity of injury. The acute radiation syndrome is characterized by an initial period of toxicity, followed by a period of latency in which there is a sense of well being, and finally overt manifestation of injury. The duration of the latent period is directly related to the duration and magnitude of exposure. Symptomatology will depend on the organ system primarily affected, which in turn is a function of dose. Human tissues most susceptible to the effects of radiation are those with a rapid turnover rate such as the hematopoietic system, the gastrointestinal system, the reproductive organs, and at very high risk levels of exposure, the central nervous system.

Radiation exposure is currently measured in grays (Gy), which have replaced 'rads'. One gray (1 Gy) = 100 rads. One gray corresponds to the absorption of energy of 1 joule per kg of tissue.

Above about 100 Gy (10 000 rads) whole-body exposure, death is certain and rapid, due to irradiation of the brain. Patients die with stupor, hyperexcitability, and coma. Sudden whole-body exposure to over 10 Gy kills within anything from a few hours to about two weeks, from radiation of the brain plus hemorrhage and circulatory shock due to necrosis of the intestinal mucosa. There is nausea, persistent vomiting, and hemorrhagic diarrhea.

Whole-body radiation with 2–10 (some say 3–4) Gy causes 50% of the exposed victims to die (LD_{50}). Death is usually within several weeks from leukopenia, acute infections and acute bowel syndrome. With specialized intensive care, the LD_{50} might be close to 5 Gy. Exposure to 2–10 Gy is not absolutely lethal, and exposure to less than about 2 Gy does not kill acutely. Such exposure levels result in nausea and vomiting and long-term leukopenia, anemia and reduced host defenses. In this range of total-body irradiation, therapeutic intervention has a direct impact on survival. Early, vigorous therapy is associated with virtually certain survival.

When radiation exposure is survived or when there is prolonged low-level radiation, as from fallout, with cumulative exposure to at least 0.5 Gy per year, there can be temporary or permanent sterility, malformation of exposed fetuses, and increased risk of cancer. Loss of hair is a specific sign of radiation injury but cannot be correlated with outcome. Local skin exposure to about 1 Gy causes a first degree burn, and to about 10 Gy a second degree burn, characterized by an exudative radiodermatitis, which leads to ulceration and infection in an already immune or compromised host.

In a nuclear power plant accident, radioactive products present in the fallout may be inhaled or ingested, thereby further compromising recovery, especially if concomitant injury exists such as burns or fractures. Contamination from fallout may linger on for generations, making world regions unsafe for people, animals and plants.

We maintain that preparation for nuclear war is senseless and dangerous. Industrial nuclear accidents, however, such as occurred at Three Mile Island, Pennsylvania (USA) and Chernobyl (USSR) have taught us that the potential for peacetime radiation exposure of large civilian populations is real. Moreover, the possibility of a nuclear device falling into the hands of terrorists is quite realistic, given the current world situation. Nuclear blackmail and the detonation of a single nuclear device over an urban area, with a resultant exposure of hundreds of thousands of people to the harmful effects of radiation fallout, should be considered as a possibility. Therefore, we advocate medical disaster preparedness and planning for this unlikely scenario of a single nuclear mass disaster.

Notwithstanding the scenario, all casualties of nuclear disasters must receive prompt and effective therapy early on. Rapid rescue and transport to specialized treatment facilities is of utmost importance. During rescue efforts close attention must be paid to exposure of rescue personnel entering the fallout area. Rescue teams must be monitored, decontaminated if necessary, and rotated periodically in order to minimize radiation exposure. Treatment of the radiation syndrome is dependent on the extent and severity of exposure and initially should be guided by symptomatology. Symptoms respond to conventional therapy.

The principles of therapy include: reverse isolation, bedrest; close monitoring of fluid and electrolyte balance; complete hematological evaluation with blood component therapy when indicated; periodic examination of bone marrow aspirates; and physical examination for early detection of acute infection with rapid initiation of high dose antibiotic therapy in the event of infection. Specifically in the gastrointestinal syndrome, prophylactic sterilization of the intestinal tract is indicated. If pancytopenia occurs, reverse isolation in a sterile room with laminar flow and ultraviolet light is indicated. All articles coming into contact with the patient must be sterile.

Precautions for personnel include screening for nosocomial infections, and change of clothes before entering patient rooms. Finally, bone marrow transplantation is indicated, but only in severe cases with exposure to lethal doses which are associated with manifestations consistent with bone marrow failure.

Cerebral trauma[63, 114, 293, 377, 378, 434, 448, 512, 539, 598, 674, 682, 736b, 790, 885, 886, 926, 930, 931]

Mortality among head-injured patients who remain unconscious for over 6 hours, once about 50%, has been reduced to about 40% with intensive care management including artificial ventilation, monitoring and control of ICP, and rapid evacuation of intracranial hematomas. The main factors causing mortality and morbidity are early post-insult arterial hypoxemia and hypotension, and petechial hemorrhages in midbrain and brainstem after acceleration/deceleration injury. Gastric ulcers[863] and other extracerebral complications can increase mortality.

General patient management should follow principles of Chapters 1, 2 and 3. A few special considerations are listed below.

When the impact of head injury results in a brief period of apnea, which may be followed by airway obstruction, a bystander should immediately use the triple airway maneuver and mouth-to-mouth (in trismus mouth-to-nose) ventilation. Hypoxemia (due to aspiration, neurogenic pulmonary edema or other factors) has frequently been encountered on arrival in the emergency room. Thus, routine oxygen inhalation is recommended as soon as possible. Definitive airway control with tracheal intubation should be accompanied by the most experienced physician available, ideally an anesthesiologist, since straining, coughing and reflex hypertension as a result of protracted intubation attempts can cause cerebrovascular engorgement with ICP rise, leading to further damage to the already mechanically injured brain. Intubation may be made more risky and difficult by stupor with restlessness, straining, trismus, seizures and vomiting. The nonexpert should try as long as possible to oxygenate by bag–mask and pharyngeal suction. The expert should skillfully perform rapid intubation, using preoxygenation by hyperventilation with 100% O_2 (bag–mask), cricoid pressure, barbiturate (or other sedative), and paralysis by rapidly acting muscle relaxant. During and after intubation, keeping $PaCO_2$ low by controlled hyperventilation and PaO_2 high, the avoidance of 'bucking', tracheobronchial clearing, and maintaining arterial normotension are all important and may be difficult to accomplish.

Intracranial hemorrhage does not produce oligemic shock, but results in coma and ICP rise, which reduce cerebral perfusion pressure and eventually lead to brain herniation and apnea. Coma can progress to brain death or a vegetative state. The latter can be permanent or reverse itself partially (Chapter 3, Tables 10–12).

'Concussion' implies no significant anatomic brain injury. Hallmarks are brief CNS depression and retrograde amnesia, headache, dizziness and nausea, without localizing signs. The pupils may be fixed and dilated in the early phase just after injury, even in salvageable patients. 'Contusion' implies more prolonged unconsciousness and often focal signs. All patients with head injury should be evaluated in the hospital emergency department and considered as possible candidates for admission.

After initial resuscitation, one should determine the level of consciousness, pupillary reaction, vital signs and extracranial injuries. A skull roentgenogram is less helpful in guiding management than clinical signs and CT imaging. Life support by experts must be uninterrupted during transport to the CT facility, etc. One must promptly recognize epidural (arterial) hemorrhage (e.g. from the sequence of 'concussion'–lucid interval–stupor–contralateral hemiparesis–ipsilateral dilated and fixed pupil). Immediate surgical intervention is indicated; the prognosis is excellent only if epidural hematoma is drained within 1–2 hours. Subdural (usually venous) hemorrhage is also life-threatening, but symptoms develop more slowly. Evacuation by emergency burr holes or craniotomy is more effective in epidural than in subdural hematoma. If this is not possible in a trauma center with neurosurgery, the general traumatology surgeon should be trained to perform these life-saving procedures. Subarachnoid hemorrhage results in bloody CSF and may not require immediate surgery. Hemorrhages within the brain substance can be recognized by CT scanning.

If the patient remains in coma after initial resuscitation, life support should be according to the guidelines of Chapter 3. Acute intracranial hypertension calls for endotracheal intubation, artificial ventilation, relaxation, osmotherapy and perhaps barbiturate (Table 6). Both mannitol i.v. and barbiturate i.v. can reverse increased ICP, but the beneficial effect of ICP control on neurologic outcome of patient groups overall is not convincing[539]. The prophylactic use of barbiturate therapy in one randomized study of comatose head injury patients throughout the first 72 hours[931] has resulted in an increased incidence of intractable hypotension and no reduction in mortality and morbidity. CBF after severe head injury followed by death or disability may be high or low[598].

The assessment of head-injured patients requires continuous monitoring and titrated life support, accompanied by ongoing reassessment to be compared with the initial clinical picture. Arterial pressure is usually high (or low in accompanying extracranial injuries) and should be controlled at normotensive or slightly below normotensive levels. Progressive bradycardia (Cushing response to increased ICP), usually accompanied by hypertension, suggests a lesion in need of surgery. Head injury tends to cause hyperthermia which should be reversed to moderate hypothermia. A simple way of following the neurologic dysfunction is use of the Glasgow coma scale (Table 9). Lumbar puncture, EEG and radiotracer techniques are not helpful in the initial management of cerebral trauma.

Head injury as well as ischemic anoxia and other brain insults can be followed by generalized seizures, which can cause asphyxia from pharyngo-laryngospasm and apnea. Neurons suffer not only from hypoxemia second-ary to impaired oxygenation during convulsions, but also from the hypoxic acidosis induced by the increased metabolic (electric) activity of neurons. Thus, management of generalized convulsions requires $IPPV/O_2$, if neces-sary with the aid of a muscle relaxant. Soon thereafter, administration of a CNS depressant such as diazepam, thiopental or pentobarbital (for rapid action), and phenobarbital or phenytoin (for prolonged effect) can minimize the electric discharges from the brain. Seizure disorders can stimulate cardiac dysrhythmias.

Spinal cord trauma[12, 22, 736a, 902, 927]

Any victim of trauma with injury above the clavicle should be suspected of having cervical spine injury. This calls for assessment, resuscitation and life support with head–neck–chest aligned in the neutral position and without moving the spine during transport. Moderate backward tilt of the head is acceptable, but maximal backward tilt, flexion or rotation of the head are prohibited. As soon as possible, with head–neck–chest aligned manually (Figs. 4 and 35), the patient should be placed on a spine board and immobilized with semi-rigid cervical collar, using sandbags and tape, for transport to the trauma center. Initial assessment should include: search for neck deformity, pain, tenderness, motor and sensory disturbances of the extremities, bladder and rectal control, and spinal shock (hypotension without tachycardia); a lateral cervical spine and chest roentgenogram; and CT scanning if available. Management includes immobilization and general life support including maintenance of arterial normotension. Experimental treatments in attempts to save integrity of the spinal cord include surgical decompression, local hypothermia, and a variety of pharmacologic and physical agents under investigation for both cerebral and spinal cord resuscitation. Since management of spine injury requires specialized knowledge and experience, these patients should be taken to spinal cord injury centers.

Thoracic trauma[22, 49, 260, 296, 368, 412, 468, 516, 552, 556, 668, 736b, 799]

Although thoracic trauma rarely requires resuscitative surgery, it is the cause of about one-fourth of trauma deaths, many of which are preventable. The predominant cause of death is progressive hypoxemia from pulmonary contusion, atelectasis, consolidation and shunting, worsened at times by flail chest and/or pneumothorax. Tension pneumothorax and cardiac tampo-nade are summarized below. For intrathoracic exsanguination cardiac arrest, see 'open-chest CPR', Chapter 2 (Fig. 51). Open pneumothorax (sucking chest wound) also leads to atelectasis and hypoxemia. The defect should be promptly closed with a sterile occlusive dressing taped on three sides, leaving the fourth side open to function as a valve. A chest tube should be placed distant from the defect (Chapter 1A, Fig. 20). Surgical closure is performed later. Massive hemothorax is usually caused by a penetrating injury, less commonly by blunt trauma. It should be detected from percussion, auscultation and a shock state. Treatment requires pleural drainage and restoration of blood volume. An autotransfusion device should be used if available. Sometimes emergency thoracotomy may be required, which should be performed by a skilled surgeon[164a, 846, 847, 902].

Flail chest was thought in the past to cause progressive hypoxemia and hypercarbia from 'pendel air'. This is now thought to be less important than pulmonary contusion and consolidation, which would require higher negative intrathoracic pressures for lung expansion than the flail chest will permit. Some patients can be managed without tracheal intubation, with titrated increase in FIO_2 by mask (perhaps with CPAP) (Fig. 22). Pain control and monitoring of blood gas values (particularly alveolar-arterial PO_2 gradient) are important. Intercostal nerve or thoracic epidural blocks should be considered. When there is significant shunting during spontaneous breathing (relatively low arterial PO_2 on constant FIO_2), controlled hyperventilation is capable of re-expanding the lungs (increasing FRC), counteracting flailing and shunting, and stabilizing the chest wall and thereby reducing pain (Moerch).

Besides flail chest and pulmonary contusion, causes of death are traumatic aortic rupture, tracheobronchial injury, and traumatic diaphragmatic hernia. They all usually require emergency surgery. Myocardial contusion requires ECG and hemodynamic monitoring and management similar to that of myocardial infarction. If the patient with crushed chest develops cardiac arrest, one should start with closed-chest CPR and switch to open-chest CPR if the closed technique fails to produce a palpable pulse, and when uncontrollable intrathoracic hemorrhage is suspected.

Tension pneumothorax is an opening into the pleural space, either through the chest wall or through the lung, with pressure in the pleural space rising above atmospheric throughout the respiratory cycle. This collapses the ipsilateral lung. Previously healthy individuals will become hypoxemic from 40–50% shunt. If the opening operates as a one-way valve, for instance in lung contusion, rupture of alveolar blebs, or air trapping in asthma or emphysema, positive-pressure ventilation or coughing can force increments of gas into the pleural space, where the gas cannot escape and a tension pneumothorax develops. Alveoli may also rupture into the pulmonary interstitial spaces, resulting in mediastinal and subcutaneous emphysema (noticed in the form of crepitation about the neck) and subserosal blebs, which can rupture secondarily into the pleural space.

Tension pneumothorax should be suspected when there is progressive difficulty in ventilating the lungs, progressive inability of the lungs to deflate passively, progressive deterioration of the circulation (decrease in venous return, arterial hypotension, tachycardia), mediastinal shift (evidenced by tracheal shift or mediastinal shift noted on chest percussion), and progressive distension of the abdomen (inversion of diaphragm or pneumoperitoneum of air dissecting from tension pneumothorax). Circulatory arrest seems to be the combined result of severe hypoxemia (compression atelectasis) and compression and kinking of bronchi and major vessels. Treatment of suspected pneumothorax consists of confirmation by needle puncture and drainage by large-bore tube (Chapter 1A, Fig. 20). When, in the presence of pulselessness, tube drainage is ineffective to relieve the tension pneumothorax, open chest cardiac resuscitation is indicated (Chapter 2).

Cardiac tamponade produces a type of obstructive shock, and should be suspected under circumstances that may disrupt the integrity of the heart wall (stab wound, gunshot wound, intracardiac needle injection, postcardiac surgery, perforation by stiff intracardiac catheter, infarcted ventricular wall). There are signs of compromised cardiac output with arterial hypotension, elevated CVP with venous distension, and pulsations, muffled heart sounds and pulsus paradoxus (during deep inhalations the arterial pressure decreases markedly). There may be substernal pain. If time permits a roentgenogram, it will show a widened heart shadow. MAP, pulse pressure and cardiac output decline, while venous pressure and heart rate increase. Death in asystole or VF is due to progressive inability of the heart to fill during diastole. The rapidity of dying depends on the speed with which blood accumulates in the pericardium. Treatment includes pericardial needle aspiration via the paraxyphoid approach, preferably under ECG monitoring. Aspiration may have to be repeated and perhaps followed by the surgical creation of a pleural-pericardial window. In pulselessness, suspicion of cardiac tamponade is an indication for open-chest CPR with opening and drainage of the pericardial sac and direct surgical control of the bleeding site.

Abdominal trauma[22, 105, 163, 164, 184, 632, 799, 901, 902]

About 25% of penetrating injuries involve the abdomen. Blunt abdominal injuries (which represent 6% of all trauma) constitute up to 25% of all trauma deaths[902].

Because of the dome shape of the diaphragm, injuries to the abdomen may involve the thorax and vice versa. One should suspect abdominal trauma from location of bruises and wounds and the type of accidents. The decision for emergency laparotomy, which may be life-saving, requires assessment of the shock state, and of the abdomen and lower part of the thorax by inspection, auscultation (bowel sounds), palpation (abdominal wall muscle guarding), percussion tenderness, rebound tenderness, and rectal and vaginal examination. There may be retroperitoneal vascular injuries or exsanguinating hemorrhage into the abdomen from the aorta or venae cavae, and less rapid bleeding from the liver, spleen or kidneys. Penetrating injury often causes hemorrhage or perforation of bowel, and is usually an indication for laparotomy. Blunt abdominal trauma is an indication for peritoneal lavage. Resuscitation should not be delayed by X-ray examinations when the patient is in shock.

Peritoneal lavage[226] is for diagnosing occult intraperitoneal bleeding and biliary or intestinal injury. It is also indicated in selected patients with penetrating injury. It should not be performed when there is free peritoneal air seen on the roentgenogram, in peritonitis, or in patients who have had previous laparotomies. Peritoneal lavage is not an innocuous procedure.

Technique of peritoneal lavage[22b]

1. Decompress the urinary bladder by catheter.
2. Decompress the stomach by gastric tube.
3. Surgically prepare the entire abdomen.
4. Inject local anesthetic in the midline one-third of the distance from umbilicus to the symphysis pubis.
5. Vertically incise skin and subcutis to fascia.
6. Incise fascia and peritoneum.
7. Insert peritoneal dialysis catheter (or regular 12–16 gauge vascular catheter), at least 8 inches long, into the peritoneal cavity (without needle or trocar; under vision).
8. Direct the peritoneal catheter toward the left or right pelvis.
9. Connect a syringe to the catheter and aspirate.
10. If blood is not obtained, instill 1 liter of lactated Ringer's solution into the peritoneal cavity.
11. Gently agitate the abdomen.
12. Allow fluid to equilibrate for 5–10 minutes and then syphon off and inspect drained fluid (color, smell).
13. Send a sample to the lab for RBC and WBC count, bacterial gram stain, and smear for fibers. A red blood cell count greater than $100\,000/mm^3$, a white cell count greater than $500/mm^3$, or presence of bile, pus, fecal material or bacteria is an indication for laparotomy.
14. Negative lavage does not rule out retroperitoneal injury. For possible pancreatic injury, determine serum amylase.

Exsanguinating intra-abdominal hemorrhage should be suspected when there is hypovolemic shock with rapid deterioration and peritoneal signs. The prehospital management might include inflation of the MAST leg and abdominal garments (Chapter 1C, Fig. 35). In the hospital, one should be ready for transthoracic temporary occlusion of the aorta before releasing the pressure suit for laparotomy and repair[858]. Anesthesia, resuscitation and resuscitative laparotomy may have to go hand in hand.

Extremity trauma[21, 22]

Patients with only fractures and soft-tissue injuries of the extremities are rarely in need of major resuscitative efforts, except for the need to prevent or immediately correct hypovolemia from major external or intra-tissue blood volume loss. This can be life-threatening in fractures of the femur (particularly bilateral), traumatic amputations, crushing trauma of the pelvis, major open fractures of any kind, and polytrauma with multiple fractures. A closed femur fracture can result in 1–2 liter internal blood loss. In general, extremity trauma should not receive priority attention during emergency resuscitation and primary survey. Immobilization of fractured extremities before moving the patient, however, is important to prevent further injury, pain, fat embolization, shock and morbidity. One can effectively improvise immobilization, even without splints. For learning immobilization with the use of air splits and lower leg traction splints, see an advanced first aid manual[25b, 126]. Resuscitation has priority over splinting!

Anesthesia in disasters

This is a major subject which is considered in another chapter of this book. Considerations of sedation, analgesia, and anesthesia (local-regional, general) must parallel the above considerations of trauma, resuscitation, and resuscitative surgery. Here are only a few comments.

The perception of trauma-induced pain depends on variable combinations of the initial painful stimulus and its psychologic modification, particularly by fear ('flight or fight'). Injured persons who appear to suffer pain should, as feasible, receive local analgesia by immobilization of fractures and other physical means, and perhaps need the use of systemic analgesics. One must consider safety before comfort. All central nervous system depressants can induce life-threatening hypotension and hypoventilation, particularly in shock. For systemic analgesia, ketamine has been suggested because of its relatively minor depressant effects on vital functions. Morphine (2 mg i.v.) or meperidine (10 mg i.v.), repeated as necessary for titration, have withstood the test of time. Fentanyl, an excellent narcotic for balanced general anesthesia with controlled ventilation, we consider contraindicated for analgesia in the spontaneously breathing patient, as it can unexpectedly induce apnea (breathholding, chest wall spasm), leading to asphyxia, even before the onset of coma.

For resuscitative minor invasive procedures (e.g. cricothyrotomy, pleural drainage, external hemostasis), no anesthesia or local anesthesia is preferred.

For resuscitative surgery, general principles of anesthesia practice prevail. Under primitive conditions, local-regional anesthesia (with the exception of spinal or epidural anesthesia), with intravenous titration of morphine, meperidine or ketamine, should be considered. Full general anesthesia for major resuscitative or definitive surgery should be, whenever possible, under the direction of a trained anesthesiologist, using standard equipment, in stationary or fully equipped mobile operating room facilities. To be prepared for sudden unexpected multiplication of operative needs in disasters, one should consider stockpiling appropriate anesthesia apparatus. This could economically include the draw-over vaporizer (for halothane-ether, or other volatile agents), the bellows system of Oxford University[501], the vaporizer-self-refilling bag–valve–mask system of Baltimore City Hospital[616, 710], or the Falkland system[383]. These devices permit the full range of analgesia–anesthesia with or without neuromuscular blockade and controlled ventilation, even in the absence of compressed gases, using air as the vehicle. Equipment and supplies for anesthesia must be compatible with those for resuscitation and transportation, including airway control, ventilation, fluid resuscitation and monitoring.

Chapter 5

Teaching of First Aid and Resuscitation

What to Teach to Whom (Table 14)

Providing society with optimal 'life supporting first aid and resuscitation', to reduce mortality and morbidity, is dependent on optimal teaching, in both quality and quantity. Every community, region and country should have an organized system for teaching, testing and evaluating impact on outcome of first aid and resuscitation knowledge and skills at all levels, ranging from the lay public to physician specialists[23b, 25a, b, 69a, c, 81, 124–127, 723, 724, 730, 779, 967].

All of the basic life support and most of the advanced and prolonged life support techniques listed in Table 14 and described in this manual have been subjected to studies that demonstrated their teachability and impact (National Institute of Health Project 1975, P. Safar, principal investigator[668, 720, 730, 736, 753, 781]). Each community must decide how to allocate its resources[602]. Data are scarce and needed on the impact that educational programs have on patient care process and outcome[153, 216, 399, 467, 485, 667, 668, 684].

Guidelines for teaching should be as uniform as possible within each country, at least for the training of nonphysicians, and should hopefully be at least similar (although not necessarily identical) throughout the world. Guidelines regarding which techniques to teach the lay public need to be clearly defined to avoid confusion; guidelines regarding which techniques to teach health care personnel (from lifeguards to physician specialists), on the other hand, require more flexibility, to facilitate updating of concepts and techniques as needed and to allow clinical judgment to optimize care. Physicians eager to advance resuscitation medicine should learn to walk before running; e.g. get first hand experience in resuscitating patients with the presently recommended basic and advanced life support methods, before experimenting with exotic new drugs.

Each agency responsible for providing guidelines on the teaching of cardiopulmonary cerebral resuscitation (CPCR) techniques will have to consider several questions:

1. Does the technique in question have documented life-saving potential?
2. What are the possible risks and complications of the technique, as

Table 14. What to teach to whom.

● should be taught
○ might be taught
— should not be taught

Phases	Steps	Measures	Lay public	Police, fireman, lifeguard	Ambulance attendant, technician	General nurse	Intensive care nurse, paramedic	Physician, medical student, dentist	Physician specialist
I BASIC LIFE SUPPORT—BLS (Emergency oxygenation)	Airway control	*Without equipment*							
		*Head-tilt	●	●	●	●	●	●	●
		*Supine aligned position	○	●	●	●	●	●	●
		*Stable side position	●	●	●	●	●	●	●
		*Triple airway maneuver (jaw-thrust)	○	○	●	●	●	●	●
		*Manual clearing of mouth and throat	●	●	●	●	●	●	●
		Back-blows—manual thrusts	○	○	○	○	○	○	●
		With equipment							
		Pharyngeal suctioning	—	○	●	●	●	●	●
		Pharyngeal intubation	—	○	●	●	●	●	●
		Esophageal obturator airway insertion	—	—	—	—	○	○	○
		Endotracheal intubation	—	—	—	—	●	●	●
		Tracheobronchial suctioning	—	—	○	○	●	●	●
		Cricothyrotomy	—	—	—	—	○	○	●
		Translaryngeal O$_2$ jet insufflation	—	—	—	—	○	○	●
		Tracheotomy	—	—	—	—	—	○	●
		Bronchoscopy	—	—	—	—	—	—	●
		Bronchodilation	—	—	—	○	○	○	●
		Pleural drainage	—	—	—	—	○	○	●
	Breathing support	*Without equipment*							
		*Mouth-to-mouth (nose) ventilation	●	●	●	●	●	●	●
		With equipment							
		Mouth-to-adjunct without O$_2$	○	●	●	●	●	●	●
		Mouth-to-adjunct with O$_2$	—	○	●	●	●	●	●
		Manual bag-mask (tube) O$_2$ ventilation	—	—	●	●	●	●	●
		Hand-triggered O$_2$ ventilation	—	—	●	●	●	●	●

Legend:
● should be taught
○ might be taught
— should not be taught

Phases	Steps	Measures	Lay public	Police, fireman, lifeguard	Ambulance attendant, technician	General nurse	Intensive care nurse, paramedic	Physician, medical student, dentist	Physician specialist
BASIC LIFE SUPPORT— continued	Circulation support	*Without equipment*							
		*Control of ext. hemorrh.	●	●	●	●	●	●	●
		*Position for shock	●	●	●	●	●	●	●
		Pulse checking	●	●	●	●	●	●	●
		Manual chest compressions —single operator	●	●	●	●	●	●	●
		—two operators	○	●	●	●	●	●	●
		With equipment							
		Mechanical chest compression	—	—	○	—	●	—	●
		Open chest cardiac compression	—	—	—	—	—	○	●
		Pressure pants (MAST trousers)	—	—	○	—	●	●	●
II ADVANCED LIFE SUPPORT—ALS (Restoration of spontaneous circulation)	Drugs and fluids	i.v. lifeline peripheral	—	—	—	○	●	●	●
		i.v. lifeline central	—	—	—	—	○	●	●
		Medications	—	—	—	●	●	●	●
	Electrocardiography	ECG monitoring	—	—	—	○	●	●	●
	Fibrillation treatment	Defibrillation	—	—	○	○	●	●	●
		Automatic defibrillation	○	○	●	●	●	●	●
III PROLONGED LIFE SUPPORT—PLS (Cerebral resuscitation and post-resuscitation Intensive therapy)	Gauging	Determine and treat cause of demise	—	—	—	—	○	●	●
		Determine salvageability	—	—	—	—	○	○	●
	Human mentation	Cerebral resuscitation	—	—	—	—	○	○	●
	Intensive care	Multiple organ support	—	—	—	—	○	○	●

* Life supporting first aid.
Based in part on education research supported by NIH contract HR 42965.

opposed to alternative techniques, and are these outweighed by the potential benefits?

3. Is the teaching of this technique compatible with local needs and resources?

4. Can the technique be taught, and will the student subsequently be able to use his skills when the need arises?

5. How long is skill retention and how frequent should be retesting and retraining?

The results of resuscitation attempts depend on the weakest step of CPCR and the weakest link in the delivery chain from the scene via transportation and the emergency department to operating room and ICU. Training of the lay public, starting in schools, for widespread availability of bystander CPR, has produced measurable improvements in outcome[769d]. For optimizing outcome results in the future, response times for BLS and ALS must be reduced as much as feasible. This should include not only BLS training of the lay public as part of LSFA and ALS delivered by MICUs, but also enhanced training programs for 'first responders', such as police, life guards, firefighters, and perhaps even taxi drivers. Novel considerations for the training of first responders are needed for the implementation of earliest possible defibrillation with the use of automatic external defibrillators[176, 219].

Guidelines are indispensable for the successful implementation of large and decentralized teaching programs, whether in hospitals, by organizations or in schools. This book, geared to international needs, contains the necessary subject matter to be considered for the formation of national guidelines. We helped the League of Red Cross Societies (LRCS) to publish a lay instructors' manual on life supporting first aid (LSFA) including CPR basic life support (BLS), to enhance the likelihood of uniform guidelines worldwide[126, 720]. For advanced and prolonged life support (ALS, PLS) by health professionals, we refer to this book for international and the American Heart Association guidelines as an example of national guidelines[23b], realizing that each country and agency should feel free to modify 'what to teach to whom' of ALS and PLS, according to their local circumstances.

How to Teach and Test Resuscitation Skills
(Tables 15–20)

Teaching the lay public

For the life-saving steps which can be learned most readily by anyone (see Fig. 60; Table 15). *The need for mass training* has been pointed out by many investigators. The sooner resuscitation is started after ventilatory or circulatory arrest, the better the chances of survival[153, 216a, 223, 471, 472, 492]. Immediate initiation of life support measures, which is highly desirable, can in most cases be achieved only through action by bystanders. The late Asmund Laerdal worked from the 1950s on convincing the medical profession about the need to teach as many lay people and professionals as possible to become effective resuscitators[443, 444]. Ideally, the whole teachable population should be taught life supporting first aid (LSFA), which in our judgment should include CPR basic life support (BLS) without equipment (single operator technique with 2:15 ratio) (Table 14), because this would yield the highest feasible salvage rates. We have shown through education research since the 1950s that direct mouth-to-mouth ventilation and CPR Steps A–B–C[73, 74, 81, 107, 472, 967] can be taught effectively to the lay public— even to school children 10–11 years old. The life-saving potential of mouth-to-mouth ventilation[471] and CPR[153] by the lay public has been demonstrated, and it has also been shown that such teaching is effective[73, 74, 107, 234, 445, 472, 744, 967].

In the USA and some other countries, campaigns to teach CPR basic life support to the public have been in progress for some years, and have resulted in the training of millions of people. By 1985, in the USA, an estimated 30 million people had had some CPR instruction[23b, 443]. In recent years, school systems have also been involved. In the future, schools should play a fundamental role in the dissemination of first aid and CPR basic life support proficiency to the public at large. School age is excellent for learning the necessary knowledge and simple psychomotor skills. Teaching school children also allows for annual retraining. Education research has shown that frequent retraining is important for retaining performance capability[23b]. There are large differences between countries in their readiness to start mass training in first aid and CPR basic life support. In countries where such training has been started on a large scale, the following evolutionary stages have been recognized[443].

1. *Medical consensus.* Today there is scientific documentation of the desirability, feasibility and safety of teaching life supporting first aid and CPR basic life support without equipment to the entire teachable population (see above). Rejecting or discouraging such teaching is not justified anywhere.

2. *Guidelines.* Guidelines for teaching and practicing first aid and resuscitation can be drawn on a national level, or derived unmodified or modified

from another country or from an international organization that represents experts in resuscitation.

3. *Public awareness.* When the importance of first aid and resuscitation by bystanders is understood by the public at large, the general response is overwhelmingly positive to accept an active role in life-threatening emergencies. The news media have helped greatly in bringing about such an understanding. For example, a Gallup poll conducted in 1977 in the USA showed that 65% of the population had heard about CPR, 54% would like to take a CPR course, and 80% would like to make CPR training a requirement for all high school students.

4. *Implementation.* Programs for training and retraining of instructors and rescuers have evolved like the branches of a tree. We recommend that all school children be required to have annual training in life supporting first aid starting at age 11 and CPR basic life support without equipment starting at age 13. In the elderly or sick trainee, there can sometimes be problems[23b, 299]. Intelligent persons often effectively improvise[472]. Therefore *some* CPR exposure for all people will probably save more lives than perfection achieved by a few[78, 446, 447, 715, 744, 753, 967]. Repetitive film viewing[78, 753] improved test performance, although not as much as manikin practice. We recommend widespread CPR skill demonstrations via television[78, 446, 447], particularly in developing countries.

Implementation of training programs will depend on available training materials and methods and instructor-coordinators (organizers) (see below).

Teaching health care personnel (Table 15, Fig. 59)

All health care personnel, from first responders, such as police, firemen and lifeguards, up to physician specialists, should be trained in life supporting first aid and CPR Steps A–B–C (basic life support) without equipment[69]. In addition, each category of personnel should be trained in steps and measures that require use of equipment, to a level decided by designated description of ability, facilities and needs of that personnel group (Table 15). All practicing physicians, dentists and nurses, including hospital physician house staff and attending staff, should be required to demonstrate proficiency annually in CPR Steps A–B–C with simple equipment items used in the hospital; and ideally also in advanced cardiac life support (ACLS)[23] and advanced trauma life support (ATLS)[22b]. They can do so by participating in resuscitation efforts on patients, with prospective review, or by passing knowledge tests and skill tests on manikins, which may or may not be preceded by a training course.

In addition, physicians and nurses working in anesthesiology, emergency departments and intensive care units should be trained in some aspects of prolonged life support, including new cerebral resuscitation measures. CPR basic, advanced and prolonged life support should be included in the curricula of all health profession schools and hospitals[56, 57, 678]. Annual retraining is necessary unless the trainee is frequently involved in actual resuscitation cases. Physicians also need frequent retraining, even in basic life support[779]. Medical students should be trained in ALS.

Teaching methodology (Table 15, Fig. 59)

In emergency resuscitation, the acquisition of knowledge per se is less important than the acquisition of psychomotor *skills*. Knowledge as the basis for appropriate use of skills and of judgment is increasingly important in advanced and prolonged life support. We have in the 1960s and 1970s used knowledge tests to develop and document the teaching impact of certain manuals[126, 697, 720], books[736] and films[292, 304, 708]. Concerning acquisition of skills in the late 1950s, studies in Baltimore[700] demonstrated that lay persons could effectively perform mouth-to-mouth ventilation on anesthetized human volunteers after merely having watched a demonstration or seen pictures. The same seems to be the case for other life supporting first aid measures[744].

When the Laerdal Resusci-Anne manikin became available in 1960, it was shown first in Norway that practicing mouth-to-mouth breathing on manikins improved performance[471, 472]. In 1964, manikin practice was also found to improve correct performance rates and to reduce potentially injurious performance rates of nonphysicians after training in CPR basic life support without equipment[967].

Selected, motivated and qualified nonphysicians should receive *instructors' courses* in CPR basic life support without equipment; and selected physicians should receive instructors' courses in the use of equipment and in advanced life support. In some countries, in addition, selected nurses and paramedic instructors have also been trained to teach a variety of advanced life support measures. For the teaching of physicians and nurses in prolonged life support (intensive therapy, including cerebral resuscitation), hospital-based guided patient care experiences are required (Table 15).

Most CPR courses given by instructors are erroneously limited by time. Individualized learning of knowledge and skills to perfection (i.e. passing tests) is more important than course hours. Also, some traditional courses given by instructors focus on lengthy lectures with slides that fail to teach the necessary skills. Most important is skill practice on manikins and on one another, coached by the instructor until perfect performance is achieved.

Individuals who have already acquired some knowledge and skills in first aid and resuscitation should not be required to take lengthy courses, but rather should be tested to determine the level of knowledge and skills already acquired. Based on test results, remedial self-training and retesting in specific areas of deficit can be provided before certification.

Teaching methods for life support comprise the following three elements:

Table 15. Preferred training methods.

● should be taught
○ might be taught
— should not be taught

Phases	Steps	Measures	Manikins	Co-students	Anesth. patients	Human corpses	Lab animals	Supervised clinical experience
I BASIC LIFE SUPPORT—BLS (Emergency oxygenation)	Airway control	*Without equipment*						
		*Head-tilt	●	○	●	○	—	●
		*Supine aligned position	○	●	○	○	—	—
		*Stable side position	○	●	○	○	—	●
		*Triple airway maneuver (jaw-thrust)	●	○	●	○	—	○
		*Manual clearing of mouth and throat	●	○	○	○	—	—
		Back blows—manual thrusts	●	○	—	○	—	—
		With equipment						
		Pharyngeal suctioning	●	—	○	○	—	○
		Pharyngeal intubation	●	—	○	○	—	●
		Esophageal obturator airway insertion	●	—	○	○	—	○
		Endotracheal intubation	●	—	●	○	●	●
		Tracheobronchial suctioning	●	—	●	○	●	●
		Cricothyrotomy	○	—	—	○	●	—
		Translaryngeal O_2 jet insufflation	○	—	—	○	●	—
		Tracheotomy	—	—	—	○	●	●
		Bronchoscopy	●	—	—	○	●	●
		Bronchodilation	—	—	—	—	●	●
		Pleural drainage	—	—	—	○	●	●
	Breathing support	*Without equipment*						
		*Mouth-to-mouth (nose) ventilation	●	—	○	—	—	—
		Mouth-to-mouth hand-head position	●	●	○	—	—	—
		With equipment						
		Mouth-to-adjunct without O_2	●	—	○	—	—	○
		Mouth-to-adjunct with O_2	●	—	○	—	—	○
		Manual bag-mask (tube) O_2 ventilation	●	—	○	—	○	○
		Hand-triggered O_2 ventilation	●	—	○	—	○	○
		Mechanical ventilation	○	—	○	—	●	●

Table 15. *(cont.)*

● should be taught
○ might be taught
— should not be taught

Phases	Steps	Measures	Manikins	Co-students	Anesth. patients	Human corpses	Lab animals	Supervised clinical experience
BASIC LIFE SUPPORT—continued	Circulation support	*Without equipment*						
		*Control of ext. hemorrh.	○	●	—	—	—	○
		*Position for shock	○	●	○	—	—	—
		Pulse checking	●	●		—	—	
		Manual chest compressions						
		—single operator	●	—	—	○	○	●
		—two operators	●	—	—	○	○	●
		With equipment						
		Mechanical chest compression	●	—	—	○	○	○
		Open chest cardiac compression	—	—	—	—	●	○
		Pressure pants (MAST trousers)	○	○	—	—	—	●
II ADVANCED LIFE SUPPORT—ALS (Restoration of spontaneous circulation)	**Drugs and fluids**	i.v. lifeline peripheral	○	○	○	○	●	○
		central	—	—	○	—	●	○
	Electrocardiography	ECG monitoring	○	—	○	—	●	●
	Fibrillation treatment	Defibrillation	○	—	—	—	●	●
III PROLONGED LIFE SUPPORT—PLS (Cerebral resuscitation and post-resuscitation intensive therapy)	Gauging	Determine and treat cause of demise						
		Determine salvageability	—	—	—	—	—	
	Human mentation	Cerebral resuscitation	—	—	—	—	○	●
	Intensive care	Multiple organ support	—	—	○	—	○	●

* Life supporting first aid.

Based in part on education research supported by NIH contract HR 42965.

Verbal instruction

This conveys the knowledge items and provides the necessary guidance of skill practice. Clarity, accuracy and repetition are necessary. In the use of self-teaching systems, instruction can be by the coordinator or from an audiotape.

Visualization

Techniques and procedures can be visualized in the form of demonstrations, blackboard drawings, printed pictures or charts, projected slides, or films. Good skill-demonstration films are useful as supplements to illustrations, to show specific techniques, preferably in slow motion. Illustrations should be correct, simple to understand, and simple to show, preferably without projection equipment. Lay persons should have pocket cards (Fig. 60).

Practice

Skill practice is the most important aspect for learning first aid and resuscitation measures. Training manikins must be used for practicing lung ventilation, chest compressions and a number of other steps, whereas some other measures can be practiced effectively on live persons, anesthetized patients, and more rarely on human corpses and laboratory animals (Table 15).

Manikins (Fig. 58) should be as realistic as practically feasible to enhance motivation and physiologically correct learning. Each student should have enough time for manikin practice to reach perfection in performance. Ideally, there should be no more than 4–6 students per manikin for any given session. Supervised manikin practice to perfection allows guidance and evaluation by the instructor while the student is practicing.

Automatic feedback from manikins by way of light signals, dials or other indicators is desirable and is essential for self-training systems. Diagrammatic records of the student's performance give information that can be studied in detail by the student and provide the evaluator with exact, objective data. Recording manikins like the widely field-tested and used Laerdal recording Resusci-Anne manikin are extremely valuable[744, 967].

CPR manikins should simulate airway obstruction with flexion of the neck, and natural chest resistance to lung inflations and chest compressions; permit the performance of jaw thrust and application of face masks without leak; display the adequacy of ventilation and sternal compressions; and have a carotid pulse that can be made to appear and disappear. Arrhythmia manikins are used for defibrillation practice.

Conscious human volunteers have been used for selected aspects of first aid and resuscitation practice. Control of external hemorrhage (using stick-on moulages), body positioning and splinting are effectively practiced on one another. Exhaled air ventilation cannot be practiced properly on human volunteers, since their airway does not obstruct with flexion of the neck, and the volunteer resists inflation attempts. On the other hand, head-tilt, jaw-thrust, opening the mouth and finger probe (without deep insertion of the finger) can be demonstrated and practiced. Similarly, while sternal compressions should not be carried out on a conscious human subject, students can demonstrate on one another the exact point for application of pressure and the proper hand position.

Unconscious humans, i.e. anesthetized patients, may be used for practicing airway control, various methods of artificial ventilation, cannulation of vessels and monitoring of vital signs. All such activities, however, should be under the strictest control and direct personal supervision of a staff anesthesiologist who assumes the responsibility for possible injuries. Supervised practice on anesthetized patients, during the time spent with an anesthesia service, is the 'ultimate' method for the acquisition of knowledge, judgment and skills with basic and advanced life support measures (except for sternal compressions which should be practiced on manikins). It is difficult to acquire resuscitation skills under controlled conditions in intensive care units or during hospital-wide resuscitation attempts, as they should be carried out by personnel already skilled in these measures.

Human corpses have been used for practicing resuscitation. In some countries consent from relatives is required. Relaxed fresh corpses are ideal, but usually not available when needed, making training programs that include corpses difficult to organize. After rigor mortis has set in, corpses are not suitable for practicing resuscitation techniques other than insertion of an endotracheal tube and resuscitative surgical procedures.

Laboratory animals have been used effectively for the demonstration and practice of certain skills and decision making, such as electrocardiography, defibrillation, drug therapy, open-chest cardiac compressions, intubation, catheterization of vessels and mechanical ventilation. The open-chest and closed-chest cardiac resuscitation training programs in the 1950s in Baltimore (Safar and Redding) and Cleveland (Beck and Leighninger) included dog laboratory demonstration and practice sessions for physicians and medical students. These sessions proved particularly valuable for demonstrating various patterns of dying, and techniques for restoration of spontaneous circulation. The dog is not suitable, however, for practicing basic life support, because its airway does not reliably obstruct with flexion of the neck. Furthermore, mouth-to-mouth ventilation is not aesthetically or practically feasible on the dog. Sternal compressions can be practiced realistically, but only on (small) flat-chested dogs. The anterior/posterior diameter of the thorax in relation to its width is greater in most dogs than in humans.

The unavailability of animal laboratories in hospitals makes it necessary to practice certain steps of advanced life support on the less realistic arrhythmia manikins. These practice sessions should include detailed demonstration and handling of the equipment and supplies on resuscitation carts used in the local hospital.

Self-training systems (Fig. 59) have many advantages over traditional lectures and instructor-coached manikin practice. People learn at individual rates; therefore, training programs should allow for individualized learning to perfection. Self-training systems should encourage students to acquire knowledge from illustrated texts, or tape-recorded lectures, or both. Self-training systems have also proved effective for the acquisition of skills in life supporting first aid[81, 107, 234] and CPR basic life support[56, 73, 74, 81, 730, 744]. Even bathroom graffiti can be used to teach CPR-BLS[309b].

Well qualified life support instructors are usually scarce, and even the greatest enthusiasts may tire of the repetitive nature of this type of teaching.

Self-training systems require coordinators to organize and control the learning laboratories. A CPR instructor-coordinator, not necessarily one with training in education, should set up the self-training laboratory, trouble shoot, answer questions, test knowledge and skills, coach to perfect performance by remedial training, retest, certify and recertify periodically.

Teaching CPR Basic Life Support Without Equipment

In the 1970s the Laerdal self-training system, which consists of flip charts, audiotapes, printed guides, a recording adult manikin and an infant manikin, was modified and found to be as effective as instructor methods in teaching CPR basic life support to lay people[73, 74] and health care personnel[730, 744] (Fig. 59). This also proved to be the case for the Laerdal life supporting first aid self-training system[107, 234], the main item of which is a special manual. Manikin practice, however, improved mouth-to-mouth performance rates. The manikin is thus desirable for learning ventilation and essential for learning sternal compressions[56, 73, 74, 81, 107, 125, 471, 744, 967].

Mouth-to-mouth risks to trainee rescuers

Preventing disease transmission via manikins[23b, 132]

With recommended decontamination of manikins, the risk of acquiring a serious infectious disease (e.g. herpes, hepatitis, AIDS, tuberculosis) from a co-trainee via a mouth-to-mouth manikin is probably almost zero. An estimated 150 million persons have had manikin CPR practice worldwide. There has never been a documented case of manikin practice having been responsible for a bacterial, fungal or viral disease (reference 23b, page 2926).

Recommendations[23b] include the following (AHA):

1. Study manikin manufacturers' sanitary recommendations.

2. Students or instructors should refrain from practice if they have skin or oral lesions, have an infectious disease, or are known to be seropositive for hepatitis B.
3. Manikin care should be according to manufacturers' instructions.
4. Minimize two-rescuer practice where there is no opportunity to disinfect the manikin between students.
5. Practice finger sweep on separate decontaminated manikins.
6. Between practicing trainees, change face shield (which is not essential) and wipe and wet surfaces for at least 30 seconds with hypochlorite (above) or 70% alcohol.
7. Emphasize thorough physical cleaning (scrubbing, wiping and inside rinsing) between classes with soap, water and hypochlorite or alcohol.
8. After each class, use sodium hypochlorite 500 p.p.m. (one-quarter cup of liquid household bleach per gallon of tap water to wipe wet surfaces and rinse lower airways for 10 minutes.

The AIDS virus is inactivated in 10 minutes by alcohol or hypochlorite. AIDS is not transmitted by casual personal contact, by touching 'contaminated' inanimate surfaces, or via air.

In view of the very low risk of transmission of very infectious disease by manikin practice, 'the lifesaving potential of CPR and broad-scale CPR training should be continued and emphasized'.

Disease transmission from patients[23b]

No transmission of hepatitis B or AIDS through mouth-to-mouth breathing has been documented. Lay persons who resuscitate persons they know should have no reluctance to perform direct exhaled air ventilation.

There is a theoretical risk of salivary transmission of AIDS. Therefore, to minimize the risk, those who may resuscitate strangers should carry a saliva-filter 'handkerchief' (Laerdal) or a mouth-to-mouth adjunct (mask or airway) with a one-way valve, and in suspicious cases wear gloves.

Teaching CPR Basic Life Support with Equipment

Use of airways, masks, bags and equipment for oxygen administration, suctioning and tracheal intubation should be taught to health professionals. Each trainee should first study illustrated texts and demonstration films, and then come to suitable learning laboratories with manikins, pictures, audiotapes and the necessary equipment and supplies. Learning the use of oxygen equipment requires the presence of a coordinator to prevent accidents. For information on training materials, instructors should contact their local Red Cross and Heart Association, and appropriate manufacturers (e.g. Laerdal, Ambu).

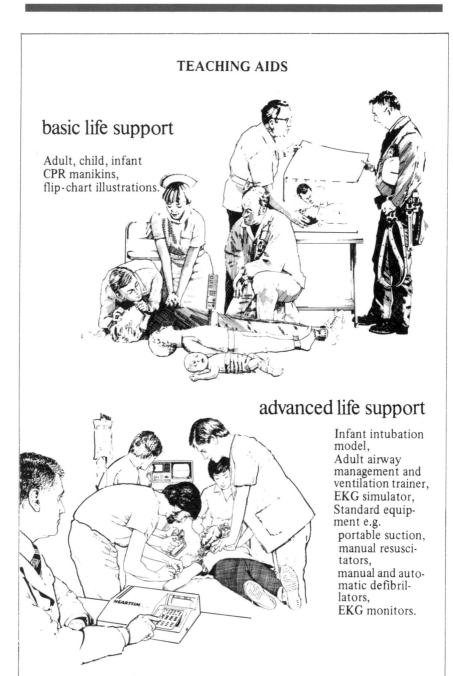

TEACHING AIDS

basic life support

Adult, child, infant
CPR manikins,
flip-chart illustrations.

advanced life support

Infant intubation
model,
Adult airway
management and
ventilation trainer,
EKG simulator,
Standard equip-
ment e.g.
  portable suction,
  manual resusci-
  tators,
  manual and auto-
  matic defibril-
  lators,
EKG monitors.

Fig. 59. Resuscitation teaching aids.

Teaching Proficiency in Endotracheal Intubation

Learning endotracheal intubation requires practice on manikins as well as on anesthetized patients. The use of human corpses and animals is optional. This author recommends the following training program:

1. Students should study an illustrated text (e.g. Chapter 1A of this manual) and then view a good intubation training film, e.g. *Endotracheal Intubation Manikin Practice*[814].

2. Ability to intubate realistic adult and infant manikins can be acquired through self-teaching or supervised practice. Not only correct tube placement, but also the correct sequence of steps and timing is necessary. Students should be able to intubate the trachea and start lung ventilation within 30 seconds.

3. Once the manikin intubation has been mastered, final training should follow, where feasible, as supervised practice on anesthetized patients under controlled conditions or field performance on patients in need of intubation, under 'hand-holding' supervision by the ambulance physician[860]. Supervised training of this type should continue until the instructor is convinced that the student clearly demonstrates ability to intubate without supervision.

Other methods for tracheal intubation skill practice include the use of monkeys and cats (which are useful for newborn intubation practice) and human corpses (Chapter 1A).

Teaching Advanced and Prolonged Life Support

Knowledge can be learned from well illustrated teaching texts. Skills of individual life support techniques can be learned from demonstration films, and supervised clinical experience of adequate duration. Practice of advanced life support measures in the learning laboratory should, if possible, include dysrhythmia recognition and the application of defibrillating electrodes on the arrhythmia manikin or other suitable training aid[23c, 131]. Training objectives, including types and numbers of exposures to clinical problems and performance of treatments, should be clearly defined. Advanced life support knowledge and skills should be tested.

Acquisition of knowledge and of judgment in clinical problem solving (e.g. which steps to use in what sequence for restoration of spontaneous circulation) can be enhanced by the use of written or computerized programmed instruction materials (algorithms). For the acquisition of advanced and prolonged life support skills, no completely effective self-training materials are available yet. There is no substitute for supervised clinical practice. For advanced and prolonged life support, including cerebral resuscitation, knowledge *can* be self-learned from teaching texts, without lectures[22, 23, 720, 736, 755d, 799], whereas skills and judgement should be acquired mainly from supervised clinical experience in anesthesiology and acute medicine. This learning can be initiated and enhanced by ACLS (AHA)[23] and ATLS (ACS)[22] self-training modules[56, 74, 744, 781]. Ideally these should be permanently set up in major emergency teaching hospitals. For ALS learning modules, new ALS manikins, arrhythmia trainers, and intubation manikins have been created by the Laerdal (Fig. 59) and Ambu companies. Automatic defibrillation should increasingly become an optional addition to BLS training[176, 219].

Testing (Tables 16–20)

Knowledge acquisition can be tested quite reliably with well designed written tests in the multiple choice format. Each question and answer pair should reflect the material actually taught in the program. *Criteria* for passing knowledge tests should be established as correct answers to a minimum number of all questions and all of a few key questions.

Psychomotor skills can be tested reliably during performances that simulate resuscitation attempts, either on manikins (e.g. CPR basic life support; endotracheal intubation) or on human volunteers (e.g. head-tilt, jaw-thrust, hand positions, hemorrhage control, body positioning). For skills not practiced on or recorded by the manikin, appropriate checklists should be used (Tables 16–20).

The *criteria for passing* skill performance tests should be established on the basis of physiologic requirements for successful resuscitation and practical considerations, which may call for more lenient criteria to be applied in the testing of lay personnel and more stringent criteria in the testing of health care personnel[23b, 73, 74, 736, 967]. For skill testing and certifying copy Tables 16–20.

For the training of millions in life supporting first aid, testing and certifying is impractical and probably not necessary. However, testing for CPR basic life support without equipment is desirable, because of the possibility of causing harm with sternal compressions when they are not needed. Testing of knowledge and skills in the use of equipment and in advanced and prolonged life support is recommended before certification.

Certification of students in life supporting first aid for the completion of a training program (without obligatory tests) is desirable. Certification in CPCR should be for the successful completion of defined knowledge and skill tests. Resuscitators and instructor-coordinators should be certified separately for CPR basic, advanced and prolonged life support (Tables 16–20).

Table 16. Skill test on *adult* manikin: checklist and passing criteria for CPR basic life support without equipment on adults (adapted from American Heart Association).

Student's name   Date   Evaluator's name

☐ Passed   ☐ Failed

INITIAL PHASE

Measures	Technique	Time
☑ Check if correct sequence	☑ Check if correct performance	☑ Check if within correct time lapse min.–max.
1 ☐ Establishing unresponsiveness	☐ Shake ☐ Shout: ☐ Call <help> ☐ Turn patient onto back if found in other position	seconds ☐ 3–5 ☐ 3–5
2 ☐ Opening airway	☐ Head tilt-chin support	☐ 3–5
☐ Establishing breathlessness	☐ Keep ear over mouth and nose and observe chest (look–listen–feel)	
3 ☐ Providing initial inflations	☐ Two times to make chest rise	☐ 4–8
4 ☐ Establishing pulselessness	☐ Palpation of the carotid pulse on near side. Maintain head tilt	☐ 5–10
☐ Activating EMS system	☐ Knows EMS phone No.	
5 ☐ Providing one-rescuer ventilation–compression	☐ Four full cycles providing a total of 60 compressions and 8 ventilations ☐ Proper rescuer posture ☐ Landmark checking each time ☐ Proper hand position ☐ Proper compression depth (4–5 cm) ☐ No bouncing. 50/50 compr./relax. ☐ Proper compressions minute rate (80–100) ☐ Adequate ventilation volume (0.8 l) ☐ Proper ratio vent: compression (2:15)	☐ 50–90
6 ☐ Checking return of spontaneous pulse and breathing	☐ Feel for carotid pulse ☐ Check for breathing	☐ 5–10

CONSECUTIVE PHASE

Pass criteria: (A variation of ± 10% is permissible).

A single rescuer proceeds as above and should perform at least 12 adequate ventilations and 60 correct compressions during initial 100 seconds.

When a *second rescuer* becomes available, two rescuer performance should provide 12 ventilations and 60 compressions per minute. One ventilation should be alternated with each five compressions.

Takeover and switching of two rescuers should be as described in Chapter 2C.

Table 17. Skill test on *infant* manikin: checklist and passing criteria for CPR basic life support without equipment on infants (adapted from American Heart Association).

Student's name   Date   Evaluator's name

☐ Passed   ☐ Failed

INITIAL PHASE

Measures	Technique	Time
☑ Check if correct sequence	☑ Check if correct performance	☑ Check if within correct time lapse min.-max.
1 ☐ Establishing unresponsiveness	☐ Shake shoulder gently ☐ Shout ☐ Call <help> ☐ Turn if necessary	seconds ☐ 3–5
2 ☐ Opening airway ☐ Establishing breathlessness	☐ Moderate head tilt ☐ Keep ear over mouth and nose and observe chest (look–listen–feel)	☐ 3–5
3 ☐ Providing initial inflations	☐ Ventilate twice to make chest rise	☐ 4–8
4 ☐ Establishing pulselessness	☐ Palpation of the brachial or femoral pulse on near side	☐ 5–10
☐ Activating EMS system	☐ Knows EMS phone No.	
5 ☐ Providing one-rescuer ventilation-compression	☐ Ten full cycles providing a total of 10 ventilations and 50 compressions ☐ Proper finger position just below midsternum ☐ Proper compression depth (1–2 cm) ☐ Proper compression rate/min (> 100) ☐ Proper ratio alternated compression: ventilation (5:1)	☐ 30–60
6 ☐ Checking return of spontaneous pulse and breathing	☐ Feel for brachial or femoral pulse ☐ Check for breathing	☐ 5–10

CONSECUTIVE PHASE

Pass criteria: (A variation of ± 10% is permissible).

The rescuer should during the initial 60 seconds provide at least 45 compressions and 12 ventilations.

Table 18. Skill test on adult manikin: checklist and passing criteria for CPR Steps A–B–C with *equipment* (RRC, Univ. Pittsburgh).

Student's name	Date	Evaluator's name

☐ Passed

☐ Failed

Measures	Technique	Time
	☑ Check if correct performance	☑ Check if within correct time lapse
Suctioning (CPR recording manikin)	☐ Assembled and tested correctly suctioning equipment ☐ Demonstrated correct oropharyngeal suctioning	seconds ☐ < 45
Pharyngeal intubation (adult intubation manikin)	☐ Inserted correctly oropharyngeal airway ☐ Inserted correctly nasopharyngeal airway	☐ < 15 ☐ < 15
O$_2$ delivery system (connect to ventilation devices below)	☐ Tightened cylinder yoke before opening valve ☐ Established correct connections to the 3 ventilation devices below ☐ Provided O$_2$ flow of 5–15 l/min to mask and bag	
Ventilation devices (CPR recording manikin)	☐ Mouth-to-mouth pocket mask Ventilated with at least three tidal volumes of 0.8 l ☐ Bag–valve–mask Ventilated with at least three tidal volumes of 0.8 l ☐ Manually triggered O$_2$ ventilator Ventilated with at least three tidal volumes of 0.8 l	☐ < 30 ☐ < 30 ☐ < 30

Table 19. Skill test on *intubation* manikins: checklist and passing criteria for endotracheal intubation manikin tests (RRC, Univ. Pittsburgh).

Student's name	Date	Evaluator's name

☐ Passed

☐ Failed

Measures	Technique	Time
	☑ Check if correct performance	☑ Check if within correct time lapse
Endotracheal intubation of *adult* manikin	☐ Checked laryngoscope light before use ☐ Checked tube patency before use ☐ Held laryngoscope correctly ☐ Used no grossly traumatic maneuver during intubation attempt ☐ Inserted tube into trachea rapidly ...... ☐ < 30 ☐ Gave first lung inflation rapidly via tube by bag–valve or mouth ...... ☐ < 60 ☐ Inflated cuff of tube correctly (with helper) ☐ Used bite-block, secured tube and connected ventilation device correctly ☐ Checked to rule out bronchial intubation	seconds
Endotracheal intubation of *infant* manikin	☐ Checked laryngoscope light before use ☐ Checked tube patency before use ☐ Held laryngoscope correctly ☐ Used no grossly traumatic maneuver during intubation attempt ☐ Inserted tube into trachea rapidly ...... ☐ < 30 ☐ Gave first lung inflation rapidly via tube (by mouth) .... ☐ < 60 ☐ Used bite-block, secured tube and connected ventilation device correctly ☐ Checked to rule out bronchial intubation	
Endotracheal suctioning (curved-tipped catheter)	☐ Used correct technique to suction each lung separately .... ☐ < 60	

Table 20. Skill test with *advanced life support* materials: checklist and passing criteria for miscellaneous advanced life support measures (RRC, Univ. Pittsburgh).

Student's name	Date	Evaluator's name

☐ Passed

☐ Failed

Measures	Technique	Time
	☑ Check if correct performance	☑ Check if within correct time lapse
Venous infusion	☐ Correctly assembled intravenous infusion and cannulation equipment	
	☐ Correctly described sites and techniques of peripheral vein cannulation	
	☐ Correctly described sites and techniques of central vein cannulation	
Drugs	☐ Correctly prepared single-dose i.v. injection of lidocaine for PVCs (pt. with pulse)	
	☐ Correctly prepared single-dose i.v. injection of epinephrine (pt. with cardiac arrest)	
	☐ Correctly prepared single-dose i.v. injection of bicarbonate (first 'blind' dose for patient with cardiac arrest)	
ECG recognition	☐ Correctly applied peripheral ECG electrodes	
(arrhythmia manikin)	☐ Correctly applied chest defibrillator-ECG monitor electrodes	
	☐ Recognized *lethal* ECG patterns (VF, VT, electric asystole, electromechanical dissociation)	☐ 15 seconds each
	Recognized *life-threatening* ECG patterns	☐ 15 seconds each
	☐ Regular sinus rhythm with multifocal PVCs	
	☐ Second degree heart block	
	☐ Third degree heart block	
Defibrillation	☐ Charged defibrillator with 200–360 J	
(arrhythmia manikin, hospital crash cart)	☐ Placed two defibrillating chest electrodes with saline pads correctly	☐ < 60 seconds
	☐ Checked for VF before countershock.	
	☐ Discharged defibrillator and kept paddles on chest to check ECG. Ordered 'hands off' before shock	
	☐ Checked pulse and continued CPR according to ECG rhythm displayed by examiner	

Chapter 6

Organization

Hospital-Wide Organization[22, 23, 227, 730]

CPCR services inside hospitals that should be in readiness 24 hours per day include: (1) basic, advanced and prolonged (cardiac and trauma) life support capability in the emergency department, ICUs and other special care units, provided by personnel of these units; (2) a hospital-wide resuscitation team which responds within seconds to calls from anywhere in the hospital, including critical care units when their staffs need help; (3) a mechanism for preventing cardiac arrest by providing life support in myocardial ischemia and infarction, in cases not requiring resuscitation (dysrhythmia recognition and control); and (4) capability to respond in a well coordinated fashion to both internal and external disasters (see below).

Every acute care hospital should have a specific multidisciplinary committee with responsibility for providing CPR services 24 hours per day and for ensuring high standards of resuscitation and intensive therapy. This committee should include at least an anesthesiologist, a cardiologist, a surgeon-traumatologist, a nurse, an administrator, and physicians representing the emergency department and ICUs. The committee should be responsible for providing: (1) written treatment protocols; (2) training and practice sessions in CPCR; (3) training in intensive therapy; and (4) periodic review of records of resuscitation attempts, with identification of mistakes and feedback to the medical personnel involved, to minimize chances of similar mistakes in the future. A separate, similar committee should address disaster preparedness.

Every general hospital with acute care facilities should provide an advanced life support unit (see below) in its emergency department, so that any patient who has symptoms suggestive of myocardial infarction or other cardiopulmonary emergency will be placed immediately on monitoring and surveillance, until a definite decision is made regarding his care. If there is a strong suspicion that the patient has had an acute myocardial infarction he/she should be transferred to the coronary care unit or ICU. During transfer the patient should be connected to a battery-operated monitor-defibrillator. If necessary, appropriate drugs should be administered en route.

Organization and mobilization of hospital personnel for CPCR calls will depend on local circumstances. One (usually chaotic) method is a *general response*, i.e. to have all physicians and nurses who hear the alert respond to it. The physician present who is most experienced in resuscitation (which is often difficult to determine or agree upon after the start of resuscitation) should take charge, since lack of team leadership is the most common cause of ineffective, incompetently carried out CPCR efforts. The team leader must define the responsibilities of those personnel who are needed and dismiss those who are not. The presence of too many medical personnel at a resuscitation can be as detrimental to the patient's care as the presence of too few.

A better plan is a *designated team response*. In this system, the committee appoints in advance team leaders to share 24 hour coverage hospital-wide, who must exercise decisive team leadership. In large hospitals with 24 hour coverage by physicians of various disciplines, members of one discipline can be chosen on the basis of their experience and availability to assume the role of team leader. This avoids the confusion which occurs at the scene when one discipline is not clearly in charge. Another approach is to select team leaders on the basis of overall expertise with CPCR rather than specialty affiliation. Team leaders should be beyond the junior house officer training status. The team (including the team leader) is usually composed of an anesthesiologist, internist (e.g. cardiologist) and surgeon (traumatologist); a resuscitation cart technician, respiratory therapist or paramedic; and at least two nurses from the arrest location. One potential problem with the designated team leader approach is variability in training and experience of house staff of various departments serving on the resuscitation team.

In emergency rooms and ICUs, team function occurs automatically, as most members are working together most of the time. Lack of skilled, knowledgeable team leadership (because of departmental territorialism), delegation of CPR efforts to inexperienced house staff, and noninvolvement of resuscitation-skilled anesthesiologists outside operating rooms have since the early 1960s led to a deterioration of the quality of CPR efforts in many hospitals, particularly outside of special care units. This trend must be reversed.

The hospital resuscitation team should be capable of performing all phases of CPCR basic and advanced life support with and without equipment. We recommend that the hospital's CPCR and trauma teams be combined. An advanced trauma life support (ATLS) team should include an internist and must also be competent in emergency cardiac care.

One method of team function is as follows. The person recognizing the emergency starts resuscitation and calls for a helper, who in turn calls the telephone operator by a pre-arranged alert number that overrides all other calls. The telephone operator pages the team by an emergency code and gives the location. This is essential to avoid delay caused by calling back for the location. The team members respond to the alert and rush to the scene. The team leader takes over ventilation or checks the adequacy of ventilation started by another person and monitors the effectiveness of chest compressions. The resuscitation cart technician who has brought the cart to the scene prepares the defibrillation ECG monitoring paddles and as soon as possible attaches the ECG limb electrodes. One nurse assists with i.v. infusions and draws up medications. The second nurse keeps records. The team leader reads the ECG, determines drug therapy and applies counter-shocks as needed, and if help is scarce inserts i.v. cannulae or performs a cut-down. Intubation should be attempted by a staff member who is skilled in the technique and who can perform it quickly. Special nurses, particularly those assigned to the emergency department and ICUs, should be trained and authorized to defibrillate and give special drugs, as preordered.

The patient should be transported from the scene of the resuscitation to the ICU only after stabilization. The traumatized patient in the emergency room should have life support ongoing, but if necessary be rushed to the operating room without waiting for stabilization, which may not be possible without resuscitative surgery. The person who initiates emergency resuscitation must ensure that the patient receives post-resuscitative intensive care. If complex post-resuscitative intensive care (e.g. brain resuscitation) is indicated, hospitals without this expertise available should seek advice by phone rather than transfer patients from one hospital to another at a time when every minute of sophisticated life support counts. Hospital ICU organization[735, 799, 828a] and ICU physician education guide-lines[717, 727, 735, 747, 799, 828b] are beyond the scope of this book.

Community-Wide Organization
(Table 21)[10, 26, 55, 216, 254, 730, 747, 1000]

CPCR capability must be part of all components of the emergency medical services (EMS) delivery system (Table 21)[26, 254, 730, 735, 747, 783]. This makes it an 'Emergency and Critical Care Medicine' (ECCM) delivery system—the implementation of 'resuscitology'[579, 746]. Such an ECCM system is only as good as its weakest component. A continuum of life-support from scene through ICU is essential[26, 497, 715, 747]. Knowledgeable, authoritative coordination of all role players and agencies involved in the EMS system, with physician leadership, is essential. Such coordination can be accomplished either through the voluntary approach via EMS (ECCM) community councils, which have evolved in the USA since 1968[26], or through local or regional governmental authority, as in many European countries[254].

Each regional system must be coordinated by an *emergency medical operations and communications center* (EMOC), staffed by experienced dispatchers who are ECCM-physicians or physician-guided paramedics or nurses. The function of such an EMOC is to appraise and respond to everyday medical emergencies, as well as disasters, by mobilizing resources outside hospitals and controlling the flow of patients to hospitals. The center, all ambulance and rescue vehicles (including helicopters), and all emergency hospitals should be linked by both special telephone lines and two-way radio-telephones. The center should be staffed by personnel capable of identifying the need for basic or advanced life support ambulances, fire department, police or rescue services, and be empowered in each case to select ambulance services and hospitals according to the needs of the patients.

The graded response of community-wide life support should start with the *lay public* being given instructions in life supporting first aid (LSFA) and CPR basic life support. This alone could save thousands of lives in many countries each year[73, 74, 81, 107, 177, 356, 492, 573, 670, 744, 967]. A single public access *telephone number* must be available to reach the EMS dispatching center (EMOC). An intriguing idea is to coach the caller by telephone how to initiate life support[59].

Ambulances[10, 21–23, 125, 254, 723, 730]

Ideally, all emergency ambulances, irrespective of staffing, should be *designed*, *equipped* and *supplied* for basic and advanced cardiac and trauma life support, according to (national) standards (mobile ICUs)[21, 23b, 723]. Even if *staffed* only by basic life support personnel, the advanced equipment should be available for doctors to use. All ambulances should be staffed for at least basic life support capability by specially trained emergency medical technicians (EMTs, EMT 1s) (basic ambulance personnel)[177, 723, 905]. A selected number of these ambulances (sufficient for 24 hour coverage of the community) should be staffed and equipped for advanced life support capability by paramedics (EMT IIs) (advanced ambulance personnel; mobile ICUs). EMTs and paramedics should follow standing treatment protocols and be guided by emergency physicians via radio; this is the prevalent pattern in the USA[125a]. In many other countries, physician-staffed ambulances are prevalent[254]; these are theoretically the ideal, if affordable, and if the physicians riding ambulances are experienced with resuscitation in the field. The advantage of physician-staffed over paramedic-staffed systems in terms of patient outcome has not been documented.

Prehospital advanced life support was pioneered in the early 1960s by physician-staffed ambulances in Czechoslovakia[784], the Soviet Union[862], Germany[10, 196, 204, 254, 255] and Ireland[611]. In the USA these services have evolved later as mobile ICUs[69a, 723] staffed by specially trained paramedics, who should be guided by physicians[69, 124–127, 153, 569, 723].

When trained lay bystanders start CPR at the scene within 4 minutes of cardiac arrest, and advanced life support ambulance personnel subsequently restart spontaneous circulation before reaching the hospital, hospital discharge of over 40% has been achieved among victims of prehospital sudden cardiac death[153, 492]. In addition, experiences in recent wars have shown that with control of hemorrhage at the scene and rapid transportation to an advanced life support surgical facility, if necessary by aircraft, mortality is measurably reduced among victims of severe trauma[908]. Therefore, ideally, each community should provide basic life support outside hospitals within 3–4 minutes, and advanced life support within 10 minutes in urban and 30 minutes in rural areas. Realistically, however, it is recognized that this goal cannot be reached in many regions of the world.

When there are basic life support ambulance personnel only, salvage rates for cardiac arrest victims have been disappointing[966]. Selected ambulances should be upgraded to advanced life support capability. An intermediate EMT I with defibrillation capability offers advantages[217, 797, 869]. Automatic defibrillation by laymen looks promising[176].

Advanced cardiac and trauma life support (ALS, ATLS) is part of the practice of medicine, even if practiced outside the hospital. ACLS-ATLS capability, however, can be achieved even by trained paramedics with little previous education, and by trained part-time practicing volunteer paramedics, provided there is strong direction by physicians[69c, 125a]. Training of ALS personnel should include standing orders and treatment protocols based on national standards[124–127]. All nonphysicians giving ALS in the field should be in radio contact with guiding ECCM physicians[124–127]. Paramedics who staff mobile ICUs should be thoroughly trained by physicians in advanced life support, and deliver treatments according to their training and standing orders for which the service's physician director is responsible. These standing orders should be modified by physician guidance via radio as needed. The degree to which paramedics should be permitted to act on their own in resuscitation cases depends on their competence and that of the physician giving the radio command[55, 125a, 569].

The physician director who is knowledgeable and skilled in the management of basic and advanced CPR should assume the medical responsibility for each basic and advanced life support ambulance service. These responsibilities include control of the quality of patient care and directly or remotely supervising the activities of paramedics[125]. Paramedics must be familiar with the use of voice and ECG telemetry equipment for advanced cardiac care[569]. (ECG telemetry, after use in a transitional time period, has been given up by most ambulance services.) Special continuing education programs for all life support unit staff are required. Nonphysician staff (paramedics and nurses) of fixed ALS units (see below) must have constant access to radio communication with the physician director, for example the one staffing the emergency medical operations center. Direction of advanced emergency cardiac care by paramedics and nurses in the field can be enhanced by the optional use of ECG telemetry. The medical director should establish a sound referral policy to have patients delivered to the most appropriate, not necessarily the nearest, hospital.

Medical control over a community's EMS system, including *pre-hospital* emergency care, both basic and advanced, requires the authority of a specifically assigned physician (medical director), who should be responsible for medical care provided by all personnel in the system[571]. This physician must take responsibility for training, certification, approval of medical equipment and supplies, approval of treatment protocols, and maintenance of quality control, which includes ongoing case reviews. Prehospital ALS must be carried out by physicians or be under the continuing direction of physicians who are experienced in emergency and resuscitative care. Physicians giving radio command should adhere as much as possible to agreed treatment protocols, to provide some uniformity in the delivery of care, which will improve the standard of overall care[125].

When the call suggests respiratory distress, unconsciousness, pulselessness, severe trauma or suspicion of heart attack, a mobile ICU should be dispatched. In some communities (e.g. Los Angeles) a two-stage response has proved practical, i.e. all calls are answered by ambulances providing basic life support only; in cases possibly requiring advanced life support, a paramedics' vehicle or a physician with special equipment in his car arrives at the scene separately; the basic life support ambulance is then used for transporting the patient to the hospital, accompanied by the physician. We rather recommend a system in which the EMOC dispatcher sends mobile ICUs with paramedics to the scene when the call suggests the possibility of an acutely life-threatening critical condition; in addition, the EMOC emergency physician director or his designate goes to the scene in the hospital-based MICU or by separate car, but only if necessary.

The use of physician-staffed *helicopter* ambulances, pioneered in Europe[254], has been on the increase in recent years, for the transport of acutely critically ill and injured patients from the scene (Maryland) of the accident, from isolated or otherwise inaccessible sites (Swiss), and from smaller hospitals to major emergency hospitals (Pittsburgh). A heliport should be established at every major emergency hospital, close enough to the emergency department to obviate the need for transfer between helicopter and special care unit by ambulance. Helicopter ambulances and fixed-wing aircraft for patient transport should have the same equipment as recommended for mobile ICU-type ambulances. For transport of critical cases, they should be staffed by paramedics, ICU-ED nurses or emergency physicians.

A comment on priorities based on cost, patient outcome data and common sense[602, 909]: A community which now provides advanced *hospital* care (e.g. cardiac, neurologic and/or transplant surgery, ICUs, CCUs), but does *not* provide *prehospital* defibrillation, medication, intubation and infusion capability, should correct this deficiency. If not, it can legitimately be blamed for 'putting the cart before the horse'. In third world countries, EMS developments must be adapted to economic realities[961].

Hospitals[22, 23, 26, 164, 730]

Life-threatening emergencies, particularly resuscitation cases, should be taken to the nearest hospital that has comprehensive emergency facilities.

These major emergency hospitals, which should also function as 'trauma centers', should be established on a regional basis. They should be staffed around the clock by teams of specialists available within minutes and should conform to the highest standards attainable within the community. Unless the patient is beginning to wake up at the scene or during transportation, it is desirable to transfer resuscitation cases to advanced hospital ICUs. Patients suspected of myocardial infarction should be admitted to the nearest hospital that can provide emergency cardiac care.

The ECCM capability of a hospital should be made known to the medical community and the public by designating the hospital as (1) a major (advanced) emergency hospital-trauma center, (2) an emergency hospital, or (3) a basic emergency facility (with advanced life support stations but not long-term intensive therapy required), or using some similar categorization. A category (2) hospital should have an ICU with basic intensive medical care, i.e. full-time staffing with specially trained nurses, a (part-time) ICU physician director and coverage by physicians from outside the ICU. A category (1) hospital, usually a 'tertiary referral facility', should receive directly from the field, cases of multitrauma and other major life-threatening emergencies with multiple organ failure. The category (1) hospital should have an advanced emergency department, operating room and ICUs (staffed by physician specialists), and be staffed around the clock with full-time physicians in-house, who are trained or in training in emergency medicine, critical care medicine (intensive care medicine) and traumatology (but not novices).

Advanced Life Support Units[23b]

Advanced life support (ALS) units (resuscitation units) may be: (1) *hospital-based* in emergency departments, ICUs or coronary care units; or (2) *outside hospitals*, as (a) *stationary* units ('life support station') in special locations such as airports or (b) *mobile* units in form of special ambulances (mobile ICUs). Widespread basic life support capability of trained members of the lay public and first responders (e.g. policemen, firemen, lifeguards) should sustain life while calling and waiting for a mobile ICU or transporting the patient to a fixed advanced life support unit.

All these units must be capable of providing basic and advanced life support (Fig. 2, Table 1), including the use of equipment, for a variety of emergencies ranging from severe trauma to sudden cardiac arrest, for infants, children and adults. The stationary unit should be located in airports, railroad stations, sport arenas, convention centers, stadiums, civic auditoriums, industrial plants, large office building complexes, and other areas with large in-transit populations. Mobile ICU ambulances staffed by paramedics can be used as stationary life support units parked temporarily at a special event.

These life support units should be able to provide advanced life support by: (1) identifying patients with cardiopulmonary emergencies; (2) administering oxygen, instituting immediate monitoring, and establishing an i.v. infusion prior to obtaining a detailed history; (3) providing continued surveillance until a professional decision on management is made; (4) stabilizing the patient's condition prior to transfer to the hospital; and (5) following guidelines on referrals, record keeping and communication[23b].

Advanced life support units should be accessible, clearly marked and staffed at all times by a team including at least two persons trained in advanced life support, one being a physician if possible. In the absence of a physician, the nonphysician personnel should be linked by two-way radio communication with a physician familiar with the unit and its standing orders. Each ALS unit must have an established referral policy (transfer agreement) to bring the patient to the most appropriate hospital, with life support continued during transportation.

The equipment, drugs and records required for ALS are basically similar, whether that life support is carried out within the hospital, in a fixed ALS station or in a mobile ICU. Personnel working in mobile ALS units, however, require additional training, since the special constraints of the work necessitate expertise in communications, ECG telemetry, rescue, extrication, emergency driving, security, local geography, crowd control and mass casualty management. Furthermore, *physicians guiding mobile ICU personnel should themselves have first-hand experience in providing advanced life support on the streets and in the field*[10, 124–127, 256, 723].

Equipment: advanced life support stations

The equipment and supplies for hospital-based, stationary and mobile ALS units should at least include basic ingredients of a hospital resuscitation cart. For intrahospital units, such carts should be provided in strategic locations, such as the emergency department, ICU, coronary care unit, operating suite, recovery room, X-ray department, cardiac catheterization laboratory, etc., and at least one cart should be mobile for hospital-wide use. Each hospital nursing station or floor should have this equipment available for use within 1–2 minutes. Ideally, not only mobile ICU ambulances but also ambulances staffed by basic life support personnel should carry ALS equipment, in case physicians or paramedics come to the scene and need it.

Equipment for fixed and mobile life support stations

1. *Equipment for CPR Steps A and B* (Chapters 1A and 1B)
Oropharyngeal and nasopharyngeal airways of all sizes (S-tubes optional)
Suction equipment

Tracheal intubation equipment; nasogastric tubes
Cricothyrotome
Translaryngeal oxygen jet insufflation set (optional)
Mouth-to-mouth pocket mask with oxygen nipple
Bag–valve–mask unit with oxygen reservoir and PEEP valve
Oxygen supply, at least in the form of two small (size E) cylinders with
  reducing valve and delivery tube, capable of supplying at least 15
  liters of oxygen per minute

2. *Equipment for CPR Step C and advanced life support* (Chapters 1C
  and 2)
Backboard for CPR; folded towels
Battery-powered (portable, direct current) defibrillator with ECG
  monitor oscilloscope, external defibrillator paddles and ECG elec-
  trodes incorporated; ECG stick-on electrodes; sterile internal
  defibrillator paddles for adults and children
Portable ECG recorder (optional) with chest leads for refined ECG
  diagnosis to be connected to the defibrillator monitor
Thoracotomy set for open-chest CPR
Long needles for pericardial and spinal taps
Sterile gloves
Blood pressure cuff and stethoscope
Venous tourniquets
Bladder catheterization set
i.v. infusion sets with normal and micro-drips, including catheter-
  inside and catheter-outside needles (plastic cannulae) sizes 14 to 22
  gauge (including long CVP catheters and CVP manometer);
  infusion stopcocks; extension tubes; swabs; tapes; scissors
Intravenous *solutions* in plastic bags, including:
(a) 5% dextrose in water
(b) lactated Ringer's, isotonic NaCl solution, or balanced isotonic salt
  solution with normal pH
(c) 5% dextrose in 0.45% sodium chloride solution
(d) a colloid solution, such as dextran 40, dextran 70, hydroxyethyl
  starch, 5% albumin in saline, plasma protein fraction or polygelatin (Hemaccel)
  (If only one solution is possible, use Ringer's.)
For the administration of drugs, an assortment of syringes and needles
For basic *trauma* life support (LSFA), sterile dressings and pressure
  bandages, scissors, tapes, sheets and blankets
For EMT *trauma* life support, cervical collar with sand bags, spine
  board (long and short), air splints, femur traction splint
For advanced *trauma* life support (ATLS), a MAST (pressure suit),
  pleural (thoracocentesis) drainage set, pericardiocentesis set, peritoneal lavage set, tracheotomy set

3. *Recommended Drugs* (Chapter 2)
epinephrine
sodium bicarbonate
norepinephrine, dopamine and dobutamine
a vasodilator (e.g. nitroprusside or nitroglycerin)
thiopental or pentobarbital; diazepam
succinylcholine
pancuronium
lidocaine
procainamide
bretylium
atropine
diphenylhydantoin
methylprednisolone or dexamethasone
furosemide or ethracrynic acid
mannitol
morphine
digoxin
verapamil or diltiazem; nimodipine or lidoflazine
calcium chloride
dextrose 20%
isoproterenol
aminophylline
metaproterenol aerosol
diphenhydramine
naloxone (Narcan)
other drugs, depending on personal preference
Prefilled syringes ready for injection are desirable. Individual-dose
vials are preferred over multiple-dose vials.

Legal Considerations[1, 23, 67, 524]

Medico-legal recommendations concerning CPR remain in flux, since the
law is often established by precedents set by lawsuits after injury, and
therefore follows rather than precedes events occurring in practice. Laws
vary greatly among states and countries. CPCR practitioners, teachers and
organizers should familiarize themselves with existing laws relevant to
resuscitation in their own jurisdiction, such as the Medical Practice Act, the
Good Samaritan Act, the definition of death, and 'living will' laws. The
views presented here are mostly those of the American Heart Association
CPR Committee legal advisers.

Fear of the law is unjustified. In the USA recovery of damages against a
physician cannot be based on an undesirable outcome alone; there must also

be proof that the physician acted negligently, and that the negligence was the cause of the patient's injury. There have, however, been many lawsuits won by patients' relatives when a hospital staff's failure to attempt resuscitation led to injury or death.

Legal advisors state that standards and guidelines for CPR are not intended to limit or inhibit persons inside or outside hospitals from providing emergency medical treatment. Since it may be unrealistic to expect immediate compliance with these standards in some circumstances, a reasonable time for implementation should be allowed. For legal considerations of initiation and termination of resuscitation efforts and orders not to resuscitate, see Chapter 3.

State laws should clarify what nonphysician health care personnel can and should do; clarify the medical practice act accordingly; give immunity (for acts in good faith and not involving gross negligence or wilful, wanton or reckless misconduct) for those certified in basic or advanced life support; make training and certification in CPR a job requirement for key health care personnel; and prevent law enforcement officers from interfering with resuscitation efforts by qualified persons. Ideally, hospitals should establish regulations to restrict hospital physician staff privileges to those who have shown the ability to render basic life support.

In most jurisdictions, there are several general laws relevant to the provision of emergency life support measures. The doctrine of *res ipsa loquitur* (the thing speaks for itself) can be explained by the example of a cardiac arrest in the operating room in which it might be assumed that negligence occurred, and that the professional must prove that negligence did not occur. The 'Good Samaritan Law' in force in most of the United States and other countries is meant to protect medical and paramedical persons from civil liability when, acting in good faith, they attempt to resuscitate a person. This includes the physician who renders help at the scene outside the hospital or walks into a hospital and is suddenly called upon to help. 'Informed consent' applies to surgical and other therapeutic procedures that may result in cardiac arrest or indeed in any untoward and undesirable result. Although it is impossible to state specifically what 'informed consent' should include, in general a physician should explain to a patient the reasonably available therapeutic options, and the risks and benefits of each. In general, there is no substitute for good communication between physician and patient or, if the patient is unconscious, his relatives. Informed consent cannot be obtained in resuscitation cases when the patient is unconscious, the relatives are not available or are in emotional shock, and special (often innovative) operative or otherwise invasive treatments are needed immediately in order to be effective. For these situations the 'emergency exception' for informed consent applies. This exception should (but in the USA does not yet) apply also to well designed and peer-reviewed clinical resuscitation research protocols[1a, b].

Hospitals and ambulance services must live up to the standards of care and practice. Although health care professionals used to be held only to prevailing community standards, there has been a strong shift in recent years toward holding them to national professional standards. If a hospital or ambulance service lacks appropriate equipment and/or resuscitative procedures, it can be held liable for falling below this standard.

Disaster Resuscitology (Table 21)[60, 117, 255, 751–756, 976]

The scope and complexity of modern disaster planning, response and analysis are too extensive to be covered here. We refer to appropriate organizations and texts[8, 60, 117, 165, 195, 255, 256, 339, 366, 367, 451, 505, 510, 526, 530, 609, 667, 755, 803, 907, 976]. This section will summarize a few topics important for resuscitation attempts in disasters.

A disaster is 'a sudden and extremely unfortunate event that affects many people'. A medical disaster is usually defined as 'an event in which the number or severity of acutely ill or injured persons exceeds the capacity of the local every day emergency medical services (EMS) system'. Disaster medicine, until recently, concerned itself mainly with public health aspects and the rehabilitation of uninjured survivors and the involved region. Over the past decade, disaster medicine has been expanded to include resuscitation (emergency resuscitation plus intensive care; i.e. CPCR phases I, II and III)[752]. With the Second World Congress on Emergency and Disaster Medicine in Pittsburgh in 1981, we introduced the term 'disaster resuscitology'[752] to indicate that dying and crippling processes of those not instantly killed in disasters deserve more attention, and that this is a new field for scholarly inquiry. Disaster-related research in the past has been mainly the domain of sociology and epidemiology. Disaster medicine with emphasis on resuscitation medicine (emergency and critical care medicine) received a strong impetus with the initiation of the Club of Mainz by the late Rudolf Frey in 1976[255]. In 1981 it was renamed the World Association for Emergency and Disaster Medicine (WAEDM), and in 1985 it initiated the *Journal of the WAEDM*[907]. Membership with Journal subscription is available to interested and involved physicians and nonphysician leaders, teachers, researchers or organizers (Secretary of the WAEDM: Dr Peter Baskett, Dept of Anaesthetics, Frenchay Hospital, Bristol BS16 1LE, England; tel. 272-565656).

When considering resuscitation responses to disasters, one must differentiate between at least three types of disaster:

1. multicasualty incidents (MCI), such as transportation accidents or fires, in which the local EMS system initiates its disaster plan, which may require help from neighboring (regional) EMS systems;
2. mass disasters, such as major earthquakes, floods and wars, which overwhelm, damage or destroy the local-regional EMS system's disaster

Table 21. Community-wide emergency and critical care medicine system (from P. Safar[26, 720, 730a]).

	Suggested physician responsibilities		
	Service components		Coordination
Components	Emergency Dept. physicians ★★★	CCM (ICU) physicians ★★★	Community Council's EM-CCM physicians ★★★
(1) Treatment at the scene recognition of the emergency and aid by bystanders*	—	—	
(2) Initiation of system by bystander**	(+)	—	(1)–(7) coordinated by (8)–(11)
(3) Resuscitation and stabilization at the scene by members of the system*	+	(+)	(8) Organization communication
			(9) Planning education evaluation
(4) Transportation with life support* Preferably by advanced life support ambulance service	+	(+)	(10) Research
			(11) Disaster plan: Hospital
(5) Treatment in the emergency dept. multidisciplinary team team leadership	+ Clinical base of ED physician	(+) Resus. only	Community National (NDMS) NDM operations center
(6) Management in the operating room by surgeons and anesthesiologists	—	(+)	Trauma hospitals Resusc. med. disaster teams = hosp. trauma teams
(7) Treatment in the ICU Major emergency hospital with advanced physician-staffed ICUs	—	+ Clinical base of ICU physician	Military–civilian collaboration Airlift-evacuation (military) International guidelines

* Prehospital physician advice and radio control of EMTs and paramedics. Presence of physician optional.

** Call mobile ICU ambulance, by universal emergency telephone number. + required; (+) optional.

*** Ideally (utopian?) the same group of resuscitologists (multidisciplinary team) would be responsible for *all* components.

For abbreviations, see Glossary

plan, which would then initiate the state or national disaster medicine system (NDMS);
3. endemic disasters, such as the interactions of starvation, infection, dehydration and revolution, usually in poor developing countries, which need long-term ongoing economic and political solutions.

Each regional EMS system, and within it each emergency (trauma) hospital, should have a plan for expanding its everyday resuscitative and trauma surgery capabilities to cope with disasters with large numbers of casualties. These regional (multicommunity), local (single-community) and hospital disaster plans must include considerations for a variety of personnel, ranging from the lay public to physician specialists, a variety of equipment and supplies (some stockpiled), and a variety of transportation systems. Helicopter ambulances in large numbers (available from the Armed Forces) are crucial since many disasters result in blocked access roads for ambulance vehicles. These plans must also include radio communications (since telephone lines may be blocked or cut), not only between emergency department physicians and ambulance personnel, but also between emergency (trauma) hospitals, and between each hospital and the Medical Disaster Operations Center, which must be linked (physically or by radio) with the overall Disaster Operations Center. Centralized coordination and authority of disaster relief efforts (starting locally, if necessary moved to regional or even state or national level)—in many countries planned as part of 'Civil Defense' (linked with the Armed Forces)—must have continuous input on needs from the disaster scene. Orders should be given jointly by the medical (emergency physician) and nonmedical (governmental) disaster operations officer.

Dying processes in disasters[165, 754, 755]

In multicasualty incidents, any kind of trauma and medical emergency may be encountered. Burns are frequent. In mass disasters, the number of dead or dying when outside help arrived have ranged from millions in plagues or world wars, via up to 100 000 in one major earthquake (e.g. China, Peru) or flood (e.g. Bangladesh), to fewer than 100 in a hurricane or fire. In mass disasters such as earthquakes, hurricanes and floods, death can be instantaneous, as from crushing of the head or chest, exsanguinating external or internal hemorrhage, or drowning. Dying can progress over minutes or hours from asphyxia or hypovolemic shock; or be delayed for days when secondary to crush syndrome or sepsis. Even potentially noncrippling head injury can cause several minutes of apnea immediately upon impact, and then upper airway soft-tissue obstruction due to coma and hypoxemia as the result of aspiration or pulmonary edema. Inhalation of smoke or toxic gas (e.g. Bhopal, India, 1984) as well as dust inhalation in earthquakes can cause rapid or slow asphyxiation from airway irritation and pulmonary damage.

Interviews of physician eyewitnesses of major earthquakes revealed that many of those who were accessible for resuscitation and who were dying slowly did so from exsanguinating external hemorrhage, shock from multiple fractures, coma with airway obstruction, internal crushing injuries, head injuries, dust inhalation, blunt chest injuries and delayed wound sepsis[751, 755].

Resuscitation potentials in disasters[165, 751, 755, 921a]

There has been a progressive decrease in the mortality of those injured in everyday emergencies, in multicasualty incidents (e.g. transportation accidents) and those injured in wars (e.g. Middle East, Vietnam), in part due to prompt application of modern resuscitation and rapid transportation. Whether this also applies to natural mass disasters, such as earthquakes, needs to be researched. In major recent earthquakes in Peru and Italy, anecdotal information obtained from involved physician survivors through interviews suggest that possibly 50% of those ultimately declared dead are not crushed to death instantaneously, but died slowly, some over minutes or hours, others within 1 week post-impact[754, 755]. It has been estimated that up to 40% of those who died slowly (approximately 20% of all who died) could have been saved if uninjured co-victims had applied life supporting first aid (LSFA) immediately, and if specialized advanced trauma life support (ATLS) medical teams had been flown to the scene within 6 hours and promptly stabilized and evacuated to trauma hospitals those in need and potentially salvageable[755]. Uninjured and lightly injured victims remained buried alive under the rubble for up to one week. Exact figures on the salvageability of earthquake victims do not exist since in general no autopsies were performed.

Realizing these postulated life saving potentials has so far been impossible for several reasons: (1) lack of LSFA training of the lay public; (2) delayed detection of buried victims (dogs and sensors arrived too late; innovative new technology is needed for the detection of alive, buried victims); (3) delayed or impossible extrication (innovative new nontraumatic airliftable extrication technology is needed); (4) delayed arrival of resuscitation medicine disaster teams to provide ATLS (they usually arrived after 48 hours, but could be effective only if in operation within 6–12 hours); (5) the erroneous concept that medical volunteers of any kind are helpful (the need is for expert teams); (6) delayed evacuation without life support, often to an inappropriate hospital; (7) lack of quantity, quality and uniformity of life-saving equipment and supplies; (8) inadequacies in communication, mutual understanding, and coordination of agencies and authorities[255, 609, 755, 976].

The suspected, but not yet proved, resuscitation potentials in mass disasters face logistic limitations. These are primarily time limits within which resuscitation can be effective. For LSFA to be effective, it must be applied within seconds to minutes; this is possible only through the actions of uninjured bystanders (co-victims). ATLS, including resuscitative surgery, should arrive within about 1 hour in order for treatment of traumatic shock to be effective. This can usually be achieved only by a local paramedic or physician-staffed ambulance service, or by military medicine. The third line of defense is surgical wound care to prevent sepsis, special procedures to preserve tissue, and advanced intensive care for prolonged shock, which are most likely to be effective if delivered within about 6 h. Some feel that ATLS teams can save lives up to 12 hours after injury.

The WAEDM[976, 977] and other international disaster medicine oriented groups[366, 367, 451, 526, 609, 907, 978] have recommended the organization, on a standby basis, at least in regions prone to mass disasters, of small scouting and research teams which could be at the scene within one hour to report via radio the need for a local, regional and/or national response, and collect information according to research protocols.

National disaster medical systems[85, 505,755, 809, 921a]

When a mass disaster, such as a major earthquake, strikes the resources of the local-regional EMS response system may be overwhelmed, damaged or destroyed. In this case a state or national disaster medical system (NDMS) response should be initiated. Such an NDMS response must be preplanned. For example, in the USA, planning of an NDMS has been going on since 1980. The system is planned for the scenario of a major earthquake anywhere in the country which would kill thousands instantaneously and generate up to 100 000 seriously injured patients requiring hospitalization. The prerecruitment of that many hospital beds from volunteering hospitals nationwide has been accomplished. This plan would also serve victims of a major conventional (not nuclear) war. NDMS planning is under the auspices of three agencies: (1) the public health service (Department of Health and Human Services, DHHS); (2) the military (Department of Defense, DOD); and (3) the Federal Emergency Management Agency (FEMA) (civil defense agency). In addition, the system calls for about 150 disaster medical response teams (we prefer to call them 'resuscitation medicine disaster teams') to be flown rapidly to the disaster site. These teams should come from trauma hospitals nearby and, if more are needed, also far away. Each team should be totally self-sustaining and small enough to fit into one large helicopter. These teams should provide ATLS in the field, stabilize and sort (triage) the victims, and manage evacuation. The NDMS plan also calls for large mobile field hospitals to follow. We applaud the field resuscitation team concept, but are skeptical about the use of field hospitals which would offer little resuscitation potential. They are too cumbersome and expensive and require over 3 days to be mobilized, transported and set up, whereas ATLS with resuscitative surgery is needed within 6–12 hours.

Rather, we suggest that NDMS planning be used to foster not only public education in LSFA, but also the establishment nationwide of advanced trauma hospitals. These hospitals would provide the experienced trauma resuscitation teams to go out and replenish their staffs from second and third call up systems, who would take care of the most serious evacuated casualties. ATLS and resuscitative surgery would be performed in some instances in the field using mobile ICUs or airlifted mobile operating room—ICU combinations[837a]. Definitive care would be in the receiving hospitals. Members of the same team should come from the same trauma hospital, as they should be used to working together.

While in industrialized countries traumatology teams are stronger in the civilian sector, in some developing countries they may primarily come from the military. Military physicians in peace time should participate in NDMS planning, and gain traumatology experience in busy civilian trauma hospitals. The NDMS also requires a large-scale air transport and evacuation plan which must rely heavily on helicopters and the armed forces. Information on NDMS planning in the USA is available[505].

The greatest obstacle to effective resuscitation response in mass disasters has been a lack of authoritative coordination of agencies and helpers. Authority for command and coordination at the disaster site should consist of at least one medical and one nonmedical (military or governmental) disaster operations officer, both working together side by side. At the disaster site they must be visibly identified.

To study and develop disaster resuscitology worldwide, the WAEDM is recommending communication between similar planning efforts in various countries. By aiming for increasing international compatibility of mass disaster plans, training of personnel, equipment, supplies and communication, aid across national borders, early enough to make an impact on life saving, might be facilitated.

International aid across borders in recent major earthquakes has been frustrated by bureaucratic obstacles posed by local governments; the arrival too late (after 48 hours) of too many well meaning volunteers who found nothing to do; and the obstruction of facilities by volunteer helpers with unneeded skills and by unneeded equipment and supplies.

Military leadership of NDMS planning and response has been recommended by many[85, 752-756, 809], since military medicine seems to be the only system always in readiness, and already funded, which has the communication facilities, short response time, trained medical personnel, necessary equipment and supplies, airlift capability, extrication and rescue technology, and authoritative leadership and organization required for resuscitating victims in mass disasters such as major earthquakes. The military is crucial for massive airlift capability to and from the scene[65a, 85, 754].

While the NDMS plan for the USA offers an opportunity to incorporate military and civilian planners and to encourage cooperation, the temptation to fully adopt the military model for combat medical care should be resisted[65a]. The military paradigm is based on amphibious assaults and battles planned six weeks to one year ahead of time, with a relatively predictable casualty load, which evolves over several days to weeks. Mass disasters such as major earthquakes, on the other hand, may involve totally unexpected thousands of casualties occurring in minutes. Clearly, the logistic and mobilization requirements are different and the greatest impact will be made by the immediate local and surrounding (regional) EMS response within minutes to a few hours, rather than the response which can be mobilized from the outside for delivery in 24–48 hours. Heavy involvement of the military, particularly military medicine, however, in NDMS planning and response is desirable for logistic, economic and humanitarian reasons.

Local disaster medical systems[117, 339]

These should be designed primarily for multicasualty incidents and include all the components of the EMS system mentioned above. The 'resuscitation medicine disaster teams' should consist of physicians, nurses and paramedics experienced in resuscitation, traumatology, anesthesia and sorting (triage). They will probably be needed in multicasualty incidents only if rapid transport with life support by paramedics to the nearest hospital cannot be accomplished. Again, a physician leader at the disaster medical operations center in the field is essential.

Individuals responsible for disaster planning in hospitals and in governmental positions, and military physicians, require extensive training and experience before they can begin to plan or mount a coherent response to a major disaster. In the USA, efforts to develop such training are currently being undertaken by the FEMA. The identified areas with which the EMS planner or incident commander must be familiar are: (1) definitions (especially multicasualty incident type disaster versus mass disaster, for that particular EMS system); (2) agency roles and responsibilities; (3) field operations and capabilities; (4) transportation needs and capabilities; (5) communications; (6) hospital capabilities and receiving/transfer functions; (7) logistic needs and capabilities; (8) interagency coordination and agreements, both prospective and operational; (9) a workable resource catalog; (10) demobilization procedures; (11) post-incident requirements; (12) structure and necessity for evaluation, training and realistic exercises; and (13) disaster research.

Sorting (triage) is to be carried out during emergency resuscitation and in several steps along the way, before and after evacuation. The lightly injured, as well as the hopelessly injured and dead, are to be ignored in mass disasters, except for pain relief. The in-between casualties are to be separated into those in whom treatment can be delayed and those who need immediate resuscitative therapy. Those stabilized are evacuated according to needs.

Nuclear disasters[142, 487, 754, 755c, 755d, 809, 908, 928]

These might happen as the result of technologic failure and human error (e.g. Three Mile Island, USA; Chernobyl, USSR) or be caused by terrorism. Nuclear accidents call for special disaster preparedness, considering the whole range from the accidental explosion of a nuclear warhead to the subtle leak of radioactive material into air, water and ground from a nuclear reactor or power plant. Explosions and fires cause blast and burn injuries combined with acute radiation. Their emergency treatment is hampered by the need to resuscitate while providing protective clothing for isolation of victims and for reverse isolation of rescuers, and the need for early decontamination. For radiation injuries, see Chapter 4.

Sudden whole body exposure to radioactive material can kill most people in the near vicinity of the accident (exposure to over 1000 rems) within hours to about 2 weeks, from cerebral radiation and hemorrhage, necrosis of the intestinal mucosa and circulatory shock. (A usual X-ray examination gives exposure to about 0.02 rem.) Those more distant (exposure to 200–1000 rems) have about a 50% chance of dying within 2–6 weeks from leukopenia, acute infections and acute bowel syndrome. Exposure to less than about 200 rems is not acutely fatal, but gives nausea and vomiting and long-term leukopenia. Prolonged low-level radiation from fallout increases the risk of cancer and malformation of offspring. Contamination may linger on for generations, making whole regions unsafe for people, animals and plants. While the half life of radioactive iodine is short, those of cesium and strontium are years, and that of plutonium is thousands of years. Thus, an important part of disaster preparedness is mass evacuation.

Nuclear war[142, 148, 452, 487, 754, 755c, 755d, 908, 928, 977]

Physicians and scientists worldwide have agreed that a nuclear war cannot remain limited and would inevitably expand into a holocaust, and that no meaningful disaster medicine planning for such an event is possible. Recommendations by the WAEDM support recommendations by the World Health Organization, the International Red Cross and other organizations.

The WAEDM states the following[977]: '(1) Disaster medical preparedness should be continued and developed for conventional wars, nuclear accidents and a single small nuclear bomb explosion (e.g. by accident or terrorism). (2) All governments and powers in possession of nuclear weapons should take initiatives to reduce and ultimately eliminate their nuclear arsenals worldwide. (3) All governments and powers currently in possession of nuclear weapons should agree not to assist, in any way, other powers at present without nuclear weapons to obtain them in the future. (4) *Any meaningful disaster medicine preparedness for a nuclear holocaust is impossible.* Such attempts at planning nuclear war medical preparedness represent an unjustifiable use of medical and financial resources. However, in the awful event of a nuclear holocaust the members would, of course, do what they could to relieve pain and suffering.'

Chapter 7

Philosophical–Ethical Conclusions
Peter Safar and Nancy Caroline

Delivery of Cardiopulmonary Cerebral Resuscitation

The phases and steps of cardiopulmonary cerebral resuscitation (CPCR) (Fig. 2, Table 1) comprise an outline of the knowledge and skills required of emergency and critical care medicine personnel. But resuscitation capability depends also on practical experience, common sense, a flexible approach to emergency situations, and rapid, titrated actions. Resuscitation, that is, should be based on science and carried out with art. The necessary appreciation of the need for speedy action and attention to technical details can be acquired only with experience and objective evaluation of one's own performance. Knowledge gained through reading and lectures does not guarantee the ability to resuscitate effectively. Nor does manikin practice, although it helps. Furthermore, emergency and long-term resuscitation are 'treatment by titration', in contradistinction to the 'treatment by prescription' of general medical practice; and therefore it cannot be assumed that the skills of resuscitation will have been learned in the course of general medical practice. For health care personnel entrusted with responsibility for resuscitation, there is no substitute for observing role models in action and gaining first-hand practical experience with patients.

Those involved in resuscitation must be able to function as team members and/or team leaders. Patient outcome after resuscitation attempts depends in part on the correct deployment of all the steps described in this book, throughout all components of the emergency and critical care medicine delivery system, prehospital and intrahospital. Too often the outcome is determined by the weakest step or component. Thus, physicians in general and anesthesiologists in particular should concern themselves with the educational and organizational aspects of resuscitation services within their hospital and community.

CPCR can make an impact not only in industrialized but also in *developing countries*, provided attention is paid to priorities of needs and cost-effectiveness. The order of priorities for new or expanding programs in recent years has often been inappropriate. We suggest considering as the highest priority, training of the lay public in life supporting first aid (LSFA) and CPR Steps A–B–C without equipment (which is inexpensive), with the development of ambulance services with the first basic and later advanced life support to follow. Then would come emergency departments and trauma surgery in hospitals with safe modern anesthesia and general recovery room-type ICUs. We would consider as the lowest priority, special hospital ICUs with computerized sophisticated equipment (which is very expensive) as they have questionable cost-effectiveness. In regions where overwhelming lethal public health problems like starvation and epidemics must receive highest priority, even emergency medicine has to receive lower priority consideration.

Ethical Questions in the Future

We discussed in Chapter 3 our thoughts on when not to resuscitate, and when and how to discontinue emergency resuscitation and long-term life support. Management of the conscious rational patient in the terminal stages of a hopeless condition should be guided primarily by the patient's wishes[929]. Management of the incompetent unresponsive patient with a hopeless condition is on the other hand one of the major emotional, ethical and legal issues in medicine today, a problem brought about in part by the advances in resuscitation technology. Under such circumstances, medical management should first of all be guided by the patient's previously stated wishes (living will) via a proxy (primary physician, relative, friend)[929]. Second, medical management of the unresponsive patient should be guided by the reliability of measurements used to determine the irreversibility of unresponsiveness (Chapter 3). Third, medical care decision-making should be based on the concept of 'appropriate level of care'[58,305,720,929]: (1) emergency resuscitation; (2) intensive therapy (prolonged, advanced life support); (3) general medical care; and (4) general nursing care. Care levels 3 and 4 may include 'letting die', i.e. passive euthanasia[46]. 'Letting die' a permanently unconscious patient represents a medical decision. It may include discontinuance of artificial ventilation, antibiotics, and artificial feeding and hydration, although the legality of discontinuing nutrition and hydration even of permanently comatose patients is still uncertain in most states in the USA. Should it also consider withdrawal of an artifical airway? Declaring as ethical the withdrawal of all forms of life support in the patient proved to be permanently unresponsive has been recommended by some of us since the beginning of modern resuscitation[631,713]. This approach has recently been accepted by medical leaders[929], and was endorsed as ethical in 1986 by the American Medical Association[24]. However, in contrast to passive euthanasia (letting die), active euthanasia (actions with the intent to kill) or assistance in suicide for the hopeless rational patient who is demanding it is in general not condoned by the medical profession or by law.

Dying and resuscitation are much less investigated than the beginning of life[727,728,746]. Breakthroughs through chance discoveries will probably be scarce since dying and the post-resuscitation syndrome are complex multifactorial phenomena. Therefore, coordinated systematic research is needed, using progressions from bench studies, via short-term mechanism-oriented laboratory studies, to long-term animal outcome studies[745, 759, 760], to multicenter randomized clinical trials. Controlled prospective clinical research in resuscitation medicine is extremely difficult, but one such program has been in existence during the recent decade[1-4, 191, 404]. The informed consent issue in clinical cardiac arrest studies could be solved ethically by including randomized, well-designed studies in the emergency exception to consent[1].

Future technologic developments in resuscitation medicine will undoubtedly create new problems. These technologic advances include emergency cardiopulmonary bypass for CPCR in cases of prolonged cardiac arrest, which will permit the reversal of prolonged cardiac arrest and the delivery of novel cerebral resuscitation methods. When should cardiopulmonary bypass be stopped in the unweanable patient? In patients on cardiopulmonary bypass after an arrest, the heart may not resume beating; if there is evidence of cerebral recovery, they might become recipients of artificial or transplanted hearts. Those who develop evidence of cerebral or brain death while on artificial circulation might become donors of still viable organs. Research into the biologic limits to the reversibility of clinical death of the entire organism, into the technologic resuscitation potentials, and into outcome predictions (as pursued at the International Resuscitation Research Center of the University of Pittsburgh) would also apply to individual organs in transplantation medicine. Prospects of suspended animation (preservation) of the entire organism in a momentarily nonreversible terminal state of an ultimately potentially salvageable individual (e.g. the mortally wounded without brain injury) might gain time to enable transportation, correction of the problem and delayed resuscitation; such a science fiction scenario could in the future become scientific fact in resuscitation.

As resuscitation research and practice progress, society will have many new questions to answer: How reliable must prognosticating methods be for the decision to let die in vegetative state? Can patients in proved cerebral death or persistent vegetative state (without total brain death) become organ donors? How can society obtain the many more donor hearts needed? How much permanent brain damage in a conscious person justifies 'letting die'? Who decides? Who is the most appropriate proxy for the unresponsive incompetent patient? How detailed must the patient's living will be for refusal to prolong dying in hopeless situations? What are the patient's rights in clinical resuscitation research[1, 2]? What are the physician's rights in clinical resuscitation research? What are experimental animals' rights in resuscitation research? Which has precedent, the physician's duty to preserve life (with what quality, what quantity) or the physician's duty to heal and alleviate pain? Who should allocate finite resources, and how? In critical care triage[305], should society determine what is fair[46], or should it be the assumed will of the patient, or the wish of family? These and other questions suggest some general guidelines for answers: it is, to begin with, the physician's duty to serve not only the individual patient but also society. Death when one's 'time has come' is a natural event for the patient and should not be considered by health professionals as a defeat or failure. The patient must have the right to decide on his/her treatments and dying. Patients deserve the consensus of three proxies: (1) the primary physician; (2) the family or friend; and (3) a resuscitation specialist. The decision-making on appropriate levels of care is a medical one; it should be guided by the patient's wish (or assumed wish), available technology, and reason and compassion—not by fear of law suits and legal precedent. The law usually lags behind society's perceptions of what is ethical.

The task of physicians and nurses involved in caring for hopeless cases includes helping the patient's family and friends by orchestrating painless dying with equanimity and dignity; this belongs to the art of medicine. Such 'good' dying of the person 'whose time has come' can and should be arranged even in the resuscitation and critical care unit setting. For example, an emergency resuscitation attempt in a very old, previously healthy person who suffers sudden cardiac death can transform an unexpected catastrophic event into 'good dying'. After restoration of spontaneous circulation and life support, and recognition of severe cardiogenic shock, the patient may temporarily recover consciousness until the loved ones can say good-bye, and then be assisted in an orderly, painless, dignified departure. For example, the skillful use of narcotics in the dying person who is not to be resuscitated can help family and friends by preventing struggling in shock and prolonged asphyxiation in pulmonary edema.

Near-death Experiences

Some mystics have sought in resuscitated persons' reported experiences a proof of 'life after death', of having seen heaven or hell[261, 555]. Many patients who recover consciousness after resuscitation from coma in a terminal state, with or without cardiac arrest, report dreams or hallucinations. Some of these have surprising similarities, such as going through a tunnel, observing yourself from the outside, meeting religious figures or loved ones, pleasant lights and sounds, and complete resignation, tranquility, and no pain. Others report unpleasant sensations. We respect those who believe that such near-death experiences are in support of life after death. Scientific evidence available, however, indicates that when there is no brain metabolism, there are no sensations or dreams. Some patients who had suffered sudden cardiac arrest (without a preceding shock state) and early prompt resuscitation with rapid recovery of consciousness reported to one of us that they experienced blackout (nothingness) and no near-death experiences. The reported near-death experiences can be explained in several ways. (1) Dreams and hallucinations occur when brain metabolism is altered by shock, trauma, toxins, drugs and so on, but not when there is zero metabolism, as in clinical death. Such altered (not zero) brain function is common, even in cardiac arrest cases, as for example due to shock (low blood flow) before the arrest and during resuscitation and recovery. (2) The hearing and feeling of persons and actions surrounding the patient (i.e. reality during dying or postanoxic recovery) is similar to the state of light anesthesia; the patient cannot see or move at will, but can hear real events.

Resuscitation and the Evolution of Man

Resuscitation should be based on science and practiced with reason and compassion. The human brain—the site of bodily integration and reactions, human mentation, feelings, values, behavior, compassion and love—must be the target organ of resuscitation. The human brain—much more vulnerable to hypoxia than the brains of less 'intelligent' species[672]—is considered by its possessors to be 'the peak of evolution destined to build this earth' (Teilhard de Chardin). Creations of the human brain, such as humanism (which includes medicine), have declared that even a single human life is of inestimable value.

Modern resuscitation has made a medical impact by saving individuals whose lives would otherwise have been cut short before their 'time to die' had come. Is this worth the effort? Can it be justified—socially, morally, economically? Is it supportive of human evolution on this earth? Certainly, as long as all life is merely viewed as species-oriented, resuscitation of a few individual humans assumes trivial significance. Where resuscitation promotes survival of the unfit, it even exerts an untoward effect on the evolution of our species. Those who argue for such resuscitative nihilism, must, however, to be consistent, condemn the endeavors of the medical arts and sciences in any form. For all of human disease and misery must then be viewed as part of nature's selective process, and medical intervention of any kind must be seen as ill advised, because it tampers with evolution. We believe, however, that those concerned about the evolution of our species would be better advised to work on eradication of war, violent crime and man-made disasters, all of which destroy primarily the young and the fit.

Few would argue that resuscitation applied without judgment and compassion is morally and economically acceptable. The debilitated elderly patient, the terminal cancer patient in intractable pain, the severely brain injured patient without prospect of human mentation—their dying should be permitted to proceed without the imposition of costly and in these instances dehumanizing life-support technology.

But what of those whose dying occurs from potentially reversible conditions imposed by the arbitrary mischances of nature, before they have had time to live 'full lives'? We consider their reanimation to the point of human mentation not only defensible but also desirable. The doctrine of natural selection must be repugnant to man as a medical professional.

Medicine represents an imposition of human values on a random universe; an assertion that compassion, reason and decency constitute a higher ethic than chance.

Research on the mechanisms of dying and its reversibility—less advanced than research on the beginnings of human life—should be fostered, not only to acquire new knowledge per se. Science, art and humanism (medicine is a mix of these three) are prime examples of increasing consciousness on this earth, and must therefore be considered positive for evolution. Bertrand Russell said 'For many only the examined life is worth living'. We want to add that 'only the examined death is worth fighting or accepting'.

Resuscitation implies a commitment on the side of life. To devote one's energies to the restoration of lives cut short before fulfillment is to declare life as intrinsically valuable—that it is worth living. Although the therapeutic impact of resuscitation may affect only a few, its moral impact may affect many, in a world where life is often regarded as cheap. The overall goal of our efforts must be restoration not only of circulatory and respiratory functions but of human mentation as well. Those who return from the shores of Lethe should be enabled to re-enter the community of the living in a manner approaching the ancient ideal:

Mens sana in corpore sano (Juvenal).

References

To limit the number of references, we regret that some additional historic and novel contributions could not be included.

1a. Abramson NS, Meisel A, Safar P: Informed consent in resuscitation research. *J Amer Med Assoc* **246:** 2828, 1981.
1b. Abramson NS, Meisel A, Safar P: Deferred consent: A new approach for resuscitation research. *J Amer Med Assoc* **255:** 2466, 1986.
2a. Abramson N, Sutton K, Safar P, et al: Neurologic recovery after cardiac arrest. *Crit Care Med*, **15:** 431, 1987 (abstract).
2b. Abramson NS, Safar P, Detre KM, et al: Neurologic recovery after cardiac arrest: effect of duration of ischemia. *Crit Care Med* **13:** 930, 1985.
3. Abramson NS, Safar P, Detre K, et al: Brain Resuscitation Clinical Trial (BRCT) I Study Group: Randomized clinical study of thiopental loading in comatose cardiac arrest survivors. *N Engl J Med* **314:** 397, 1986.
4. Abramson NS, Detre K, Hedstand U, et al: Brain Resuscitation Clinical Trial (BRCT) II Study Group: Methodology of the BRCT II: Post-cardiac arrest calcium entry blocker (lidoflazine) administration. *Proceedings, 7th European Congress of Anaesthesiology*, Vienna, 1986. Vienna, W. Maudrich, 1986.
5. Adams AP, Henville JD: A new generation of anesthetic ventilators: The Pneupac and Penlon A–P. *Anaesthesia* **32:** 34, 1977.
6. Adelson L: A clinicopathologic study of the anatomic changes in the heart resulting from cardiac massage. *Surg Gyn Obst* **104:** 513, 1957.
7. Adelson L, Hoffman W: Sudden death from coronary artery disease: A statistical study. *J Amer Med Assoc* **176:** 129, 1961.
8. Adler J (Ed): *Proceedings International Symposium on Disaster Medicine*, Jerusalem, Israel, 1984. International publication (JA, Shaare-Zedek Hospital, Jerusalem, Israel).
9. Ahnefeld FW, Halmagyi M, Uberla K: Untersuchungen zur Bewertung Kolloidaler Volumunenersatzmittel. *Anaesthesist* **14:** 137, 1965.
10. Ahnefeld FW, Dick W, Kilian J, Schuster HP: *Notfallmedizin*. Klinische Anaesthesiologie und Intensivtherapie. Vol. 30. Heidelberg, Springer-Verlag, 1986.
11. Albin MS, Bunegin L, Helsel P, et al: DMSO protects brain against experimental pressure induced focal ischemia. *Crit Care Med* **4:** 251, 1980 (abstract).
12. Albin MS: Acute spinal cord trauma: In: *Textbook of Critical Care*. WC Shoemaker, WL Thompson, PR Holbrook (Eds). Philadelphia, WB Saunders, 1984, p. 928.
13. Alderman EL: Analgesics in the acute phase of myocardial infarction. *J Amer Med Assoc* **220:** 1646, 1974.
14. Aldrete JA, Romo-Salas F, Jankowsky L, et al: Effect of pretreatment with thiopental and phenytoin on postischemic brain damage in rabbits. *Crit Care Med* **7:** 466, 1979.
15. Alfonsi G, Gilbertson L, Safar P, et al: Cold water drowning and resuscitation in dogs. *Anesthesiology* **57:** A80, 1982 (abstract).
16a. Alifimoff JK, Safar P, Bircher N, et al: Cardiac resuscitability and cerebral recovery after closed-chest, MAST augmented and open-chest CPR. *Anesthesiology* **53:** S151; **53:** S147, 1980 (abstracts).
16b. Alifimoff JK, Safar P, Bircher NG: Opening the chest to keep the brain alive in prolonged cardiopulmonary resuscitation. *J World Assoc Emerg Disaster Med* 1/Suppl I: 233, 1985.
17. Allen GS, Ahn HS, Preziosi TJ, et al: Cerebral arterial spasm—a controlled trial of nimodipine in patients with subarachnoid hemorrhage. *N Engl J Med* **308:** 619, 1983.

18. Altemeier WA, Todd J: Studies on the incidence of infection following open-chest cardiac massage for cardiac arrest. *Ann Surg* **158:** 596, 1963.
19. Althaus U, Aeberhard P, Schupbach P, et al: Management of profound accidental hypothermia with cardiorespiratory arrest. *Ann Surg* **195:** 492, 1982.
20. Ambersen WR, Flecksner J, Steggerda FR, et al: On use of Ringer–Locke solutions containing hemoglobin as a substitute for normal blood in mammals. *J Cell Compar Physiol* **5:** 359, 1934.
21. American Academy of Orthopedic Surgeons, Committee on Injuries: *Emergency Care and Transportation of the Sick and Injured.* 2nd ed, 1984. American Academy of Orthopaedic Surgeons, 430 North Michigan Ave, Chicago, IL 60611, USA.
22a. American College of Surgeons: *Early Care of the Injured Patient.* Philadelphia, WB Saunders, 1980.
22b. American College of Surgeons Committe on Trauma (Collicott PE, et al): *Advanced Trauma Life Support Course for Physicians, 1984.* American College of Surgeons, 55 East Erie Street, Chicago, IL, 60611, USA.
23a. American Heart Association (AHA) and National Academy of Sciences-National Research Council (NAS-NRC): Standards for Cardiopulmonary Resuscitation (CPR) and Emergency Cardiac Care (ECC). *J Amer Med Assoc* **198:** 372, 1966; **227** (Suppl): 833, 1974; **244** (Suppl): 453, 1980.
23b. American Heart Association (AHA) 1985 National Conference (Montgomery WH, Chairman; Donegan J; McIntyre KM; Albarran-Sotelo R; Jaffe AS; Ornato JP; Paraskos JA; et al): Standards and guidelines for cardiopulmonary resuscitation (CPR) and emergency cardiac care (ECC). *J Amer Med Assoc* **255**(Suppl): 2841, 1986.
23c. American Heart Association (AHA): *Advanced Cardiac Life Support Manual, 1981, 1983.* American Heart Assoc, 7320 Greenville Ave, Dallas, TX 75231, USA.
24. American Medical Association (AMA): *Guidelines for Foregoing Life Supporting Treatment in Permanent Coma, 1986.* American Medical Association, 535 N Dearborn Street, Chicago, IL 60010, USA.
25a. American Red Cross: *Standard First Aid and Personal Safety.* 2nd ed. Garden City, NY, Doubleday, 1979.
25b. American Red Cross: *Advanced First Aid and Emergency Care.* 2nd ed. Garden City, NY, Doubleday, 1979.
26. American Society of Anesthesiologists, Committee on Acute Medicine (Safar P, Chairman): Community-wide emergency medical services. *J Amer Med Assoc* **204:** 595, 1968.
27. Ames A, Wright RL, Kowada M, et al: Cerebral ischemia. The no-reflow phenomenon. *Am J Pathol* **52:** 637, 1968.
28. Ames A III, Nesbett FB: Pathophysiology of ischemic cell death. I. Time of onset of irreversible damage; importance of the different components of the ischemic insult. *Stroke* **14:** 219, 1983.
29. Anderson JL, Roder HE, Green LS: Comparative effects of beta-adrenergic blocking drugs on experimental ventricular fibrillation threshold. *Am J Cardiol* **51:** 1196, 1983.
29a. Angelos M, Reich H, Safar P, et al: Neurologic outcome after 10 min cardiac arrest plus 10 min CPR, and resuscitation with cardiopulmonary bypass, in dogs. *Ann Emerg Med* **16:** 515, 1987 (abstract).
30. Apgar V: A proposal for a new method of evaluation of the newborn infant. *Anesth Analg* **32:** 260, 1953.
31. Arena J: Management of specific poisonings. In: *Principles and Practice of Emergency Medicine.* G Schwartz, P Safar, JH Stone, et al (Eds). Philadelphia, WB Saunders, 1986, p 1700.
32. Arfors KE, Hillered L: Oxygen radicals and biological injury. In: *Protection of Tissues Against Hypoxia.* A Wauquier, M Borgers, WK Amery (Eds). New York, Elsevier, 1982, p 223.
33. Artz CP, Moncrief JA, Pruitt BA: *Burns, A Team Approach.* Philadelphia, WB Saunders, 1979.

34. Asmussen E, Hahn-Petersen A, Rosendal T: Air passage through the hypopharynx in unconscious patients in the prone position. *Acta Anaesth Scand* **3:** 123, 1959.
35. Astrup J, Moller-Sorenson P, Rahbeck-Sorenson H: Inhibition of cerebral oxygen and glucose consumption in the dog by hypothermia, pentobarbital and lidocaine. *Anesthesiology* **55:** 263, 1981.
36. Astrup P: The quantitative determination of surplus amounts of acid or base in the human body. K Mellemgaard, P Astrup (Eds). *Scand J Clin Lab Invest* **12:** 187, 1960.
37. Atcheson SG, Fred HL: Complications of cardiac resuscitation. *Am Heart J* **89:** 263, 1975.
38. Auerbach PS, Geehr EC: Inadequate oxygenation and ventilation using the esophageal gastric tube airway in the prehospital setting. *J Amer Med Assoc* **250:** 3067, 1983.
38a. Ayres SM: Ventricular function. In: *Textbook of Critical Care*. WC Shoemaker, WL Thompson, PR Holbrook (Eds). Philadelphia, WB Saunders, 1984, p. 333. Chapter 49.
39. Babbs CF, Abendschein DR, Tacker WA, et al: Subject dependent factors in ventricular defibrillation. *Med Instrum* **10:** 52, 1976.
40. Babbs CF, Yim GKW, Whister SJ, et al: Elevation of ventricular fibrillation threshold in dogs by antiarrhythmic drugs. *Am Heart J* **98:** 345, 1979.
41. Babbs CF, Redding JF, Safar P, et al (Eds): Cardiopulmonary Resuscitation. Third Purdue Conference Proceedings. (a) *Crit Care Med* **8:** 117, 1980. (b) *Med Instrum* **14:** 1, 1980.
42. Babbs CF, Bircher N, Burkett DE, et al: Effect of thoracic venting on arterial pressure and flow during external cardiopulmonary resuscitation in animals. *Crit Care Med* **9:** 785, 1981.
43. Babbs CF: Role of iron ions in the genesis of reperfusion injury following successful cardiopulmonary resuscitation: preliminary data and biochemical hypothesis. *Ann Emerg Med* **14:** 777, 1985.
44. Bachman L, Downes JJ, Richards CC, et al: Organization and function of an intensive care unit in a children's hospital. *Anes Analg Curr Res* **46/5:** 570, 1967.
45. Baethmann A, Go KG, Unterberg A (Eds): *Mechanisms of Secondary Brain Damage*. New York, Plenum Press, 1986.
46. Baier K: The ethics of passive euthanasia. *Crit Care Med* **4:** 317, 1976.
47. Baird RG, Dela Rocha AG, Miyagishima RT: Assisted circulation following myocardial infarction: A review of 25 patients treated before 1971. *Can Med Assoc J* **107:** 287, 1972.
48. Baker CC, Caronna JJ, Trunkey DD: Neurologic outcome after emergency room thoracotomy for trauma. *Amer J Surg* **139:** 677, 1980.
49. Baker CC, Thomas AM, Trunkey DD: The role of emergency room thoracotomy in trauma. *J Trauma* **20:** 848, 1980.
50. Barach AL, Martin J, Eckman M: Positive pressure respiration and its application to the treatment of acute pulmonary edema. *Ann Intern Med* **12:** 754, 1938.
51. Barber RE, Lee J, Hamilton WK: Oxygen toxicity in man: A prospective study in patients with irreversible brain damage. *N Engl J Med* **283:** 1478, 1970.
52. Bar-Joseph G, Safar P, Stezoski SW, et al: (a) Irreversible hemorrhagic shock model in the monkey. *J World Assoc Emerg Disaster Med* **1,** Suppl I: 169, 1985. (b) Survival after severe hemorrhagic shock in monkeys. *Anesthesiology* **57:** 97, 1982 (abstract). (c) Stroma-free hemoglobin, hydroxyethyl starch, lactated Ringers, or blood, for severe prolonged hemorrhagic shock in monkeys. *Crit Care Med* **11:** 219, 1983 (abstract).
53. Barnett WM, Alifimoff JK, Paris PM, et al: Comparison of open-chest cardiac massage techniques in dogs. *Ann Emerg Med* **15:** 408, 1986.
54. Bartlett RH, Gazzaniga AB: Extracorporeal circulation for cardiopulmonary failure. *Curr Prob Surg* **15/5:** 1, 1978.
55. Baskett PJF, Diamond AW, Cochrane DF: Urban mobile resuscitation: training and service. *Brit J Anaesth* **48:** 377, 1976.
56. Baskett PJF, Lawler PGP, Hudson RBF, et al: Resuscitation teaching room in a district general hospital. *Brit Med J* **1:** 568, 1976.

57. Baskett PJF: Aspects of cardiopulmonary resuscitation. *WFSA Lectures*; JSM Zorab, J Moyers (Eds) **2:** 75, 1984.

58. Baskett PJF, Sowden GR, Robins DW: Ethics in resuscitation. *Amer J Emerg Med* **2:** 273, 1984.

59. Baskett PJF, Carss A, Withers DA: Resuscitation by telephone. *J Brit Assoc Immed Care (BASICS)* 7/2: 46, 1984.

60a. Baskett PJF, Duerner P (Eds): Airport and aircraft disasters. *J World Assoc Emerg Disaster Med* 1/2, 1985.

60b. Baskett PJF, Fisher J (Eds): Proceedings of the Fourth World Congress on Emergency and Disaster Medicine, Brighton, UK, 1985. *J World Assoc Emerg Disaster Med* 3/1, 1987.

60c. Baskett PJF, Weller R (Eds): *Medicine for Disasters*. Bristol, J Wright, 1987.

61. Beck CS, Pritchard H, Feil SH: Ventricular fibrillation of long duration abolished by electric shock. *J Amer Med Assoc* **135:** 985, 1947.

62. Beck CS, Leighninger DS: Death after a clean bill of health. *J Amer Med Assoc* **174:** 133, 1960.

63. Becker DP, Miller JD, Ward JD, et al: The outcome from severe head injury with early diagnosis and intensive management. *J Neurosurg* **47:** 491, 1977.

64. Beckstead JE, Tweed WA, Lee J, et al: Cerebral blood flow and metabolism in man following cardiac arrest. *Stroke* **9:** 569, 1978.

65. Beecher H (Chairman, Harvard Medical School Ad Hoc Committee to examine the definition of brain death): A definition of irreversible coma. *J Amer Med Assoc* **205:** 337, 1968.

65a. Bellamy RF: The causes of death in conventional warfare—implications for combat casualty care research. *Milit Med* **149:** 55, 1984.

66. Bendixen HH, Egbert LD, Hedley-Whyte J, et al: *Respiratory Care*. St. Louis, CV Mosby, 1965.

67. Benesch K, Abramson N, Grenvik A (Eds): *Medico-Legal Aspects of Critical Care*. Rockville, MD, Aspen, 1986.

68. Benitz WE, Sunshine P: Neonatal resuscitation. In: *Current Therapy in Neonatal-Perinatal Medicine 1985–1986*. NM Nebon (Ed). Philadelphia, BC Decker, 1986.

69a. Benson DM, Esposito G, Dorsch J, et al: Mobile intensive care by 'unemployable' blacks trained as emergency medical technicians (EMTs) in 1967–69. *J Trauma* **12:** 408, 1971.

69b. Benson DM, Stewart C: Inadequacy of pre-hospital emergency care. *Crit Care Med* **1:** 130, 1973.

69c. Benson DM, Weigel J: Advanced life support by volunteer fire department ambulance personnel. *J Am Coll Emerg Physicians* **4:** 119, 1975.

70. Benzer H, Frey R, Huegin W, et al (Eds): *Textbook of Anesthesiology and Resuscitation* (in German). 5th Ed, Heidelberg, Springer-Verlag, 1982.

71. Berenyi KJ, Wolk M, Killip T: Cerebrospinal fluid acidosis complicating therapy of experimental cardiopulmonary arrest. *Circulation* **52:** 319, 1975.

72. Berg RA: Emergency infusion of catecholamines into bone marrow. *Am J Dis Child* **138:** 810, 1984.

72a. Bergmann H: Organisation eines flaechendeckenden Notarztwagensystems in Oester-reich. *Oest Aerzteztg* **41:** 15, 1986.

73. Berkebile P, Benson D, Ersoz C, et al: Public Education in Heart–Lung Resuscitation. Evaluation of three self-training methods in teenagers. (a) *Crit Care Med* **1:** 115, 1973. (b) *Proc National Cnf on CPR 1973*, Dallas, Amer Heart Assoc, 1975. (c) *Crit Care Med* **4:** 134, 1976 (abstract).

74. Berkebile P: Education in cardiopulmonary-cerebral resuscitation using self-training methods. *J World Assoc Emerg Disaster Med* 1/Suppl I: 75, 1985.

75. Bigelow WG, Lindsay WK, Greenwood WF: Hypothermia: Its possible role in cardiac surgery. *Ann Surg* **132:** 849, 1950.

76a. Bindslev L, Eklund J, Norlander O, et al: Treatment of acute respiratory failure by extracorporeal CO_2 elimination performed by surface heparinized artificial lung. *Anaesthesiology* **67**: 117, 1987.

76b. Bing RJ: Cardiac metabolism. In: *Cardiac Diagnosis and Treatment*. NO Fowler (Ed). 3rd ed. Hagerstown, MD, Harper & Row, 1980, p 281.

77. Birch LH, Kenney LJ, Doornbos F, et al: A study of external cardiac compression. *J Mich St Med Soc* **61**: 1346, 1962.

78. Bircher NG, Safar P, Stewart R: A comparison of standard, MAST-augmented, and open-chest CPR in dogs. *Crit Care Med* **8**: 147, 1980.

79. Bircher N, Safar P: Comparison of standard and 'new' closed-chest CPR and open-chest CPR in dogs. *Crit Care Med* **9**: 384, 1981.

80. Bircher N, Safar P, Eshel G et al: Cerebral and hemodynamic variables during cough-induced CPR in dogs. *Crit Care Med* **10**: 104, 1982.

81. Bircher N, Safar P: Life-supporting first aid (LSFA) and infant CPR (ICPR) self-training in children. *Crit Care Med* **11**: 251, 1983 (abstract).

82a. Bircher N, Safar P: Open-chest cardiopulmonary resuscitation: An old method whose time has returned. *Amer J Emerg Med* **2**: 568, 1984.

82b. Bircher N, Safar P: Manual open-chest cardiopulmonary resuscitation. *Ann Emerg Med* **13**: 770, 1984.

83. Bircher N, Safar P: Cerebral preservation during cardiopulmonary resuscitation. *Crit Care Med* **13**: 185, 1985.

84. Bircher NG, Safar P: Intracranial pressure and other variables during simultaneous ventilation-compression cardiopulmonary resuscitation. In: *Intracranial Pressure VI*. JD Miller, GM Teasdale, JO Rowan, et al (Eds), p 747. Berlin/Heidelberg, Springer-Verlag, 1986.

85. Bisgard JC: The role of the military in international military-civilian collaboration for disaster medicine in the USA. *J World Assoc Emerg Disaster Med* **1/1**: 21, 1985.

86. Bishop R, Weisfeldt ML: Sodium bicarbonate during cardiac arrest. Effect of arterial pH, PCO_2 and osmolality. *J Amer Med Assoc* **235**: 506, 1976.

87. Bjork RJ, Snyder BD, Champion BC, et al: Medical complications of cardiopulmonary arrest. *Arch Int Med* **142**: 500, 1982.

88. Black PM: Predicting the outcome from hypoxic-ischemic coma: Medical and ethical implications. *J Amer Med Assoc* **254**: 1215, 1985.

89. Blalock A: *Principles of Surgical Care, Shock and Other Problems*. St. Louis, Mosby, 1940.

90. Bleyaert AL, Nemoto EM, Safar P, et al: Thiopental amelioration of brain damage after global ischemia in monkeys. *Anesthesiology* **49**: 390, 1978.

91. Bleyaert AL, Sands PA, Safar P, et al: Augmentation of post-ischemic brain damage by severe intermittent hypertension. *Crit Care Med* **8**: 41, 1980.

92. Bleyaert A, Safar P, Nemoto E, et al: Effect of post-circulatory-arrest life-support on neurological recovery in monkeys. *Crit Care Med* **8**: 153, 1980.

93. Boehm R: Ueber Wiederbelebung nach Vergiftungen und Asphyxie. *Arch Exp Pathol Pharmakol* **8**: 68, 1878.

94. Boidin MP: Airway patency in the unconscious patient. *Brit J Anesth* **57**: 306, 1985.

95. Borgers M, Thone F, VanReempts J, et al: The role of calcium in cellular dysfunction. *Amer J Emerg Med* **2**: 154, 1983.

96. Boyan CT: Cold or warmed blood for massive transfusions. *Ann Surg* **160**: 282, 1964.

97. Bozhiev AA, Tolova SV, Trubina E: Peculiar features of resuscitation with the use of extracorporeal circulation. *Kardiologiia* **14**: 101, 1976 (in Russian).

98. Bozza-Marrubini M: Classifications of coma. *Intensive Care Med* **10**: 217, 1984.

99. Brader E, Klain M, Safar P, et al: High frequency jet ventilation vs. IPPV for CPR in dogs. *Crit care Med* **9**: 162, 1981 (abstract).

100. Brader E, Jehle D, Safar P: Protective head cooling during cardiac arrest in dogs. *Ann Emerg Med* **14**: 510, 1985 (abstract).

101. Brantigan CO, Grow JB: Cricothyroidotomy: Elective use in respiratory problems requiring tracheotomy. *J Thorac Cardiovasc Surg* **71:** 72, 1976.
102. Braunwald E (Ed): *Heart Disease: A Textbook of Cardiovascular Medicine.* Philadelphia, WB Saunders, 1980.
103. Braunwald E: Mechanism of action of calcium-channel-blocking agents. *N Engl J Med* **307:** 1618, 1982.
104. Braunwald E, Kloner RA: Myocardial reperfusion. A double edged sword? *J Clin Invest* **76:** 1713, 1985.
105. Breinton M, Miller SE, Lim RC, et al: Acute abdominal aortic injuries. *J Trauma* **22/6:** 481, 1982.
106. Breivik H, Safar P, Sands P, et al: Clinical feasibility trials of barbiturate therapy after cardiac arrest. *Crit Care Med* **6:** 227, 1978.
107. Breivik H, Ulvik NM, Blikra G, et al: Life-supporting first aid self-training. *Crit Care Med* **8:** 659, 1980.
108. Brierley JB, Meldrum BS, Brown AW: The threshold and neuropathology of cerebral anoxic-ischemic cell change. *Arch Neurol* **29:** 367, 1973.
109. Brillman JA, Sanders AB, Otto CW, et al: Outcome of resuscitation from fibrillatory current using epinephrine and phenylephrine in dogs. *Crit Care Med* **13:** 912, 1985.
110. Brinkmeyer S, Safar P, Motoyama E, et al: Superiority of colloid over electrolyte solution for fluid resuscitation. *Crit Care Med* **9:** 369, 1981.
111. Brodersen P, Jorgensen EO: Cerebral blood flow and oxygen uptake, and cerebrospinal fluid biochemistry in severe coma. *J Neurol Neurosurg Psychiatry* **37:** 384, 1974.
112. Brophy TO'R: Complications of endotracheal intubation. *WFSA Lectures*; JSM Zorab, J Moyers (Eds) **2:** 275, 1984.
113. Brown DC, Lewis AJ, Criley JM: Asystole and its treatment: the possible role of the parasympathetic nervous system in cardiac arrest. *J Amer Coll Em Phys* **8:** 448, 1979.
113a. Brown CG, Werman HA, Davis EA, et al: The effects of graded doses of epinephrine on regional myocardial blood flow during cardiopulmonary resuscitation in swine. *Circulation* **75:** 491, 1987.
114. Bruce DA, Gennarelli TA, Langfitt TW: Resuscitation from coma due to head injury. *Crit Care Med* **6:** 254, 1978.
115. Buchaner M, Schreinemachers D, Visscher MB: Effect of bretylium tosylate on ventricular fibrillation threshold. *Arch Intern Med* **124:** 95, 1969.
116. Bulkley GB: The role of oxygen free radicals in human disease processes. *Surgery* **94:** 407, 1983.
117. Burkle FM Jr, Sanner PH, Wolcott BW (Eds): *Disaster Medicine.* New York, Medical Examination, 1984.
118. Byrne D, Pass HI, Neely WA, et al: External versus internal cardiac massage in normal and chronically ischemic dogs. *Am Surg* **46:** 657, 1980.
119. Caldwell G, Millar G, Quinn E, et al: Simple mechanical methods of cardioversion: a defence of the precordial thump and cough version. *Brit Med J (Clin Res)* **291:** 627, 1985.
120. Cantadore R, Vaagenes P, Safar P, et al: Cardiopulmonary bypass for resuscitation after prolonged cardiac arrest in dogs. *Ann Emerg Med* **13:** 398, 1984 (abstract).
121. Cantadore R, Vaagenes P, Safar P, et al: Post-resuscitation syndrome: Cardiovascular-metabolic-pulmonary derangements after prolonged cardiac arrest and intensive care in dogs. *Proceedings 7th European Congress of Anaesthesiology*, Vienna 1986. Vienna, W Maudrich, 1986.
122. Cantu R, Ames A, DiGancinto G: Hypotension: A major factor limiting recovery from cerebral ischemia. *J Surg Res* **9:** 525, 1969.
123. Carden NL, Steinhaus JE: Lidocaine resuscitation in cardiac ventricular fibrillation. *Circ Res* **4:** 680, 1956.
124. Caroline NL: Medical care in the streets. *J Amer Med Assoc* **237:** 43, 1977.
125a. Caroline NL: *Emergency Care in the Streets.* Boston, Little Brown, 1979, 1983, 1987.
125b. Caroline NL: *Ambulance Calls. Review Problems in Emergency Care.* Boston, Little Brown, 1980, 1987.

125c. Caroline NL: *Emergency Medical Treatment. A Text for EMT-As and EMT-Intermediates.* Boston, Little Brown, 1982, 1987.

126. Caroline NL: *Life Supporting Resuscitation and First Aid: A manual for instructors of the lay public.* Guidelines of the League of Red Cross and Red Crescent Societies (LRCS) and the World Federation of Societies of Anaesthesiologists (WFSA), 1984. Geneva, LRCS, 17 Chemin des Crets, 1211 Geneva 19, Switzerland.

127. Caroline NL: Emergency medical services (EMS) lessons for worldwide health care (1981). *J World Assoc Emerg Disaster Med* 1/Suppl I:67, 1985.

128. Carroll R, Hedden M, Safar P: Intratracheal cuffs: performance characteristics. *Anesthesiology* 31: 275, 1969.

129. Carroll RG, Kamen JM, Grenvik A, et al: Recommended performance specifications for cuffed endotracheal and tracheostomy tubes: A joint statement of investigators, inventors, and manufacturers. *Crit Care Med* 1: 155, 1973.

130. Carson BS, Lasry BW, Bowes WA, et al: Combined obstetric and pediatric approach to prevent meconium aspiration syndrome. *Am J Obstet Gynecology* 126: 712, 1976.

131. Carveth SW, Burnap TK, Bechtel J, et al: Training in advanced cardiac life support. *J Amer Med Assoc* 235: 2311, 1976.

132a. Center for Disease Control (Atlanta, GA, USA): (1) Recommendations for decontaminating manikins used in cardiopulmonary resuscitation. *Hepatitis Surveillance Report* 42: 34, 1978. (2) Recommendations for preventing transmission of infection with Human T-Lymphotropic Virus Type III/Lymphadenopathy-Associated Virus in the workplace. *Morbidity and Mortality Weekly Report* 34(45): 681, 1985. CDC, 1600 Clifton Road, NE, Atlanta, GA 30333, USA.

132b. Center for Disease Control (Atlanta, GA, USA): Task Force report on acquired immune deficiency syndrome (AIDS). *New Engl J Med* 309: 740, 1983.

133. Cerchiari E, Hoel TM, Safar P, et al: Effect of anoxic reperfusion, superoxide dismutase and deferoxamine therapy on cerebral blood flow and metabolism and somato-sensory evoked potentials after asphyxial cardiac arrest in dogs. *Crit Care Med* 14: 390, 1986 (abstract). *Stroke*, in press, Dec 1987.

134. Cerchiari EL, Klein E, Safar P, et al: Cardiovascular component of the post-resuscitation syndrome after cardiac arrest in dogs. Proc. International Resuscitation Research Symposium: The Reversibility of Clinical Death, May 2–4, 1987, Pittsburgh PA, USA. *Crit Care Med*, in press (abstract).

135. Cerchiari E, Sclabassi R, Safar P, et al: Post-cardiac arrest predictive correlations with outcome, of cerebral electrophysiologic and clinical recovery patterns in dogs. In preparation.

136. Chaillou A: *La serum-thérapie et le tubage du larynx dans les croups diphtériques.* Paris, 1895.

137. Chameides L, Brown GE, Raye JR, et al: Guidelines for defibrillation in infants and children: Amer Heart Assoc Target Activity Group: CPR in the young. *Circulation* 56(Suppl): 502A, 1977.

138. Champion HR, Sacco W, Carnazzo AJ, et al: The trauma score. *Crit Care Med* 9: 672, 1981.

139. Chandra N, Rudikoff MT, Weisfeldt ML: Simultaneous chest compression and ventilation at high airway pressure during cardiopulmonary resuscitation. *Lancet* i: 175, 1980.

140. Chandra N, Snyder LD, Weisfeldt ML: Abdominal binding during cardiopulmonary resuscitation in man. *J Amer Med Assoc* 246: 351, 1981.

140a. Chandra N: New techniques of cardiopulmonary resuscitation. In: *Cardiopulmonale und cerebrale Reanimation (CPCR).* W Mauritz, K Steinbereithner, Eds. Vienna, Verlag Wilhelm Maudrich, 1987.

141. Chapman JH, Menapace FJ, Howell RR: Ruptured aortic valve cusp: A complication of the Heimlich maneuver. *Ann Emerg Med* 12: 446, 1983.

142. Chazov EI: Nuclear war, the ultimate disaster. *J World Assoc Emerg Disaster Med* 1/1: 5, 1985.

143. Chernow B, Holbrook P, D'Angona DS Jr, et al: Epinephrine absorbed after intratracheal administration. *Anesth Analg* 63: 829, 1984.

144. Chernow B, Lake CR (Eds): *The Pharmacologic Approach to the Critically Ill Patient.* Baltimore, Williams & Wilkins, 1983.
145. Cheung JY, Bonventre JV, Malis CD, et al: Calcium and ischemic injury. *New Engl J Med* **314:** 1670, 1986.
146. Chow MSS, Ronfeld RA, Ruffett D, et al: Lidocaine pharmacokinetics during cardiac arrest and external cardiopulmonary resuscitation. *Am Heart J* **102:** 799, 1981.
147. Cingolani HE, Faulkner SL, Mattiazzi AR, et al: Depression of human myocardial contractility with 'respiratory' and 'metabolic' acidosis. *Surgery* **77:** 427, 1975.
148. Civil Defense Office, Bern: The civil defense system of Switzerland. *J World Assoc Emerg Disaster Med* **1/1:** 12, 1985.
149. Clements JA: Pulmonary surfactant. *Amer Rev Resp Dis* **101,** 984, 1970.
150. Clemmesen C, Nilsson E: Therapeutic trends in the treatment of barbiturate poisoning. *Clin Pharmacol Ther* **2:** 220, 1961.
151. Cleveland JC: Complete recovery after cardiac arrest for three hours. *N Engl J Med* **284:** 334, 1971.
152. Clusin WT, Bristow MR, Baim DS, et al: The effects of diltiazem and reduced serum ionized calcium on ischemic ventricular fibrillation in the dog. *Circ Res* **50:** 518, 1982.
153. Cobb LA, Werner JA, Trobaugh GB: Sudden cardiac death. 1 A decade's experience with out-of-hospital resuscitation. 2 Outcome of resuscitation: Management and future directions. *Modern Concepts of Cardiovasc Dis (Amer Heart Assoc)* **49:** 1, 37, 1980.
154. Cole S, Corday E: Four-minute limit for cardiac resuscitation. *J Amer Med Assoc* **161:** 1454, 1956.
155. Collinsworth KA, Kalman SM, Harrison DC: The clinical pharmacology of lidocaine as an anti-arrhythmic drug. *Circulation* **40:** 1217, 1974.
156. Comroe JH, Dripps RD, Dumke PR, et al: Oxygen toxicity: the effect of inhalation of high concentrations of oxygen for 24 hours on normal men at sea level and at a simulated altitude of 18 000 feet. *J Amer Med Assoc* **128:** 710, 1945.
157. Comroe JH, Dripps RD: Artificial respiration. *J Amer Med Assoc* **130:** 381, 1946.
158a. Conn AW, Edmonds JF, Barker GA: Near drowning in cold fresh water: Current treatment regimen. *Can Anaesth Soc J* **25:** 259, 1978.
158b. Conn AW, Edmonds JF, Barker GA: Cerebral resuscitation in near-drowning. *Paediatr Clin North Am* **4:** 127, 1979.
159. Cooper MA: Lightening injuries: Prognostic signs for death. *Ann Emerg Med* **9:** 134, 1980.
160. Cordero L, Hon EH: Neonatal bradycardia following nasopharyngeal stimulation. *J Pediatrics* **78:** 441, 1971.
161. Council of National Cooperation in Aquatics: *The New Science of Skin and Scuba Diving.* New York, Association Press, 1970.
162. Cournand A, Morley HL, Werko L, et al: Physiological studies of the effects of intermittent positive pressure breathing on cardiac output in man. *Amer J Physiol* **152:** 162, 1948.
163. Cowley RA, Trump BF (Eds): *Pathophysiology of Shock, Anoxia, and Ischemia.* Baltimore, Williams & Wilkins, 1981.
164a. Cowley RA, Dunham CM: *Shock Trauma/Critical Care Manual.* Initial Assessment and Management. Baltimore, University Park Press, 1982.
164b. Cowley RA: The total emergency medical system for the state of Maryland. *Maryland State Med J*, July 1975.
165. Cowley RA, Ramzy AI, McAllister P (Eds): Focus on disasters. Proceedings of the Second International Assembly on Emergency Medical Services, Baltimore, April 1986. *J World Assoc Emerg Disaster Med* **2/1–4,** 1986.
166. Crafoord C: Pulmonary ventilation and anaesthesia in major chest surgery. *J Thorac Surg* **9:** 237, 1940.
167. Crampton RS, Aldrich RF, Stillerman R, et al: Prehospital CPR in acute myocardial infarction. *N Engl J Med* **286:** 1320, 1972.
168. Cranford R: Termination of treatment in persistent vegetative state. *Seminars Neurol* **4/1:** 36, 1984.

169. Crile GW, Dolley DH: An experimental research into the resuscitation of dogs killed by anesthetics and asphyxia. *J Exp Med* **8:** 713, 1906.
170. Criley JM, Blaufuss AJ, Kissel GL, et al: Cough-induced cardiac compression: self-administered form of cardiopulmonary resuscitation. *J Amer Med Assoc* **236:** 1246, 1976.
171. Criley JM, Niemann JT, Rosborough JP, et al: Modifications of cardiopulmonary resuscitation based on the cough. *Circulation* 74(suppl IV):42, 1986.
172. Croom EW: Rupture of stomach after attempted Heimlich maneuver. *J Amer Med Assoc* **250:** 2602, 1983.
173. Crowell JW, Jones CE, Smith EE: Effects of allopurinol on hemorrhagic shock. *Amer J Physiol* **16:** 744, 1969.
174. Crul JF, Neursing BTJ, Zimmerman AHE: The ABC sequence of cardiopulmonary resuscitation. *J World Assoc Emerg Disaster Med* 1/Suppl I:236, 1985.
175. Cullen JP, Aldrete JA, Jankovsky L, et al: Protective action of phenytoin in cerebral ischemia. *Anesth Analg* **58:** 165, 1979.
176a. Cummins RO, Eisenberg MS, Bergner L, et al: Sensitivity, accuracy and safety of an automatic external defibrillator: Report of a field evaluation. *Lancet* **ii:** 318, 1984.
176b. Cummins RO, Eisenberg MS, Graves JR, et al: Automatic external defibrillators used by emergency medical technicians: A controlled clinical trial. *Crit Care Med* **13:** 945, 1985.
177. Cummins RO, Eisenberg MS: Prehospital cardiopulmonary resuscitation. *J Amer Med Assoc* **253:** 2408, 1985.
178. Dahl CF, Ewy GA, Warner ED, et al: Myocardial necrosis from direct current countershock. *Circulation* **50:** 956, 1974.
179. Damir EA, Axelrod AY: Pathophysiological basis of choosing anaesthesia according to vital indices in patients in terminal states. In: *Osnovy Reanimatologii.* Moscow, 1966, p 284 (in Russian).
180. Dauchot P, Gravenstein JS: Bradycardia after myocardial ischemia and its treatment with atropine. *Anesthesiology* **44:** 501, 1976.
181. Dawes GS: *Foetal and Neonatal Physiology.* Chicago, Yearbook Med Publ, 1968.
182. Dawidson I, Haglind E, Gelin LE: Hemodilution and oxygen transport to tissue in shock. *Acta Chir Scand Suppl* **489:** 245, 1979.
183a. Day R, Crelin ES, DuBois AB: Choking: The Heimlich abdominal thrust vs. back blows: An approach to measurement of inertial and aerodynamic forces. *Pediatrics* **70,** 113, 1982.
183b. Day R: Differing opinions on the emergency treatment of choking. *Pediatrics* **71:** 976, 1983.
184. Defore WW Jr, Mattox KL, Jordan GL Jr, et al: Management of 1590 consecutive cases of liver trauma. *Arch Surg* **11:** 493, 1976.
185. Del Guercio LRM, Feins NR, Cohn JD, et al: A comparison of blood flow during external and internal cardiac massage in man. *Circulation* **30:** 63, 1964; 31/32 (suppl. 1): 171, 1965.
186. Del Maestro RF: An approach to free radicals in medicine and biology. *Acta Physiol Scand* **492:** 153, 1980.
187. Dembo DH: Calcium in advanced life support. *Crit Care Med* **9:** 358, 1981.
188. Demopoulos HB, Flamm ES, Pietronigro DD, et al: The free radical pathology and the microcirculation in major central nervous system disorders. *Acta Physiol Scand* **492**(Suppl): 91, 1980.
189. Deshmukh H, Weil MH, Swindall A, et al: Echocardiographic observations during cardiopulmonary resuscitation: A preliminary report. *Crit Care Med* **13:** 904, 1985.
190. DeSilva RA, Hennekens CH, Lown B, et al: Lignocaine prophylaxis in acute myocardial infarction: An evaluation of randomized trials. *Lancet* **ii:** 855, 1981.
191. Detre K, Abramson N, Safar P, et al: Collaborative randomized clinical study of cardiopulmonary-cerebral resuscitation. *Crit Care Med* **9:** 395, 1981.
192. DeVenuto F (Ed): Symposium issue. Acellular oxygen-delivering resuscitation fluids. *Crit Care Med* **10:** 237, 1982.

193. Diack AW, Welborn WS, Rullman RG, et al: An automatic cardiac resuscitator for emergency treatment of cardiac arrest. *Med Instrum* **13:** 78, 1979.

194. Dick W, Ahnefeld FW: Proposals for standardized tests of manually operated resuscitators for respiratory resuscitation. *Resuscitation* **4:** 149, 1975.

195. Dick W, Hirlinger WK, Mehrkens HH: Intramuscular ketamine: an alternative pain treatment for use in disasters? *Emergency and Disaster Medicine.* C Manni, SI Magalini (Eds). Heidelberg, Springer-Verlag, 1985, p 167.

196. Dick WF: Mobile intensive care unit. *J World Assoc Emerg Disaster Med* 1/Suppl I: 139, 1985.

197. Dikshit K, Vyden JK, Forrester JS, et al: Renal and extrarenal hemodynamic effects of furosemide in congestive heart failure after acute myocardial infarction. *N Engl J Med* **288:** 1087, 1973.

198. Ditchey RV, Winkler JV, Rhodes CA: Relative lack of coronary blood flow during closed-chest resuscitation in dogs. *Circulation* **66:** 297, 1982.

199. Ditchey RV, Lindenfeld JA: Potential adverse effects of volume loading on perfusion of vital organs during closed-chest resuscitation. *Circulation* **69:** 181, 1984.

200. Don Michael TE, Lambert EH, Mehran A: Mouth-to-lung airway for cardiac resuscitation. *Lancet* **2:** 1329, 1968

201. Don Michael TA: The role of the esophageal obturator airway in cardiopulmonary resuscitation. *Circulation* 74(suppl IV):134, 1986.

202. Donegan JH (Ed): *Cardiopulmonary Resuscitation: Physiology, Pharmacology, and Practical Application.* Springfield, IL, Charles C. Thomas, 1982.

203. Dorrance GM: On the treatment of traumatic injuries of the lungs and pleurae. *Surg Gynecol Obstet* **11:** 160, 1910.

204. Dortmann C, Croh R, Frey R: Der Mainzer Notarztwagen. *Anaesthesist* **19:** 212, 1970.

205. Downes JJ, Wood DW, Harwood I, et al: Intravenous isoproterenol infusion in children with severe hypercapnia due to status asthmaticus: Effects on ventilation, circulation, and clinical score. *Crit Care Med* **1:** 63, 1973.

206. Downs JB, Kleir EF, Desautels D, et al: Intermittent mandatory ventilation: A new approach to weaning patients from mechanical ventilators. *Chest* **64:** 331, 1973.

207. Draper WB, Whitehead RW: The phenomenon of diffusion respiration. *Anesth Analg* **28:** 307, 1949.

208. Dripps RD, Kirby CK, Johnson J, et al: Cardiac resuscitation. *Ann Surg* **127:** 592, 1948.

209. Dripps RD, Eckenhoff JE, Vandam LR: *Introduction to Anesthesia.* Philadelphia, WB Saunders, 1957, 1982.

210. Dunn P: Localization of the umbilical catheter by post-mortem measurement. *Arch Dis Child* **41:** 61, 1966.

211. Durrer JD, Lie KI, van Capelle JL, et al: Effect of sodium nitroprusside on mortality in acute myocardial infarction. *N Engl J Med* **306:** 1121, 1982.

212. Eckenhoff JE: Some anatomic considerations of the infant larynx influencing endotracheal anesthesia. *Anesthesiology* **12:** 401, 1951.

213. Edgren E, Terent H, Hedstrand U, et al: Cerebral spinal fluid markers in relation to outcome in patients with global cerebral ischemia. *Crit Care Med* **11:** 4, 1983.

214a. Edgren E, Sutton K, Abramson NS, et al: Early predictors of poor neurologic outcome in comatose cardiac arrest survivors. *Anesthesiology* **85:** A88, 1986 (abstract).

214b Edgren E: The Prognosis of Hypoxic-Ischaemic Brain Damage Following Cardiac Arrest. PhD Thesis, University of Uppsala, Sweden. *Acta Universitatis Upsaliensis* **89:** 44, 1987.

215. Einthoven W, Fahr G, DeWaart A: On the direction and manifest size of the variations of potential in the human heart and on the influence of the position of the heart on the form of the electrocardiogram. *Pfluegers Arch Ges Physiol* **150:** 275, 1913 (in English: *Amer Heart J* **40:** 163, 1950).

216a. Eisenberg MS, Bergner L, Hallstrom A: Cardiac resuscitation in the community: Importance of rapid provision and implications for program planning. *J Amer Med Assoc* **241:** 1905, 1979.

216b.   Eisenberg MS, Hallstrom A, Bergner L: Long-term survival after out-of-hospital cardiac arrest. *N Engl J Med* **306:** 1340, 1982.

216c.   Eisenberg MS, Bergner L, Hallstrom AP: *Sudden Cardiac Death in the Community.* New York, Praeger, 1984.

217.   Eisenberg MS, Copass MK, Hallstrom AP: Treatment of out-of-hospital cardiac arrest with rapid defibrillation by emergency medical technicians. *New Engl J Med* **302:** 1379, 1980.

218.   Eisenberg MS, Bergner L, Hallstrom A: Epidemiology of cardiac arrest and resuscitation in children. *Ann Emerg Med* **12:** 672, 1983.

219.   Eisenberg MS, Cummins RO, Moore J, et al: Use of automatic external defibrillators in the home. *Crit Care Med* **13:** 946, 1985.

220.   Elam JO, Brown ES, Elder JD, Jr: Artificial respiration by mouth-to-mask method. A study of the respiratory gas exchange of paralyzed patients ventilated by operator's expired air. *N Engl J Med* **250:** 749, 1954.

221.   Elam JO, Greene DG, Brown ES, et al: Oxygen and carbon dioxide exchange and energy cost of expired air resuscitation. *J Amer Med Assoc* **167:** 328, 1958.

222.   Elam JO, Greene DG, Schneider MA, et al: Head-tilt method of oral resuscitation. *J Amer Med Assoc* **172:** 812, 1960.

223.   Elam JO, Greene DG: Mission accomplished: successful mouth-to-mouth resuscitation. *Anesth Analg* **40:** 440, 578, 672, 1961.

224.   Elam JO, Ruben AM, Greene DG: Mouth-to-nose resuscitation during convulsive seizures. *J Amer Med Assoc* **176:** 565, 1961.

225.   Elam JO: The intrapulmonary route for CPR drugs. In: *Advances in Cardiopulmonary Resuscitation.* P Safar, JO Elam (Eds). New York, Springer-Verlag 1977, Chapter 21.

226.   Elam JO, ViaReque E, Rattenborg CC: Esophageal electrocardiography and low energy ventricular defibrillation. In: *Advances in Cardiopulmonary Resuscitation.* P Safar, JO Elam (Eds). New York, Springer-Verlag, 1977, Chapter 26.

227.   Eltringham RJ, Baskett PJF: Experiences with a hospital resuscitation service. *Resuscitation* **2:** 57, 1973.

228.   Engstrom CG: The clinical application of prolonged controlled ventilation. *Acta Anaesth Scand* Suppl 13, 1963.

229.   Epstein MF: Resuscitation: In: *Schaffer's Diseases of the Newborn.* ME Avery, HW Taeusch, Jr (Eds). Philadelphia, WB Saunders, 1984, p 100.

230.   Ernster L: Oxygen as an environmental poison. *Chemica Scripta* **26:** 525, 1986.

231.   Eross B: Nonslipping, nonkinking airway connections for respiratory care. *Anesthesiology* **34:** 571, 1971.

232.   Eshani A, Ewy GA, Sobel BE: Effects of electrical countershock on serum creatinine phosphokinase (CPK) isoenzyme activity. *Am J Cardiol* **37:** 12, 1976.

233.   Esmarch JF: *The Surgeon's Handbook on the Treatment of Wounded in War.* New York, Schmidt, 1878, p 113.

234.   Esposito G, Safar P, Medsger A: Life supporting first aid (LSFA) self-training for the public. *J World Assoc Emerg Disaster Med* 1/Suppl I: 91, 1985.

235.   Ewy GA, Hellman DA, McClung S, et al: Influence of ventilation phase on transthoracic impedance and defibrillation effectiveness. *Crit Care Med* **8:** 164, 1980.

236.   Ewy GA, Dahl CF, Zimmerman M, et al: Ventricular fibrillation masquerading as ventricular standstill. *Crit Care Med* **12:** 41, 1981.

237.   Ewy GA: Electrical therapy for cardiovascular emergencies. *Circulation* **74**(suppl IV) 111, 1986.

238.   Fairley HB: The Toronto General Hospital respiratory unit. *Anaesthesia* **16:** 267, 1961.

239.   Feustel PJ, Ingvar MC, Severinghaus JW: Cerebral oxygen availability and blood flow during middle cerebral artery occlusion: effects of pentobarbital. *Stroke* **12:** 858, 1981.

240.   Fink BR: The etiology and treatment of laryngeal spasm. *Anesthesiology* **17:** 569, 1956.

240a.   Firt P, Hejhal L: Treatment of severe hemorrhage. *Lancet* **273:** 1132, 1957.

241.   Fischer EG, Ames A: Studies on mechanisms of impairment of cerebral circulation following ischemia: effect of hemodilution and perfusion pressure. *Stroke* **3:** 538, 1972.

242. Fisher J, Vaghaiwalla F, Tsitlik J, et al: Determinations and clinical significance of jugular venous valve competence. *Circulation* **65:** 188, 1982.

243. Flagg PJ: *The Art of Resuscitation*. New York, Reinhold, 1944.

244. Flameng W, Daenen W, Borgers M, et al: Cardioprotective effects of lidoflazine during 1-hour normothermic global ischemia. *Circulation* **64:** 796, 1981.

245. Flameng W, Xhonneux R, Borgers M: Myocardial protection in open-heart surgery. In: *Protection of Tissues against Hypoxia*. A Wauquier, M Borgers M, WK Amery (Eds). Amsterdam/New York, Elsevier, 1982, p. 403.

246. Fleckenstein A: *Calcium Antagonism in Heart and Smooth Muscle. Experimental Facts and Therapeutic Potentials*. New York, John Wiley, 1983.

246a. Fleischer JE, Lanier WL, Milde JH, et al: Effect of lidoflazine on cerebral blood flow and neurologic outcome when administered after complete cerebral ischemia in dogs. *Anesthesiology* **66:** 304, 1987.

247. Foldes FF: *Muscle Relaxants in Anesthesiology*. Springfield, IL, Charles C Thomas, 1957.

248. Foldes FF, Swerdlow M, Siker ES: *Narcotics and Narcotic Antagonists*. Springfield, IL, Charles C Thomas, 1964.

249. Forbes WH: Carbon monoxide. In: *Artificial Respiration*. JL Whittenberger (Ed). New York, Hoeber (Harper and Row), 1962, p 194.

250. Forrester JS, Diamond G, Chatterjee K, et al: Medical therapy of acute myocardial infarction by application of hemodynamic subsets. *N Engl J Med* **295:** 1356 and **295:** 1404, 1976.

251. Francis GS, Sharma B, Hodges M: Comparative hemodynamic effects of dopamine and dobutamine in patients with acute cardiogenic circulatory collapse. *Amer Heart J* **103:** 995, 1982.

252. Frey R, Jude J, Safar P: External cardiac resuscitation. Indication, technique and results. *Deutsche Med Wchschr* **17:** 857, 1962.

253. Frey R, Eyrich K, Lutz H, et al: *Infusionstherapie*. Munich, Aesopus Verlag, 1974.

254. Frey R, Nagel E, Safar P (Eds): Mobile intensive care units. Advanced emergency care delivery systems. Symposium Mainz 1973. *Anesthesiology and Resuscitation* Vol. 95. Heidelberg, Springer-Verlag, 1976.

255. Frey R: The Club of Mainz for improved worldwide emergency and critical care medicine systems and disaster preparedness. *Crit Care Med* **6:** 389, 1978.

256. Frey R, Safar P (Eds): Proceedings of the First World Congress on Emergency and Disaster Med (Club of Mainz), Mainz, 1977. (Vol. 1) *Types and Events of Disasters. Organization in Various Disaster Situations.* (Vol. 2) *Resuscitation and Life Support, Relief of Pain and Suffering. Disaster Medicine.* Heidelberg, Springer-Verlag, 1980.

256a Frey R, Huegin W, Mayrhofer O: *Lehrbuch der Anaesthesiologie und Wiederbelebung*. 5th Ed. Berlin, Springer-Verlag, 1982.

257. Freye E: Cardiovascular effects of high dosages of fentanyl, meperidine, and naloxone in dogs. *Anesth Analg* **53:** 40, 1974.

258. Fridovich I: Superoxide radical: an endogenous toxicant. *Ann Rev Pharmacol Toxicol* **23:** 239, 1983.

259. Frumin MJ, Epstein RM, Cohen G: Apneic oxygenation in man. *Anesthesiology* **20:** 789, 1959.

260. Fulton FL: Penetrating wounds of the heart. *Heart and Lung* **7/2:** 262, 1978.

261. Gallup G: *Adventures in Immortality*. New York, McGraw-Hill, 1982.

262. Gamelli R, Saucier J, Browdie D: An analysis of cerebral blood flow, systemic base deficit accumulation, and mean arterial pressure as a function of internal cardiac massage rates. *Amer Surg* **45:** 26, 1979.

263. Garfein OB (Ed): Clinical pharmacology of cardiac antiarrhythmic agents. *Ann New York Acad Sci* **432:** 1, 1984.

264. Gascho JA, Crampton RS, Sipes JN, et al: Energy levels and patient weight in ventricular defibrillation. *J Amer Med Assoc* **242:** 1380, 1979.

265. Gattinoni L, Kolobow T, Tomminson T, et al: Low frequency positive pressure ventilation with extracorporeal carbon dioxide removal (LFPPV-ECCO$_2$R): An experimental study. *Anes Analg* **57:** 470, 1978.

266. Gauger GE: What do 'fixed, dilated pupils' mean? *N Engl J Med* **284:** 1105, 1971.

267a. Geddes LA, Tacker WA, Rosborough JP, et al: Electrical dose for ventricular defibrillation of large and small animals using precordial electrodes. *J Clin Invest* **53:** 310, 1974.

267b. Geddes LA, Tacker WA, Cabler P, et al: The decrease in transthoracic impedance during successive ventricular defibrillation trials. *Med Instrum* **9:** 179, 1975.

268. Geehr EC, Lewis FR, Auerbach PS: Failure of open-heart massage to improve survival after prehospital nontraumatic cardiac arrest. *N Engl J Med* **314:** 1189, 1986.

269. Gelin LW, Solvell L, Zederfeldt A: The plasma volume expanding effect of low viscous dextran and macrodex. *Acta Chir Scand* **122:** 309, 1969.

270. Gelin LE: Reaction of the body as a whole to injury. *J Trauma* **10:** 932, 1970.

271. Gerst PH, Fleming WH, Malm Jr: Increased susceptibility of the heart to ventricular fibrillation during metabolic acidosis. *Circ Res* **19:** 63, 1966.

272. Geyer RP, Monroe RG, Taylor K: Survival of rats having red cells totally replaced with emulsified fluorocarbon. *N Engl J Med* **289:** 1077, 1973.

273. Gibbon JH Jr: Application of mechanical heart and lung to cardiac surgery. *Minn Med* **37:** 171, 1954.

274. Gillespie NA: *Endotracheal Anesthesia*. Madison, WI, University of Wisconsin Press, 1950.

275. Gilroy J, Barnhart MI, Meyer JS: Treatment of acute stroke with dextran 40. *J Amer Med Assoc* **210:** 293, 1969.

276. Ginsberg MD, Myers RE: The topography of microvascular perfusion in the primate brain following total circulatory arrest. *Neurology* **22:** 998, 1972.

277. Gisvold SE, Safar P, Rao G, et al: Prolonged immobilization and controlled ventilation do not improve outcome after global brain ischemia in monkeys. *Crit Care Med* **12:** 171, 1984.

278. Gisvold SE, Safar P, Hendrickx HHL, et al: Thiopental treatment after global brain ischemia in pigtail monkeys. *Anesthesiology* **60:** 88, 1984.

279. Gisvold SE, Safar P, Saito R, et al: Multifaceted therapy after global brain ischemia in monkeys. *Stroke* **15:** 803, 1984.

280. Gisvold SE, Safar P, Alexander H, et al: Cardiovascular tolerance of thiopental anesthesia for brain resuscitation in monkeys. *Acta Anaesth Scand* **29(3):** 339: 1985.

281. Gold HK, Leinbach RC, Saunders CA: Use of sublingual nitroglycerin in congestive failure following acute myocardial infarction. *Circulation* **46:** 839, 1972.

282. Goldberg LI, Hseih YY, Resnekov L: Newer catecholamines for treatment of heart failure and shock: An update on dopamine and a first look at dobutamine. *Prog Cardiovasc Dis* **19:** 327, 1977.

283. Goldberger E: Modes of cardiac pacing. In: *Treatment of Cardiac Emergencies*. St. Louis, CV Mosby, 1977, p. 219.

284. Goldstein A, Wells BA, Keats AS: Increased tolerance to cerebral anoxia by pentobarbital. *Arch Intern Pharmacodynamie Thérapie* **161:** 138, 1966.

285. Goldstein RA, Passamani ER, Roberts R: A comparison of digoxin and dobutamine in patients with acute infarction and cardiac failure. *N Engl J Med* **303:** 846, 1980.

286. Gomes JAC, Hariman RI, Kang PS, et al: Programmed electrical stimulation in patients with high-grade ventricular ectopy: Electrophysiologic findings and prognosis for survival. *Circulation* **70:** 43, 1984.

287. Goodman LS, Gilman A: *The Pharmacological Basis of Therapeutics*. New York, MacMillan, 1985.

288. Gordon AS, Sadove MS, Raymon F, et al: Critical survey of manual artificial respiration. *J Amer Med Assoc* **147:** 1444, 1951.

289. Gordon AS, Frye CW, Gittelson L, et al: Mouth-to-mouth versus manual artificial respiration for children and adults. *J Amer Med Assoc* **167:** 320, 1958.

290. Gordon AS, Belton MK, Ridolpho PF: Emergency management of foreign body airway obstruction. Comparison of artificial cough techniques, manual extraction maneuvers, and simple mechanical devices. In: *Advances in Cardiopulmonary Resuscitation*. P Safar, JO Elam (Eds). New York, Springer-Verlag, 1977, p 39.

291. Gordon AS: Improved esophageal obturator airway and new esophageal gastric tube airway. In: *Advances in Cardiopulmonary Resuscitation*. P Safar, JO Elam (Eds). New York, Springer-Verlag, 1977, p 58.

292. Gordon AS: CPR training films. (a) *Breath of Life (Steps A and B)*; (b) *Pulse of Life (Steps A, B and C)*; (c) *Prescription for Life (Steps A–D)*; and (d) *Life in the Balance (Cardiac Care Unit)*. Amer Heart Assoc, 7320 Greenville Ave, Dallas, TX 75231, USA, 1960s; 1980s. Also from: Pyramid Films, Box 1048, Santa Monica, CA 90406, USA, 1986.

293. Gordon E: Controlled respiration in the management of patients with traumatic brain injuries. *Acta Anaesth Scand* **15:** 193, 1971.

294. Grace WJ, Chadbourn JA: The first hour in acute myocardial infarction. *Heart Lung* **3:** 736, 1974.

295. Grace WJ, Kennedy RJ, Nolte CT: Blind defibrillation. *Amer J Cardiol* **34:** 115, 1974.

296. Graham JG, Mattox KL, Beall AC Jr: Penetrating trauma of the lung. *J Trauma* **19:** 665, 1979.

296a. Graham DI: The pathology of brain ischemia and possibilities for therapeutic intervention. *Brit J Anaesth* **57:** 3, 1985.

297. Greenbaum DM, Millen JE, Eross B, et al: Continuous positive airway pressure without tracheal intubation in spontaneously breathing patients. *Chest* **69:** 615, 1976.

298. Greenbaum DM: Secondary cardiac dysrhythmias. *Heart Lung* **6:** 308, 1977.

299. Greenberg M: CPR: A report of observed medical complications during training. *Ann Emerg Med* **12:** 194, 1983.

300. Greenberg RP, Ward JD, Lutz H, et al: Advanced monitoring of the brain. Brain Failure and Resuscitation. *Clinics in Crit Care Med*. A Grenvik, P Safar (Eds). New York, Churchill Livingstone, 1981.

301. Gregory GA, Kitterman JA, Phibbs RH, et al: Treatment of idiopathic respiratory distress syndrome with continuous positive airway pressure. *N Engl J Med* **284:** 1333, 1971.

302. Gregory GA: Resuscitation of the newborn. In: *Textbook of Critical Care*. WC Shoemaker, WL Thompson, PR Holbrook (Eds). Philadelphia, WB Saunders, 1984, p 19. Chapter 3.

303. Grenvik A: Respiratory, circulatory, and metabolic effects of respirator treatment: a clinical study in postoperative thoracic surgical patients. *Acta Anaesth Scand* (Suppl) **19:** 1, 1966.

304. Grenvik A, Safar P: Teaching films on life support techniques in intensive care. Film 1: *Respiratory Failure: Diagnosis and Airway Care*. Film 2: *Respiratory Failure: Prolonged Artificial Ventilation*. Film 3: *Monitoring and Support of Circulation*. Film 4: *General Care and Central Nervous System Monitoring*. 1970. Univ Pittsburgh Center for Instructional Resources, Pittsburgh, PA 15260, USA (Historic films).

305. Grenvik A, Powner DJ, Snyder JV, et al: Cessation of therapy in terminal illness and brain death. *Crit Care Med* **6:** 284, 1978.

306. Grenvik A, Safar P (Eds): *Brain Failure and Resuscitation*. Clinics in Critical Care Medicine. New York, Churchill Livingstone, 1981.

307. Grenvik A: Brain death and permanently lost consciousness. In: *Textbook of Critical Care*. WC Shoemaker, WL Thompson, PR Holbrook (Eds) Philadelphia, WB Saunders, 1984, p 968.

308. Grenvik A, Hardesty R, Griffith B, et al: Multiple organ procurement by interhospital transfer of heartbeating cadavers. *Transplantation Proc* **16:** 251, 1984.

309. Grillo HC, Cooper JD, Geffin B, et al: A low pressure cuff for tracheostomy tubes to minimize tracheal injury: A comparative clinical trial. *J Thorac Cardiovasc Surg* **62:** 898, 1971.

309a. Guerci AD, Shi AY, Levin H, et al: Transmission of intrathoracic pressure to the intracranial space during cardiopulmonary resuscitation in dogs. *Circ Res* **56:** 20, 1985.

309b. Grogono AW, Jastremski MS, Nugent W: Educational graffiti: better use of the bathroom wall. *J World Assoc Emerg Disaster Med* **1** (Suppl 1):93, 1985.

310. Guildner CW: Resuscitation—opening the airway. *J Amer Coll Emerg Phys* **5:** 588, 1976.
311. Guildner CW, Williams D, Subitch T: Emergency management for airway obstruction by foreign material. In: *Advances in Cardiopulmonary Resuscitation.* P Safar, JO Elam (Eds). New York, Springer-Verlag, 1977, p 51.
312. Gurvich NL, Yuniev SG: Restoration of a regular rhythm in the mammalian fibrillating heart. *Amer Rev Sov Med* **3:** 236, 1946.
313. Gurvitch AM, Romanova NP, Mutuskina EA: Quantitative evaluation of brain damage resulting from circulatory arrest to the central nervous system or the entire body: I. Electroencephalographic and histological evaluation of the severity of permanent post-ischaemic damage. *Resuscitation* **1:** 205, 1972.
314. Gurvitch AM, Mutuskina EA, Novoderzhkina IS: Quantitative evaluation of brain damage in dogs resulting from circulatory arrest to the central nervous system of the whole animal: II. Electroencephalographic evaluation during early recovery of the gravity and reversibility of post-ischaemic cerebral damage. *Resuscitation* **1:** 219, 1972.
315. Gurvitch AM: Determination of the depth and reversibility of postanoxic coma in animals. *Resuscitation* **3:** 1, 1974.
316. Gutgesell HP, Tacker WA, Geddes WA, Geddes LA, et al: Energy dose for ventricular defibrillation of children. *Pediatrics* **6:** 898, 1976.
317. Guyton AC: *Physiology of the Human Body.* Philadelphia, WB Saunders, 1985.
318. Hake TG: Studies on ether and chloroform from Prof. Schiff's physiological laboratory. *Practitioner* **12:** 241, 1874.
319. Hakim AM, Moss G: Cerebral effects of barbiturate. Shift from 'energy' to 'synthesis' metabolism for cellular viability. *Surg Forum* **27:** 497, 1976.
320. Hallenbeck JM, Leitch DR, Dutka AJ, et al: Prostaglandin I_2, indomethacin, and heparin promote postischemic neuronal recovery in dogs. *Ann Neurol* **12:** 145, 1982.
321. Hallenbeck JM, Dutka AJ, Tanishima T, et al: Polymorphonuclear leukocyte accumulation in brain regions with low blood flow during the early post-ischemic period. *Stroke* **17:** 246, 1986.
322. Hamm CW, Opie LH: Protection of infarcting myocardium by slow channel inhibitors. Comparative effects of verapamil, nifedipine, and diltiazem in the coronary-ligated, isolated working rat heart. *Circ Res* **52** (Suppl I): 129, 1983.
323. Hammargren Y, Clinton JE, Ruiz E: A standard comparison of esophageal obturator airway and endotracheal tube ventilation in cardiac arrest. *Ann Emerg Med* **14:** 953, 1985.
324. Harris CS, Baker SP, Smith GA, et al: Childhood asphyxiation by food. A national analysis and overview. *J Amer Med Assoc* **251:** 2231, 1984.
325. Harris LC, Kirimli B, Safar P: Augmentation of artificial circulation during cardiopulmonary resuscitation. *Anesthesiology* **28:** 730, 1967.
326. Harris LC, Kirimli B, Safar P: Ventilation-cardiac compression rates and ratios in cardiopulmonary resuscitation. *Anesthesiology* **28:** 806, 1967.
327. Harrison EE, Amey BD: Use of calcium in electromechanical dissociation. *Ann Emerg Med* **13:** 844, 1984.
328. Haugen RK: The cafe coronary. Sudden death in restaurants. *J Amer Med Assoc* **186:** 142, 1963.
329. Hect HH, Hutter OF: Action of pH on cardiac Purkinje fibers. *Fed Proc* **23:** 157, 1964.
330. Hedden M, Ersoz CJ, Safar P: Tracheoesophageal fistulas following prolonged artificial ventilation via cuffed tracheostomy tubes. *Anesthesiology* **31:** 281, 1969.
331. Hedden M, Ersoz CJ, Donnelly WH, et al: Laryngotracheal damage after prolonged use of orotracheal tubes in adults. *J Amer Med Assoc* **207:** 703, 1969.
332. Hedges JR, Barsan WB, Doan LA, et al: Central versus peripheral intravenous routes in cardiopulmonary resuscitation. *Amer J Emerg Med* **2:** 385, 1984.
333. Heiberg J: A new expedient in administering chloroform. *Med Times Gazette*, January 10, 1874.
334. Heimlich HJ: A life-saving maneuver to prevent food choking. *J Amer Med Assoc* **234:** 398, 1975.

335. Heimlich HJ, Hoffmann KA, Canestri FR: Food-choking and drowning deaths prevented by external subdiaphragmatic compresson: Physiological basis. *Ann Thorac Surg* **20:** 188, 1975.
336. Heimlich HJ: Subdiaphragmatic pressure to expel water from the lungs of drowning persons. *Ann Emerg Med* **10:** 476, 1981.
337. Hekmatpanah J: Cerebral blood flow dynamics in hypotension and cardiac arrest. *Neurology* **23:** 174, 1973.
338. Hendrickx H, Safar P, Rao GR, et al: Asphyxia, cardiac arrest and resuscitation in rats. I. Short-term recovery. *Resuscitation* **12:** 97, 1984. II. Long-term behavioral changes. *Resuscitation* **12:** 117, 1984.
339. Herman RE: *Disaster Planning for Local Government.* New York, Universe Books, 1982.
340. Hess D, Baran C: Ventilatory volumes using mouth-to-mouth, mouth-to-mask and bag valve mask techniques. *Amer J Emerg Med* **3:** 292, 1985.
341. Hess D, Kapp A, Kurtek W: The effect of the rescuer breathing supplemental oxygen during exhaled air ventilation. *Respiratory Care* **30:** 691, 1985.
342. Heymans C: Survival and revival of nervous tissue after arrest of the circulation. *Physiol Rev* **30:** 325, 1950.
343. Hilberman M, Maseda J, Stinson EB, et al: The diuretic properties of dopamine in patients after open-heart operation. *Anesthesiology* **61:** 489, 1984.
344. Hill JD, DeLevall MR, Fallat RJ, et al: Acute respiratory insufficiency: Treatment of prolonged extracorporeal oxygenation. *J Thorac Cardiovasc Surg* **64:** 551, 1972.
345. Hillered L, Ernster L: Respiratory activity of isolated rat brain mitochondria following in vitro exposure to oxygen radicals. *J Cereb Blood Flow Metab* **3:** 207, 1983.
346. Hillered L, Ernster L, Arfors K: Brain ischemia and oxygen radicals. In: *3rd International Symposium on Cerebral Ischemia.* J Geelen (Ed). Amsterdam, Elsevier Biomedical Press, 1984.
347. Hingson RA: Western Reserve anesthesia machine, oxygen inhalator and resuscitator. *J Amer Med Assoc* **167:** 1077, 1958.
348. Hoel TM, Safar P, Kazziha S, et al: General and neurologic recovery after 10 minutes ventricular fibrillation cardiac arrest in dogs treated with intravenous lidocaine post-arrest. In preparation.
349. Hoff JT: Resuscitation in focal brain ischemia. *Crit Care Med* **6:** 245, 1978.
350. Holbrook PR, Yeh HC: Outcome evaluation in critical care medicine. In: *Textbook of Critical Care.* WC Shoemaker, WL Thompson, PR Holbrook (Eds). Philadelphia, WB Saunders, 1984, p 1025. Chapter 122.
351a. Holmdahl MH: Pulmonary uptake of oxygen, acid–base metabolism, and circulation during prolonged apnea. *Acta Chir Scand* (Suppl) **212:** 1, 1956.
351b. Holmdahl MH. Control of acidosis in status asthmaticus with THAM. *1st Scand Soc Anesth Mtg,* Gausdal, Norway, 1958.
352. Holmdahl MH: Respiratory care unit. *Anesthesiology* **23:** 559, 1962.
353. Hooker DR, Kouwenhoven WB, Langworthy OR: Effect of alternating electrical currents on the heart. *Amer J Physiol* **103:** 444, 1933.
354. Horowitz LN, Josephson ME, Kastor JA: Intracardiac electrophysiologic studies as a method for the optimization of drug therapy in chronic ventricular arrhythmia. *Prog Cardiovasc Dis* **23:** 81, 1980.
355. Hosobuchi Y, Baskin DS, Woo SK: Reversal of postischemic neurologic deficit in gerbils by the opiate antagonist naloxone. *Science* **215:** 69, 1982.
356. Hossli G: Die Behandlung des Bewusstlosen durch den praktischen Arzt. *Z Aerztl Fortbild* **51:** 955, 1962.
357. Hossmann KA, Kleihues P: Reversibility of ischemic brain damage. *Arch Neurol* **29:** 375, 1973.
358. Hossmann KA: Review: Treatment of experimental cerebral ischemia. *J Cereb Blood Flow Metab* **2:** 275, 1982.
359. Hossmann KA: Animal experimental models and treatment of cerebral ischemia. *Maladies et Medicaments/Drugs and Diseases* **1:** 13, 1984.

360. Houle DB, Weil MH, Brown EB Jr, et al: Influence of respiratory acidosis on ECG and pressor responses to epinephrine, norepinephrine and metaraminol. *Proc Soc Exp Biol Med* **94**: 561, 1957.

361. Howland WS, Schweizer O: Physiologic compensation for storage lesion of banked blood. *Anesth Analg* **44**: 8, 1965.

362. Huch A, Huch R, Lübbers DW: Quantitative polarographische Sauerstoff druckmessung auf der Kopfhaut des Neugeborenen. *Arch Gynaek* **207**: 443, 1969.

363. Huguenard P: Artificial hibernation. *Anaesthesist* **1**: 33, 1953.

364. Ibsen B: The anaesthetist's viewpoint on treatment of respiratory complications in poliomyelitis during the epidemic in Copenhagen, 1952. *Proc R Soc Med* **47**: 72, 1954.

365. Ikada S, Yanai N, Ischikawa S: Flexible bronchofiber scope. *Keio J Med* **17**: 2, 1968.

366. International Committee of the Red Cross (ICRC). *Bulletin*. ICRC, 17 Ave de la Paix, 1202 Geneva, Switzerland (Tel. 41-22-346001). (See also LRCS.)

367. International Physicians for the Prevention of Nuclear War (IPPNW). *Newsletter*. IPPNW, 225 Longwood Ave, Boston, MA 02115, USA (Tel. 617/738-9404).

368. Ivatury RR, Shah PM, Ito K, et al: Emergency room thoracotomy for the resuscitation of patients with 'fatal' penetrating injuries of the heart. *Ann Thorac Surg* **32**: 377, 1981.

369. Jackson C: The technique of insertion of intratracheal insufflation tubes. *Surg Gynecol Obstet* **17**: 507, 1913.

370. Jackson D, Friday K, Wilson NJ, et al: Calcium ionophore antagonists and the impaired reperfusion phenomenon following total cerebral ischemia (TCI). *Crit Care Med* **10**: 206, 1982 (abstract).

371. Jacobs HB: Emergency percutaneous transtracheal catheter and ventilator. *J Trauma* **12**: 50, 1972.

372. Jacoby JJ, Hamelberg W, Ziegler CH, et al: Transtracheal resuscitation. *J Amer Med Assoc* **162**: 625, 1956.

373. Jaffe AS, Roberts R: The use of intravenous nitroglycerin in cardiovascular disease. *Pharmacotherapy* **2**: 273, 1982.

373a. Jaffe AS: Cardiovascular pharmacology I. *Circulation* **74**(suppl IV): 70, 1986.

374. James SL, Weisbrot IM, Prince CE, et al: The acid–base status of human infants in relation to birth asphyxia and the onset of respiration. *J Pediatr* **52**: 379, 1958.

375. James SL: Emergencies in the delivery room. In: *Behrman's Neonatal–Perinatal Medicine*. AA Fanaroff, RJ Martin, IR Kerkatz (Eds). St Louis, CV Mosby, 1983.

375a. Jastremski MS, Vaagenes P, Sutton K, et al: Early glucocorticoid treatment does not improve neurologic recovery from global brain ischemia. *Ann Emerg Med* **16**: 500, 1987 (abstract).

376. Javid M: Urea—new use of an old agent. Reduction of intracranial and intraocular pressure. *Surg Clin North Amer* **38**: 907, 1958.

377. Jennett B, Bond M: Assessment of outcome after severe brain damage: a practical scale. *Lancet* **i**: 480, 1975.

378. Jennett B, Teasdale G, Galbraith S, et al: Severe head injuries in three countries. *J Neurol Neurosurg Psychiatry* **40**: 291, 1977.

379. Jesudian MCS, Hanson RR, Keenan RL, et al: Bag–valve–mask ventilation; two rescuers are better than one: Preliminary report. *Crit Care Med* **13**: 122, 1985.

380. Johnson J, Kirby CK: *Surgery of the Chest*. Chicago, Year Book Medical Pub, 1964.

381. Jorgensen EO, Malchow-Moller A: Cerebral prognostic signs during cardiopulmonary resuscitation. *Resuscitation* **6**: 217, 1978.

382. Jorgensen EO, Malchow-Moller A: Natural history of global and critical brain ischemia. Parts I, II, III. *Resuscitation* **9**: 133, 1981.

383. Jowitt MD: Resuscitation and anesthesia in a battle situation: the Falkland Islands Campaign. *J World Assoc Emerg Disaster Med* **1**: 43, 1985.

384. Jude JR, Kouwenhoven WB, Knickerbocker GG: Cardiac arrest: report of application of external cardiac massage on 118 patients. *J Amer Med Assoc* **178**: 1063, 1961.

385. Jude JR, Elam JO: *Fundamentals of Cardiopulmonary Resuscitation*. Philadelphia, FA Davis, 1965.

386. Jurkiewicz J: The effect of haemodilution on experimental brain edema. *Europ J Intensive Care Med* **3:** 167, 1977.
387. Kaback KR, Sanders AB, Meislin HW: MAST suit update. *J Amer Med Assoc* **252:** 2598, 1984.
388. Kagstroem E, Smith ML, Siesjo BK: Local cerebral blood flow in the recovery period following complete cerebral ischemia in the rat. *J Cereb Blood Flow Metab* **3:** 170, 1983.
389. Kalimo H, Garcia JH, Kamijyo Y, et al: The ultrastructure of 'brain death'. II. Electron microscopy of feline cortex after complete ischemia. *Virchows Archiv (B) Cell Pathology* **25:** 207, 1977.
390. Kamen JD, Wilkinson CJ: A new low pressure cuff for endotracheal tubes. *Anesthesiology* **34:** 482, 1971.
391. Kamm G, Graf-Baumann T (Eds): *Anaesthesia Notebook for Medical Auxiliaries*. Berlin, Springer-Verlag, 1982.
392. Kampschulte S, Morikawa S, Safar P: Recovery from anoxic encephalopathy following cardiac arrest. *Fed Proc* **28:** 522, 1969 (abstract).
393. Kampschulte S, Smith J, Safar P: Oxygen transport after cardiopulmonary resuscitation. *Anaesth Reanimation* **30:** 95, 1969 (in German).
394. Kampschulte S, Marcy J, Safar P: Simplified physiologic management of status asthmaticus in children. *Crit Care Med* **1:** 69, 1973.
395. Kampschulte S, Safar P: Development of multidisciplinary pediatric intensive care unit. *Crit Care Med* **1:** 308, 1973.
396. Kantrowitz A, Tjonneland S, Freed PS, et al: Initial clinical experience with intraaortic balloon pumping in cardiogenic shock. *J Amer Med Assoc* **203:** 113, 1968.
397. Kaplan BC, Civetta JM, Nagel EL, et al: The Military Anti-Shock Trouser in civilian pre-hospital emergency care. *J Trauma* **13:** 843, 1973.
398. Katz L, Vaagenes P, Safar P, et al: Brain resuscitative potential of methylprednisolone after asphyxial cardiac arrest in rats. *Anesthesiology* **63:** A111, 1985 (abstract).
399. Kaye W, Mancini ME, Rallis SF, et al: Can better basic and advanced cardiac life support improve outcome from cardiac arrest? *Crit Care Med* **13:** 916, 1985.
400. Kazda S, Mayer D: Postischemic impaired reperfusion and tissue damage: consequences of a calcium-dependent vasospasm? In: *Calcium Entry Blockers and Tissue Protection*. T Godfraind, PM Vanhoutte, S Govoni, et al (Eds). New York, Raven Press, 1985, p 129.
401. Keen WW: A case of total laryngectomy (unsuccessful) and a case of abdominal hysterectomy (successful), in both of which massage of the heart for chloroform collapse was employed, with notes of 25 other cases of cardiac massage. *Ther Gaz* **28:** 217, 1904.
402. Keenan RL, Boyan CP: Cardiac arrest due to anesthesia. Study of incidence and causes. *J Amer Med Assoc* **253:** 2373, 1985.
403. Keith A: Mechanisms underlying the various methods of artificial respiration. *Lancet* **13:** 747, 1909.
404. Kelsey SK, Abramson NS, Detre K, et al: Randomized clinical study of cardiopulmonary resuscitation: Design, methods and patient characteristics. *Amer J Emerg Med* **4:** 72, 1986.
405. Kennedy JW, Ritchie JL, David KB, et al: The Western Washington randomized trial of intracoronary streptokinase in acute myocardial infarction. *N Engl J Med* **309:** 1477, 1983 and **312:** 1073, 1985.
406. Keren A, Tzivoni D, Gavish D, et al: Etiology, warning signs, and therapy of torsade de pointes. *Circulation* **64:** 1167, 1981.
406a. Kern KB, Sanders AB, Badylak SF, et al: Long-term survival with open-chest cardiac massage after ineffective closed-chest compression in a canine preparation. *Circulation* **75:** 498, 1987.
406b. Kern KB, Carter AB, Showen RL, et al: Twenty-four hour survival in a canine model of cardiac arrest comparing three methods of manual cardiopulmonary resuscitation. *J Am Coll Cardiol* **7:** 859, 1986.

406c. Keszler H, Winoto K, Nemoto E: A reliable dog model of cardiac arrest and resuscitation. *Crit Care Med* **8:** 242, 1980 (abstract).
407. Kirby RR, Downs JB, Civetta JM, et al: High level positive end-expiratory pressure (PEEP) in acute respiratory insufficiency. *Chest* **67:** 156, 1975.
408. Kirby RR, Smith RA, DeSautels DA: *Mechanical Ventilation.* New York, Churchill Livingstone, 1985.
409. Kirimli B, Harris LC, Safar P: Drugs in cardiopulmonary resuscitation. *Acta Anaesth Scand* (Suppl) **23:** 255, 1966.
410. Kirimli B, Kampschulte S, Safar P: Cardiac arrest from exsanguination in dogs. Evaluation of resuscitation methods. *Acta Anaesth Scand* (Suppl) **29:** 183, 1968.
411. Kirimli B, Kampschulte S, Safar P: Resuscitation from cardiac arrest due to exsanguination. *Surg Gynecol Obstet* **129:** 89, 1969.
412. Kirsh MM, Behrendt DM, Orringer MB, et al: The treatment of acute traumatic rupture of the aorta: a ten year experience. *Ann Surg* **184:** 308, 1976.
413. Kirstein A: Autoskopie des Larynx und der Trachea. *Berl Klin Wochenschr* **32:** 475, 1895.
414. Kitterman JA, Phibbs RH, Tooley WH: Catheterization of umbilical vessels in newborn infants. *Pediatr Clin North Amer* **17:** 895, 1970.
415. Klain M, Smith RB: High frequency percutaneous transtracheal jet ventilation. *Crit Care Med* **5:** 280, 1977.
416. Klain M, Keszler H, Brader E: High frequency jet ventilation in CPR. *Crit Care Med* **9:** 421, 1981.
417. Klain M: High-frequency ventilation. In: *Textbook of Critical Care.* WC Shoemaker, WL Thompson, PR Holbrook (Eds) Philadelphia, WB Saunders, 1984, p 323.
418. Klatzo I: Brain edema following brain ischemia and the influence of therapy. *Brit J Anaesth* **57:** 18, 1985.
419. Klaus MH, Fanaroff AA: *Care of the High Risk Neonate.* Philadelphia, WB Saunders, 1979.
420. Klein NA, Siskind SJ, Frishman WH: Hemodynamic comparison of intravenous amrinone and dobutamine in patients with chronic congestive heart failure. *Amer J Cardiol* **48:** 170, 1981.
421. Kochanek PM, Dutka AJ, Hallenbeck JM: Indomethacin, prostacyclin and heparin improve postischemic cerebral blood flow without affecting early postischemic granulocyte accumulation. *Stroke* **18:** 634, 1987.
422. Koch-Weser J: Drug therapy: Bretylium. *N Engl J Med* **300:** 473, 1979.
423. Koehler RC, Chandra N, Guerci AD, et al: Augmentation of cerebral perfusion by simultaneous chest compression and lung inflation with abdominal binding following cardiac arrest in dogs. *Circulation* **67:** 266, 1983.
424. Koehler RC, Michael JR, Guerci AD, et al: Beneficial effect of epinephrine infusion on cerebral and myocardial blood flows during CPR. *Ann Emerg Med* **8:** 744, 1985.
425. Kofke WA, Nemoto EM, Hossmann KA, et al: Monkey brain blood flow and metabolism after global brain ischemia and post-insult thiopental therapy. *Stroke* **10:** 554, 1979.
426. Kolobow T, Gattinoni L, Tomlinson T, et al: Control of breathing using an extracorporeal membrane lung. *Anesthesiology* **46:** 138, 1977.
427. Koster RW, Dunning AJ: Intramuscular lidocaine for prevention of lethal arrhythmias in the prehospital phase of acute myocardial infarction. *N Engl J Med* **313:** 1105, 1985.
428. Kouwenhoven WB, Milner WR: Treatment of ventricular fibrillation using a capacitor discharge. *J Appl Physiol* **7:** 253, 1954.
429. Kouwenhoven WB, Jude JR, Knickerbocker GG: Closed-chest cardiac massage. *J Amer Med Assoc* **173:** 1064, 1960.
430. Kouwenhoven WB: The development of the defibrillator. *Ann Intern Med* **71:** 449, 1969.
431. Kovach AGB, Sandor P: Cerebral blood flow and brain function during hypotension and shock. *Ann Rev Physiol* **38:** 571, 1976.
432. Kraven T, Rush BF, Ghosh A, et al: Correlation of survival and metabolic response produced by ATP-MgCl₂ in hemorrhagic shock. *Circ Shock* **6:** 186, 1979.

433. Kreiselman J: A new resuscitation apparatus. *Anesthesiology* **4:** 608, 1943.
434. Krenn J, Steinbereithner K, Sporn P, et al: The value of routine respiratory treatment in severe brain trauma. In: *Advances in Neurosurgery*, Vol. 3, H Penzholz, M Brock, J Hamer (Eds). Berlin, Springer-Verlag, 1975, p 134.
435. Kristoffersen MB, Rattenborg CC, Holaday DA: Asphyxial death: the roles of acute anoxia, hypercarbia and acidosis. *Anesthesiology* **28:** 488, 1967.
436. Kucher R: Krankengut, Ergebnisse, Aufbau und Organisation der Intensivbehandlungsstation der I. Chir Univ-Klinik Wien. In: *Probleme der Intensivbehandlung*. K Horatz, R Frey (Eds). Heidelberg, Springer-Verlag, 1968.
437. Kuhn F: *Die perorale Intubation*. Berlin, S Karger, 1911.
438. Kuhn GJ, White BC, Swetman RE, et al: Peripheral vs. central circulation times during CPR: A pilot study. *Ann Emerg Med* **10:** 417, 1981.
439. Kuhns DB, Kaplan S, Basford RE: Hexachlorocyclohexanes, potent stimuli of O_2^- production and calcium release in human polymorphonuclear leukocytes. *Blood* **68:** 535, 1986.
440. Kuller L, Cooper M, Perper J, et al: Epidemiology of sudden death. *Arch Intern Med* **129:** 714, 1972.
441. Kupersmith J, Antman EM, Hoffman BF: In vivo electrophysiological effects of lidocaine in canine acute myocardial infarction. *Circ Res* **36:** 84, 1975.
442. Laborit H, Huguenard P: *Practice of Hibernation Therapy in Surgery and Medicine* (French). Paris, Masson, 1954.
443. Laerdal AS: Adapting first aid to actual needs. *J World Assoc Emerg Disaster Med* 1/Suppl I: 63, 1985.
444. Laerdal T: Experience in teaching cardiopulmonary resuscitation (CPR) in the USA and in Europe. *J World Assoc Emerg Disaster Med* 1/Suppl I: 64, 1985.
445. Lane J (Ed): *Reanimacao* (Portuguese). Rio de Janeiro, Guanabara Koogan, 1981 (in Portuguese).
446. Lane JC: Cardiopulmonary resuscitation training in developing regions (1981). *J World Assoc Emerg Disaster Med* 1/Suppl I: 88, 1985.
447. Lane JC, Nagase Y: Feasibility of teaching resuscitation by television in Brazil. *J World Assoc Emerg Disaster Med* 1/Suppl I: 89, 1985.
448. Langfitt TW: Increased intracranial pressure. In: *Neurologic Surgery*. JP Youmans (Ed). Philadelphia, WB Saunders, 1973.
449. Lawin P: *Praxis der Intensivbehandlung*. Stuttgart, Thieme, 1975, 1981.
450. Lawson NW, Butler GH III, Roy CT: Alkalosis and cardiac arrhythmias. *Anesth Analg* **52:** 951, 1973.
451. League of Red Cross Societies (LRCS). *Weekly News*. LRCS, PO Box 276, 17 Chemin des Crets, 1211 Geneva 19, Switzerland (Tel. 41-22-345580). (See also Kisselev AK: The LRCS. *J World Assoc Emerg Disaster Med* 1/1: 3, 1985).
452. Leaning J, Keyes L (Eds): *The Counterfeit Ark: Crisis Relocation for Nuclear War*. Cambridge, Ballinger Publishing Company, 1984.
453. Ledingham IM: Central rewarming systems for treatment of hypothermia. *Lancet* **5:** 1168, 1980.
454. Ledingham IM, Macdonald AL, Douglas IHS: Monitoring of ventilation. In: *Textbook of Critical Care*. WC Shoemaker, WL Thompson, PR Holbrook (Eds). Philadelphia, WB Saunders, 1984.
455. Lee HR, Blank WS, Massion WH, et al: Venous return in hemorrhagic shock after application of Military Anti-Shock Trousers. *Amer J Emerg Med* **1:** 7, 1983.
456. Lee SK, Vaagenes P, Safar P, et al: Effect of cardiac arrest time on the cortical cerebral blood flow generated by subsequent standard external CPR in rabbits. *Ann Emerg Med* **13:** 385, 1984 (abstract).
457. Leighninger DS: Contributions of Claude Beck. Historic vignette. In: *Advances in Cardiopulmonary Resuscitation*. P Safar, JO Elam (Eds). New York, Springer-Verlag, 1977, p 259.
458. Lemire JG, Johnson AL: Is cardiac resuscitation worthwhile? A decade of experience. *New Engl J Med* **286:** 970, 1972.

459. Lesser R, Bircher N, Safar P, et al: Venous valving during standard cardiopulmonary resuscitation (CPR). *Anesthesiology* **53:** S153, 1980 (abstract).

460. Lesser R, Bircher N, Safar P, et al: Sternal compression before ventilation in cardiopulmonary resuscitation. *J World Assoc Emerg Disaster Med* 1/Suppl I: 239, 1985.

461. Levine DG, Schwartz GR, Ungar JR: Drug abuse. In *Principles and Practice of Emergency Medicine*. G Schwartz, P Safar, J Stone, et al (Eds). Philadelphia, WB Saunders, 1986, p 1744.

462. Levine R, Gorayeb M, Safar P, et al: Cardiopulmonary bypass after cardiac arrest and prolonged closed-chest CPR in dogs. *Ann Emerg Med* **16:** 620, 1987.

463. Levine S: Anoxic-ischemic encephalopathy in rats. *Am J Pathol* **36:** 1, 1960.

464. Levy DE, Brierley JB: Delayed pentobarbital administration limits ischemic brain damage in gerbils. *Ann Neurol* **5:** 59, 1979.

465. Levy DE, Bates D, Caronna JJ, et al: Prognosis in nontraumatic coma. *Ann Int Med* **94:** 293, 1981.

466. Levy DE, Caronna JJ, Singer BH, et al: Predicting outcome from hypoxic-ischemic coma. *J Amer Med Assoc* **253:** 1420, 1985.

467. Liberthson RR, Nagel EL, Hirschman JC, et al: Prehospital ventricular fibrillation. Prognosis and follow-up course. *N Engl J Med* **291:** 317, 1974.

468. Liedtke AJ, DeMuth WE: Nonpenetrating cardiac injuries: a collective review. *Amer Heart J* **86:** 687, 1973.

469. Lin SR, O'Connor MJ, Fischer HW, et al: The effect of combined dextran and streptokinase on cerebral function and blood flow after cardiac arrest: an experimental study on the dog. *Invest Radiol* **13:** 490, 1978.

470. Lin MR, Nemoto EM, Kessler PD: Alterations in whole brain cyclic AMP and cerebral cortex Na-inducible cyclic AMP in rats during and after complete global ischemia. In: *Brain Protection: Morphological, Pathophysiological and Clinical Aspects*. K Wildemann, S Hoyer (Eds). New York, Springer-Verlag, 1983, p 55.

471. Lind B: Teaching mouth-to-mouth resuscitation in primary schools. *Acta Anesth Scand* (Suppl) **9:** 63, 1961.

472. Lind B, Stovner J: Mouth-to-mouth resuscitation in Norway. *J Amer Med Assoc* **185:** 933, 1963.

473. Lind B, Snyder J, Kampschulte S, et al: A review of total brain ischemia models in dogs and original experiments on clamping the aorta. *Resuscitation* **4:** 19, 1975.

474. Lind B, Snyder J, Safar P: Total brain ischemia in dogs: Cerebral physiological and metabolic changes after 15 minutes of circulatory arrest. *Resuscitation* **4:** 97, 1975.

475. Lindholm CE: Prolonged endotracheal intubation. *Acta Anaesth Scand* (Suppl) **33:** 1, 1969.

476. Lindholm CE, Carroll RG: Evaluation of tube deformation pressure in vitro. *Crit Care Med* **3:** 196, 1975.

476a. Lindner KH, Ahnefeld FW, Rossi R: Azidoseausgleich bei Reanimation. In: *Cardiopulmonale und cerebrale Reanimation (CPCR)*. W. Mauritz, K Steinbereithner, Eds. Vienna, Verlag Wilhelm Maudrich, 1987.

477. Livesay JJ, Follette DM, Fey KH, et al: Optimizing myocardial supply/demand balance with adrenergic drugs during cardiopulmonary resuscitation. *J Thorac Cardiovasc Surg* **76:** 244, 1978.

478. Longstreth T, Clayson KJ, Sumi SM: Cerebrospinal fluid and serum creatine kinase BB activity after out-of-hospital cardiac arrest. *Neurology* **31:** 455, 1981.

479. Longstreth WT, Diehr P, Inui TS: Prediction of awakening after out-of-hospital cardiac arrest. *N Engl J Med* **308:** 1378, 1983.

480. Longstreth WT: High blood glucose level on admission and poor neurologic recovery after cardiac arrest. *Ann Neurol* **15:** 59, 1984.

481. Lorkovic H: Influence of changes in pH on the mechanical activity of cardiac muscle. *Circ Res* **19:** 711, 1966.

482. Lown B, Marcus F, Levine HD: Digitalis and atrial tachycardia with block. *N Engl J Med* **260:** 301, 1959.

483. Lown B: Comparison of AC and DC electroshock across the closed chest. *Amer J Cardiol* **10**, 223, 1962.

484. Lown B: The philosophy of coronary care. *Arch Klin Med* **216**: 201, 1969.

485. Lown B, Wolff M: Approaches to sudden death from coronary heart disease. *Circulation* **44**: 130, 1971.

486. Lown B, Crampton RS, DeSilva RA, et al: The energy for ventricular fibrillation—too little or too much? *N Engl J Med* **298**: 1252, 1978.

487. Lown B: Physicians and nuclear war. (a) *N Engl J Med* **246**: 2331, 1981. (b) *J World Assoc Emerg Disaster Med* **1**: 8, 1985.

488. Lucas SK, Schiff HV, Flaherty JT, et al: The harmful effects of ventricular distension during postischemic reperfusion. *Ann Thorac Surg* **32**: 486, 1981.

489. Luce JM, Ross BK, O'Quinn RJ, et al: Regional blood flow during cardiopulmonary resuscitation in dogs using simultaneous and non-simultaneous compression and ventilation. *Circulation* **67**: 258, 1983.

490. Ludwig S, Kettrick RG, Parker M: Pediatric cardiopulmonary resuscitation. *Clin Pediatr* **23**: 71, 1984.

491. Lund I, Lind B (Eds): International Symposium on Emergency Resuscitation. Oslo, Norway, 1967. *Acta Anaesth Scand* (Suppl) **29**, 1968. (See also ref. 631.)

492. Lund I, Skulberg A: Cardiopulmonary resuscitation by lay people. *Lancet* **ii**: 702, 1976.

493. Lundberg N: Continuous recording and control of ventricular fluid pressure in neurosurgical practice. *Acta Psychiatr Neurol Scand* **36**(Suppl 149), 1960.

494. Lunde P: Ventricular fibrillation after intravenous atropine for treatment of sinus bradycardia. *Acta Med Scand* **199**: 369, 1976.

495. Lundy JS, Adams RC: Thiopental sodium intravenous anesthesia. *Army Med Bulletin* **63**: 90, 1942.

496. Lunkenheimer PP, Rafflenbuel W, Keller H, et al: Application of transtracheal pressure oscillations as a modification of 'diffusion respiration'. *Brit J Anaesth* **44**: 627, 1972.

497. Lust P: Resuscitation in the pre-hospital phase. Continuum of physician leadership from scene to intensive care unit (1981). *J World Assoc Emerg Disaster Med* **1**/Suppl. I: 127, 1985.

498. Maass: Die Methode der Wiederbelebung bei Herztod nach Chloroformeinathmung. *Berlin Klin Wochschr* **29**: 265, 1892.

499. Macewen W: Clinical observations on the introduction of tracheal tubes by the mouth instead of performing tracheotomy or laryngotomy. *Brit Med J* **2**: 163, 1880.

500. Macintosh RR: A new laryngoscope. *Lancet* **i**: 205, 1943.

501a. Macintosh RR: Oxford inflating bellows. *Brit Med J* **ii**: 202, 1953.

501b. Macintosh RR: A plea for simplicity. *Brit Med J* **ii**: 1054, 1955.

502. MacKenzie GJ, Taylor SH, McDonald AH, et al: Hemodynamic effects of external cardiac compression. *Lancet* **i**: 1345, 1964.

503. MacMurdo SD, Nemoto EM, Nikki P, et al: Brain cyclic-AMP and possible mechanisms of cerebrovascular dilatation by anesthetics in rats. *Anesthesiology* **55**: 435, 1981.

504. Magill IW: Endotracheal anesthesia. *Amer J Surg* **34**: 450: 1936.

505. Mahoney LE (Chairman): National Disaster Medical System (NDMS) USA planning committee. Division of Emergency Coordination, United States Public Health Service, 5600 Fishers Lane, Room 4-81, Rockville, MD, 20857, USA, 1984.

506. Maier GW, Tyson GS Jr, Olsen CO, et al: The physiology of external cardiac massage: High impulse cardiopulmonary resuscitation. *Circulation* **70**: 86, 1984.

507. Malmcrona R, Schroeder G, Werlio L: Hemodynamic effects of metaraminol. *Amer J Cardiol* **13**: 10, 1964.

508. Maloney JV Jr, Smyth CM, Gilmore JP, et al: Intra-arterial and intravenous infusion: a controlled study of their effectiveness in the treatment of experimental hemorrhagic shock. *Surg Gynecol Obstet* **97**: 529, 1953.

508a. Maningas PA, DeGuzman LR, Tillman FJ, et al: Small-volume infusion of 7.5% NaCl in 6% dextran 70 for the treatment of severe hemorrhagic shock in swine. *Ann Emerg Med* **15**: 1131, 1986.

509. Manni C, Magalini SI, Scrascia E (Eds): *Total Parenteral Alimentation.* New York, American Elsevier, 1976.

510. Manni C, Magalini SI (Eds): *Emergency and Disaster Medicine.* Proceedings of the Third World Congress on Emergency and Disaster Med (Club of Mainz), Rome, 1983. Heidelberg, Springer-Verlag, 1985.

511. Marshall LF, Shapiro HM, Rauscher A, et al: Pentobarbital therapy for intracranial hypertension in metabolic coma. Reye's syndrome. *Crit Care Med* **6**: 1, 1978.

512. Marshall LF, Smith RW, Shapiro HM: The outcome with aggressive treatment in severe head injuries. II. Acute and chronic barbiturate administration in the management of head injury. *J Neurosurg* **50**: 26, 1979.

513. Marta JA, Davis HS, Eisele JH: Vagomimetic effects of morphine and innovar in man. *Anesth Analg* **52**: 817, 1973.

514. Massumi RA, Mason DT, Amsterdam EA, et al: Ventricular fibrillation and tachycardia after intravenous atropine for treatment of bradycardias. *N Engl J Med* **287**: 336, 1972.

515. Mattar JA, Weil MH, Shubin H, et al: Cardiac arrest in the critically ill: II. Hyperosmolal states following cardiac arrest. *Amer J Med* **56**: 162, 1974.

516. Mattox KL, Espada R, Beall AC: Performing thoracotomy in the emergency center. *J Amer Coll Emerg Phys* **3**: 13, 1974.

517. Mattox KL, Beall AC: Resuscitation of the moribund patient using portable cardiopulmonary bypass. *Ann Thorac Surg* **22**: 436, 1976.

518. Mattox KL, Feliciano DV: Role of external cardiac compression in truncal trauma. *J Trauma* **22**: 934, 1982.

518a. Mauritz W, Steinbereithner K (Eds): *Cardiopulmonale und cerebrale Reanimation (CPCR).* Vienna, Verlag Wilhelm Maudrich, 1987.

519. Mayrhofer O: Die Intensivabteilungen am neuen Klinikum der Universitaet Wien. In: Aktuelle Probleme der Intensivbehandlung, In: *Intensivmedizin, Notfallmedizin, Anaesthesiologie Vol. 12.* P. Lawin, Ed. Stuttgart, Thieme, 1978.

520. McCabe CJ, Browne BJ: Esophageal obturator airway, ET tube, and pharyngeal-tracheal lumen airway. *Amer J Emerg Med* **4**: 64, 1986.

521. McCord JM: Oxygen-derived free radicals in postischemic tissue injury. *N Engl J Med* **312**: 159, 1985.

522. McGrath RB: Gastroesophageal lacerations. A fatal complication of closed chest cardiopulmonary resuscitation. *Chest* **83**: 571, 1983.

523. McGregor M: The nitrates and myocardial ischemia, editorial. *Circulation* **66**: 689, 1982.

524. McIntyre KM: Medicolegal aspects of CPR and ECC. In: *Advanced Cardiac Life Support Manual.* Dallas, Amer Heart Assoc, 1981, 1983.

525. McNamara J, Mollot M, Dunn R, et al: Effect of hypertonic glucose in hypovolemic shock in man. *Ann Surg* **176**: 247, 1972.

526. Medecine Sans Frontières: Reports on disaster relief actions by physicians. 68 Blvd St Marcel, 75005 Paris, France. Tel. 33-1-47072929.

527. Meisel A, Grenvik A, Pinkus RL, et al: Hospital guidelines for deciding about life-sustaining treatment: Dealing with health 'limbo'. *Crit Care Med* **14**: 239, 1986.

528. Melker RJ: Alternative methods of ventilation during respiratory and cardiac arrest. *Circulation* **74**(suppl IV): 63, 1986.

529. Melker RJ: Asynchronous and other alternative methods of ventilation during CPR. *Ann Emerg Med* **13**: 758, 1984.

530. Melton RJ, Riner RM: Revising the rural hospital disaster plan: a role for the EMS system in managing the multiple casualty incident. *Ann Emerg Med* **10**: 39, 1981.

531. Messmer K (Ed): Hemodilution, a symposium. *Anaesthesist* **25**: 123, 1976.

532. Meuret GH, Themann H: Calcium antagonism in cardiopulmonary resuscitation. *J World Assoc Emerg Disaster Med* **1**: 224, 1985.

533. Meyer M (Ed): Special symposium issue. Proceedings International Symposium on Acute Respiratory Insufficiency, Potsdam, East Germany, 1980. *Anaesth Reanimatologie* **6**, 1981.

534. Michael JR, Guerci AD, Koehler RC, et al: Mechanisms by which epinephrine augments cerebral and myocardial perfusion during cardiopulmonary resuscitation in dogs. *Circulation* **69**: 822, 1984.

534a. Michael JR, Guerci AD, Koehler RC, et al: Mechanisms by which epinephrine augments cerebral and myocardial perfusion during cardiopulmonary resuscitation in dogs. *Circulation* **69**: 822, 1984.

535. Michenfelder JD, Theye RA: The effects of anesthesia and hypothermia on canine cerebral ATP and lactate during anoxia produced by decapitation. *Anesthesiology* **33**: 430, 1970.

536. Michenfelder JD, Milde HJ, Sundt TM: Cerebral protection by barbiturate anesthesia. Use after middle cerebral artery occlusion in Java monkeys. *Arch Neurol* **33**: 345, 1976.

537. Mikulic E, Cohn JN, Franciosa JA: Comparative hemodynamic effects of inotropic and vasodilator drugs in severe heart failure. *Circulation* **56**: 528, 1977.

538. Milai AS, Davis G, Safar P: Simplified apparatus for IPPB aerosol therapy. *Anesthesiology* **26**: 362, 1965.

539. Miller JD: Barbiturate and raised intracranial pressure. *Ann Neurol* **6**: 189, 1979.

540. Miller JR, Meyers RE: Neuropathology of systemic circulatory arrest in adult monkeys. *Neurology* **22**: 888, 1972.

541. Miller J, Trech D, Horwitz L, et al: The precordial thump. *Ann Emerg Med* **13**: 791, 1984.

542. Miller RD (Ed): *Anesthesia* (2nd edn). New York, Churchill Livingstone, 1986.

543. Miller RR, Awan NA, Joyce JA, et al: Combined dopamine and nitroprusside therapy in congestive heart failure: Greater augmentation of cardiac performance by addition of inotropic stimulation to afterload reduction. *Circulation* **55**: 881, 1977.

544. Miller WF, Sproule BJ: Successful use of intermittent inspiratory positive pressure oxygen breathing in pulmonary edema. *Dis Chest* **35**: 469, 1959.

545. Miller WF: Aerosol therapy in acute and chronic respiratory disease. *Arch Intern Med* **131**: 148, 1973.

546. Minuck M, Sharma PG: Comparison of THAM and sodium bicarbonate in resuscitation of the heart after ventricular fibrillation in dogs. *Anesth Analg* **56**: 38, 1977.

547. Mirowski M, Reid PR, Mower MM, et al: Termination of malignant ventricular arrhythmias with an implanted automatic defibrillator in human beings. *N Engl J Med* **303**: 322, 1980.

548. Mirowski M, Reid PR, Winkle RA, et al: Mortality in patients with implanted automatic defibrillators. *Ann Int Med* **98**: 585, 1983.

549. Miyake T, Kinoshita K, Ishii N: First report of an experimental study in dogs of cerebral cardiopulmonary resuscitation (CPCR). *Resuscitation* **10**: 105, 1982.

550. Modell JH, Davis JH: Electrolyte changes in human drowning victims. *Anesthesiology* **30**: 414, 1969.

551. Modell JH: Near drowning. *Circulation* **74**(suppl IV): 27, 1986.

552. Moerch ET, Avery EE, Benson DW: Hyperventilation in the treatment of crushing injuries of the chest. *Surg Forum* **6**: 270, 1956.

553. Mollaret P, Goulon M: Le coma depasse (Mémoire préliminaire). *Rev Neurol* **101**: 3, 1959.

554. Montgomery WH (Chairman): 1985 National Conference on Standards and Guidelines for Cardiopulmonary Resuscitation and Emergency Cardiac Care. *J Amer Med Assoc* **255**(Suppl): 2841, 1986.

555. Moody R: *Life After Life*. New York, Bantam, 1976.

556. Moore EE, Moore JB, Galloway AC: Post-injury thoracotomy in the emergency room: A critical evaluation. *Surgery* **86**: 500, 1979.

557. Moore FD, Lyons JH, Pierce EC, et al: *Post-Traumatic Pulmonary Insufficiency*. Philadelphia, WB Saunders, 1969.
558. Moossy J, Reinmuth OM (Eds): *Cerebrovascular Diseases* (12th Research Conference). New York, Raven Press, 1981.
559. Moossy J: Pathologic studies—an essential guide (1981). *J World Assoc Emerg Disaster Med* 1/Suppl I: 18, 1985.
560. Moossy J: Pathology of ischemic cerebrovascular disease. In: *Neurosurgery*. RH Wilkins, SS Rengachary (Eds). New York, McGraw-Hill, 1985, p 1193.
561. Morikawa S, Safar P: Mouth-to-nose resuscitation. *Acta Anaesth Scand*, Suppl 9: 70, 1961.
562. Morikawa S, Safar P, DeCarlo J: Influence of head position upon upper airway patency. *Anesthesiology* 22: 265, 1961.
563. Morioka T, Teresaki H, et al: Extracorporeal lung assist (ECLA) without intubation. Personal communication, 1984.
564. Mueller H: Treatment of acute myocardial infarction. In: *Textbook of Critical Care*. WC Shoemaker, WL Thompson, PR Holbrook (Eds). Philadelphia, WB Saunders, 1984, p 403. Chapter 59.
565. Muendich K, Hoflehner G: Ventilation bronchoscopy. *Anaesthesist* 2: 121, 1953.
566. Mukharji J, Rude RE, Poole WK, et al: Risk factors for sudden death after acute myocardial infarction: Two-year follow-up. *Amer J Cardiol* 54: 31, 1984.
567. Mullie A, Lust P, Penninckx J, et al: Monitoring of cerebro-spinal fluid enzyme levels in postischemic encephalopathy after cardiac arrest. *Crit Care Med* 9: 399, 1981.
568. Mushin WW, Rendell-Baker L, Thompson PW, et al: *Automatic Ventilation of the Lungs*. 2nd ed, Philadelphia, FA Davis, 1969.
569. Nagel EL, Hirschman JC, Nussenfeld SR, et al: Telemetry-medical command in coronary and other mobile emergency care systems. *J Amer Med Assoc* 214: 332, 1970.
570. Nagel EL, Fine EG, Krisher JP, et al: Complications of CPR. *Crit Care Med* 9: 424, 1981 (abstract).
571. Nagel EL: Perspectives (and physician leadership) of emergency medical services (EMS) (1981). *J World Assoc Emerg Disaster Med* 1/Suppl I: 110, 1985.
572. Naito R, Yokoyama K: On the perfluorodecalin/phospholipid emulsion as the red cell substitute. In: *Proceedings of the 10th International Nutrition Symposium on PFC Artificial Blood*. Kyoto, Green Cross, 1975, p 55.
573. Nancekievill D: On-site management and treatment of motor car racing casualties. *J World Assoc Emerg Disaster Med* 1/3: 326, 1985.
574. Narayan RK, Kishore PRS, Becker DP, et al: Intracranial pressure: to monitor or not to monitor. *J Neurosurg* 56: 650, 1982.
575. National Institute of General Medical Sciences (USA): Second Conference on Supportive Therapy in Burn Care. *J Trauma* 21: Aug Suppl, 1981.
576. Nayler WG, Poole-Wilson PA, Williams A: Hypoxia and calcium. *J Mol Cell Cardiol* 11: 683, 1979.
577. Negovsky VA: *Resuscitation and Artificial Hypothermia (USSR)*. New York, Consultants Bureau, 1962.
578. Negovsky VA: Reanimatology—The Science of Resuscitation. In: *Cardiac Arrest and Resuscitation*. H Stephenson (Ed). St Louis, CV Mosby, 1974.
579. Negovsky VA: Reanimatology today: some scientific and philosophic considerations. *Crit Care Med* 10: 130, 1982.
580. Negovsky VA, Gurvitch AM, Zolotokrylina ES: *Postresuscitation Disease*. Amsterdam, Elsevier, 1983.
581. Nemoto EM, Bleyaert AL, Stezoski SW, et al: Global brain ischemia: A reproducible monkey model. *Stroke* 8: 558, 1977.
582. Nemoto EM: Pathogenesis of cerebral ischemia-anoxia. *Crit Care Med* 6: 203, 1978.
583. Nemoto EM, Erdman NW, Strong E, et al: Regional brain PO_2 after global ischemia in monkeys: evidence for regional differences in critical perfusion pressures. *Stroke* 10: 44, 1979.

584. Nemoto EM, Shiu GK, Nemmer JP, et al: Free fatty acid accumulation in the pathogenesis and therapy of ischemic-anoxic brain injury. *Amer J Emerg Med* 1: 175, 1983.

585. Niemann JT, Rosborough J, Hausknecht M, et al: Cough-CPR. Documentation of systemic perfusion in man and in an experimental model: A 'window' to the mechanism of blood flow in external CPR. *Crit Care Med* 8: 141, 1980.

586. Niemann JT: Differences in cerebral and myocardial perfusion during closed-chest resuscitation. *Ann Emerg Med* 13: 849, 1984.

587. Niemann JT, Rosborough JP, Ung S, et al: Hemodynamic effects of continuous abdominal binding during cardiac arrest and resuscitation. *Amer J Cardiol* 53: 269, 1984.

588. Niemann JT, Criley JM, Rosborough JP, et al: Predictive indices of successful cardiac resuscitation after prolonged arrest and experimental cardiopulmonary resuscitation. *Ann Emerg Med* 14: 521, 1985.

589. Niemann JT, Haynes KS, Garner D, et al: Postcountershock pulseless rhythms: response to CPR, artificial cardiac pacing, and adrenergic agonists. *Ann Emerg Med* 15: 112, 1986.

589a. Niemann JT, Rosborough JP, Niskanen RA: Mechanical 'cough' cardiopulmonary resuscitation during cardiac arrest in dogs. *Amer J Cardiol* 55: 199, 1985.

590. Nilsson E: On treatment of barbiturate poisoning. A modified clinical aspect. *Acta Med Scand* (Suppl) 253: 1, 1951.

591. Nims RG, Conner EH, Botelho SY, et al: Comparison of methods for performing manual artificial respiration on apneic patients. *J Appl Physiol* 4: 486, 1951.

592. Nobel J, et al: In: *Health Devices.* (a) Manually operated resuscitators 1: 13, 1971. (b) Defibrillators 1: 109, 1971; 2: 87, 1973; 1: 117, 1973. (c) External heart compressors 2: 136, 1973. Publ. Emergency Care Research Institute, 5200 Butler Pike, Plymouth Meeting, PA 19462, USA.

593. Nordstroem CH, Rehncrona S, Siesjo BK: Restitution of cerebral energy state, as well as of glycolytic metabolites, citric acid cycle intermediates and associated amino acids after 30 minutes of complete ischemia in rats anesthetized with nitrous oxide or pentobarbital. *J Neurochem* 30: 479, 1978.

594. Norlander OP: The use of respirators in anesthesia and surgery. *Acta Anaesth Scand* (Suppl) 30, 1968.

595. Norlander OP, William-Olsson G, Norden I, et al: Integrated display system for patient data monitoring. *Progress in Anaesthesiology.* Proceedings of the Fourth World Congress of Anaesthesiologists, London, 1968. Amsterdam, Excerpta Medica, 1970.

596. Nunn JF: *Applied Respiratory Physiology: With Special Reference to Anaesthesia.* London, Butterworths, 1975.

597. Nussmeier NA, Arlund C, Slogoff S: Neuropsychiatric complications after cardiopulmonary bypass: cerebral protection by a barbiturate. *Anesthesiology* 64: 165, 1986.

598. Obrist WD, Langfitt TW, Jaggi JL, et al: Cerebral blood flow and metabolism in comatose patients with acute head injury. *J Neurosurg* 61: 241, 1984.

599. Ohomoto T, Mura I, Konno S: A new method of external cardiac massage to improve diastolic augmentation and prolong survival time. *Ann Thorac Surg* 21: 284, 1976.

600. Olson DW, Thompson BM, Darin JC, et al: A randomized comparison study of bretylium tosylate and lidocaine in resuscitation of patients from out-of-hospital ventricular fibrillation in a paramedic system. *Ann Emerg Med* 13: 807, 1984.

601. Orlowski JP: Optimal position for external cardiac massage in infants and children. *Crit Care Med* 12: 224, 1984.

602. Ornato JP, Craren EJ, Nelson N, et al: The economic impact of cardiopulmonary resuscitation and emergency cardiac care programs. *Cardiovasc Rev Rep* 4: 1083, 1983.

603. O'Rourke GW, Greene NM: Autonomic blockade and the resting heart rate in man. *Amer Heart J* 80: 469, 1970.

604. Otto CW, Yakaitis RW: Comparison of dopamine, dobutamine, and epinephrine in CPR. *Crit Care Med* 9: 366, 1981.

605. Otto CW, Yakaitis RW, Redding JS, et al: Spontaneous ischemic ventricular fibrillation in dogs: A new model for the study of cardiopulmonary resuscitation. *Crit Care Med* **11:** 883, 1983.

606. Otto CW, Eisenberg MS, Bircher NG (Eds): Wolf Creek Conference on CPR Research No. 3, 1985. *Crit Care Med* **13:** 881, 1985 (see also Wolf Creek No. 1, 1975, ref. 734a; and No. 2, 1980, ref. 660).

606a. Otto CW: Cardiovascular pharmacology II: the use of catecholamines pressor agents, digitalis, and corticosteroids in CPR and emergency cardiac care. *Circulation* 74(suppl IV): 80, 1986.

607. Palmer E: The Heimlich maneuver misused. *Curr Prescribing* **5:** 45, 1979.

608. Palmer RF, Lasseter KC: Sodium nitroprusside. *N Engl J Med* **292:** 294, 1975.

609. Pan American Health Organization (PAHO): *Medical Supply Management after Natural Disaster*, 1983. PAHO, 525 25th St. NW, Washington, DC 20037, USA. Tel. 202/861-4325 (Dr C DeVille).

610. Pantridge JF, Geddes JS: Cardiac arrest after myocardial infarction. *Lancet* **i:** 807, 1966.

611. Pantridge JF, Geddes JS: A mobile intensive care unit in the management of myocardial infarction. *Lancet* **ii:** 271, 1967.

612. Pantridge JR, Adgey AAJ, Webb SW, et al: Electrical requirements for ventricular defibrillation. *Brit Med J* **2:** 313, 1975.

613. Papper EM, Bradley SE: Hemodynamic effects of intravenous morphine and pentobarbital sodium. *J Pharmacol Expert Therap* **74:** 319, 1942.

613a. Paraskos JA: Cardiovascular pharmacology III: atropine, calcium, calcium blockers, and β-blockers. *Circulation* 74(suppl IV): 86, 1986.

614. Parrillo JE, Ayres SM (Eds): *Major Issues in Critical Care Medicine*. Baltimore, Williams & Wilkins, 1984.

615. Patrick EA: Choking: A questionnaire to find the most effective treatment. *Emergency* **12:** 59, 1980.

616. Pearson J, Safar P: General anesthesia with minimal equipment. *Anesth Analg* **40:** 644, 1961.

617. Pearson JW, Redding JS: Influence of peripheral vascular tone on cardiac resuscitation. *Anesth Analg* **44:** 746, 1965.

618. Peirce EC: Extracorporeal circulation for open heart surgery. Springfield, IL, Charles C Thomas, 1969.

619. Peleska B: Transthoracic and direct defibrillation. *Rozhl Chir (CSSR)* **36:** 731, 1957.

619a. Penlington GN: *Anaesthesia* **29:** 494, 1974.

620. Pennington JE, Taylor J, Lown B: Chest thump for reverting ventricular tachycardia. *N Engl J Med* **283:** 1192, 1970.

621. Pennock JL, Pierce WS, Waldhausen JA: Quantitative evaluation of left ventricular bypass in reducing myocardial ischemia. *Surgery* **79:** 523, 1976.

622. Petty TL, Ashbaugh DG: The adult respiratory distress syndrome. *Chest* **60:** 233, 1971.

623. Phillips OC, Frazier TM, Graff TD, et al: The Baltimore Anesthesia Study Committee: Review of 1024 post-operative deaths. *J Amer Med Assoc* **174:** 2015, 1960.

624. Phillips SJ, Ballentine B, Sionine D, et al: Percutaneous initiation of cardiopulmonary bypass. *Ann Thorac Surg* **36:** 223, 1983.

625. Pike FH, Guthrie CC, Stewart GN: Studies in resuscitation. 1. The general conditions affecting resuscitation and the resuscitation of the blood and of the heart. *J Exp Med* **10:** 371, 1908.

626. Pinsky MR, Summer WR: Cardiac augmentation by phasic high intrathoracic pressure support in man (PHIPS). *Chest* **84:** 370, 1983.

627. Pinsky MR, Matuschak GM, Bernardi L, et al: Hemodynamic effects of cardiac-cycle specific increases in intrathoracic pressure. *J Appl Physiol* **60:** 604, 1986.

628. Plum F (Ed): Symposium on brain ischemia. *Arch Neurol* **29:** 1, 1973.

629. Plum F, Posner JB: *The Diagnosis of Stupor and Coma*. Philadelphia, FA Davis, 1980.

630. Pontoppidan H, Geffin B, Lowenstein E: Acute respiratory failure in the adult. *New Engl J Med* **287**: 690, 1972.

631. Poulsen H (Ed): International Symposium on Emergency Resuscitation, Stavanger, Norway, 1960. *Acta Anaesth Scand* (Suppl) **9**, 1961. (See also ref. 491.)

632. Powell DC, Bivins BA, Bell RM: Diagnostic peritoneal lavage. *Surg Gynecol Obstet* **155**: 257, 1982.

633. Powell WF, Ozdil T: A translaryngeal guide for tracheal intubation. *Anesth Analg* **46**: 231, 1967.

634. President's Commission (USA) for the Study of Ethical Problems in Medicine and Biomedical and Behavioural Research: Guidelines for the Determination of Death. *J Amer Med Assoc* **246**: 2184, 1981.

635. President's Commission (USA) for the Study of Ethical Problems in Medicine and Biomedical and Behavioural Research: *Deciding to Forego Life-Sustaining Treatment.* Government Printing Office, Washington, DC, 1983, p 232.

636. Pretto E, Kazziha S, Safar P: Enhanced myocardial resuscitability by lidoflazine postischemia in isolated perfused rat heart preparation. *Anesthesiology* **63**: A118, 1985 (abstract).

637. Pretto E, Safar P, Saito R, et al: Cardiopulmonary bypass after prolonged cardiac arrest in dogs. *Ann Emerg Med* **16**: 611, 1987.

638. Prevost JL, Battelli F: On some effects of electrical discharges on the hearts of mammals. *Compt Rend Acad Sci (Paris)* **129**: 1267, 1899.

639. Price DJ, Knill-Jones R: The prediction of outcome of patients admitted following head injury in coma with bilateral fixed pupils. *Acta Neurochir* (Suppl) **28**: 179, 1979.

639a. Prior PF: EEG monitoring and evoked potentials in brain ischaemia. *Brit J Anaesth* **57**: 63, 1985.

640. Proctor E: Closed-chest circulatory support by pump oxygenator in experimental ventricular fibrillation at normal temperature. *Thorax* **21**: 385, 1966.

641. Pulsinelli W, Brierley J, Plum F: Temporal profile of neuronal damage in a model of transient forebrain ischemia. *Ann Neurol* **11**: 491, 1982.

642. Raj PP, Forestner J, Watson TD, et al: Techniques for fiberoptic laryngoscopy in anesthesia. *Anesth Analg* **53**: 708, 1974.

643. Ralston SH, Babbs CF, Niebauer MJ: Cardiopulmonary resuscitation with interposed abdominal binding during cardiac arrest and resuscitation. *Amer J Cardiol* **53**: 269, 1984.

644. Ralston SH, Tacker WA, Showen L, et al: Endotracheal versus intravenous epinephrine during electromechanical dissociation with CPR in dogs. *Ann Emerg Med* **14**: 1044, 1985.

645. Raphael LD, Mantle JA, Moraski RE, et al: Quantitative assessment of ventricular performance in unstable ischemic heart disease by dextran function curves. *Circulation* **55**: 858, 1977.

646. Rattenborg CC: Effect of bicarbonate and THAM on apnea-induced hypercarbia. In: *Advances in Cardiopulmonary Resuscitation.* P Safar (Ed). New York, Springer-Verlag, 1977, p 128. Chapter 20.

647. Ravitch MM, Lane R, Safar P, et al: Lightning stroke. Recovery after cardiac massage and prolonged artificial respiration. *N Engl J Med* **264**: 36, 1961.

648a. Redding J, Voigt C, Safar P: Drowning treated with IPPB. *J Appl Physiol* **15**: 849, 1960.

648b. Redding J, Voigt C, Safar P: Treatment of seawater aspiration. *J Appl Physiol* **15**: 1113, 1960.

648c. Redding J, Cozine RA: Restoration of circulation after fresh water drowning. *J Appl Physiol* **16**: 1071, 1961.

649. Redding JS, Cozine RA, Voigt GC, et al: Resuscitation from drowning. *J Amer Med Assoc* **178**: 1136, 1961.

650. Redding JS, Cozine R: A comparison of open-chest and closed-chest cardiac massage in dogs. *Anesthesiology* **22**: 280, 1961.

651. Redding JS, Pearson JW: Resuscitation from asphyxia. *J Amer Med Assoc* **182:** 283, 1962.
652. Redding JS, Pearson JW: Evaluation of drugs for cardiac resuscitation. *Anesthesiology* **24:** 203, 1963.
653. Redding JS, Asuncion JS, Pearson JW: Effective routes of drug administration during cardiac arrest. *Anesth Analg* **46:** 253, 1967.
654. Redding J, Pearson JW: Resuscitation from ventricular fibrillation. *J Amer Med Assoc* **203:** 93, 1968.
655. Redding JS: Abdominal compression in CPR. *Anesthesiology* **50:** 668, 1971.
656. Redding JS: Precordial thumping during cardiac resuscitation. In: *Advances in Cardiopulmonary Resuscitation.* P Safar, J Elam (Eds). New York, Springer-Verlag, 1977, p 87.
657. Redding JS: Drug therapy during cardiac arrest. In: *Advances in Cardiopulmonary Resuscitation.* P Safar, J Elam (Eds). New York, Springer-Verlag, 1977, p 113.
658. Redding JS: The choking controversy: critique of evidence on the Heimlich maneuver. *Crit Care Med* **7:** 745, 1979.
659. Redding JS, Haynes RR, Thomas JD: 'Old' and 'new' CPR manually performed in dogs. *Crit Care Med* **9:** 386, 1981.
660. Redding JS (Ed): Wolf Creek Conference on CPR Research No. 2, 1980. *Crit Care Med* **9:** 357, 1981 (see also Wolf Creek No. 1, 1975, ref. 734a and No. 3, 1985, ref. 606).
661. Reedy DP, Little JR, Capraro JA, et al: Effects of verapamil on acute focal cerebral ischemia. *Neurosurgery* **12:** 272, 1983.
662. Rehncrona S, Mela L, Siesjo BK: Recovery of brain mitochondrial function in the rat after complete and incomplete cerebral ischemia. *Stroke* **10:** 437, 1979.
663. Rehncrona S, Rosen I, Siesjo BK: Excessive cellular acidosis: An important mechanism of neuronal damage in the brain? *Acta Physiol Scand* **110:** 435, 1980.
663a. Reich H, Angelos M, Safar P et al: Failure of a multifaceted anti-reoxygenation injury (anti-free radical) therapy to ameliorate brain damage after ventricular fibrillation cardiac arrest of 20 min in dogs. Proc. International Resuscitation Research Symposium 1987, Pittsburgh PA, USA. *Crit Care Med,* in press (abstract).
664. Reichek N: Long-acting nitrates in the treatment of angina pectoris. *J Amer Med Assoc* **236:** 1399, 1976.
665. Resnekov L: Calcium antagonist drugs—myocardial preservation and reduced vulnerability to ventricular fibrillation. *Crit Care Med* **9:** 360, 1981.
666. Reuler JB: Hypothermia: Pathophysiology, clinical settings, and management. *Ann Intern Med* **89:** 519, 1978.
667. Ricci EM: A model for evaluation of disaster medicine (1981). *J World Assoc Emerg. Disaster Med* 1/Suppl I: 30, 1985.
668. Ricci EM, Malloy CL, Safar P: Impact evaluation of a community-wide resuscitation training program. *J World Assoc Emerg Disaster Med* 1/Suppl I: 54, 1985.
669. Richardson JD, Adams L, Flint LM: Selective management of flail chest and pulmonary contusion. *Ann Surg* **196:** 481, 1982.
669a. Ringer S: A further contribution regarding the influence of the different constituents of the blood on the contraction of the heart. *J Physiol* **4:** 29, 1882.
670. Ritter G, Goldstein S, Leighton R, et al: The effect of bystander CPR and arrival time on successful out-of-hospital resuscitation. *Amer J Emerg Med* **2:** 358, 1984 (abstract).
671. Roberts JR, Greenberg MI, Knaub M, et al: Blood levels following intravenous and endotracheal epinephrine administration. *J Amer Coll Emerg Phys* **8:** 53, 1979.
672. Robin ED: The evolutionary advantages of being stupid. *Perspectives Biol Med* **16:** 369, 1972/3.
673. Robin ED, Cross CE, Zelis R: Pulmonary edema. *N Engl J Med* **288:** 239 (part I) and **288:** 292 (part II), 1973.
674. Rockoff MA, Marshall LF, Shapiro HM: High-dose barbiturate therapy in humans: A clinical review of 60 patients. *Ann Neurol* **6:** 194, 1979.
674a. Rogers MC, Nugent SK, Stidham GL: Effects of closed-chest cardiac massage on intracranial pressure. *Crit Care Med* **7:** 454, 1979.

675. Rosborough JP, Hausknecht M, Niemann JT, et al: Cough-supported circulation. *Crit Care Med* **9:** 371, 1981.

676. Rosborough JP, Niemann JT, Criley JM, et al: Lower abdominal compression with synchronized ventilation: A CPR modality. *Circulation* **64:** 303, 1981.

677. Rose DM, Colvin SB, Culliford AT, et al: Long-term survival with partial left heart bypass following perioperative myocardial infarction and shock. *J Thorac Cardiovasc Surg* **83:** 483, 1982.

678. Rose W: Education and training of medical students and physicians in emergency medicine in the DDR (GDR) (1981). *J World Assoc Emerg Disaster Med* 1/Suppl I: 101, 1985 (abstract).

679. Rosen M, Hillard EK: The use of suction in clinical medicine. *Brit J Anaesth* **32:** 486, 1960.

680. Rosomoff HL: Protective effects of hypothermia against pathological processes of the nervous system. *Ann NY Acad Sci* **80:** 475, 1959.

681. Rosomoff HL, Shulman K, Raynor R, et al: Experimental brain injury and delayed hypothermia. *Surg Gynecol Obstet* **110:** 27, 1960.

682. Rossanda M, Selenati A, Villa C, et al: Role of automatic ventilation in treatment of severe head injuries. *J Neurosurg Sciences* **17:** 265, 1973.

683. Rossen R, Cabat H, Anderson JP: Acute arrest of cerebral circulation in man. *Arch Neurol* **50:** 510, 1943.

684. Roth R, Stewart RD, Rogers K, et al: Out-of-hospital cardiac arrest: Factors associated with survival. *Ann Emerg Med* **13:** 237, 1984.

685. Rotheram EB, Safar P, Robin ED: CNS disorder during mechanical ventilation in chronic pulmonary disease. *J Amer Med Assoc* **189:** 993, 1964.

686. Rowbotham ES, Magill I: Anaesthetics in the plastic surgery of the face and jaws. *Proc R Soc Med* **14:** 17, 1921.

687. Royal Colleges of the United Kingdom: Diagnosis of brain death. *Brit Med J* **ii:** 1187, 1976.

688. Ruben H: Combination resuscitator and aspirator. *Anesthesiology* **19:** 408, 1958.

689. Ruben H, Elam JO, Ruben AM, et al: Investigation of upper airway problems in resuscitation. *Anesthesiology* **22:** 271, 1961.

690. Ruben H, Knudsen EJ, Carugati G: Gastric inflation in relation to airway pressure. *Acta Anaesth Scand* **5:** 107, 1961.

691. Ruben H, MacNaughton FI: The treatment of food-choking. *Practitioner* **221:** 725, 1978.

692. Rude RE, Muller JE, Braunwald E: Efforts to limit the size of myocardial infarcts. *Ann Intern Med* **95:** 736, 1981.

693. Rudikoff MT, Maughan WL, Effron M, et al: Mechanisms of blood flow during cardiopulmonary resuscitation **61:** 345, 1980.

694. Ruskin JN, McGovern B, Garan H, et al: Antiarrhythmic drugs: A possible cause of out-of-hospital cardiac arrest. *N Engl J Med* **309:** 1302, 1983.

695. Ruskin JN: Ventricular extrasystoles in healthy subjects. *N Engl J Med* **312:** 238, 1985.

696. Russell ES: Cardiac arrest: A. Survival after 2½ hours open-chest cardiac massage; and B. Survival after closed-chest cardiac massage. *Can Med Assoc J* **87:** 512, 1962.

697. Safar P, McMahon M: Resuscitation of the unconscious victim. A manual. Baltimore, MD, Fire Department, 1957; and Springfield, IL, Charles C Thomas, 1959, 1961.

698. Safar P: Mouth-to-mouth airway. *Anesthesiology* **18:** 904, 1957.

699. Safar P, Escarraga L, Elam J: A comparison of the mouth-to-mouth and mouth-to-airway methods of artificial respiration with the chest-pressure arm-lift methods. *N Engl J Med* **258:** 671, 1958.

700. Safar P: Ventilatory efficacy of mouth-to-mouth artificial respiration. Airway obstruction during manual and mouth-to-mouth artificial respiration. *J Amer Med Assoc* **167:** 335, 1958.

701. Safar P, Park CJ: Aesthetic mouth-to-tracheotomy tube breathing. *Anesthesiology* **19:** 802, 1958.

702.   Safar P: Ventilating bronchoscope. *Anesthesiology* **19:** 407, 1958.
703.   Safar P: The failure of manual artificial respiration. *J Appl Physiol* **4:** 84, 1959.
704.   Safar P, Aguto-Escarraga L, Chang F: A study of upper airway obstruction in the unconscious patient. *J Appl Physiol* **14:** 760, 1959.
705.   Safar P, Redding J: 'Tight jaw' in resuscitation. *Anesthesiology* **20:** 701, 1959.
706a. Safar P, Aguto-Escarraga L, Drawdy L, et al: Wiederbelebung I und II. *Anaesthesist* **8:** 228, 231, 1959.
706b. Safar P, Aguto-Escarraga L, Drawdy L, et al: The resuscitation dilemma. *Anesth Analg* **38:** 394, 1959.
707.   Safar P, Escarraga LA: Compliance in apneic anesthetized adults. *Anesthesiology* **20:** 283, 1959.
708a. Safar P: *Introduction to Respiratory and Cardiac Resuscitation. A Documentary Film of Human Volunteer Research.* Produced by US Walter Reed Army Institute of Research, Washington, DC, USA. Army film PMF5349, 1960. Available from: Univ Pittsburgh Center for Instructional Resources, Pittsburgh, PA 15260, USA.
708b. Safar P: *Introduction to Prolonged Artificial Ventilation. A Documentary Film of Patient Research.* Produced by Walter Reed Army Institute of Research, Washington, DC, USA. Army film PMF5348, 1960. Available from: Univ Pittsburgh Center for Instructional Resources, Pittsburgh, PA 15260, USA.
709a. Safar P, Brown TC, Holtey WH, et al: Ventilation and circulation with closed chest cardiac massage in man. *J Amer Med Assoc* **176:** 574, 1961.
709b. Safar P, Brown TC, Holtey WJ: Failure of closed-chest cardiac massage to produce pulmonary ventilation. *Dis Chest* **41:** 1, 1962.
710.   Safar P, Gedang I: Inexpensive system for the administration of ether. *Anesthesiology* **22:** 323, 1961.
711.   Safar P, DeKornfeld TJ, Pearson JW, et al: Intensive care unit. *Anaesthesia* **16:** 275, 1961.
712.   Safar P, Berman B, Diamond E, et al: Cuffed tracheostomy tube vs. tank respirator for prolonged artificial ventilation. *Arch Phys Med Rehabil* **43:** 487, 1962.
713.   Safar P (Chairman): International Symposium (1962) on *Resuscitation: Controversial Aspects.* Anesthesiology Monograph and Resuscitation Series, Vol. 1. Heidelberg, Springer-Verlag, 1963.
714.   Safar P, Kunkle H: Long-term resuscitation in intensive care units (National Research Council Symposium). *Anesthesiology* **25:** 216, 1964.
715.   Safar P: Community-wide cardiopulmonary resuscitation. *J Iowa Med Soc* Nov: 629, 1964.
716.   Safar P, Tenicela R: High altitude physiology in relation to anesthesia and inhalation therapy. *Anesthesiology* **25:** 515, 1964.
717.   Safar P: The anesthesiologist as 'intensivist'. In: *Science and Practice in Anesthesia.* JE Eckenhoff (Ed). Philadelphia, Lippincott, 1965.
718.   Safar P (Ed): *Respiratory Therapy.* Philadelphia, FA Davis, 1966, p 265.
719.   Safar P, Pennickx J: Cricothyroid membrane puncture with special cannula. *Anesthesiology* **28:** 943, 1967.
720.   Safar P: *Cardiopulmonary Cerebral Resuscitation.* Prepared for the World Federation of Societies of Anaesthesiologists. 1st ed, 1968; 2nd ed, 1981; 3rd ed, 1988. Stavanger, A Laerdal; London Philadelphia Toronto, WB Saunders.
721.   Safar P, Grenvik A: Critical care medicine: organization and staffing intensive care units. *Chest* **59:** 535, 1971.
722.   Safar P: Some central nervous system considerations in resuscitation and intensive care. Proceedings, 5th International Anaesthesie Postgraduate Course (O. Mayrhofer, Chairman), Univ. Vienna, Austria. *Vienna, Mediz Akad Wien Publ,* Sept. 1971.
723a. Safar P, Brose RA: Ambulance design and equipment for resuscitation. *Arch Surg* **90:** 343, 1965.
723b. Safar P, Esposito G, Benson DM: Ambulance design and equipment for mobile intensive care. *Arch Surg* **102:** 163, 1971.

723c. Safar P, Esposito G, Benson DM: Emergency medical technicians as allied health professionals. *Anesth Analg* **51:** 27, 1972.

724. Safar P (Chairman): *Proceedings, 1st–10th International Symposia on Emergency and Critical Care Medicine*, Univ Pittsburgh, 1967–1976. Pittsburgh, Univ Cont Educ Publ.

725. Safar P, Grenvik A, Smith J: Progressive pulmonary consolidation: Review of cases and pathogenesis. *J Trauma* **12:** 955, 1972.

726. Safar P, Nemoto EM, Severinghaus JW: Pathogenesis of central nervous system disorder during artificial hyperventilation in compensated hypercarbia in dogs. *Crit Care Med* **1/1:** 5, 1973.

727. Safar P: Critical care medicine—quo vadis: *Crit Care Med* **2:** 1, 1974.

728. Safar P: On the philosophy, physiology, history and future of resuscitation. *Anaesthesist* **23/12:** 507, 1974 (in German; English version available from author).

729. Safar P: Pocket mask for emergency artificial ventilation and oxygen inhalation. *Crit Care Med* **2:** 273, 1974.

730a. Safar P (Ed): *Public Health Aspects of Critical Care Medicine and Anesthesiology.* Philadelphia, FA Davis, 1974.

730b. Safar P: Health care delivery problems and goals: a personal philosophic appraisal. In: *Public Health Aspects of Critical Care Medicine and Anesthesiology.* P Safar (Ed). Philadelphia, FA Davis, 1974. Chapter 1.

730c. Safar P, Benson DM, Esposito G, et al: Emergency and critical care medicine: local implementation of national recommendations. In: *Public Health Aspects of Critical Care Medicine and Anesthesiology.* P Safar (Ed). Philadelphia, FA Davis, 1974. Chapter 4 (see also Chapter 6).

730d. Safar P, Benson DM, Berkebile PE, et al: Teaching and organizing cardiopulmonary resuscitation. In: *Public Health Aspects of Critical Care Medicine and Anesthesiology.* Philadelphia, FA Davis, 1974. Chapter 7.

731. Safar P, Grenvik A: Speaking cuffed tracheostomy tube. *Crit Care Med* **3:** 23, 1975.

732. Safar P, Lind B: Triple airway maneuver, artificial ventilation and oxygen inhalation by mouth–to–mask and bag–valve–mask techniques. *Proc National Conf on CPR 1973*, Dallas. Amer Heart Assoc, 1975, p 49.

733. Safar P, Stezoski SW, Nemoto EM: Amelioration of brain damage after 12 minutes cardiac arrest in dogs. *Arch Neurol* **33:** 91, 1976.

734a. Safar P, Elam J (Eds): Advances in Cardiopulmonary Resuscitation. Wolf Creek Conference on CPR Research No. 1, 1975. New York, Springer-Verlag, 1977 (see also Wolf Creek No. 2, 1980, ref. 660 and No. 3, 1985, ref. 606).

734b. Safar P: Resuscitation of the arrested brain. In: *Advances in Cardiopulmonary Resuscitation.* P Safar, J Elam (Eds). New York, Springer-Verlag, 1977, p 177. Chapters 27–29.

734c. Safar P: From back-pressure arm-lift to mouth-to-mouth, control of airway, and beyond. Historic vignette. In: *Advances in Cardiopulmonary Resuscitation.* P Safar, J Elam (Eds). New York, Springer-Verlag, 1977, p 266.

735. Safar P, Grenvik A: Organization and physician education in critical care medicine. *Anesthesiology* **47:** 82, 1977.

736a. Safar P: The mechanisms of dying and their reversal. In: *Principles and Practice of Emergency Medicine.* G Schwartz, P Safar, J Stone, et al (Eds). Philadelphia, WB Saunders, (1978), 1986. Chapter 1.

736b. Safar P, Caroline N, et al: Pathophysiology of vital organ systems failure. In: *Principles and Practice of Emergency Medicine.* G Schwartz, P Safar, J Stone, et al (Eds). Philadelphia, WB Saunders, (1978), 1986. Chapters 2–8.

736c. Safar P, Caroline N: Respiratory care techniques and strategies. In: *Principles and Practice of Emergency Medicine.* G Schwartz, P Safar, J Stone, et al (Eds). Philadelphia, WB Saunders, (1978), 1986. Chapter 11.

737. Safar P, (Ed): Brain resuscitation. Special symposium issue. *Crit Care Med* **6:** 199, 1978.

738. Safar P: Editorial. Brain resuscitation in metabolic-toxic infectious encephalopathy. *Crit Care Med* **6:** 68, 1978.
739. Safar P: Pathophysiology and resuscitation after global brain ischemia. In: *Management of Acute Intracranial Disasters.* RB Trubuhovich (Ed). Boston, Little Brown, 1979, p 239.
740. Safar P: Amelioration of postischemic brain damage with barbiturates. *Stroke* **15:** 1, 1980.
741. Safar P: Steroids in brain insults (a partial review). In: *Critical Care Medicine.* SA Villazon, JLB Llamosa, PL Hervella, et al (Eds). Amsterdam, Excerpta Medica, 1980, p 164.
742. Safar P, Bleyaert A, Nemoto E, Stezoski W: Treatment of hypoperfusion after global brain ischemia in dogs and monkeys. *Circ Shock* **7:** 200, 1980 (abstract).
743. Safar P: Resuscitation after brain ischemia. In: *Brain Failure and Resuscitation.* A Grenvik, P Safar (Eds). Clinics in Critical Care Medicine. New York, Churchill Livingstone, 1981, p 155.
744. Safar P, Berkebile P, Scott MA, et al: Education research on life-supporting first aid (LSFA) and CPR self-training systems (STS). *Crit Care Med* **9:** 403, 1981.
745. Safar P, Gisvold SE, Vaagenes P, et al: Long-term animal models for the study of global brain ischemia. In: *Protection of Tissues Against Hypoxia.* A Wauquier, M Borgers, WK Amery (Eds). Amsterdam, Elsevier, 1982, p 147.
746. Safar P: Reanimatology—The science of resuscitation (editorial). *Crit Care Med* **10:** 134, 1982.
747. Safar P: The critical care medicine continuum from scene to outcome. In: *Major Issues in Critical Care Medicine.* JE Parrillo, SM Ayres (Eds). Baltimore, Williams & Wilkins, 1984, p 71.
748. Safar P, Cantadore R, Vaagenes P: Prolonged cardiovascular system (CVS) failure after cardiac arrest (CA) and cardiopulmonary resuscitation (CPR) in dogs. *Circ Shock* **13:** 70, 1984 (abstract).
749. Safar P: Effects of postresuscitation syndrome on cerebral recovery from cardiac arrest. Review and hypotheses. *Crit Care Med* **13:** 932, 1985.
750. Safar P: Long-term animal outcome models for cardiopulmonary-cerebral resuscitation research. *Crit Care Med* **13:** 936, 1985.
751. Safar P: Resuscitation potentials in mass disasters. (a) In: Mobile ICUs (1973). *Anesthesiology and Resuscitation* Vol. 95. R Frey, E Nagel, P Safar (Eds). Heidelberg, Springer-Verlag, 1976. (b) In: *Resuscitation and Life Support in Disasters* (1977). Disaster Medicine Vol. 2. R Frey, P Safar (Eds). Heidelberg, Springer-Verlag, 1980. (c) In: Emergency and Disaster Medicine (1st R Frey memorial lecture, 1983). C Manni, SI Magalini (Eds). New York, Springer-Verlag, 1985, p. 28. (d) In: *J World Assoc Disaster Med* 1/1, 1985; 1/Suppl I, 1985; 2/1, 1986.
752. Safar P (Ed): Disaster Resuscitology. Proceedings of the Second World Congress on Emergency and Disaster Medicine (Club of Mainz), Pittsburgh, PA, USA, 1981. *J World Assoc Emerg Disaster Med* 1/Suppl I, 1985, p 159.
753. Safar P: The potential impact of cardiopulmonary cerebral resuscitation (CPCR) education (1981). *J World Assoc Emerg Disaster Med* 1/Suppl I: 70, 1985.
754a. Safar P (Ed): Military and disaster medicine. *J World Assoc Emerg Disaster Med* 1/1, 1985.
754b. Safar P: Prevention of nuclear war and disaster preparedness. *J World Assoc Emerg Disaster Med* 1/1: 18, 1985.
755a. Safar P, Ramos V, Mosquera J, et al: Anecdotes on resuscitation potentials following the earthquake of 1970 in Peru. *J World Assoc Emerg Disaster Med* **3:** 124, 1987.
755b. Safar P, Kirimli N, Agnes A, Magalini S: Anecdotes on resuscitation potentials following the earthquake of 1980 in Italy. Proc. Fourth World Congress on Emergency and Disaster Medicine, June 1985, Brighton, UK (abstract).
755c. Safar P: Resuscitation potentials in mass disasters. *J World Assoc Emerg Disaster Med* **2:** 34, 1986.

755d. Safar P, Pretto E, Bircher N: Disaster resuscitology including management of severe trauma. In: *Medicine for Disasters*, Baskett P, Weller R (Eds). John Wright, Bristol, in press.

756. Safar P, Silverstein ME: Panels on (a) emergency and disaster medicine and civil defense in nuclear war; (b) questions for military medicine; and (c) prescriptions against roots of wars. *Proceedings, IPPNW Congress*, Cologne, Germany, 1986. (Reprints from authors.)

757. Safar P: Physiologic basis of cardiopulmonary–cerebral resuscitation. In: *Cardiopulmonale und cerebrale Reanimation (CPCR)*. W Mauritz, K Steinbereithner (Eds). Vienna, Verlag Wilhelm Maudrich, 1987.

758. Safar P et al.: Emergency cardiopulmonary bypass for resuscitation from prolonged cardiac arrest. Invited review for *J Amer Med Assoc*, in preparation.

758a. Safar P: A personal history of cardiopulmonary-cerebral resuscitation. Invited review for *J Amer Med Assoc*, in preparation.

759. Safar P: Cerebral resuscitation after cardiac arrest. A review. *Circulation* 74 (suppl IV): 138, 1986.

760a. Safar P: Reversibility of clinical death in animal outcome models: the myth of the 5 minute limit. *Ann Emerg Med* 16: 514, 1987 (abstract).

760b. Safar P, Breivik H, Abramson N, et al: Reversibility of clinical death in patients: the myth of the 5 minute limit. *Ann Emerg Med* 16: 495, 1987 (abstract).

760c. Safar P, Grenvik A, Abramson N, et al (Eds): *International Resuscitation Research Symposium on the Reversibility of Clinical Death*, May 1987. *Crit Care Med*, 1988.

760d. Safar P, White B, Cummins R: Cardiopulmonary-cerebral resuscitation: Biologic limits and therapeutic potentials. Invited review for *Science*, in preparation.

761. Saito Y, Teresaki H, Otsu T, et al: Extracorporeal lung assist (ECLA) with a single catheter in puppies. *Crit Care Med* 13: 501, 1985.

762. Saklad M, Gulati R: Adaptation of Ambu respirator for high oxygen concentration. *Anesthesiology* 24: 877, 1963.

763. Salem MR, Wong AY, Mani M: Efficacy of cricoid pressure in preventing gastric inflation during bag–mask ventilation in pediatric patients. *Anesthesiology* 40: 96, 1974.

764. Samuelson T, Doolittle W, Hayward J, et al: Hypothermia and cold water near drowning: Treatment guidelines. *Alaska Med* 24: 106, 1982.

765a. Sanders AB, Kern KB, Ewy GA, et al: Improved resuscitation from cardiac arrest with open chest massage. *Ann Emerg Med* 13: 672, 1984.

765b. Sanders AB, Kern KB, Ewy GA: Time limitations for open-chest cardiopulmonary resuscitation from cardiac arrest. *Crit Care Med* 13: 897, 1985.

765c. Sanders AB, Kern KB, Atlas M, et al: Importance of the duration of inadequate coronary perfusion pressure on resuscitation from cardiac arrest. *J Amer Coll Cardiol* 6: 113, 1985.

766. Sanna G, Arcidiacano R: Chemical ventricular defibrillation of the human heart with bretylium tosylate. *Amer J Cardiol* 39: 982, 1973.

767. Sasahara AA, Cannilla JE, Morse RL, et al: Clinical and physiologic studies in pulmonary thromboembolism. *Amer J Cardiol* 20: 10, 1967.

768. Sassano J, Eshel G, Safar P, et al: Hyperthermic cardiac arrest in monkeys. *Crit Care Med* 9: 409, 1981.

769. Sassano J: The rapid infusion system. In: *Hepatic Transplantation: Anesthetic and Perioperative Management*. PM Winter, YG Kang (Eds). New York, Praeger, 1986 (*see also* ref. 970a).

770. Schanne FAX, Kane AB, Young EE, et al: Calcium dependence of toxic cell death: a final commmon pathway. *Science* 206: 700, 1979.

771. Scheidt S, Wilner G, Mueller H, et al: Intra-aortic balloon counterpulsation in cardiogenic shock. Report of a co-operative clinical trial. *N Engl J Med* 288: 979, 1973.

772. Schelton RL, Bosma JF: Maintenance of the pharyngeal airway. *J Appl Physiol* 17: 208, 1962.

773. Schiff M: Ueber direkte Reizung der Herzoberflaeche. *Arch Ges Physiol* 28: 200, 1882.

774. Schocket E, Rosenblum R: Successful open cardiac massage after 75 minutes of closed massage. *J Amer Med Assoc* **200:** 333, 1967.
775. Schofferman J, Oill P, Lewis AJ: The esophageal obturator airway. A clinical evaluation. *Chest* **69:** 67, 1976.
775a. Scholten DJ, Vaagenes P, Safar P, et al: Failure of a resuscitation drug combination to ameliorate brain damage after cardiac arrest in dogs. 1985, intramural publication.
776. Schuder JC, Rahmoeller GA, Stoeckle H: Transthoracic ventricular defibrillation with triangular and trapezoidal waveforms. *Circ Res* **19:** 689, 1966.
777. Schuster DP, Snyder JV, Klain M: High frequency ventilation during oleic acid induced pulmonary edema in dogs. *Anesth Analg* **61:** 735, 1982.
778. Schwartz AC: Neurological recovery after cardiac arrest: Clinical feasibility trial of calcium blockers. *Amer J Emerg Med* **3:** 1, 1985.
779. Schwartz AJ, Orkin FK, Ellison N: Anesthesiologists' training and knowledge of basic life support. *Anesthesiology* **50:** 191, 1979.
780. Schwartz G, Safar P, Stone J, et al (Eds): *Principles and Practice of Emergency Medicine.* Philadelphia, WB Saunders, 1986.
780a. Sclabassi RJ, Hinman CL, Kroin JS, et al: A non-linear analysis of afferent modulatory activity in the cat somatosensory system. *Electroencephalogr Clin Neurophysiol* **60:** 444, 1985.
781. Scott MA, Safar P, Berkebile P, et al: Cardiopulmonary resuscitation basic and advanced life support self-training systems for paramedical and medical personnel. Disaster Resuscitology (1981). *J World Assoc Emerg Disaster Med* 1/Suppl I: 96, 1985.
782. Secher O, Wilhjelm B: The protective action of anesthetics against hypoxia. *Can Anaesth Soc J* **15:** 423, 1968.
783. Seeley S: *Accidental Death and Disability: The Neglected Disease of Modern Society.* Committee on Trauma and Committee on Shock, Division of Medical Sciences, 1966. National Academy of Sciences, National Research Council, 2101 Constitution Ave, Washington, DC, USA, 20418.
784. Sefrna B: Analgesia in mass accidents. In: *Disaster Medicine: Resuscitation and Life Support. Relief of Pain and Suffering.* R Frey, P Safar (Eds). Berlin, Springer-Verlag, 1980.
784a. Sefrna B, Pokorny J: The physician-staffed ambulance service of Prague, C.S.S.R., 1960s. In preparation for *J. World Assoc Emerg Disaster Med.*
784b. Seidel JS: A needs assessment of advanced life support and emergency medical services in the pediatric patient: state of the art. *Circulation* 74(suppl IV): 129, 1986.
785. Sellick BA: Cricoid pressure to control regurgitation of stomach contents during induction of anesthesia. *Lancet* **ii:** 404, 1961.
786. Severinghaus JW, Bradley AF: Electrode for blood PO_2 and PCO_2 determinations. *J Appl Physiol* **13:** 515, 1958.
787. Severinghaus J: Blood gas concentrations. In: *Handbook of Physiology,* Vol. II, Section 3, Respiration. Washington, Am Physiol Soc, 1965, p 1475. Chapter 61.
788. Severinghaus JW, Stafford M, Bradley AF: $tcPCO_2$ electrode design, calibration and temperature gradient problems. *Acta Anaesth Scand* **68:** 118, 1978.
789. Shalit MN, Bellar AJ, Feinsod M, et al: The blood flow and oxygen consumption of the dying brain. *Neurology* **20:** 740, 1970.
790. Shapiro HM: Intracranial hypertension. Therapeutic and anesthetic considerations. *Anesthesiology* **43:** 445, 1975.
791. Sharp JT: The effect of body position on lung compliance in normal subjects and in patients with congestive heart failure. *J Clin Invest* **38:** 659, 1959.
792. Shea SR, MacDonald JR, Gruzinski G: Pre-hospital endotracheal tube airway or esophageal gastric tube airway: A critical comparison. *Ann Emerg Med* **14:** 102, 1985.
793. Shibolet S, Lancaster MC, Dannon Y: Heat stroke: A review. *Aviation Space Envir Med* **47:** 280, 1976.
794. Shimazu S, Shatney CH: Outcomes of trauma patients with no vital signs on hospital admission. *J Trauma* **23:** 213, 1983.
795. Shiu GK, Nemmer JP, Nemoto EM: Reassessment of brain free fatty acid liberation

during global ischemia and its attenuation by barbiturate anesthesia. *J Neurochem* **40:** 880, 1983.

796. Shoemaker WC: Comparison of the relative effectiveness of whole blood transfusions and various types of fluid therapy in resuscitation. *Crit Care Med* **4:** 71, 1976.

797. Shoemaker WC, Appel PL, Waxman KL, et al: Clinical trial of survivors cardiorespiratory pattern as therapeutic goals in critically ill post-operative patients. *Crit Care Med* **10:** 398, 1982.

798. Shoemaker WC, Appel PL, Bland R: Use of physiologic monitoring to predict outcome and assist in clinical decisions in the critically ill post-operative patient. *Amer J Surg* **146:** 43, 1983.

799. Shoemaker WC, Grenvik A, Thompson WL, Holbrook PR (Eds): *The Society of Critical Care Medicine: Textbook of Critical Care*. Philadelphia, WB Saunders, 1984, 2nd ed, 1988.

800. Shoemaker WC: Pathophysiology and therapy of shock syndromes. In: *Textbook of Critical Care*. WC Shoemaker, WL Thompson, PR Holbrook (Eds). Philadelphia, WB Saunders, 1984, p 52. Chapter 11.

801. Shoemaker WC, Tremper KK: Transcutaneous PO_2 PCO_2 monitoring in the adult. In: *Textbook of Critical Care*. WC Shoemaker, WL Thompson, PR Holbrook (Eds). Philadelphia, WB Saunders, 1984.

802a. Shubin H, Weil MH: Shock associated with barbiturate intoxication. *J Amer Med Assoc* **215:** 265, 1971.

802b. Shubin H, Weil MH, Nishijima H: Bacterial shock. In: *Critical Care Medicine Handbook*. MH Weil, H Shubin (Eds). New York, JN Kolen, 1974, p 189.

803. Shyngle JA, Sodipo JOA: Disaster preparedness in Nigeria (1981). *J World Assoc Emerg Disaster Med* 1/Suppl I: 335, 1985.

804. Siebke H, Rod T, Breivik H: Survival after 40 minutes submersion without cerebral sequelae. *Lancet* **i:** 1275, 1975.

805. Siesjo BK: *Brain Energy Metabolism*. Chichester, John Wiley, 1978.

806. Siesjo BK: Cell damage in the brain: A speculative synthesis. *J Cereb Blood Flow Metab* **1:** 155, 1981.

807. Siesjo BK, Wieloch T: Cerebral metabolism in ischemia: neurochemical basis for therapy. *Brit J Anaesth* **57:** 47, 1985.

808. Siggaard-Anderson O: Blood acid–base alignment nomogram. Scales for pH, PCO_2, base excess of whole blood of different hemoglobin concentration, plasma bicarbonate and plasma total CO_2. *Scand J Clin Lab Invest* **15:** 211, 1963.

809. Silverstein ME: National Disaster Medical System (NDMS) Planning for the USA. *J World Assoc Emerg Disaster Med* **1:** 39, 1985.

810. Singh BN, Ellrodt G, Peter CT: Verapamil: A review of its pharmacological properties and therapeutic use. *Drugs* **15:** 169, 1978.

811. Singh NP: Transtracheal jet ventilation as a new technique and experiences with ketamine and propandid in India. In: *Anesthesiology*. (WFSA Congress Kyoto, 1972). M Miyazaki (Ed). Amsterdam, Excerpta Medica, 1973, p 160.

812. Sjostrand U (Ed): Experimental and clinical evaluation of high frequency positive pressure ventilation. *Acta Anaesth Scand* **64:** 1, 1977.

813. Sladen A, Aldredge CF, Albarran R: PEEP vs. ZEEP in the treatment of flail chest injuries. *Crit Care Med* **1:** 187, 1973.

814. Sladen A: Endotracheal intubation—A training demonstration film using intubation manikin, 1977. Laerdal Medical, Armonk, New York 10504, USA.

815. Sladen A: Acid base balance. In: *Advanced Cardiac Life Support Manual*. Dallas, Amer Heart Assoc, 1981, 1983.

816. Sloviter HA, Petokovic M, Ogoshi S, et al: Dispersed fluorochemicals as substitutes for erythrocytes in intact animals. *J Appl Physiol* **27:** 666, 1969.

817. Smetana J, Racenberg E, Juna S: Resuscitation of the heart; experimental study and clinical experience. *Rev Czech Med* **7:** 65, 1961.

818. Smith AL, Hoff JT, Nielson SL: Barbiturate protection against cerebral infarction. *Stroke* **5:** 1, 1974.

819. Smith AL, Marque JJ: Anesthetics and cerebral edema. *Anesthesiology* **45:** 64, 1976.

820. Smith DS, Rehncrona S, Siesjo BK: Inhibitory effects of different barbiturates on lipid peroxidation in brain tissue in vitro: Comparison with the effects of promethazine and chlorpromazine. *Anesthesiology* **53:** 186, 1980.

821. Smith J, Penninckx JJ, Kampschulte S, et al: Need for oxygen enrichment in myocardial infarction, shock, and following cardiac arrest. *Acta Anaesth Scand* (Suppl) **29:** 127, 1968.

822. Smith JP, Bodai BI, Aubourg R, et al: A field evaluation of the esophageal obturator airway. *J Trauma* 23: 317, 1983.

823. Smith RB, Schaer WB, Pfaeffle H: Percutaneous transtracheal ventilation for anesthesia and resuscitation: a review and report of complications. *Can Anaesth Soc J* **22:** 607, 1975.

824. Snyder BD, Ramirez-Lessepas M, Sukhum P, et al: Failure of thiopental to moderate global anoxic injury. *Stroke* **10:** 135, 1979.

825. Snyder JV, Nemoto EM, Carroll RG, et al: Global ischemia in dogs: intracranial pressures, brain blood flow and metabolism. *Stroke* **6:** 21, 1975.

826. Snyder JV, Powner DJ, Grenvik A: Neurologic intensive care. In: *Anesthesia and Neurosurgery.* JE Cottrell (Ed). St Louis, Mosby, 1980, 1986.

827. Snyder JV (Ed): *Oxygen Transport in the Critically Ill.* Chicago, Year Book Medical, 1986.

828a. Society of Critical Care Medicine (SCCM) (USA): Guidelines for organization of critical care units. *J Amer Med Assoc* **222:** 1532, 1972.

828b. Society of Critical Care Medicine (SCCM) (USA): Guidelines for training of physicians in critical care medicine. *Crit Care Med* **1:** 39, 1973.

829. Sodi-Pallares D, Bisteni A, DeLeon JP, et al: Polarizing solution in myocardial infarction. *Amer J Cardiol* **21:** 275, 1968.

830. Southwick FS, Dalglish PH: Recovery after prolonged asystolic cardiac arrest in profound hypothermia. A case report and literature review. *J Amer Med Assoc* **243:** 1250, 1980.

831. Sowden GR, Baskett PJF, Robins DW: Factors associated with survival and eventual cerebral status following cardiac arrest. *Anaesthesia* **39:** 39, 1984.

832. Spear JF, Moore EN, Gerstenblith G: Effect of lidocaine on the ventricular fibrillation threshold in the dog during acute ischemia and premature ventricular contractions. *Circulation* **46:** 65, 1972.

833. Spence M: Organization for intensive care. *Med J Australia* **1:** 795, 1967.

834. Spence M: Severe intracranial infections. In: *Management of Acute Intracranial Disasters.* RV Trubuhovich (Ed). Boston, Little Brown, 1979, p 285.

835. Spoerel WE, Narayanan PS, Singh NP: Transtracheal ventilation. *Br J Anaesth* **43:** 932, 1971.

836. Sprung C, Grenvik A (Eds): Invasive procedures in critical care. *Clinics in Critical Care Medicine.* New York, Churchill Livingstone, 1985.

837. Stajduhar K, Steinberg R, Sotosky M, et al: Cerebral blood flow (CBF) and common carotid artery blood flow (CCABF) during open chest cardiopulmonary resuscitation (OCCPR) in dogs. *Anesthesiology* **59:** A117, 1983 (abstract).

837a. Star LD, Abelson LC, DelGuercio LRM, et al: Mobilization of trauma teams for aircraft disasters. *Aviation Space Envir Med* 51/11: 1261, 1980.

838. Stark MF, Rader B, Sobol BJ, et al: Cardiovascular hemodynamic function in complete heart block and the effect of isopropyl norepinephrine. *Circulation* **17:** 526, 1950.

839. Steen PA, Tinker JH, Pluth JR, et al: Efficacy of dopamine, dobutamine, and epinephrine during emergency cardiopulmonary bypass in man. *Circulation* **57:** 378, 1978.

840. Steen PA, Milde JH, Michenfelder JD: No barbiturate protection in a dog model of complete cerebral ischemia. *Ann Neurol* **5:** 343, 1979.

841. Steen PA, Michenfelder JD, Milde JH: Incomplete versus complete cerebral ischemia: Improved outcome with a minimal blood flow. *Ann Neurol* **6:** 389, 1979.

842. Steen PA, Soule EH, Michenfelder JD: Detrimental effect of prolonged hypothermia in rats and monkeys with and without regional cerebral ischemia. *Stroke* **10:** 522, 1979.

843. Steen PA, Newberg LA, Milde JH, et al: Nimodipine improves cerebral blood flow and neurologic recovery after complete cerebral ischemia in the dog. *J Cereb Blood Flow Metab* **3:** 38, 1983.

844. Steen PA, Newberg LA, Milde JH, et al: Cerebral blood flow and neurologic outcome when nimodipine is given after complete cerebral ischemia in the dog. *J Cereb Blood Flow Metab* **4:** 82, 1984.

845. Steen PA, Gisvold SE, Milde JH, et al: Nimodipine improves outcome when given after complete cerebral ischemia in primates. *Anesthesiology* **62:** 406, 1985.

846. Steichen F, Dargan EL, Perlman DM, et al: A graded approach to the management of penetrating wounds of the heart. *Arch Surg* **103:** 572, 1971.

847. Steichen FM: Traumatic hemopericardium, cardiac tamponade, and suture of penetrating heart wounds. *Surgical Rounds,* Jan, 1986, p 88.

848. Steinbereithner K, Schindler I, Mauritz W, Sporn P: Kontraindikationen—Abbruch der Reanimation. In: *Cardiopulmonale und cerebrale Reanimation (CPCR).* W Mauritz, K Steinbereithner (Eds). Vienna, Verlag Wilhelm Maudrich, 1987.

849. Steinbereithner K, Bergman NH (Eds): Intensiv Therapie (in German). Stuttgart, G Thieme, 1982. (1st ed, R Kucher, K Steinbereithner (Eds), 1972.)

850. Steinman AM: Cardiopulmonary resuscitation and hypothermia. *Circulation* **74:**(suppl IV): IV–29, 1986.

851. Stephenson HE Jr, Reid LC, Hinton JW: Some common denominators in 1200 cases of cardiac arrest. *Ann Surg* **137:** 731, 1953.

852. Stephenson HE Jr: *Cardiac Arrest and Resuscitation.* St Louis, CV Mosby, 1974.

853. Stephenson HE Jr: *Immediate Care of the Acutely Ill and Injured.* St. Louis, CV Mosby, 1974.

854. Stept WJ, Safar P: Cardiac resuscitation following two hours of cardiac massage and 42 countershocks. *Anesthesiology* **27:** 97, 1966.

855. Stept WJ, Safar P: Rapid induction/intubation for prevention of gastric content aspiration. *Anesth Analg* **49:** 633, 1970.

856. Stewart GN, Guthrie C, Burns RI: The resuscitation of the central nervous system of mammals. *J Exper Med* **8:** 289, 1906.

857. Stewart JS: Management of cardiac arrest with special reference to metabolic acidosis. *Brit Med J* **i:** 476, 1964.

858. Stewart RD: CPR in prehospital care. *Topics Emerg Med* **1:** 1, 1979.

859. Stewart RD: Tactile orotracheal intubation. *Ann Emerg Med* **13:** 175, 1984.

860. Stewart RD, Paris PM, Stoy WA, et al: Field endotracheal intubation by paramedical personnel. Success rates and complications. *Chest* **85:** 341, 1984.

861. Stoelting RK: Endotracheal intubation. In: *Anesthesia.* RD Miller (Ed). New York, Churchill Livingstone, 1986, p 523. Chapter 16.

862. Storey PB: Emergency medical services in the USSR. In: *Principles and Practice of Emergency Medicine.* G Schwartz, P Safar, J Stone, et al (Eds). Philadelphia, WB Saunders, 1986, p 666. Chapter 31.

863. Stremple JF: Stress ulceration—revisited. *Surgical Rounds* **2/12:** 40, 1979.

864. Stuckey JH, Newman MM, Dennis C: The use of the heart lung machine in selected cases of acute myocardial infarction. *Surg Forum* **8:** 342, 1957.

865. Stueven HA, Tonsfeldt DJ, Thompson BM, et al: Atropine in asystole: Human studies. *Ann Emerg Med* **13:** 815, 1984.

866. Stueven HA, Thompson B, Aprahamian C, et al: The effectiveness of calcium chloride in refractory electromechanical dissociation. *Ann Emerg Med* **14:** 626, 1985.

867. Stueven HA, Thompson B, Aprahamian C, et al: Lack of effectiveness of calcium chloride in refractory asystole. *Ann Emerg Med* **14:** 630, 1985.

868. Stullken EH, Sokol MD: The effects of heparin on recovery from ischemic brain injuries in cats. *Anesth Analg* **55:** 683, 1976.
869. Stults KR, Brown DD, Schug VL, et al: Prehospital defibrillation performed by emergency medical technicians in rural communities. *New Engl J Med* **310:** 219, 1984.
870. Sundt R, Naltz AG, Sayre GP: Experimental cerebral infarction. Modification by treatment with hemodiluting, hemoconcentrating and dehydrating agents. *J Neurosurg* **26:** 46, 1967.
871. Suter PM, Fairley HB, Isenberg MD: The optimum end-expiratory airway pressure in patients with acute pulmonary failure. *N Engl J Med* **292:** 284, 1975.
872. Swan HJC, Ganz W, Forresters J, et al: Catheterization of the heart in man with use of a flow-directed balloon-tipped catheter. *N Engl J Med* **283:** 447, 1970.
873. Swann HG, Brucer M: The cardiorespiratory and biochemical events during rapid anoxic death. *Tex Rep Biol Med* **7:** 511, 1949.
874. Sykes MK, Ahmed N: Emergency treatment of cardiac arrest. *Lancet* **ii:** 347, 1963.
875. Symon L: Flow thresholds in brain ischaemia and the effects of drugs. *Brit J Anaesth* **57:** 34, 1985.
876. Szmolenszky T, Szoke P, Halmagyi G, et al: Organ blood flow during external heart massage. *Acta Chir Acad Sci Hung* **15:** 283, 1974.
877. Tacker WA Jr, Wey GA: Emergency defibrillation dose: Recommendations and rationale. *Circulation* **60:** 223, 1979.
878. Tacker WA, Niebauer MJ, Babbs CF, et al: The effect of newer antiarrhythmic drugs on defibrillation threshold. *Crit Care Med* **8:** 177, 1980.
879. Takahashi Y, Campbell CD, Laas J, et al: Reduction of myocardial infarct size in swine: A comparative study of intraaortic balloon pumping and transapical left ventricular bypass. *Ann Thoracic Surg* **32:** 475, 1981.
880. Takaori M, Safar P: Treatment of massive hemorrhage with colloid and crystalloid solution. *J Amer Med Assoc* **199:** 297, 1967.
881. Takaori M, Safar P: Critical point in progressive hemodilution with hydroxyethyl starch. *Kawasaki Med J* **2:** 211, 1976.
882. Taussig HB: Death from lightning and the possibility of living again. *Amer Sci* **57:** 306, 1969.
883. Taylor GJ, Tucker WM, Greene HL, et al: Importance of prolonged compression during cardiopulmonary resuscitation in man. *New Engl J Med* **296:** 1515, 1977.
884. Taylor GJ, Rubin R, Tucker WM, et al: External cardiac compression: A randomized comparison of mechanical and manual techniques. *J Amer Med Assoc* **240:** 644, 1978.
885. Teasdale G, Jennett B: Assessment of coma and impaired consciousness. A practical scale. *Lancet* **ii:** 81, 1974.
886. Teasdale G, Galbraith S: Head trauma and intracranial hemorrhage. In: *Brain Failure and Resuscitation.* Clinics in Critical Care Medicine. A Grenvik, P Safar (Eds). New York, Churchill Livingstone, 1981.
887. Tedeschi CG, White CW Jr: Morphologic study of canine hearts subjected to fibrillation, electrical defibrillation and manual compression. *Circulation* **9:** 916, 1954.
888. Telivuo L, Maamies T, Siltanen P, et al: Comparison of alkalizing agents in resuscitation of the heart after ventricular fibrillation. *Ann Chir Gynaecol Finn* **57:** 221, 1968.
889. Thaler MM, Stobie GH: An improved technic of external cardiac compression in infants and young children. *New Engl J Med* **269:** 606, 1963.
890. Thevenet A, Hodges PC, Lillehei CW: The use of a myocardial electrode inserted percutaneously for control of complete atrioventricular block by an artificial pacemaker. *Dis Chest* **34:** 621, 1958.
891. Thomas ED, Ewy GA, Dahl CD, et al: Effectiveness of direct current defibrillation: Role of paddle electrode size. *Amer Heart J* **93:** 463, 1977.
891a. Thompson WL: Recognition, treatment, and prevention of poisoning. In: *Textbook of Critical Care.* WC Shoemaker, WL Thompson, PR Holbrook (Eds). Philadelphia, WB Saunders, 1984, p 801. Chapter 99.

892. Thompson WL: Rational use of albumin and plasma substitutes. *Johns Hopkins Med J* **136:** 220, 1965.

893. Thrower WB, Darby TD, Aldinger EE: Acid–base derangements and myocardial contractility. *Arch Surg* **82:** 56, 1961.

894. Tisherman S, Chabal C, Safar P, et al: Resuscitation of dogs from cold-water submersion using cardiopulmonary bypass. *Ann Emerg Med* **14:** 389, 1985.

895. Todd MM, Chadwick HS, Shapiro HM, et al: The neurologic effects of thiopental therapy following experimental cardiac arrest in cats. *Anesthesiology* **57:** 76, 1982.

895a. Todd MM, Dunlop BJ, Shapiro HM, et al: Ventricular fibrillation in the cat: A model for global cerebral ischemia. *Stroke* **12:** 808, 1981.

896. Todres ID, Rogers MC: Methods of external cardiac massage in the newborn infant. *J Pediatr* **86:** 781, 1975.

897. Torpey DJ: Resuscitation and Anesthetic Management of Casualties. *J Amer Med Assoc* **202:** 955, 1967.

898. Tossach WA: A man dead in appearance recovered by distending the lungs with air. In: *Medical Essays and Observations*. London, Caldell and Balfour, a, 1744, pt 605–608; b, 1771, pp 108–111.

899. Towne WD, Geiss WP, Yanes HO, et al: Intractable ventricular fibrillation associated with profound accidental hypothermia—successful treatment with partial cardiopulmonary bypass. *New Engl J Med* **287:** 1135, 1972.

900. Trubuhovich RV (Ed): Management of acute intracranial disasters. *Internat Anesth Clinics* **17/2–3,** 1979.

901. Trunkey DD, Shires GT, McClelland R: Management of liver trauma in 811 consecutive patients. *Ann Surg* **179:** 722, 1974.

902. Trunkey DD, Lewis FR: *Current Therapy of Trauma 1984–1985*. Philadelphia, BC Decker, 1984.

903. Turks LM, Glenn WW: Cardiac arrest—results of attempted resuscitation in 42 cases. *N Engl J Med* **251:** 795, 1954.

904. Tuttle RR, Mills J: Dobutamine: Development of a new catecholamine to selectively increase cardiac contractility. *Circ Res* **36:** 185, 1975.

905. Tweed WA, Bristow G, Donen N: Resuscitation from cardiac arrest: Assessment of a system providing only basic life support outside of hospital. *Can Med Assoc J* **122:** 297, 1980.

906. Tzivoni D, Keren A, Cohen AM, et al: Magnesium therapy for torsades de pointes. *Amer J Cardiol* **53:** 528, 1984.

907. United Nations Disaster Relief Organization (UNDRO). *UNDRO News*. UNDRO, Palais des Nations, 1211, Geneva 10, Switzerland. Tel. 41-22-310211.

908. United States Department of Defense. *Emergency War Surgery*. First US Revision of the Emergency War Surgery NATO Handbook. Washington DC, US Government Printing Office, 1975.

909. Urban N, Bergner L, Eisenberg MS: The costs of a suburban paramedics program in reducing deaths due to cardiac arrest. *Med Care* **19:** 379, 1981.

910a. Vaagenes P, Kjekshus TK, Torvik A: The relationship between cerebrospinal fluid creatine-kinase and morphological changes in the brain after transient cardiac arrest. *Circulation* **61:** 1194, 1980.

910b. Vaagenes P, Urdal P, Melvoll R, et al: Enzyme level changes in the cerebrospinal fluid of patients with acute stroke. *Arch Neurol* **43:** 357, 1986.

910c. Vaagenes P, Cantadore R, Diven W, et al: Prediction of brain damage by brain enzyme levels in cerebrospinal fluid in dogs after cardiac arrest. *Anesthesiology* **61:** A145, 1984 (abstract).

911. Vaagenes P, Cantadore R, Safar P, et al: Amelioration of brain damage by lidoflazine after prolonged ventricular fibrillation cardiac arrest in dogs. *Crit Care Med* **12:** 846, 1984.

912a. Vaagenes P, Cantadore R, Safar P, et al: Effect of lidoflazine on neurologic outcome after cardiac arrest in dogs. *Anesthesiology* **52:** A100, 1983 (abstract).

912b. Vaagenes P, Cantadore R, Safar P, et al: The effect of lidoflazine and verapamil on neurologic outcome after 10 minutes ventricular fibrillation cardiac arrest in dogs. *Crit Care Med* **12:** 228, 1984 (abstract).

913. Vaagenes P, Safar P, Cantadore R, et al: Outcome trials of free radical scavengers and calcium entry blockers after cardiac arrest in two dog models. *Ann Emerg Med* **15:** 665, 1986 (abstract).

914. Valentine PA, Frew JL, Mashford ML, et al: Lidocaine in the prevention of sudden death in the prehospital phase of acute infarction. *N Engl J Med* **291:** 1327, 1974.

915. VanHarreveld A, Ochs S: Cerebral impedance changes after circulatory arrest. *Amer J Physiol* **187:** 180, 1957.

916. VanHoutte PM, VanNeuten JM: The pharmacology of lidoflazine. *R Soc Med Int Cong Symp Series* **29:** 61, 1980.

917. VanHoutte PM (Ed): Symposium Issue. Calcium entry blockers and the cardiovascular system. *Fed Proc* **40:** 2581, 1981.

918. Van Neuten JM, VanHoutte PM: Improvement of tissue perfusion with inhibitors of Ca^{2+} influx. *Biochem Pharmacol* **29:** 479, 1980.

919. Vatner SF, Baig H: Comparison of effects of Quabain and isoproterenol on ischemic myocardium of conscious dogs *Circulation* **58:** 654, 1978.

920. Venus B, Jacobs HK, Mathru M: Hemodynamic responses to different modes of mechanical ventilation in dogs with normal and acid aspirated lungs. *Crit Care Med* **8:** 620, 1980.

921. Vesalius A: *De corporis humani fabrica.* Libri Septem. 1543; Cap IXX 1555.

921a. Villazon-Sahagun A: Mexico City earthquake: medical response. *J World Assoc Emerg Disaster Med* **1/4:** 15, 1986.

922. Visintine RE, Baick CH, Ruptured stomach after Heimlich maneuver. *J Amer Med Assoc* **234:** 415, 1975.

923. Vollmer TP, Stewart RD, Paris PM, et al: Guided orotracheal intubation using a lighted stylet. *Ann Emerg Med* **13:** 404, 1984, (abstract).

924. VonEuler US: Identification of the sympathomimetic ergone in adrenergic nerves of cattle (Sympathin-N) with laevo-noradrenaline. *Acta Physiol Scand* **16:** 63, 1948.

925. Voorhees WD, Ralston FH, Babbs CF: Regional blood flow during CPR with abdominal counterpulsation in dogs. *Amer J Emerg Med* **2:** 123, 1984.

926. Vries JK, Becker DP, Young HF: A subarachnoid screw for monitoring intracranial pressure. *J Neurosurg* **39:** 416, 1973.

927. Wagner FC: Management of acute spinal cord injury. *Surg Neurol* **7:** 346, 1977.

928. Wald N: Radiation injury. In: *Cecil Textbook of Medicine.* Philadelphia, WB Saunders, 1982, p 2228. Chapter 520.

929. Wanzer SH, Adelstein SJ, Cranford RE, et al: The physician's responsibility toward hopelessly ill patients. *New Engl J Med* **310:** 955, 1984.

930. Ward JD, Becker DP: Head trauma. In: *Textbook of Critical Care.* WC Shoemaker, WL Thompson, PR Holbrook (Eds). Philadelphia, WB Saunders, 1984, p 926. Chapter 104.

931. Ward JD, Becker DP, Miller DJ, et al: Failure of prophylactic barbiturate coma in the treatment of severe head trauma. *J Neurosurg* **62:** 383, 1985.

932. Warner DS, Deshpande JK, Wieloch T: The effect of isoflurane on neuronal necrosis following near-complete forebrain ischemia in the rat. *Anesthesiology* **64:** 19, 1986.

933. Warner ED, Dahl C, Ewy GA: Myocardial injury from transthoracic defibrillation countershock. *Arch Pathol* **99:** 55, 1975.

934. Waters RM: Resuscitation: artificial circulation by means of intermittent high pressure chest inflation with oxygen. A preliminary report. *Anesth Analg Bull* October 1921, p 15.

935. Waters RM, Rovenstein EA, Guedel AE: Endotracheal anesthesia and its historical development. *Anesth Analg* **12:** 196, 1933.

936. Waxman MB, Wald RW, Sharma AD, et al: Vagal techniques for termination of paroxysmal supraventricular tachycardia. *Amer J Cardiol* **46:** 655, 1980.

937.   Weale FE, Rothwell-Jackson RL: The efficiency of cardiac massage. *Lancet* **i**: 990, 1962.

938.   Weaver WD, Cobb LA, Copass MK, et al: Ventricular defibrillation—A comparative trail using 175-J and 320-J shocks. *N Engl J Med* **307**: 1101, 1982.

939.   Weaver WD, Copass MK, Cobb L: Improved neurologic recovery and survival after early defibrillation. *Circulation* **69**: 943, 1984.

940.   Wechsler RL, Dripps RD, Kety SS: Blood flow and oxygen consumption of the human brain during anesthesia produced by thiopental. *Anesthesiology* **12**: 308, 1953.

941.   Wecht C, Grenvik A, Safar P, et al: *Determination of Brain Death*. Bull Allegheny Co Med Soc (Pittsburgh, PA, USA), Jan 25, 1969.

942.   Wei JY, Green HL, Weisfeldt ML: Cough facilitated cardioversion of ventricular tachycardia. *Amer J Cardiol* **45**: 174, 1980.

943.   Weil MH, Shubin H (Eds): *Diagnosis and Treatment of Shock*. Baltimore, Williams & Wilkins, 1967.

944.   Weil MH, Shubin H: The 'VIP' approach to the bedside management of shock. *J Amer Med Assoc* **207**: 337, 1969.

945.   Weil HM, Henning RJ: New concepts in the diagnosis and fluid treatment of circulatory shock. *Anesth Analg* **58**: 124, 1979.

946.   Weil MH, Grundler W, Rackow EC, et al: Blood gas measurements in human patients during CPR. *Chest* **86**: 282, 1984.

947.   Weil MH, Ruiz CE, Michaels S, et al: Acid–base determinants of survival after CPR. *Crit Care Med* **13**: 893, 1985.

948.   Weil MH, Rackow EC: Cardiovascular system failure. In: *Principles and Practice of Emergency Medicine*. GR Schwartz, P Safar, JH Stone, et al (Eds). Philadelphia, WB Saunders, 1986, p 86. Chapter 3.

948a.   Weil MH, Rackow EC, Trevino R, et al: Difference in acid–base state between venous and arterial blood during CPR. *New Engl J Med* **315**: 153, 1986.

949.   Weiser FM, Adler LN, Kuhn LA: Hemodynamic effects of closed and open chest cardiac resuscitation in normal dogs and those with acute myocardial infarction. *Amer J Cardiol* **10**: 555, 1962.

950.   Weisfeldt ML, Chandra N, Fisher J, et al: Mechanisms of perfusion in cardiopulmonary resuscitation. In: *Textbook of Critical Care*. WC Shoemaker, WL Thompson, PR Holbrook (Eds). Philadelphia, WB Saunders, 1984, p 31. Chapter 5.

951.   Weisfeldt ML, Bishop RL, Greene HL: Effects of pH and PCO_2 on performance of ischemic myocardium. In: *Recent Advances in Studies on Cardiac Structure and Metabolism*, Vol. 10. PE Roy, G Roma (Eds). Baltimore, University Park Press, 1975, p 355.

952.   Weiss AT, Lewis BS, Halon DA, et al: The use of calcium with verapamil in the management of supraventricular tachyarrhythmias. *Int J Cardiol* **4**: 275, 1983.

953.   Wells BA, Keats AS, Cooley DA: Increased tolerance to cerebral ischemia produced by general anesthesia during temporary carotid occlusion. *Surgery* **54**: 216, 1963.

954.   Werner JA, Greene H, Janko CL, et al: Visualization of cardiac valve motion during external chest compression using two-dimensional echocardiography. Implications regarding the mechanism of blood flow. *Circulation* **63**: 1414, 1981.

955.   Werner JZ, Safar P, Bircher NG, et al: No improvement in pulmonary status by gravity drainage or abdominal thrusts after sea water near drowning in dogs. *Anesthesiology* **57**: A81, 1982 (abstract).

956.   White BC, Petinga TJ, Hoehner PJ, et al: Incidence, etiology, and outcome of pulseless idioventricular rhythm treated with dexamethasone during advanced CPR. *J Amer Coll Emerg Phys* **8**: 188, 1979.

957.   White BC, Gadzinski DS, Hoehner PJ, et al: Effect of flunarizine on canine cerebral cortical blood flow and vascular resistance post-cardiac arrest. *Ann Emerg Med* **11**: 110, 1982.

958.   White BC, Winegar CD, Wilson RF, et al: Possible role of calcium blockers in cerebral

resuscitation: A review of the literature and synthesis for future studies. *Crit Care Med* **11:** 202, 1983.

959. White BC, Aust SD, Arfors KE, et al: Brain injury by ischemic anoxia—hypothesis. A tale of two ions? *Ann Emerg Med* **13:** 862, 1984.

960. White RD: Cardiovascular pharmacology. Part I. In: *Advanced Cardiac Life Support Manual.* Dallas, Amer Heart Assoc, 1981, 1983.

961. White RD, Lane JC, Tincani AJ, et al: Ambulance design and economic realities in the third world. *J Emerg Med Serv* **10:** 53, 1984.

962. White RJ: Hypothermic preservation and transplantation of brain. *Resuscitation* **4:** 197, 1975.

963. Wiggers CJ: The physiological bases for cardiac resuscitation from ventricular fibrillation. Method for serial defibrillation. *Amer Heart J* **20:** 413, 1940.

964. Wiklund PE: Design of recovery room and ICU. *Anesthesiology* **26:** 667, 1965.

965. Wilder RJ, Weir D, Rush BF, et al: Methods of coordinating ventilation and closed-chest cardiac massage in the dog. *Surgery* **53:** 186, 1963.

966. Wilder RJ, Jude JR, Kouwenhoven WB: Cardiopulmonary resuscitation by trained ambulance personnel. *J Amer Med Assoc* **190:** 531, 1964.

966a. Wilson RF: Trauma. In: *Textbook of Critical Care.* WC Shoemaker, WL Thompson, PR Holbrook (Eds). Philadelphia, WB Saunders, 1984, p 877. Chapter 102.

967. Winchell SW, Safar P: Teaching and testing lay and paramedical personnel in cardiopulmonary resuscitation. *Anesth Analg* **45:** 441, 1966.

968. Winegar CP, Henderson O, White BC, et al: Early amelioration of neurologic deficit by lidoflazine after fifteen minutes of cardiopulmonary arrest in dogs. *Ann Emerg Med* **12:** 471, 1983.

969. Winter PM, Gupta RK, Michaliski AH, et al: Modification of hyperbaric oxygen toxicity by experimental venous admixture. *J Appl Physiol* **23:** 954, 1967.

970. Winter PM, Miller NJ: Oxygen toxicity. In: *Textbook of Critical Care.* WC Shoemaker, WL Thompson, PR Holbrook (Eds). Philadelphia, WB Saunders, 1984.

970a. Winter PM, Kang YG: *Hepatic Transplantation: Anesthetic and Perioperative Management.* New York, Praeger, 1986.

971. Wise BL, Chater M: Use of hypertonic mannitol solution to lower CSF pressure and decrease brain bulk in man. *Surg Forum* **12:** 398, 1961.

972. Wise G, Sutter R, Burkholder J: The treatment of brain ischemia with vasopressor drugs. *Stroke* **4:** 135, 1972.

973. Wolfe KB: Effect of hypothermia in cerebral damage resulting from cardiac arrest. *Amer J Cardiol* **6:** 809, 1960.

974. Wolfson SK, Inouye WY, Kavianian A, et al: Preferential cerebral hypothermia for circulatory arrest. *Surgery* **57:** 846, 1965.

975. Wolfson SK, Yonas H, Gur D: Local cerebral blood flow imaging with stable xenon. In: *Noninvasive Diagnostic Techniques in Vascular Disease.* EF Burnstein (Ed), 3rd ed. St. Louis, CV Mosby, 1985, p 269.

975a. Wolfson SK, Safar P, Reich H, et al: Patterns of cerebral blood flow determined by the stable xenon/CT technique in dogs after global ischemia. Proc. International Resuscitation Research Symposium, 1987, Pittsburgh PA, USA. *Crit Care Med,* in press (abstract).

976. World Association for Emergency and Disaster Medicine (WAEDM). Office: P Baskett (Hon Sec), Frenchay Hospital, Department of Anaesthetics, Bristol BS16 1LE, UK (Tel. 44-272-701212. Journal WAEDM from RA Cowley, MIEMSS, 22 South Greene St., Baltimore MD 21201, USA. Telephone: 301-528-6846).

977. World Association for Emergency and Disaster Medicine (WAEDM): Resolutions concerning disaster medicine and nuclear war. *J World Assoc Emerg Disaster Med* **1:** 15, 1985.

978. World Health Organization (WHO): *Reports and Resolutions Concerning Emergency Medical Services, Nuclear War, etc.* WHO, Ave Appia, 12H Geneva 27 Switzerland (Tel. 41-22-912111).

979. Yakaitis RW, Redding JS: Precordial thumping during cardiac resuscitation. *Crit Care Med* **1:** 22, 1973.

980. Yakaitis RW, Otto CW, Blitt CD: Relative importance of alpha and beta adrenergic receptors during resuscitation. *Crit Care Med* **7:** 293, 1979.

981. Yashon D, Wagner FC Jr, Massopust LC Jr, et al: Electrocortigraphic limits of cerebral viability during cardiac arrest and resuscitation. *Amer J Surg* **121:** 728, 1971.

982. Yatsu FM, Diamond I, Graziana C, et al: Experimental brain ischemia: protection from irreversible damage with a rapid-acting barbiturate (methohexital). *Stroke* **3:** 726, 1972.

983. Yatsu FM: Cardiopulmonary-cerebral resuscitation (editorial to Abramson, et al). *N Engl J Med* **314:** 440, 1986.

984. Zapol WM, Schneider R, Snider M, et al: Partial bypass with membrane lungs for acute respiratory failure. *Int Anesthesiol Clin* **14:** 119, 1976.

985. Zaritsky AL, Chernow B: Catecholamines, sympathomimetics. In: *The Pharmacologic Approach to the Critically Ill Patient.* B Chernow, CR Lake (Eds). Baltimore, Williams & Wilkins, 1983, pp 481–510. Chapter 27.

985a. Zaritsky A: Advanced pediatric life support: state of the art. *Circulation* **74**(suppl IV): 124, 1986.

986. Zelis R, Mansour EJ, Capone RJ, et al: The cardiovascular effects of morpine. The peripheral capacitance and resistance vessels in human subjects. *J Clin Invest* **54:** 1247, 1974.

987. Zell SC, Kurtz KJ: Severe exposure hypothermia: A resuscitation protocol. *Ann Emerg Med* **14:** 339, 1985.

988. Zesas DG: Ueber Massage des freigelegten Herzens beim Chloroformkollaps. *Zentralbl Chir* **23:** 588, 1903.

989. Zideman DA: Cardiopulmonary resuscitation—the need for national surveys. *J World Assoc Emerg Disaster Med* **1/3:** 291, 1985.

990. Zimmerman AN, Hulsmann WC: Paradoxical influence of calcium ions on the permeability of the cell membrane of the isolated rat heart. *Nature* **211:** 646, 1966. (See also The calcium paradox. *Eur Heart J* **4:** Suppl 14, 3, 1983).

991. Zimmerman JM, Spencer FC: The influence of hypothermia on cerebral injury resulting from circulatory occlusion. *Surg Forum* **9:** 216, 1958.

992. Zimmerman RA: Radiology of brain failure. In: *Brain Failure and Resuscitation.* Clinics in Critical Care Medicine. A Grenvik, P Safar (Eds). New York, Churchill Livingstone, 1981.

993. Zindler M, Dudziak R, Pulver KG: Artificial hypothermia (in German). In: *Anesthesiologie und Wiederbelebung.* R Frey, et al (Eds). Heidelberg, Springer-Verlag, 1971, p 353. Chapter C/12/c.

994. Zipes DP, Gilmour RF: Calcium antagonists and their potential role in the prevention of sudden coronary death. *Ann NY Acad Sci* **382:** 258, 1982.

995. Zoll PM, Linenthal AJ, Norman LR: Treatment of unexpected cardiac arrest by external stimulation of the heart. *N Engl J Med* **254:** 541, 1956.

996. Zoll PM, Linenthal AJ, Gibson W et al.: Termination of ventricular fibrillation in man by externally applied electric countershock. *N Engl J Med* **254:** 727, 1956.

997. Zoll PM, Linenthal AJ: Long-term electrical pacemakers for Stokes–Adams disease. *Circulation* **92:** 341, 1960.

998. Zoll PM, Belgard AH, Weintraub MJ, et al: External mechanical cardiac stimulation. *N Engl J Med* **294:** 1274, 1976.

999. Zoll PM, Zoll RH, Falk RH, et al: External noninvasive temporary cardiac pacing: clinical trials. *Circulation* **71:** 937, 1985.

1000. Zorab J, Baskett P: *Immediate Care.* Philadelphia, WB Saunders, 1977.

Glossary

Abbreviations, Definitions, Normal Values

Conventional values or SI (Système International d'Unites, World Health Organization), See *New Engl J Med* **314:** 39, 1986

A	Step A of CPCR = Airway control
A	Ampere(s) (electric current = V/Ω)
AA	Arachidonic acid (a free fatty acid)
a.c.	Alternating electric current
Acidemia	Arterial pH < 7.35
Acidosis	Reduced pH (tissues)
ACS	American College of Surgeons (see References)
ACT	Activated clotting time (normal 90–140 s). For monitoring heparin requirement during CPB (ACT usually maintained ≥ 400 s)
ACTH	Adrenocorticotropic hormone
ADO	Apneic diffusion oxygenation
ADP	Adenosine diphosphate
AED	Automatic external defibrillation
AHA	American Heart Association (see References)
AID	Automatic internal defibrillation
AIDS	Acquired immune deficiency syndrome, caused by HIV
Albumin	Serum albumin (normal 3.5–5.0 g/dl)
Alkalemia	Arterial pH > 7.45
Alkalosis	Increased pH (tissues)
ALS, ACLS, ATLS	Advanced (Cardiac, Trauma) Life Support, i.e. CPCR Steps ABC + DEF
AMA	American Medical Association (see references)
AMI	Acute myocardial infarction
AMP	Adenosine monophosphate
Amylase	Normal serum amylase 4–25 U/ml
Anoxia	No oxygen
AP	Arterial pressure, mmHg (see MAP). Also atmospheric (barometric) pressure. Also airway pressure (see BP)
Apnea	No breathing movements
ARC	American Red Cross (see References)
ARDS	Adult respiratory distress syndrome (shock lung, progressive pulmonary consolidation)
ARI (ARF)	Acute respiratory insufficiency (failure)
Arterial O_2 content	CaO_2 (normal 20 ml/dl)
Arterial O_2 transport	$\dot{C}aO_2$ (normal 1 L/min for 70 kg adult) = cardiac output (i.e. $\dot{Q}_T$) (normal 5 L/min) × arterial O_2 content (i.e. CaO_2) (normal 20 ml/dl)
ASA	American Society of Anesthesiologists (see references)
ASAT	Aspartate aminotransferase (cytosolic enzyme). Normal value in CSF < 30 U/L, see CPK
Asphyxia	Hypoxemia + hypercarbia (result of airway obstruction or apnea)
Asystole	Cessation of circulation with heart at standstill (not pumping) =

	mechanical asystole. Electric asystole = pulselessness without ECG complexes. See EMD
ATA	Atmosphere absolute = 1 atm at sea level (760 mmHg)
Atm, atm	Atmospheric pressure (normal at sea level 760 mmHg). 1 atm = 14.7 psi
ATN	Acute tubular necrosis of the kidneys
ATP	Adenosine triphosphate (tissue energy charge)
ATPS	Ambient temperature and pressure saturated with water vapor
AV	Assisted ventilation (augmentation of spontaneous breathing)
A-V Block	Atrio-ventricular block of the heart
B	Step B of CPCR = Breathing Control. Also: 'Blood'
BBB	Blood–brain barrier
BD	Brain death (= permanent functional silence of entire brain, including brain stem and medulla = coma depasse). See also PVS
BE/BD	Base excess/Base deficit of blood (normal 0 ± 3 mEq/L)
Bilirubin	Normal serum bilirubin < 1 mg/dl
BLS, BCLS, BTLS	Basic (Cardiac, Trauma) Life Support, i.e. CPCR Steps ABC
BP	Blood pressure = arterial pressure, mmHg (see MAP). Also atmospheric (barometric) pressure (normal at sea level 760 mmHg)
Bradypnea	Decreased respiratory frequency (f < 6/min)
BSEP, AEP	Brain stem (auditory) evoked potentials (CNS)
BT	Bleeding time (normal 3–9.5 min)
BTPS	Body temperature (37°C) and pressure saturated with water vapor (47 mmHg)
BUN	Blood urea nitrogen (normal 8–25 mg/dl = 2.9–8.9 mmol/L)
BV	Blood volume (= Q) (normal 8–10% of body weight in kg)
BW	Body weight in kg
C	Step C of CPCR = Circulation Control (cardiac and fluid resuscitation)
C	Compliance = distensibility, i.e. static volume change per unit pressure change of lungs or thorax or both (normal C of lungs plus thorax = 50–100 ml/cmH$_2$O in apnea and anesthesia)
c	Capillaries
°C	Degree Celsius (centigrade) = T. See also °F. 0°C (freezing water) = 32°F. 100°C (boiling water) = 222°F
CA	Cardiac arrest
[Ca^{2+}]	Calcium ion concentration (normal total serum calcium level 2.1–2.6 mmol/L = 8.5–10.5 mg/dl; normal ionized Ca^{++} = 50–60% of total)
$\dot{C}aO_2$	Arterial O$_2$ transport = CaO_2 × C.O. (normal 1 L/min)
CaO_2	Arterial O$_2$ content (normal 20 ml/dl)
$C(a-\bar{v})O_2$	Arterial–mixed venous O$_2$ content difference (normal 5 ml/dl blood)
CBF	Cerebral blood flow (normal 50 ml/100 g brain per min)
CBV	Cerebral blood volume
cc	cubic centimeter(s) (= ml)
CC	Closing capacity, i.e. lung closing volume (CV) including RV
CCM	Critical Care Medicine
CCU	Coronary (cardiac) Care Unit
$C\bar{c}vO_2$	Mixed cerebral venous (sagittal sinus, jugular bulb) O$_2$ content
Cdyn	Dynamic compliance = C measured during breathing
Cholesterol	Normal serum value 120–220 mg/dl (3.1–5.7 mmol/L)
CL	Clot lysis (whole blood). Normal no clot lysis in 24 h
[Cl$^+$]	Chloride ion concentration (normal serum chloride level 100–106 mEq/L = mmol/L)

CMRO$_2$ (G) (L)	Cerebral metabolic rate for O$_2$, glucose, or lactate = CBF × Ca − cv O$_2$ (or G) (or L) (normal CMRO$_2$ = 1.5 μ moles/g brain per min O$_2$ consumption; CMRG = 0.25 μ moles/g brain per min glucose consumption; CMR L = 0.023 μ moles/g brain per min lactate production)
CNS	Central nervous system
CO	Carbon monoxide. Normal blood CO Hb < 5% at total Hb
C.O.	Cardiac output = $\dot{Q}_T$ = total body blood flow (normal 5 L/min for 70 kg adult)
CO$_2$	Carbon dioxide. See PCO$_2$
Coag	Coagulation screening tests: See BT and whole blood CT, CR, CL, ACT. Also PT, PTT, FSP, TT, Pl, Pl agg, Fib.
COP	Colloid osmotic pressure = oncotic pressure (normal plasma COP = 25 mmHg)
COPD (COLD)	Chronic obstructive pulmonary (lung) disease, i.e. emphysema–chronic bronchitis–asthma
CorPP	Coronary perfusion pressure = diastolic aortic pressure − diastolic RAP (normal > 80 mmHg; minimal requirement for viability ≈ 30 mmHg)
CPAP	Continuous positive airway pressure = SB with EPAP and PEEP
CPB	Cardiopulmonary bypass (artificial extracorporeal circulation and oxygenation)
CPC	Cerebral Performance Categories #1 (best)–#5 (worst). Patient outcome evaluation. See OPC
CPK (= CK)	Creatine phosphokinase (cytosolic enzyme). CPK-BB = brain specific CPK (normal CSF CPK-BB values in patients < 5 U/L). Increasing CSF CPK-BB values > 20 U/L at 48 h post-CA with coma help predict PVS). Normal serum CPK < 250 U/L; CPK-MB = myocardium specific CPK (normal serum values < 10 U/L, variable with method). See also CSF ASAT and LDH
CPR, CPCR	Cardio-pulmonary resuscitation, cardio-pulmonary-cerebral resuscitation = Steps ABC (BLS) + DEF (ALS) + GHI (PLS)
CPP	Cerebral perfusion pressure = MAP minus mean ICP (or cerebral venous pressure, whichever is higher) (normal > 80 mmHg; minimal requirement for viability ≈ 30 mmHg)
CPPV	Continuous positive pressure (controlled) ventilation (IPPV + PEEP)
CR	Clot retraction (whole blood). Normal 50–100%/2 h
Cr	Creatinine = renal function value (normal serum creatinine 0.6–1.5 mg/dl)
CRPD (CRLD)	Chronic restrictive pulmonary (lung) disease, i.e. fibrosis
CS	Cardiogenic shock. Also (electric) countershock for defibrillation
CSF	Cerebrospinal fluid. Normal CSF pressure < 15 mmHg. Normal lumbar CSF protein 15–50 mg/dl (albumin 11–48 mg/dl), glucose 50–75 mg/dl
CT	Computerized tomography (roentgenology)
CT	Clotting time (whole blood). Normal 5–12 min
CV	Closing volume, i.e. % of expiratory VC above RV where during exhalation intrapulmonary airways begin to close (normal: 10% in youth, 40% in old age)
CV	Controlled ventilation (artificial ventilation). See IPPV, CPPV, MV
C$\bar{v}$O$_2$	Mixed venous O$_2$ content (normal 15 ml/dl)
CVP	Central venous pressure (normal 3–10 mmHg)
CVR	Cerebral vascular resistance (i.e. CPP/CBF) (normal 200 mmHg/CBF in ml per g brain per min)

Cyanosis	Blueish discoloration of mucous membranes and/or skin, due to excessive amount of reduced Hb
D	Step D of CPCR = Drugs and fluids
d	day(s)
d.c.	Direct electric current
DIC	Disseminated intravascular coagulation
dl	deciliter (= 100 ml)
Dyspnea	Subjective sensation of difficult or labored breathing
E	Step E of CPCR = Electrocardiography (ECG = EKG)
E	Elastance; elastic resistance (reciprocal of compliance)
EAA	European Academy of Anesthesiology
ECC	Emergency Cardiac Care. Also External cardiac (chest) compressions
ECCM	Emergency and Critical Care Medicine
ECF	Extracellular fluid (normal ECF in liters = 20–30% of BW in kg)
ECG (EKG)	Electrocardiogram (-graph)
ECMO, ECLA	Extracorporeal membrane oxygenation (-lung assist)
ED, ER	Emergency department, emergency room
EEG	Electroencephalogram (-graph)
e.g.	For example
EM	Emergency Medicine
EMD	Electromechanical dissociation, i.e. mechanical asystole with ECG complexes present (not VF, VT) = mechanical (without electrical) asystole
EMOC	Emergency Medical Operations Center
EMS	Emergency Medical Services (systems)
EMT	Emergency medical technician(s) (ambulance) = basic life support (BLS) ambulance personnel
Eq	Equivalent. See mEq
ERV	Expiratory reserve volume of lungs (normal approx. 1.5 L). see TLC
EP	Evoked (electric) potentials (CNS)
EPAP	Expiratory positive airway pressure = SB with EPAP
F	Step F of CPCR = Fibrillation treatment, i.e. (electric) defibrillation
f	Frequency (rate) of breathing, breaths/min (normal f for SB = 12–20/min)
°F	Degree Fahrenheit. See also °C. 32°F = 0°C. °F = 32 + (°C × 1.8). 212°F = 100°C
FC	Fluorocarbon(s). O_2 carrying plasma substitute
Fe	Iron. Fe^{++} or Fe^{+++} = ionized iron. Normal serum iron 50–150 $\mu g/dl$ = 9–27 $\mu mol/L$
FEMA	Federal Emergency Management Agency (USA)
FEV_1	Forced Expiratory Volume, timed for first second, i.e. spirometric expiratory VC (normal FEV_1 = > 80% of total FEV; normal FEV total = > 80% of predicted FEV)
FFA	Free fatty acid(s) = products of cell membrane lipid peroxidation
Fib	Fibrinogen = Clotting factor I in plasma (normal: 150–350 mg/dl = 4–10 $\mu mol/L$)
FIO_2	Fraction (concentration) of inhaled O_2. FIO_2 of air = 0.21 (= 21%). FIO_2 = 100% used for 100% O_2 test (i.e. PaO_2 < 600 mmHg reflects shunting, $\dot{Q}s/\dot{Q}_T$; PaO_2 = 100 mmHg with FIO_2 = 100% reflects $\dot{Q}s/\dot{Q}_T$ of approximately 50%)
$FICO_2$	Fraction (concentration) of inhaled CO_2. Normal $FICO_2$ = 0.03% Zero

FLR	Free lipid radicals
FRC	Functional residual capacity of lungs = RV + ERV (normal approx. 2.5 L). See TLC
FRS	Free radical scavengers (e.g. SOD)
FSP	Fibrin split products (normal, negative reaction at > 1 : 4 dilution)
G	Step G of CPCR = Gauging (evaluation). Steps GHI = PLS
g, gm	gram(s). (See mg)
GCS	Glasgow coma score
GI	Gastrointestinal
Glob	Serum globulin (normal 2.3–3.5 g/dl)
Gluc	Glucose (normal blood glucose fasting 70–110 mg/dl = 3.9–5.6 mmol/L)
H	Step H of CPCR = Humanizing (cerebral resuscitation). Steps GHI = PLS
h	hour(s)
[H$^+$]	Hydrogen ion concentration. See pH
Hb	Hemoglobin content in blood (normal 12–18 g/dl = 7.4–11.2 mmol/L)
HBO	Hyperbaric oxygenation
[HCO$_3^-$]	Bicarbonate ion concentration, calculated from PCO_2 and pH (normal in arterial blood = 24 mEq/L)
Hct	Hematocrit (normal 37–52%)
HF(J)V	High frequency (jet) ventilation
HFO	High frequency oscillation
HFPPV	High frequency positive pressure ventilation
HIV	Human immune deficiency virus. Can cause AIDS
HR	Heart rate (normal 50–90/min at rest)
H$_2$O	Water
H$_2$O$_2$	Hydrogen peroxide
HX	Hypoxanthine
Hypercarbia	= hypercapnea, $PaCO_2$ > 45 mmHg; result of hypoventilation
Hypocarbia	= hypocapnea, $PaCO_2$ < 35 mmHg; result of hyperventilation
Hypoxemia	Arterial PO_2 < 75 mmHg
Hypoxia	Reduced oxygen
I	Step I of CPCR = Intensive care (prolonged life support, PLS). Steps GHI = PLS
i.a.	intra-arterial
IAC-CPR	Intermittent abdominal compression CPR
IAV, IDV	Intermittent assisted (demand) ventilation
i.c.	intracardiac. Also intracellular
IC	Inspiratory capacity of lungs (= 'sighing volume') = TV + IRV (normal 3.5 L)
ICF	Intracellular fluid volume (normal 50% of BW in L)
ICP	Intracranial pressure (normal < 20 mmHg)
ICU	Intensive care unit
i.e.	*id est* (that is)
IF	Inspiratory force
i.f.	interstitial fluid
i.m.	intramuscular
IMV	Intermittent mandatory ventilation, i.e. SB with superimposed CV (IPPV or CPPV) at slow rate
i.p.	intraperitoneal

IPPB	Intermittent positive pressure (assisted) breathing (artificial ventilation)
IPPV	Intermittent positive pressure (controlled) ventilation (artificial ventilation)
IRC	International Red Cross (see references). For armed conflicts, Geneva-based
IRV	Inspiratory reserve volume of lungs (normal approx. 3 L). See TLC
ISS	Isotonic (0.9%) sodium chloride solution
i.v.	intravenous
IVC-SVC	Inferior (superior) vena cava
IVP	Intraventricular pressure ($=$ ICP)
J	Joule(s) $=$ watt(s) $\times$ second(s) $=$ electric energy $=$ work
$[K^+]$	Potassium ion concentration (normal serum potassium level 3.5–5.0 mEq/L $=$ mmol/L)
kg	kilogram(s). (See also mg)
kPa	kilopascal (pressure, tension). 1 kPa $=$ 7.5 mmHg $=$ 7.5 torr. 5.3 kPa $=$ 40 mmHg (normal $PaCO_2$). 13.3 kPa $=$ 100 mmHg
L, l	Liter(s). 1 liter $=$ 1000 ml
Lact (La)	Arterial blood lactate concentration (normal 1 mEq/L $=$ 9 mg/dl)
LAP	Left atrial pressure $\approx$ PAOP (normal 10[6–12] mmHg)
LDH	Lactate dehydrogenase (cytosolic enzyme). Normal serum LDH value 45–90 U/L. Normal CSF LDH value $<$ 60 U/L. See CPK
Leu	Leukocyte(s). See WBC(s)
LRCS	(International) League of Red Cross and Red Crescent Societies (see References). Federation of national Red Cross Societies
LSFA	Life Supporting First Aid ($=$ BCLS $+$ BTLS without equipment)
LT	Leukotriene(s)
MAP	Mean arterial pressure (normal 95 $\pm$ 10 mmHg)
MAST	Military (medical) anti-shock trousers; pressure suit. $=$ PASG
MCI	Multicasualty incident (medical disaster).
MD	Medical doctor. Also, mass disaster (see also MCI)
MEFR (PEFR)	Maximum (peak) expiratory flow rate. The highest forced expiratory flow measured with a peak flow meter (normal $>$ 500 L/min)
mEq, mOsm	milliEquivalent $=$ grams of solute in 1 ml of a 'normal' solution. milliOsmol $=$ 1/1000 of an osmole $=$ standard unit of osmotic pressure $=$ gram molecular weight (gMW) of a substance: the number of particles or ions into which a substance dissociates in 1 L solution. Osmolality of a solution depends on concentration of solute per unit of solvent
mg	milligram(s). 1 kg $=$ 1000 g. 1 g $=$ 1000 mg. 1 mg $=$ 1000 μg. 1 μg $=$ 1000 ng ($=$ 1 millionth of a gram). 1 ng $=$ 1000 pg (picograms) ($=$ 1 billionth of a gram). 1 pg $=$ 1 trillionth of a gram ($= 10^{-12}$ g).
μg	microgram(s). (See mg)
$[Mg^{++}]$	Magnesium ion concentration (normal serum magnesium level 1.5–2.0 mEq/L $=$ 0.8–1.3 mmol/L)
MICU	Mobile intensive care unit(s) (advanced life support ambulances)
min	minute(s)
ml	milliliter(s) $=$ cc (cubic centimeter).
mm	millimeter(s)
mM	millimole(s) $=$ 1/1000 of a mole. 1 mM $=$ 1000 μm. Mole: that amount of a chemical compound whose mass in grams is equivalent

	to its formula mass (gram molecular weight). See mOsm.
μm	micromole(s)
MMFR	Maximal mid-expiratory flow rate
mmHg	millimeters of mercury (pressure, tension). 1 mmHg = 1 torr = 0.133 kPa
MV	Mechanical ventilation (artificial ventilation by machine [ventilator]). See CV, IPPV, CPPV.
MV	Minute volume (of breathing) = TVs × f
MW	Molecular weight
[Na$^+$]	Sodium ion concentration (normal serum sodium level 135–145 mEq/L = mmol/L)
NaCl	Sodium chloride
NaHCO$_3$	Sodium bicarbonate
NDMS	National Disaster Medical System(s)
NEEP	Negative end-expiratory pressure. See CV, PNPV.
ng	nanogram(s). (See also mg)
NMR	Nuclear magnetic resonance (imaging, spectroscopy). = MRI
normal	'normal' solution = a solution containing in each 1000 ml 1 gram equivalent weight of the active substance
NRC/NAS	National Research Council/National Academy of Sciences (USA) (see References)
NSS	Normal (0.9%) Sodium chloride solution
O (Ω)	Ohm(s) (electric resistance = V/A)
O$_2$	Oxygen (21% in air). See also FIO_2
O$_2^-$	Superoxide radical
O$_2$ Consumption	$\dot{V}O_2$ (normal about 250 ml/min for 70 kg adult)
O$_2$uc	O$_2$ utilization coefficient (= O$_2$ consumption/arterial O$_2$ transport). Normal approx. 0.25.
OCCPR	Open-chest CPR
OH$^\cdot$	Hydroxyl radical
Osm	Osmolality (normal serum osmolality 280–296 mOsm/kg water). See milliosmol, mEq, mOsm
OPC	Overall Performance Categories #1 (best)–#5 (worst). Patient outcome evaluation. See CPC.
P	Pressure. Also plasma.
π	pi (Greek P) = oncotic (colloid osmotic) pressure
P-50	Blood PO_2 at 50% O$_2$ saturation of Hb, signifying the position of the HbO$_2$ dissociation curve (HbO$_2$ affinity) (normal P-50 27 mmHg)
Pa	Pascal (pressure), see kPa
$PACO_2$, PAO_2	Alveolar PCO_2 ($\approx PaCO_2$). Alveolar PO_2 (normal 100 mmHg) $PAO_2 = FIO_2$(PB-47) $- PaCO_2$/R
$P(A-a)O_2$	Aveolar – arterial O$_2$ tension (pressure) gradient (normal $P(A-a)O_2$ with FIO_2 100% = < 100 mmHg; increase reflects pulmonary shunting). See $\dot{Q}_S/\dot{Q}_T$. $P(A-a)O_2 = FIO_2$ (PB $- PaCO_2 - 47$) $- PaO_2$
$PaCO_2$	Arterial CO$_2$ tension (pressure) (normal 35–45 mmHg = 4.7 – 6.0 kPa)
PaO_2	Arterial O$_2$ tension (pressure) (normal 75–100 mmHg = 10 – 13 kPa with $FIO_2 = 21\%$. PaO_2 500–600 mmHg with $FIO_2 = 100\%$). [If $PaO_2 = 100$ mmHg with $FIO_2 = 100\%$ .... $\dot{Q}_S/\dot{Q}_T$ is approx. 50%]
PAP	Pulmonary artery pressure (normal 25/10 mmHg; mean 15 mmHg)
PASG	Pneumatic anti-shock garment = MAST

PAWP, PCWP, PAOP   Pulmonary artery wedge pressure (normal 10 [6–12] mmHg). Reflects left atrial pressure (= capillary wedge pressure) (= pulmonary artery occlusive pressure)

PB   Barometric pressure = BP = AP

PBSS   Pittsburgh brain stem score

$P\bar{c}\bar{v}O_2$ Mixed cerebral venous (sagittal sinus, jugular bulb) PO_2 (normal 30–40 mmHg)

PE   Pulmonary edema. Fluid movement across capillary walls = K(filtration coefficient, i.e. membrane permeability) × c([Pc – Pif] + [πif – πc]) and lymphatic drainage

PEEP   Positive end expiratory pressure. See CPPV and SB-CPAP.

$PETCO_2$ End tidal CO_2 tension (pressure) ($\approx PaCO_2$) (normal $PETCO_2$ 35–45 mmHg)

PG   Prostaglandin(s)

pg   picogram(s). (See also mg)

pHa   negative logarithm of hydrogen ion concentration in arterial blood (normal 7.35–7.45). pH = pK (i.e. 6.1) + log [HCO_3^-]/[H_2CO_3], i.e. the Henderson–Hasselbalch equation

PH_2O Water vapor pressure (normal in alveoli 47 mmHg at 37°C)

PIO_2 Inhaled O_2 tension (pressure)

PL   Phospholipids of membranes

Pl   Platelet count in whole blood (normal 150 000–350 000/mm^3)

Pl Aggr   Platelet aggregation (normal full response to ADP, epinephrine, collagen)

PLS   Prolonged Life Support, i.e. CPCR Steps GHI

PM   Paramedics (ambulance) = advanced life support (ALS) ambulance personnel

PNPV   Positive-negative pressure (controlled) ventilation

p.o.   *per os* (by mouth)

ppm   Parts per million

prn   *pro re necessita* (as needed)

Prot   Serum protein(s), total (normal 6.0–8.4 g/dl)

PRS   Post-resuscitation syndrome

psi   pounds per square inch. 14.7 psi = 1 atmosphere

PSVT   Paroxysmal supraventricular tachycardia(s) (ECG)

Pt   Patient(s)

PT   Prothrombin = clotting factor II (normal 60—140%) Normal prothrombin time < 2 s deviation from control (70–100%)

PTT   Partial thromboplastin time, activated (normal 25–38 s)

PVC   Premature ventricular contraction(s) (ventricular extrasystoles)

$P\bar{v}CO_2$ Mixed venous PCO_2 (normal 45–50 mmHg)

PVR   Pulmonary vascular resistance = PAP – LAP/cardiac output (normal 75–150 dynes s cm^{-5})

PVS   Persistent vegetative state (= cerebral [cortical] death = apallic syndrome = coma prolongé). See also BD

$\dot{Q}_S/\dot{Q}_T$ Blood flow shunted through nonventilated alveoli, in % of total C.O. (normal < 5%). Shunt equation for $FIO_2 = 100\%$: $\dot{Q}_S/\dot{Q}_T = Cc'O_2 - CaO_2/Cc'O_2 - C\bar{v}O_2$. (where $Cc'O_2$ is end-capillary O_2 content, which is [1.34 × Hb cont.] × [HbO$_2$ Sat] + PAO_2[0.0031])

$\dot{Q}_T$ Cardiac output = C.O. (normal 5 L/min in 70 kg resting adult)

RAP   Right atrial pressure $\approx$ CVP (normal 3–10 mmHg)

RBCs   Red blood corpuscles (normal erythrocyte count 4.2–5.9 million/mm^3). RBC sedimentation rate, normal 1–20 mm/h

RQ   Respiratory exchange ratio (respiratory quotient), i.e. $\dot{V}CO_2/\dot{V}O_2$ (normal 0.8)

RRC	International Resuscitation Center, Pittsburgh, PA, USA
RV	Residual volume of lungs (normal approx. 1 L). See TLC.
S	Serum
s,sec	second(s)
SaO_2	Arterial HbO_2 saturation (normal 96–100%)
SAP	Systemic arterial pressure (normal 90–100 mmHg mean)
SB	Spontaneous breathing
SB – CPAP (EPAP)	Spontaneous breathing with continuous (expiratory) positive airway pressure
SECPR	Standard external CPR
SEP	Somatosensory evoked potentials (CNS)
SFH	Stroma-free hemoglobin. O_2 carrying plasma substitute.
SG	Specific gravity
SGOT	Serum glutamic-oxaloacetic transaminase, liver function test (normal 10–40 IU/L)
SGPT	Serum glutamic pyruvic transaminase, liver function test (normal 5–35 IU/L)
Shunt	$\dot{Q}_S/\dot{Q}_T$
SOD	Superoxide dismutase (natural free radical scavenger)
SPP	Systemic perfusion pressure = MAP – CVP (or RAP)
stat	*statim* (immediately)
STPD	Standard temperature (0°C) and pressure (760 mmHg), dry
SV	Stroke volume (heart) = C.O./HR
SVC-CPR	Simultaneous ventilation-compression CPR ('new' CPR)
SVC, IVC	Superior (inferior) vena cava
SVR, TPR	Systemic vascular resistance (total peripheral resistance) = MAP – RAP/cardiac output (normal 700–1400 dynes s cm – 5)
T	Temperature, in °C
Tachypnea	Increased respiratory frequency (f > 30/min)
THAM	Tris buffer
TLC	Total lung capacity (RV + ERV + TV + IRV) (normal approx. 6 L). VC = ERV + TV + IRV. IC = TV + IRV.
torr	Torricelli, unit of pressure. 1 torr = 1 mmHg = 0.133 kPa
TPA	Total parenteral alimentation (i.v. feeding)
TPR	Total peripheral resistance = SVR
TT	Thrombin time (normal, control ± 5 s). Normal control = 12–18 s
TV	Tidal volume of lungs (normal approx. 0.5 [0.4–1.0] L). See TLC
TX	Thromboxane(s)
U, UF	Urine. Urine flow
UA	Uric acid
UK	United Kingdom
USA	United States of America
USSR	Union of Soviet Socialist Republics
V	Volt(s) (electric tension = A × Ω)
$\dot{V}_A$	Alveolar ventilation per min (BTPS) = $\dot{V}_E - (V_D \times f)$ (normal approx. 5 L/min)
VC	Vital capacity of lungs (ERV + TV + IRV) (normal approx. 5 L)
V_D	Dead space (BTPS), i.e. anatomic dead space (normal approx. 2 ml/kg BW) plus alveolar dead space (normal zero)
V_D/V_T	Dead space/tidal volume ratio (normal 0.3)
$\dot{V}_E$	Minute volume (BTPS) = $V_T \times f$ (normal approx. 8 l/min)
VEP	Visual evoked potentials (CNS)

VF	Ventricular fibrillation
$\dot{V}O_2$, $\dot{V}CO_2$	Oxygen consumption (CO_2 production) per min (STPD) = cardiac output times arteriovenous O_2 (CO_2) content difference (normal $\dot{V}O_2$ = about 250 ml/min for 70 kg adult)
$\dot{V}/\dot{Q}$	Pulmonary ventilation/perfusion ratio (normal approx. 1)
VT	Ventricular tachycardia
W	Watt(s) (electric power = V $\times$ A)
WAEDM	World Association for Emergency and Disaster Medicine (see References)
W s	Watts $\times$ seconds = joules (J) = electric energy. Power $\times$ time = work.
WBCs	White blood corpuscles. Normal leukocyte count 4300–10 800/mm^3)
WFSA	World Federation of Societies of Anaesthesiologists (see References)
X, XD, XO	Xanthine, xanthine dehydrogenase, xanthine oxidase
ZEEP	Zero end expiratory pressure (= IPPV)

Table 22. Suggested case report form for cardiopulmonary cerebral resuscitation attempt (P. Safar, WFSA-CPR Committee).

Complete one form for each patient. Insert data or check what is applicable.

Reporting physician, name . . . .

phone number . . . .

Hospital, name . . . .

address (incl. city, country) . . . .

Patient, name . . . .

hospital number . . . .

Age (years) . . . .

Male ☐   Female ☐

Date of arrest   month ☐☐, day ☐☐, year ☐☐☐☐

Location of arrest: outside hospital ☐ in hospital: Operating room ☐
Emergency Department ☐
ICU-CCU ☐
Other location ☐

IMMEDIATELY PRE-ARREST
No background disease, healthy ☐

With background disease   ☐
if yes, state disease . . . .

ARREST
Cause of arrest . . . .

Estimated duration of insult:	min:sec
Cardiac arrest (no pulse) without CPR	:
Arrest with CPR-ABC	:
Severe hypotension or hypoxemia without CPR-ABC	:

Continued on next page

Table 22. (*cont.*)

RESUSCITATION (check all applicable)

Mouth-to-mouth/nose	☐	Electric countershock	☐
Other IPPV method	☐	Drugs during CPR-ABC	☐
Tracheal intubation	☐	Successful restoration of	
Ext. cardiac compression	☐	spontaneous circulation yes	☐
Open-chest cardiac massage	☐	no	☐
ECG taken during arrest	☐		
if yes—VF	☐	if yes, was patient admitted to ICU? yes	☐
asystole	☐	no	☐
QRS complexes	☐		

POST-ARREST (follow for at least 4 weeks or until earlier death)

Patient followed over . . . . days/weeks/months/years (check)

Recovered consciousness: yes ☐ no ☐

 if yes, ... min/hours/days (check) after restoration of spontaneous circulation

Discharged from hospital . . . . days post-arrest

 discharged alive ☐ dead ☐

If discharged alive, is still alive . . . . days/weeks/months/years post-arrest (check)

 died after discharge . . . . days/weeks/months/years post-arrest

 (check)

If died, cause of death. . . . .

PERFORMANCE CAPABILITY (check one for each time)

Times:	Pre-arrest	Best while in hospital	At time of discharge from hospital	Best after discharge from hospital
1. Normal	☐	☐	☐	☐
2. Conscious, moderately disabled because of:				
(a) Brain dysfunction:	☐	☐	☐	☐
(b) Other organ system dysfunction	☐	☐	☐	☐
3. Conscious, severely disabled because of:				
(a) Brain dysfunction:	☐	☐	☐	☐
(b) Other organ system dysfunction	☐	☐	☐	☐
4. Unconscious (not brain death), vegetative	☐	☐	☐	☐
5. Brain death, death	☐	☐	☐	☐
6. Under anesthesia	☐	☐	☐	☐

Comments:

1

IF UNCONSCIOUS ——
(no response to shouting and touching)

(A)irway

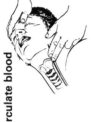

Tilt Head back
Support chin
Hear, feel air flow
at mouth and nose

If Tilt inadequate,
add Open Mouth
and Thrust Jaw

2

IF NOT BREATHING ——

(B)reathe

Mouth-mouth   or   Mouth-nose

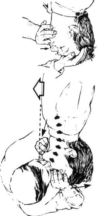

Inflate until chest moves.
Let exhale passively.

If pulse —— Continue 12/min

3

IF NO PULSE ——

(C)irculate blood

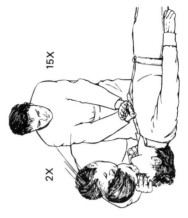

ALTERNATE:

Compressing chest 15X (2 per sec)
and
Inflating lungs 2X (2 sec each)

Continue 15 : 2

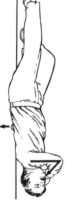

15X

2X

Compress chest at lower half of sternum
Call for Help

IF FOREIGN MATTER ——

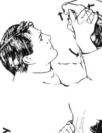

or

or

Clear Mouth and Throat

IF UNCONSCIOUS AND BREATHING ——

Turn to Stable Side Position.

Other arm behind back

Hand under cheek   Lower knee flexed

—— Keep Head Tilted Back.

If BLEEDING externally ——

COMPRESS wound until bleeding stops.

Elevate wound if possible.

Apply clean cloth or pressure bandage if possible.

Place victim horizontal.

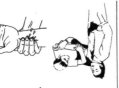

If in SHOCK and CONSCIOUS ——

place victim horizontal.

Elevate legs.

Search for external bleeding.

Control bleeding with pressure.

Suspect shock if pale, cold, clammy, restless or apathetic — or if pulse weak.

Do not leave. Call for help.

During extrication and rescue hold head-neck straight (no turning, no flexing).

From
CARDIOPULMONARY CEREBRAL RESUSCITATION
By Peter Safar, MD and N. Bircher, MD Saunders Publ. 1987

© Illustrations Laerdal Medical, 1987

IMPORTANT INFORMATION

● If I am a rescuer

GET HELP

Call Ambulance: _____

Call Hospital to take victim: _____

● If I am a victim

My special medical condition is:

My blood group is:

My physician: _____

Please also notify: _____

If I am unconscious and if resuscitated my physicians agree that I will remain permanently unconscious ——

I do not want dying prolonged with intensive care (check) ☐

I wish to donate my organs to save another person (check) ☐

Victim's signa. _____

Witness signa. _____

Instruction
LIFE SUPPORTING FIRST AID - CPR
by the

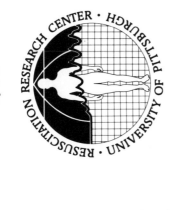

RESUSCITATION RESEARCH CENTER · UNIVERSITY OF PITTSBURGH

3434 Fifth Avenue
Pittsburgh PA 15260 USA

World Federation of Societies of Anaesthesiologists, Secretariat: Dept. Anaesthesia Frenchay Hospital, Bristol BS 161 LE England. Phone: 272-565656.
World Association for Emergency and Disaster Medicine, Secretariat: Dept. Anaesthesia Frenchay Hospital, Bristol BS 161 LE England. Phone: 272-565656.
League of Red Cross and Red Crescent Societies, 17 Chemin de Crets, Box 327, 1211 Geneva 19 Switzerland, Phone:22-345580.

Sponsoring organization:

Index

Page numbers in **bold** refer to main entries. Page numbers in *italics* refer to illustrations.

A, *see* Airway control
A-B-C sequence, *see* Basic life support
Abbreviations, *see Glossary*
Abdomen, exsanguinating hemorrhage into, 122, 214–215, 302–303, 336–337
Abdominal aorta, palpation of pulse in, 99–100, 283
Abdominal pressure to force air or water out of stomach, 75, 280, 296, 311
Abdominal restraint during CPR, 114–115
Abdominal thrusts (Heimlich maneuver), 12, 26, **27–28**
  in infants and children, *30*, 281, 284, 285
  techniques of, *28, 29*
Abdominal trauma, 325, **335–337**
  exsanguinating intra-abdominal hemorrhage, 214–215, 336–337
  peritoneal lavage, 336
Acetazolamide, 241
Acid-base status
  control of, 240–241
  severe disturbances causing cardiac arrest, 307–308
Acidemia, control of, 145, 150, 151, 241, 307
Acute myocardial infarction, *see* Myocardial infarction
Adenosine triphosphate (ATP), 259
Adrenaline, *see* Epinephrine
Advanced life support (ALS, CPR steps D-E-F), 3, 5, 9–10, **127–225**
  ambulance personnel providing, 363–364
  American Heart Association guidelines, 12
  equipment for units providing, 367–369
  teaching, 341, 342, 344, 347, 352, 354, 359
  units, 360, 366–367
Advanced trauma life support (ATLS), 10–11, **119–122,** 127, 320–324
  in mass disasters, 374, 375
  teams, 361
AIDS, risk of transmission of, 12, 173, 350–351
Air embolism, cerebral, in divers, 312

Air transport, 365, 376
Airway control (CPR step A), 3, 4, **16–67**
  history of, 8
  in trauma victims, 17, 75–76, 322, 323, 331
  see also Tracheal intubation; Tracheotomy; Triple airway maneuver; *other specific maneuvers*
Airway obstruction, 300
  bronchodilation and clearing, 64
  bronchoscopy for, 62
  causes, 15
  clearing by suction, 32–33
  complete, 15, 16, 301
  cricothyrotomy for, 59, *61*
  diagnosis of, 16
  in infants and children, *30*, 280–281, 284–285
  manual clearing of, 12, **25–31,** 284–285
  in neonates, 287, 288
  partial, 15–16, 300
  translaryngeal oxygen jet insufflation in 59–61
  triple airway maneuver in, 22
Airways (artificial)
  esophageal gastric tube, 37
  esophageal obturator, insertion of, **37–39,** *38*
  pharyngeal, *see* Pharyngeal tubes
Albumin, human serum, 174–175
Alcohol intoxication, 318
Alkalemia, 241, 307
Allen's test, 136
Allopurinol, 258, 260
ALS, *see* Advanced life support
Alveolar anoxia, 299–300
Alveolar hypoxia, 300
Alveolar ventilation, adequacy of, 94
Ambu infant bag-mask-oxygen units, 288
Ambulance personnel
  advanced trauma life support (ATLS) by, 119, 320, 364
  defibrillation by, 116, 364
  training in first aid and resuscitation, 340–341, 363–364

Ambulances, **363–365**, 379–380
  external CPR in, 116–117
  helicopter, 365, 373
  mobile intensive care units (ICUs), 363,
    364, 365, 366–367
American College of Surgeons (ACS),
  advanced trauma life support
  (ATLS) course, 320–321
American Heart Association (AHA), 9,
  284–285, 295–296
  CPR standards of 1985, 11–12
Aminophylline, 64, 315
AMPLE history in trauma, 324
Amrinone, 157
Anaphylaxis, 319–320
Anesthesia
  cardiac arrest related to, 317–318
  in disasters, 337–338
  in field conditions, apparatus for, 84, 338
  malignant hyperpyrexia in, 306–307
  'therapeutic', 246, 260
Anesthetized patients, teaching first aid and
    resuscitation on, 346–347, 349
Angina, relief of, 164
Animal models for evaluation of post
    cardiac arrest brain-orientated
    therapy 251
Animals, laboratory, teaching first aid and
    resuscitation on, 346–347, 349–350
Anoxia, alveolar, 299–300
Antecubital veins, 129, **130–131**
Anticholinesterases, intoxication with,
    318–319
Antitoxin sera, anaphylactic reactions to,
    319
Aorta, abdominal, palpation of pulse,
    99–100, 283
Apallic syndrome, *see* Vegetative state,
    persistent
Apgar scoring system, 287
Apnea, 1, 300
  after cardiac arrest, 98, 99
  recognition of airway obstruction in,
    16
  sudden, causing asphyxia, 301, 308
Apneic diffusion oxygenation, 301
Arrhythmias, *see* Dysrhythmias
Arsenic poisoning, 319
Arterial catheterization, 94, **136–138**
  complications, 138
  of femoral artery, 137, *139*
  in neonates, 289
  of radial artery, 136–137
  sampling technique, 137–138
  in small children and infants, 137

Arterial pressure
  monitoring, **143–144**
  post-resuscitation control of, 241–242,
    245, 246, 248
  see also Hypertension; Hypotension
Arterial puncture, 136
Asphyxia, 98, **300–301**
  neonatal, 287, 288–290
Aspiration of foreign matter, *see* Foreign
    matter, aspiration of
Assisted ventilation (AV), 21, 68, *71*
Asthmatic crisis, *see* Status asthmaticus
Asystole, **181–182, 198**
  ECG patterns of, *182, 192*
  electric, 98, 178, 181, *192*, 198
  mechanical, *see* Electromechanical
    dissociation
  treatment of, 145, **148**, 149, 198
Atherosclerosis, maximum backward tilt of
    head in, 294–295
ATLS, *see* Advanced trauma life support
Atracurium, 169
Atrial fibrillation, 186, *189*, 299
Atrial flutter, *188*
Atrial tachycardia, paroxysmal (PAT),
    184–185
Atrial tachydysrhythmias, propranolol for,
    165
Atrioventricular blocks, 98, 181, 182,
    187–188
  first-degree, 187, *190–191*
  pacing in, *see* Pacing, cardiac
  second-degree Mobitz type I
    (Wenckebach), 187, 188, *190–191*
  second-degree Mobitz type II, 187, 188,
    190–191
  third degree (complete), 187, 188,
    190–191
  treatment of, 158, 159, 160, 187, 188
Atropine, **159**
  in bradycardia, 159, 187, 188, 191, 299
  in myocardial infarction, 159, 187–188
  in pediatric resuscitation, 286
  routes of administration, 132, 218
Autolysis of tissues, 232
AVPU neurologic evaluations, 323

B, *see* Breathing support
Back blows, 11, 26, 27, 28–29
  in infants and children, *30*, 281, 284–285
  techniques of, *28, 29*
Back-pressure arm-lift (prone) method of
    emergency artificial ventilation
    (Holger-Nielson), 68

Backboards (spine boards)
for extrication of shocked patients, 124
for moving patients with CPR, 116
for suspected spinal injuries, 312, 323, 333
Bag-valve-mask (-oxygen) units, self-refilling, *82*, **83–85**, 219
modifications for special uses, 84
for neonates or infants, *282*, 288
technique of use, 84, 85
Balloon counterpulsation, intra-aortic, 222, 243, 297
Barbiturates, **166–167**
in head trauma, 254, 255–256, 259, 332
intoxication, 167, 318
post cardiac arrest, for brain resuscitation, 231, 253, **254–256**, 259, 317–318
Base deficit, 151, 289
in hemodilution, 173
Base excess, *140*, 151
Basic cardiac life support (BCLS), 10
Basic life support (BLS, CPR steps A-B-C), 3, *4*, 9, **107–118**
ambulance personnel providing, 116–117, 363, 364
American Heart Association recommendations, 11–12
C-A-B sequence, 117–118, 291, 294
combinations of ventilation and cardiac compressions, 107–114
drugs used during, 145–148, 154
in infants and children, 280–281, *282*, 283–284
monitoring effectiveness of, 114
recommended techniques of, 111–114
teaching, 340–341, 342, 343, 379
with equipment, 344, 346–347, 351–353, 357
without equipment, 343, 346–347, 350, 355–356
Basic trauma life support (BTLS), 10, 119, 320
see also First aid, life supporting
Basilic vein, *130–131*, 134
Baxter formula, 328
BCLS (basic cardiac life support), 10
Beclomethasone aerosol, 64
Benzodiazepines, 167
Beta-blockers, 165
Bird mark VIII ventilator, 88
Blood
sampling via catheters, 137–138
whole, for transfusion, 173, 175, 177
Blood flow

produced by direct internal cardiac compression, 213, 217
produced by external cardiac compression, 101–102
Blood gases, 94, 240–241
arterial sampling for, 136–138, 289
Blood pressure, *see* Arterial pressure; Central venous pressure; Pulmonary artery occlusion pressure
Blood transfusions, 172, 175–176, 302, 326
disadvantages of, 173–174
intra-arterial, 172, 303
BLS, *see* Basic life support
Brachial artery, palpation of pulse, 99, *282*, 283
Bradycardia, 181
drug treatment in, 158, 159, 188, 191, 299
emergency pacing in, 114, 211–212, 292–294
of heart block, 181, 182, 187
junctional (nodal), 188
sinus, 183, *184–185*, 188
see also Atrioventricular blocks; Pacing, cardiac
Brain damage
in carbon monoxide poisoning, 316–317
evaluation of, 266–268
in neonates, 287, 290
prediction of, 266, 271
socioeconomic impact, 229, 277
see also Coma; Head trauma; Post-resuscitation syndrome; Vegetative state, persistent
Brain death
criteria, 273–276
definition of, 272
during emergency resuscitation, 269, 270–271
terminating life support in, 249, 272–276, 277
Brain-orientated therapy, post-resuscitation, 3, *5*, 229–232, **238–260**
areas of research in, 231–232, 251
barbiturates, 254–256, 259
calcium entry blockers, 161–162, 256–257, 259
corticosteroids, 163, 247, 248
etiology-specific combination therapies, 258–259
free radical scavengers, 257–258, 259
history, 230
miscellaneous measures, 259–260
objectives of, 245
promotion of reperfusion, 252–254

Brain-orientated therapy, *contd*
  special therapeutic potentials, 231, 244, 251–259
  stabilization of extracerebral organs, 238–244
  standard measures, 244, 245–250
  see also Coma; Intensive therapy
Breathing, spontaneous, augmentation of, 21, 68, *71*
  see also SB-CAP *and* SB-PAP
Breathing support (CPR step B), 3, *4*, **68–97**
Bretylium, 145, 147, 148, **153–154**, 193
Bronchial intubation, inadvertant, 57
Bronchitis, with asphyxiation, 64
Bronchodilation therapy, 64, 84, 315
Bronchoscopes
  flexible fiberoptic, 62
  rigid tube, 43, 62
Bronchoscopy for clearing tracheobronchial tree, 62
Bronchospasm, 300, 315
Brooke airways, 79
BTLS, *see* Basic trauma life support
Burns, **327–329**
  assessment of, 327, 328
  from electric shock, 308

C, *see* Circulation support
C-A-B sequence in witnessed cardiac arrest, 117–118, 291, 294
Calcium
  administration, 132, **159–160**
    in pediatric resuscitation, 286
  serum levels, cardiac function and, 307
Calcium entry blockers, **160–162**
  in cardiac arrest, 160–161
  dangerous effects, 161
  for post-CPR cerebral resuscitation, 161–162, 231, 253, **256–257**, 259–286
Caloric (oculovestibular) reflex, 265, 266, 271
Capnography, 139–141
Carbon dioxide
  continuous end-tidal monitoring (capnography), 139–141
  electrodes for blood gas analysis, 138, 141
Carbon dioxide tension (PCO_2)
  arterial, 94, 240–241, 246, 248
  methods of measurement, 138–142
  transcutaneous, 141–142
  see also Hypercarbia
Carbon monoxide poisoning, 316–317
Cardiac arrest
  anesthesia-related, 317–318
    animal models, 251
    case report form, *440–441*
    causes of, 98, 280, 307
    development of, 2
    diagnosis of, 1, 99–100
    ECG patterns in, 178, 181–182, *182*
    exsanguination, 302–303
    fluid administration after, 171, 173
    hypothermia with, 214, 219, 304–305
    irreversible (cardiac death), 269–270
    ischemic-anoxic insult, evaluation of, 261–263
    length of time of, 98–99, 225, 231
    in neonates, 289–290
    outcome
      evaluation of, 266–268
      prediction of, 266
    post-resuscitation syndrome, 98, 231, 232–237
    post-resuscitation therapy, 238–239
      see also Intensive therapy
    primary, 1–2, 98
    secondary, 2, 98, 273
    unwitnessed, 214
      defibrillation in, 145, 148, 204
      drug treatment in, 145, **148**
    witnessed, **291–294**
      C-A-B sequence in, 117–118, 291, 294
      cough CPR in, 147, 291–292
      drug treatment in, 145, **147**
      immediate defibrillation in, 102, 127, 145, 147, 204, 207, 291, 294
      precordial thumping in, 292–294
Cardiac (chest) compression: lung inflation ratios, 11, 77–78, 107, *108*, *109*
  in infants and children, *282*, 284
Cardiac (chest) compression (external), 9, **101–106**
  blood flow rates produced by, 101–102
  for cardiac pacing, 114, 292–293
  complications, 295
  history, 8
  in infants and children, 105, 106, *282*, 283–284
  mechanisms of blood flow during, 101
  in neonates, 289
  techniques of, 102–106, *103*, *104*
Cardiac compressions, open-chest (direct), 102
  advantages of, 9–10, 213, 217
  technique of, *216*, 217–218
Cardiac death (irreversible cardiac arrest), 269–270
  sudden, prevention of, 296–299

Cardiac dysrhythmias, life-threatening, 183–198
Cardiac output, 95
  measurement of, 241
  post-cardiac arrest, *235*
Cardiac resuscitation, *see* Circulation support
Cardiac tamponade, 214, **335**
Cardiogenic shock, 222, 243, **297**
Cardiopulmonary bypass, emergency, 10, 102, 127, **219–222**, 259, 260
  apparatus for, *221*
  ethical problems, 381
  possible technique of, 221–222
  in pulmonary embolism, 219, 315
Cardiopulmonary cerebral resuscitation (CPCR)
  case report form, *440–441*
  delivery of, 379–380
  evolution (natural selection) and, 383–384
  future ethical problems, 380–382
  history, 3–4
  legal considerations, 369–371
  organization of services, 360–378
  phases and steps, 5, *6–7*, 9–12
  trauma-orientated, 10–11
  see also Brain-orientated therapy, post-resuscitation; Cardiopulmonary resuscitation
Cardiopulmonary resuscitation (CPR)
  A-B-C, *see* Basic life support
  American Heart Association (AHA) recommendations, 11–12, 295–296
  apparent brain death during, 269, 270–271
  combinations of ventilation and cardiac compressions, 107–114
  complications and pitfalls, 294–296
  cough, 147, **291–292**
  D-E-F, *see* Advanced life support
  ECG monitoring during, 178, 179–180
  importance of time, 98–99, 225, 231
  in intubated patients, 110, 112
  machines (chest thumpers), 117
  monitoring effectiveness of, 114
  one operator, 11, 107, *108*, 110, **111**
  open-chest, 118, 127, **212–219**
    advantages of, 213, 217
    history, 212–213
    indications, 214–215
    intracardiac injection of drugs, 132, 218
    technique of, *215*, *216*, 217–219
  outcome, evaluation of, 266–268
  outside the hospital, 116–117
  pediatric, 279–286

simplified technique, 113
simultaneous ventilation-compression (SVC-CPR), 102, 114–116
standard external, 101–118
switching between two operators, 113–114
teaching, *see* Teaching first aid and resuscitation
terminating, 269–271
transition from one to two operators, 113
two operator, 11, **107–110**, *109*, 112
when not to start, 269
Cardiothoracic surgery, barbiturate anesthesia in, 255
'Cardiovascular collapse', 198
Cardiovascular stimulants, 154–155
Cardiovascular support, post-resuscitation, 241–243
Cardioversion, synchronized, 197, 209, 285
Carinal reflex, 265
Carotid artery
  blood flow produced by external cardiac compressions, 101
  palpation of pulse, *99*, 100, 114, 283
Catalase, 258
Central venous catheterization, 130, **132–134**, 241
  complications, 295
Central venous pressure (CVP), 133, 241
  for guiding fluid administration, 173, 242
  monitoring, 143–144
Cephalic vein, *130–131*, 134
Cerebral acidosis induced by sodium bicarbonate, 307
Cerebral air embolism in divers, 312
Cerebral alkalosis due to hyperventilation, 307–308
Cerebral blood flow (CBF)
  measuring, 250
  post-cardiac arrest, *235*
  produced by external cardiac compressions, 101–102
Cerebral death, 272, 276
Cerebral edema, control of, 163, 166, 245–247, 253
Cerebral electrical impedance, 250
Cerebral metabolism
  measures to reduce, 253, 254
  measuring, 250
Cerebral performance categories, 249, 267, 268
Cerebral perfusion pressure, maintenance of, 245
Cerebral reoxygenation injury after cardiac arrest, 233, *236–237*

Cerebral reperfusion failure, post-
   resuscitation, 232–233, *234, 235*
   therapies counteracting, 252–254
Cerebral resuscitation, *see* Brain-orientated
   therapy, post-resuscitation
Cerebral trauma, *see* Head trauma
Cerebrospinal fluid, *see* CSF
Cervical spine trauma, 322, 323, **333**
   airway control in, 17, 22, 76
   in drowning victims, 312
   head turning, 25
   positioning of patient, 19, 295, 333
Chest compressions, *see* Cardiac (chest)
   compressions (external)
Chest deformities, open-chest CPR in, 214
Chest injuries, 10, **333–335**
Chest-pressure arm-lift (supine) method of
   emergency artificial ventilation
   (Silvester), 68
Chest thrusts, 27, **28,** 29, 281
   in infants and children, 284, 285
Chest thumpers (external CPR machines),
   117
Chest thumping, *see* Precordial thumping
Children, **279–286**
   arterial catheterization, 137
   bronchoscope sizes, 43
   crichothyrotomy, 60
   defibrillation in, 203, 285
   determination of pulselessness, 99–100,
      283
   drugs for resuscitation in, 285–286
   exhaled air ventilation in, 77, *282,* 283
   external cardiac compressions in, 105,
      106, *282,* 283–284
   laryngoscope blade sizes, 43
   manual clearing of airway obstruction,
      29, *30,* 281, 284–285
   tracheal intubation in, 55, 281
   tracheal tubes for, 41, 42, 44, 55
   tracheostomy tubes, 42
Chin support (chin lift), head-tilt by, 17,
   18
Chlorpromazine, 254, 258
Circulation support (CPR step C), 3, *4,*
   98–125
   in trauma victims, 119–124, 322–323
Clinical death, 1, 2, 272
Clotting tests, 176
CNS depressants, poisoning with, 167
Coagulation problems after blood
   transfusions, 176
Cocaine
   overdose, 318
   for topical anesthesia, 53

Colloid osmotic pressure of plasma, 135,
   174, 242
Colloid plasma substitutes, 172, 174–175,
   177, 326, 328
Coma
   after cardiac arrest, 98, 99, 232, 238
   evaluation of outcome, 266–268
   in head trauma, 331
   intensive care guidelines for, 245–250
   irreversible, *see* Vegetative state,
      persistent
   obstructive asphyxia in, 15, 300
   predicting outcome, 266
   scoring (evaluation of depth of), 249, 262,
      263–265
   'therapeutic', 246, 260
Community-wide organization of
   emergency delivery systems, 290–
   291, 362–363, 372
Concussion, 331–332
Consciousness, return of, after cardiac
   arrest, 238
Consent, informed, 370
Contusion, brain, 332
Convulsions (seizures)
   in head trauma, 333
   prevention or control of, 166–167, 168,
      246, 248, 255
Corneal reflex in coma, 265
Coronary artery angioplasty, emergency,
   299
Coronary artery bypass, emergency, 299
Coronary artery disease, 296
   risk factors for, 296–297
Coronary blood flow produced by external
   cardiac compressions, 102
Corpses, human, teaching first aid and
   resuscitation on, 344–345, 349
Corticosteroids, **163**
   post CPR, 163, 247, 248
   in status asthmaticus, 163, 315
Cough cardiopulmonary resuscitation
   (CPR), 147, **291–292**
Coughing in airway obstruction, 281
CPAP (continuous positive airway
   pressure), spontaneous breathing
   with, *see* SB-CPAP
CPPV (continuous positive pressure
   ventilation, IPPV plus PEEP), 21,
   69–70, *71*
   in neonates, 289
   for open-chest CPR, 216, 219
   in pulmonary edema, 313
Creatine phosphokinase (CPK-BB) in CSF,
   249, 250, 266, 278

Cricoid pressure
  during positive pressure inflations, 20, 75, 283
  during tracheal intubation, 48
Cricothyrotomy, 27, 31, **59,** *61*
Critical care triage, 276, 277
Croup, 280–281
Crowing, 16
Cryoprecipitate, 175
CSF (cerebrospinal fluid)
  creatine phosphokinase (CPK-BB), 249, 250, 266, 278
  pH, 246, 250, 259
CT scanning
  in head trauma, 332
  in persistent vegetative state, 278
CVP, *see* Central venous pressure
Cyanide poisoning, 319
Cyanosis, 99, 288

D, *see* Drugs and fluids
D-E-F, *see* Advanced life support
Death
  biologic (panorganic), 272
  brain, *see* Brain death
  cardiac, 269–270
  causes of preventable or reversible sudden, 1, 2
  cerebral, 272, 276
  clinical, 1, 2, 272
  near-death experiences, 382–383
  'social', *see* Vegetative state, persistent
  from trauma, causes of, 320
  see also Dying *and* Euthanasia
Decamethonium, 168
Decompression, rapid, in high altitude flying, 299, 300
Decompression sickness in divers, 312
Deferoxamine, 253
Defibrillation (electric), 12, 114, **199–225**
  a.c. (alternating current) shock, 202–203
  by ambulance personnel, 116, 364
  automatic external, 209–210
  automatic internal (implanted), 210–211
  d.c. (direct current) shock, 202–203
  ECG monitoring for, 204, 205
  empirical, 207, 291
  energy requirements, 200–201, 203, 205
  facilitation by bretylium, 154
  history, 8
  indications, 199
  in infants and children, 203, 285
  internal direct, 202–203, *215,* 218–219
  lidocaine and, 152
  myocardial damage due to, 202–203

  recommendations to improve success of, 209
  synchronized cardioversion, 197, 209, 285
  technique of, **204–207,** *206,* 208
  training in, 352
  in unwitnessed cardiac arrest, 145, 148, 204
  using esophageal-to-chest surface electrodes, 207
  in witnessed cardiac arrest, 102, 127, 145, 147, 204, 207, 291, 294
Defibrillators, 178, **203–204**
  automatic external, *210*
  energy output, 200–201
  paddles, 203–204
  placement of, *206*
Dentists, teaching first aid and resuscitation to, 340–341, 346
Department of Transportation (US), 320
Developing countries, CPCR services in, 379–380
Dexamethasone, 163, 248, 315
Dextrans, 175
Dextrose (glucose) infusions, 171, 303–304
  hypertonic, 175, 259, 327
Diamorphine, *see* Heroin
Diarrhea, oral fluid therapy in, 176
Diazepam, 167, 246, 248
Digitalis, **162**
Diltiazem, 160–161, 256, 257
Diphenylhydantoin, *see* Phenytoin
Disaster medical response teams, 375–376, 377
Disaster resuscitology, 371
Disasters, **371–378**
  anesthesia in, 337–338
  dying processes in, 373–374
  endemic, 373
  local disaster medical systems, 377
  mass, 269, 371–373
    oral fluid therapy in, 176
  multicasualty incidents, 269, 371, 377
  national disaster medical systems, 375–377
  nuclear, 329, 330, 377–378
  resuscitation potentials in, 374–375
  resuscitation triage in, 269, 377
Diuretics, 166, 249
Divers, hyperbaric injuries to, 312
Dobutamine, 154, 155, **157,** 297
  in pediatric resuscitation, 286
Dogs, teaching first aid and resuscitation on, 349
Doll's eye (oculocephalic) reflex, 265, 266, 271

Dopamine, 154, 155, **156–157**
  in cardiogenic shock, 156, 297
  in pediatric resuscitation, 286
Dorsal venous arch, *130–131*
Drowning, **310–312**
  cold water, 305, 311
  fresh water, 310–312
  near-, 64, 310–311
  sea water, 310–312
Drugs, **145–170**
  after restoration of spontaneous
    circulation, 148
  anaphylactic reactions, 319
  central venous route, 134
  during CPR steps A-B-C, 145–148
  intoxication, 318–319
  intracardiac injection, 132, 218
  intramuscular route, 132
  intratracheal instillation, 132
  intravenous route, 129–130
  physician's emergency kit, 170
  for resuscitation in infants and children,
    285–286
Drugs and fluids (CPR step D), 3, 5, 127,
  129–177
  see also Drugs *and* Fluid resuscitation
Dying
  care during, 382
  processes, in disasters, 373–374
  research needs, 380–381
  see also Death *and* Euthanasia
Dysrhythmias, cardiac, life-threatening,
  183–198

E, *see* Electrocardiography
Earthquakes, 373, 374, 376
ECG, *see* Electrocardiography
EEG, (electroencephalography)
  during cardiopulmonary resuscitation
    (CPR), 270
  for evaluation of coma, 266
  post-resuscitation monitoring, 249, 250
Elder valve, *87*
Electric countershock, *see* Defibrillation
Electric shock, 98, **308–310**
  from lightning, 308
  high voltage, 199–200, 308, 309–310
  low voltage (household a.c. current), 199,
    308, 309
  treatment of victims of, 309
'Electrical therapy', 199
Electrocardiography (ECG, CPR step E), 3,
  5, 127, **178–198**
  defibrillation and, 178, 204, 205

during cardiopulmonary resuscitation
  (CPR), 178, 180
long-term monitoring, 179, 241
patterns of cardiac arrest, 181–182,
  269–270
patterns of life-threatening dysrhythmias,
  183–198
techniques of, 178–180
telemetry, 180, 364
Electrodes for blood gas and pH analysis,
  138, 141
Electrolyte disturbances, cardiac arrest due
  to, 307
Electrolyte solutions for fluid replacement,
  172, 174
Electromechanical dissociation (EMD,
  mechanical asystole), 98, 178,
  181–182, 198
  ECG patterns of, *182*
  treatment of, 145, **148**, 149, 160, 182, 198
Elevation of bleeding sites, 120
Emergency and Critical Care Medicine
  (ECCM) delivery systems, 362, 372
Emergency medical operations and
  communications center (EMOC],
  362–363
Emergency medical services (EMS)
  community-wide organization of, 9,
    362–363
  disaster planning, 373, 377
  medical control of, 364–365, 372
  for neonatal intensive care, 290–291
Emergency medical technicians (EMTs),
  363
Emphysema
  severe, with barrel chest, 214
  Venturi mask in, 94
Encephalitis, 247, 250, 255–256
Endotracheal intubation, *see* Tracheal
  intubation
Ephedrine, 158
Epidural hematoma, 11, 323–324, 332
Epiglottis, airway obstruction by, 15
Epiglottitis, 62, 280–281
Epinephrine (adrenaline), 12, 129, **149**
  in CPR steps A-B-C, 118, 145–146, 147,
    148, 149
  in exsanguination cardiac arrest, 302
  intracardiac injection of, 132, 218
  in neonates, 290
  in pediatric resuscitation, 285–286
  routes of administration, 129, 132, 134
Esophageal gastric tube airway, 37
Esophageal obturator airways, insertion of,
  37–39, *38*

Esophageal stethoscope, 50, 178
Esophageal-to-chest surface electrodes, defibrillation using, 207
Esophagus, inadvertant intubation of, 57
Ethacrynic acid, 166
Ethical problems, future, 380–382
Euthanasia
    active, 380
    passive ('letting die'), 380, 381, 382
        in persistent vegetative state, 276–278
Exhaled air ventilation, 12, 20–21, **75–80**
    history, 7–8
    in infants and children, 77, *282*, 283, 288
    techniques of, *76*, 77–78, *81*
    in tracheotomized and laryngectomized patients, 76
    transmission of disease via, 12, 350–351
    see also Mouth-to-mouth ventilation; Mouth-to-nose ventilation *and* Mouth-to-adjunct ventilation
Expiratory reserve volume (ERV), *142*
Expiratory retardation, 68, *71*
Exsanguination cardiac arrest, 302–303
External jugular vein, puncture and catheterization of, 129–130, 133
Extracellular fluid volume, 172
Extracorporeal lung assist (ECLA), 223–224
Extracorporeal membrane oxygenation (ECMO), **222–223**, 224
    indications, 223
Extremity trauma, 120, **337**
Extubation, tracheal, 56
Eye movements in coma, 266
Eye opening in coma, 264
Eyelash reflex in coma, 265

F, *see* Fibrillation treatment
Face masks
    Laerdal pocket masks, 79–80, *81*
    for SB-PAP, 73
Family
    certification of brain death and, 276
    of patients in persistent vegetative state, 277
Femoral artery
    catheterization, 137, *139*
    intra-arterial pressure monitoring via, 143–144
    palpation of pulse, 99, 283
Femoral vein, puncture and catheterization of, 130

Femur, fractures of, blood loss in, 337
Fentanyl, 52, 165, 337
    overdose, 318
Fiberoptic bronchoscopes, 62
Fiberoptic laryngoscopic tracheal intubation, 55
Fibrillation treatment (CPR step F), 3, 5, 127, **199–225**
    see also Defibrillation
Finger sweeping, *25*, *26*, 281, 284
Firemen, teaching first aid and resuscitation to, 340–341, 344
First aid, life supporting (LSFA), 3, 10, **119**, 320–322
    in mass disasters, 374–375
    teaching, **339–359**, 379
    see also Teaching first aid and resuscitation
'Fist' pacing, *see* Precordial thumping, repetitive
Flail chest, 334
Fluid resuscitation, **171–177**
    in burn injury, 327, 328
    choice of fluids, 173–176
    history, 7
    in neonates, 289
    objectives during administration, 171
    oral therapy, 176
    routes of administration, 129–134
    in traumatic hypovolemic shock, 10–11, 323, 325–327
    volumes required, 171, 172
    see also Intra-arterial infusions; Intravenous infusions
Flunarizine, 161, 256, 257
Fluorocarbons, 176, 327
Fluosol, 176
Foot, veins of dorsum of, *130–131*
Forced expiratory volume (FEV), *142*, 143
Foreign matter
    airway obstruction by, 12, 15, 300
        clearing by suction, 32–33
        manual clearing of, *25–31*, 281, 284–285
    aspiration of
        bronchodilation and clearing of airways, 64
        bronchoscopy for, 62
Fractures of extremities, 337
Free radical scavengers, 231, 253, **257–258**, 259
Free radicals, formation of, post-resuscitation, *236–237*
Functional residual capacity (FRC), *142*
Furosemide, 166

G, *see* Gauging
Gag reflex, 265
Gallamine, 168, 169
Gas
  inhalation of oxygen-free, 299–300
  mixtures with reduced oxygen
    concentration, 300
Gasping
  in cardiac arrest, 98, 99
  in cough CPR, 292
Gastric intubation, 50, **57–58**, 243, 323
Gastrointestinal system, post-resuscitation
    support, 243, 244
Gastrointestinal trauma, 325
Gauging (CPR step G), 3, 5, 229
Gelatin solutions, 175
Glasgow coma scale, 262, 263, 264
Glasgow outcome categories, 266–268
Glasgow-Pittsburgh coma scale, 262, 263,
    264–265
Glasgow-Pittsburgh outcome categories,
    267, 268
Glucose (dextrose) solutions, 171, 303–304
  hypertonic, 175, 259, 327
Glutathione, 258
Glutethimide overdose, 318
Glyceryl trinitrate, *see* Nitroglycerin
'Good Samaritan Law', 370
Guedel tubes, *see* Pharyngeal tubes
Gurgling, 16

H, *see* Human mentation
Halothane, brain resuscitation and, 256, 260
Hand, veins of dorsum of, 129, *130–131*
Head, backward tilt of, 15, **17**, *18*, 22, 77
  in cervical spine injury, 22, 295, 333
  complications and pitfalls, 294–295
  in infants and children, 280
Head trauma, 320, 323, 325, **331–333**
  esophageal obturator airways and, 39
  Glasgow coma scale, 263
  intensive therapy in, 245–246, 247
  protective effects of barbiturates in, 254,
    255–256, 259, 332
  tracheal intubation in, 40, **51**, 52, 331
Heart block, *see* Atrioventricular blocks
Heart rate in neonates, 288–289
Heat cramps, 306
Heat exhaustion, 306
Heat stroke (heat pyrexia), 306
Heimlich maneuver, *see* Abdominal thrusts
Helicopters
  ambulances, 365, 373
  for evacuation of disaster victims, 376
Hematocrit, reduced, *see* Hemodilution

Hemodilution
  intracarotid hypertensive, 231, 252, 259
  normovolemic, 173, 252, 259, 326
Hemoglobin, stroma-free, 176, 327
Hemorrhage
  exsanguination cardiac arrest, 302–303
  external, control of, 120, *121*, 322, 323,
    324
  in extremity trauma, 120, 337
  fluid resuscitation in, 172–173, 174, 302,
    323, 326–327
  internal, management of, 120–122,
    214–215, 322–323, 336–337
  intracranial, *see* Intracranial hemorrhage
  traumatic, emergency management of, 10,
    11, **119–125**
Hemothorax, 334
Heparinization, post-resuscitation, 253, 259,
    260
Hepatitis, risks of transmission, 12, 173,
    350–351
Heroin
  for analgesia, 166
  overdose, 318
Herpes, risks of transmission, 12, 350–351
High altitude, alveolar hypoxia at, 300
High-frequency jet ventilation (HFJV), **89–
    90**, *91*, 240
  advantages and disadvantages, 90
  during external CPR, 116
  transtracheal, 90, *91*
Holger-Nielsen (back-pressure arm-lift,
    prone) method of emergency
    artificial ventilation, 68
Hospitals
  advanced life support units in, 360,
    366–367
  with emergency services, regional
    organization of, 365–366
  field, 375
  organization of CPCR services within,
    360–362
  resuscitation carts, 367
  resuscitation teams, 361–362
  transfer of disaster victims to, 376
Human mentation (CPR step H), 3, 5, 229
Humidification of inspired gases, 64, 92
Hydrochloric acid, administration of, 241
Hydroxyethyl starch, 175
Hydroxyl radicals (OH·), **236–237**, 257, 258
Hyperbaric injuries to divers, 312
Hyperbaric oxygenation, 96
Hypercapnia, *see* Hypercarbia
Hypercarbia, 300, 308
  diagnosis of, 16, 94

without hypoxemia, 301
Hyperglycemia, 304
Hyperpotassemia (hyperkalemia), cardiac
    arrest due to, 307
Hyperpyrexia, malignant, during
    anesthesia, 306–307
Hypertension
    acute myocardial infarction with, 298
    post cardiac arrest, 146, 245, 248, 252,
       259
Hyperthermia, 247, 306–307
Hypertonic glucose, 175, 259, 327
Hypertonic saline solutions, 174, 326, 328
Hyperventilation
    for acidemia of cardiac arrest, 145, 150,
       151
    cerebral alkalosis due to, 307–308
    in cerebral trauma, 246
Hypnotic drugs, overdose of, 318
Hypoglycemia, 303–304
Hypotension
    acute myocardial infarction with, 297
    in neonates, 289
    see also Shock
Hypothermia, **304–305**
    accidental (without submersion), 305
    for brain resuscitation, 249, 253–254, 259
    cardiac arrest with, 214, 219, 304–305
    during cold water drowning, 305, 311
    induced, in surgical patients, 305
    rewarming methods, 305
Hypoventilation, 300
Hypovolemic shock
    in burn injury, 327–328
    fluid administration in, 171–173, 326–327
    in heat exhaustion, 306
    oral fluid therapy in, 176
    in trauma 10–11, 119, 323, **325–327**
Hypoxia, 16, 94, 300
    cardiac arrest due to, 98, 301
    in head trauma, 331
    hypercarbia without, 301
Hypoxia, alveolar, 300

I, *see* Intensive therapy
Immobilization
    or fractured extremities, 337
    post-resuscitation, 246, 248, 259
    of trauma victims, 323, 333
IMV (intermittent mandatory ventilation),
    21, 68, *71*
    post-resuscitation, 94, 239–240
Indomethacin, 260
Infants, **279–286**
    arterial catheterization, 137

bronchoscope sizes, 43
    cricothyrotomy, 61
    defibrillation in, 203, 285
    determination of pulselessness, 99–100,
       283
    drugs for resuscitation in, 285–286
    exhaled air ventilation in, 77, *282*, 283
    external cardiac compressions in, 106,
       282, 283–284
    laryngoscope blade sizes, 43
    manikins, 356
    manual clearing of airway obstruction,
       30, 281, 284–285
    tracheal intubation in, 55, 281
    tracheal tubes for, 41, 42, 44, *45*, 55
    tracheostomy tubes, 42
    see also Neonatal resuscitation
Infection control, post-resuscitation, 244
Informed consent, 370
Infusions
    drug administration via, 169
    intra-arterial, 138, 172, 303
    intravenous, *see* Intravenous infusions
Insect poisons (stings), anaphylactic
    reactions to, 319
Inspiratory capacity (IC), *142*
Inspiratory reserve volume (IRV), *142*
Instructors in first aid and resuscitation,
    training of, 345
Insulin, 259
Intensive care units (ICUs)
    in developing countries, 380
    mobile, 363, 364, 365, 366–367
    triage of patients in, 276, 277
Intensive therapy (CPR step I), 3, 5, 229,
    238–250
    blood gases and acid-base status 240–241
    cardiovascular support, 241–243, 244
    gastrointestinal system support, 243, 244
    history, 3, 230
    infection control, 244
    for neonates and children, 290–291
    pulmonary support, 239–240, 242
    renal system support, 243, 244
    stabilization of extracerebral organs,
       238–244
    see also Brain-orientated therapy,
       post-resuscitation
Intermittent mandatory ventilation, *see*
    IMV
Internal jugular vein, catheterization of,
    130, 133, 134, *135*
International Red Cross, 285
Intra-aortic balloon counterpulsation, 222,
    243, 297

Intra-arterial infusions, 138, 172, 303
Intracardiac injection of drugs, 132, 218
Intracarotid hypertensive hemodilution, 231, 252, 259
Intracranial hemorrhage, 247, 248, 323–324, 331, 332
Intracranial pressure (ICP)
  control of, 245, 247–250, 332
  monitoring, 247, 248, 250
  post-cardiac arrest, *235*
Intramuscular administration of drugs, 132
Intrapulmonary administration of drugs, 132
Intratracheal instillation of drugs, 132
Intravenous cannulation, peripheral, 129–130, 326
  choice of veins, 12, 129–130
  by cut-down, 130, 326
  technique of, *130–131*
Intravenous infusions, 171–173
  apparatus for, *130–131*
  in cardiogenic shock, 297
  choice of fluids, 173–176
  choice of veins for, 129–130
  in exsanguination cardiac arrest, 302
  objectives of, 171
  post-resuscitation, 243, 248
  rapid administration technique, 171–172
  in status asthmaticus, 316
  for titrated drug administration, 169
  in traumatic hypovolemic shock, 10–11, 323, 325–327
  volumes required, 171, 172
  see also Fluid resuscitation
Intubation, tracheal, *see* Tracheal intubation
IPPB (intermittent positive pressure breathing), 21, 68, *71*
IPPV (intermittent positive pressure ventilation), 68, *71*, 94–95
  in asthmatic crisis, 64
  circulatory depression in, 69
  complications and pitfalls, 69, 294–295
  during external CPR in intubated patients, 110
  emergency, 20–21, 68, **75–89**, 94
  high-frequency, 89–90, 116, 240
  indications for, 69, 97
  in neonates, 288–289
  plus PEEP, *see* CPPV
  prolonged, 69, 88
  weaning, 72, 96, 240
  see also Exhaled air ventilation
Iron chelators, 253
Isoflurane for brain resuscitation, 256, 260

Isoprenaline, *see* Isoproterenol
Isoproterenol, 154, **158–159**
  in bradycardia of heart block, 158, 187, 188, 191
  in pediatric resuscitation, 286
Isotonic saline, 172, 174, 326

Jaw lift technique, thumb-, *23*, 24
Jaw-thrust (forward displacement of mandible), 15, 17, 22, *23*, 24
  mouth-to-mask ventilation and, 79–80
Jaw-thrust maneuver, *see* Triple airway maneuver
Jet insufflation, translaryngeal oxygen, 27, 31, **59–61, 89**
Jet ventilation, high-frequency, *see* High-frequency jet ventilation
Jugular vein
  external, puncture and catheterization of, 129–130, 133
  internal, cannulation of, 130, 133, 134, *135*
Junctional (nodal) rhythms, 186–187, *189*

Ketamine analgesia, 337
Kidneys, acute tubular necrosis of (ATN), 324

Laerdal infant bag-mask-oxygen units, 288
Laerdal pocket masks, 79–80, *81*
Laerdal pressure drainings, 121
Laerdal recording Resusci-Anne manikin, 348
Laerdal self-training system, 350
Laerdal Silicon Resuscitators, *82*, 84
Laryngectomized patients, emergency mouth-to-stoma ventilation in, 76
Laryngoscope blades, 41–44, *45*, 55
Laryngoscopy
  in airway obstruction, 27
  anatomical views during, *46*
  fiberoptic, for tracheal intubation, 55
  for insertion of gastric tube, 58
  for nasotracheal intubation, 53, 55
  for orotracheal intubation, *46–47*, **48–49**, 55
Laryngospasm, 15, 300
  postextubation, 56
Laryngotracheobronchitis, 62
Lay public
  first aid and resuscitation skills to be taught to, 11, 27, 107, 340–341, 363, 379

teaching resuscitation skills to, 343–346, 350

see also First aid, life supporting

League of Red Cross Societies (LRCS), 342

Legal implications of CPCR, 369–371

'Letting die', *see* Euthanasia, passive

Lidocaine (lignocaine), 51, **152–153**
  for anesthesia of upper airways, 51–52
  in CPR steps A-B-C, 145, 146, 147, 148
  in pediatric resuscitation, 286
  for premature ventricular complexes (PVCs), 152, 193, 299
  routes of administration, 132, 218
  side-effects, 152–153
  technique of administration, 153
  in ventricular tachycardia (VT), 197, 299

Lidoflazine, 161–162, 253, 256, 257

Life support
  advanced, *see* Advanced life support
  basic, *see* Basic life support
  prolonged, *see* Prolonged life support

Life supporting first aid, *see* First aid, life supporting

Lifeguards, teaching first aid and resuscitation to, 340–341, 346

Lightning shocks, 308

Lignocaine, *see* Lidocaine

Lipid radicals, free (FLR), *236–237*

Liver function, post-resuscitation monitoring, 243, 244

Local anesthetics
  cerebral metabolism and, 253
  overdose, 153, 318

Lodoxamide, 253, 258

LSFA, *see* First aid, life supporting

Lung rupture
  complicating positive pressure inflation, 69, 295
  translaryngeal oxygen jet insufflation and, 60

Lung volumes, measurement of, 142–143

Magnesium chloride ($MgCl_2$), 259

Magnesium serum levels, cardiac function and, 307

Mandible, forward displacement of, *see* Jaw-thrust

Manikins, 345, 348, 350
  Laerdal recording Resusci-Anne, 348
  measures taught using, 346–347
  prevention of disease transmission via, 12, 350–351
  for teaching endotracheal intubation, 353, 358
  testing skills using, 355–358

Mannitol osmotherapy, 249, 253

Masks, *see* Face masks

Mass spectrometry, 141

MAST, *see* Military (medical) antishock trousers

Maxillofacial trauma, airway control in, 323

Maximum mid-expiratory flow rate (MMFR), 142–143

Meconium obstructing airways in neonates, 288

Medic Alert bracelets or necklaces, 125

Meperidine (pethidine), 165, 337

Metabolic acidemia, 241

Metabolic alkalemia, 150, 241

Metaproterenol, 64, 315

Metaraminol, 154, **157–158**

l-Methionine, 258

Methoxamine, 154

Methylprednisolone, 163, 248, 315

Meuller maneuver, 292

Military (medical) antishock trousers (MAST, PASG), 119, **120–122**, 323
  deflation of, 121–122
  during external CPR, 115
  in intra-abdominal hemorrhage, 122 214–215, 302–303, 336–337
  technique of application, *122*

Military medicine, national disaster organization and, 376–377

Mobitz type I AV block, 187, 188, *190–191*

Mobitz type II AV block, 187, 188, *190–191*

Morphine, **165**, 298, 299, 313, 337

Motor responses in coma, 264

Motor vehicle accidents, 280

Mouth
  forcing open, techniques of, 25, *26*
  opening of, in triple airway maneuver, 15, 22
  suctioning of, 33

Mouth-to-adjunct ventilation, 34, **79–80**, *81*, 351
  using S-shaped pharyngeal tubes, *35, 36*, 79

Mouth-to-mouth plus nose ventilation in infants, 77, *282, 283*, 288

Mouth-to-mouth ventilation, 24, 68, **75–78**
  in drowning or near-drowning victims, 311–312
  history, 3–4
  teaching, 340, 343, 346, 350
  technique of, *20, 76*, 77–78
  transmission of disease via, 12, 350–351

Mouth-to-nose ventilation, 24, **75–78**
  technique of, *20, 76*, 78

Mouthpieces for SB-PAP, 73
Multicasualty incidents, 269, 371, 377
  see also Disasters
Muscle relaxants, 51, **168–169**, 245–246, 248
Myocardial infarction, 98, **296–299**
  with acute pulmonary edema, 298
  drug treatment in, 159, 165, 187–188, 297, 298
  fluid administration after, 171, 173, 297
  with hypertension, 298
  with hypotension, 297
  prevention of sudden cardiac death in, 298–299
Myocardial ischaemia, 296–299

Naloxone, 260, 286
Narcotic analgesics, **165–166**, 337
  overdose, 318
Nasal masks for SB-PAP, 73
Nasal passage, obstruction of, 15
Nasogastric tubes, insertion of, 57–58
Nasopharyngeal sunctioning, 33, 287
Nasopharyngeal tubes, 34, 36
  technique of insertion, *35*, 36
Nasotracheal intubation
  blind, 53
  complications of, 57
  fiberoptic laryngoscopic, 55
  technique of **53**
Nasotracheal suction, blind, 32, 33
National disaster medical systems, 375–377
Near-death experiences, 382–383
Near-drowning, 64, 310–311
Neck lift, head-tilt by, 17, *18*
Neck trauma, see Cervical spine trauma
Nembutal, *see* Pentobarbital
Neonatal resuscitation, 280, *282*, **286–291**
  equipment required, 290
  see also Infants
Neurologic evaluation
  in coma, 262, 263–265, 266
  of trauma victims, 323
Neurosurgery, barbiturate anesthesia in, 255
Nifedipine, 161–162, 256, 257
Nimodipine, 161, 162, 256, 257
Nitrogen narcosis, 312
Nitroglycerin, 163, **164**, 298
Nitroprusside, 163, **164**
Noradrenaline, *see* Norepinephrine
Norepinephrine, 154, **155–156**, 297
  in pediatric resuscitation, 286
Normosol, 174
Novocain, *see* Procaine

Nuclear disasters, 329, 330, 377–378
Nuclear war, 330, 378
Nurses, teaching first aid and resuscitation to, 340–341, 346–347

Oculocephalic (doll's eye) reflex, 265, 266, 271
Oculovestibular (caloric) reflex, 265, 266, 271
One operator CPR 11, **107**, *108*, 110, **111**
  switching between operators, 113–114
  transition to two operators, 113
Oral fluid therapy, 176
Oropharyngeal suctioning, 32, 33, 288
Oropharyngeal tubes (airways)
  Guedal type, 34, *35*, 36
    technique of insertion, *35*, 36
  S-shaped, 34, *35*, 36
Orotracheal intubation
  complications of, 57
  fiberoptic laryngoscopic, 55
  tactile digital, 54
  technique of, *46–47*, **48–50**
  transillumination, 54
Orotracheal tubes, sizes of, 42
Osmotherapy, 249, 253, 259
Overall performance categories, 249, 267, 268
Oximetry, non-invasive (pulse), 141
Oxygen
  -carrying blood substitutes, 176, 327
  electrodes 138
  -free gas, inhalation of, 299–300
  gas mixtures with reduced concentration of, 300
Oxygen administration, 21, **92–94**, 298
  in acute pulmonary edema, 312–313
  adjustable-pressure automatic oxygen-powered ventilators, 88
  delivery systems, 92–94
  during mouth-to-mouth ventilation, 79
  at high altitude, 96
  in high pressure conditions, 96
  high-frequency jet ventilation, **89–90**, *91*, 116
  hyperbaric, 96
  manually triggered oxygen-powered ventilators, 86, *87*
  in neonates, *282*, 288–289
  post-resuscitation, 239–240, 246
  selection of techniques, 94–97
  spontaneous breathing with positive airway pressure (SB-PAP) for, 72–74, 93

translaryngeal jet insufflation, 27, 31,
  59–60, *61*, 89
  via Laerdal pocket masks, 79–80, *81*, 93
  via self-refilling bag-valve-mask units, *82*,
  83–85, 93, *282*, 288
Oxygen consumption ($\dot{V}O_2$), 241
  in hypothermia, 304–305
Oxygen content
  of arterial blood (CaO_2), 97, 138, 241
  of mixed venous blood (CvO_2), 138, 241
Oxygen-powered ventilators
  adjustable-pressure automatic, 88
  manually triggered, **86**, *87*
Oxygen radicals (O_2^-), *236–237*, 257, 258
Oxygen saturation, measurement of, 141
Oxygen tension (PO_2)
  arterial (PaO_2), 70, 94
    post-resuscitation, 246, 248
    for selection of ventilation patterns, 96
  measurement of, 138
  mixed venous (PvO_2), 70, 96, 173
  transcutaneous (tcPO_2), 141–142
Oxygen transport, arterial, 95
Oxygenation
  apneic diffusion, 301
  assessment of adequacy of, 94, 95, 96
  emergency, 9, **68–97**
  extracorporeal membrane, *see*
    Extracorporeal membrane
    oxygenation
  100% oxygen test, 96
  see also Oxygen administration
Oxygenators, portable emergency pump,
  219

Pacemakers, cardiac
  ECG rhythms of, *192*
  types of, 212
Pacing, cardiac
  emergency, **211–212**
  external cardiac compressions, 114,
    292–293
  external electric, 187, 188, 191, 211
  'fist' (precordial thumping), 187, 191,
    211, 292–294
  transthoracic wire, 211
  transvenous, 187, 211, 212, 243
Packed red blood cells, 175–176, *177*
Painful stimuli, reactions of comatose
  patients to, 264, 271
Pancuronium, 168, 169
Paramedics trained in advanced life
  support, 119, 364
PASG, *see* Military (medical) antishock
  trousers

PCO_2, *see* Carbon dioxide tension
Peak flowmeters, 143
Pediatric cardiopulmonary resuscitation,
  279–286
  see also Children *and* Infants
PEEP (positive end-expiratory pressure),
  20, 68, **69–72**, *71*
  with high-frequency jet ventilation, 90
  indications for, 69–70
  optimization of, 70, 96
  post-resuscitation, 239–240
  valves for SB-PAP, 73
  see also CPPV
Pentobarbital, 166–167
  in brain resuscitation, 249, 254–256
  for control of seizures and restlessness,
    166–167, 168, 246, 248
Pentothal, *see* Thiopental
Performance categories
  cerebral, 249, 267, 268
  overall, 249, 267, 268
Peripheral resistance, 97
Peritoneal lavage for diagnosis of
  intra-abdominal injury, 336
Persistent vegetative state, *see* Vegetative
  state, persistent
Pethidine (meperidine), 165, 337
pH
  of arterial blood, 240–241, 246, 248,
    307
  of CSF, 246, 250, 259
  electrodes, 138
  see also Acid-base status
Pharyngeal suctioning, 32, 33
Pharyngeal tubes (airways), 34, *35*, 36
  S-tubes, exhaled air ventilation using, *35*,
    79
  technique of insertion, **34–36**, *35*
Phenothiazines, overdose of, 318
Phenoxybenzamine, 260
Phenylephrine, 254
Phenytoin (diphenylhydantoin), **167–168**
  for brain resuscitation, 253, 256, 259
  for control of seizures and restlessness,
    246, 248
Phlebotomy, 298
Physicians
  in ambulances, 363
  emergency drug kit, 170
  responsibilities for emergency medical
    services, 364, 367, 372
  training in first aid and resuscitation,
    119–120, 320, 340–341, 344–345
Pittsburgh brain stem score (PBSS), 262,
  263, 265

Plasma
  colloid osmotic pressure, 135, 174, 242
  colloid substitutes, 172, 174–175, 177,
    326, 328
  fresh frozen, 175, 177
  pooled, 175
  protein fractions, 174–175
Plasmanate, 174–175
Pleural drainage, 64–67, 70
  technique of, *65*, **66–67**
Pneumatic anti-shock garment (PASG), *see*
  Military (medical) antishock trousers
Pneumothorax
  open, 333–334
  tension, 64, 295, **334–335**
  pleural drainage in, *65*, 66–67, 70
Pneupac ventilator, 88
PNPV (positive-negative pressure
  (controlled) ventilation), 68, *71*
PO_2, *see* Oxygen tension
Poisoning, 318–319
Police, teaching first aid and resuscitation
  to, 340–341, 346
Polycythemia in neonates, 288
Polytrauma, severe, 324–325
Position
  for external cardiac compressions, 104
  for shock, *123*, 124
  stable side, *18*, **19**, 124
  supported supine aligned, *18*, **19**, 124
  Trendelenburg, 124
  upright, CPR in, 116, 310
Positive airway pressure (PAP) with
  spontaneous breathing, *see* SB-PAP
Post-resuscitation syndrome, 98, 231,
  232–237
  cerebral reoxygenation injury of, 233,
    236–237
  cerebral reperfusion failure of, 232–233,
    234, *235*
Post-resuscitative brain-orientated therapy,
  see Brain-orientated therapy,
  post-resuscitation
Potassium chloride, administration of, 241
Potassium serum levels, cardiac function
  and, 307
Precordial thumping (chest thumping)
  repetitive (fist pacing), 187, 191, 211,
    292–294
  in witnessed cardiac arrest, 147, 205–206,
    292–294, *293*
Premature atrial contractions (complexes,
  PACs), *184–185*, 186
Premature junctional (nodal) rhythms,
  186–187, *189*

Premature ventricular contractions
  (complexes, PVCs), 152, 165, **193**,
    194–195, 299
  treatment of, 193
Pressure on bleeding points
  manual, 120, *121*
  using dressings, 120, *121*
Procainamide, **153**, 193, 197
Procaine, **153**
Prolonged life support (PLS, CPR steps
  G-H-I), 3, 5, 10, 12, **227–278**
  teaching, 341, 342, 344, 347, 352–354
  termination of, 272–276
  see also Brain-orientated therapy,
    post-resuscitation; Intensive therapy
Promethazine, 258
Pronestyl, *see* Procainamide
Propranolol, **165**
Prostacyclin, 12, 260
Pulmonary artery catheterization, **134–136**
  indications, 134
  technique of, 135–136
Pulmonary artery occlusion (wedge)
  pressure (PAOP, PAWP), 134, 155,
    241
  for guiding fluid administration, 173, 242,
    297
  normal range, 134–135
Pulmonary artery pressure (PAP), 134, 241
Pulmonary edema
  acute, **312–314**
  acute myocardial infarction with, 298
  in burn injury, 328
  fluid administration and, 174
  neurogenic, 325
  oxygen administration in, 72, 313
  prevention of, 242–243
  treatment of, 165, 166, 243, 313–314
Pulmonary embolism, 214, 219, **314–315**
Pulmonary support, post-resuscitation,
  239–240, 242
Pulse
  monitoring by tissue oximeters, 141
  palpation of, 99–100, 283
Pulsus irregularis perpetuus, 186
Pupils
  dilation of, 98, 100, 270
  reactivity of, 100, 114, 266
Puritan (Bennett) Resuscitator (PMR-2), 83

Quinidine, 153

Radial artery
  catheterization, 136–137

intra-arterial pressure monitoring via,
143–144
palpation of pulse, 99
puncture, 136
Radiation, low-level, prolonged exposure
to, 330, 378
Radiation injuries, 329–331, 378
Radiation sickness (acute radiation
syndrome)
symptoms of, 329–330
treatment of, 330–331
Radio
for communication in disasters, 373
physicians guiding resuscitation via, 364,
367
Red blood cells, packed, 175–176, 177
Renal failure, acute, causes of, 243
Renal system, post-resuscitation support,
243, 244
Rescue
of drowning victims, 312
of nuclear disaster casualties, 330
of trauma victims, 322
'Rescue breathing' 75
Rescue pull, 123–124, 321
technique of, *123*
Residual volume (RV), *142*
Respiratory acidemia, 241
Respiratory alkalemia, 240, 241
Respiratory distress syndrome
adult (ARDS), 324
neonatal, SB-PAP in, 72
Respiratory stimulants, 286
Restlessness, control of, 166, 246, 248
Resuscitation carts, hospital, 367
Resuscitation Council (UK), 284–285
Resuscitation medicine disaster teams,
375–376, 377
Resuscitation teams, hospital, 361–362
Ringer's solution, 172, 174, 177, 326
lactated, 174, 328
Robertshaw valve, *87*
Ruben-Ambu self-refilling bag-valve-mask
unit, *82*

S-tubes for exhaled air ventilation, 34, *35*,
36, 79
Salicylate overdose, 319
Saline solutions
hypertonic, 174, 326, 328
isotonic, 172, 174, 326
with normal pH, 174
Saphenous vein
cut-down, 130
great, *130–131*

small, *130–131*
SB-CPAP (spontaneous breathing with
continuous positive airway pressure),
72–73, *74*, 93, 240, 313
SB-PAP (spontaneous breathing with
positive airway pressure), **72–74**, 84
advantages and disadvantages, 73–74
equipment for, 73, *74*
function of, 72–73
in neonates, 72, 289
School children, teaching first aid and
resuscitation to, 343, 346
Scuba divers, hyperbaric injuries to, 312
Sedation for tracheal intubation of
conscious patients, 52
Seizures, *see* Convulsions
Septic shock, corticosteroids for, 163
Shock, **325–327**
anaphylactic, 319–320
cardiogenic, 222, 243, **297**
classification of, 325
definition of, 124, 325
fluid replacement in, 172–173, 326–327
of heat stroke (heat pyrexia), 306
hypovolemic, *see* Hypovolemic shock
in neonates, 290
traumatic, 122–124, 322–323, 325–326
'Shock lung', 324
Siggaard-Anderson nomogram, *140*, 151
Sighing (intermittent deep lung inflations),
69
Silvester (chest-pressure arm-lift, supine)
method of emergency artificial
ventilation, 68
Simultaneous ventilation-compression
cardiopulmonary resuscitation (SVC-
CPR), 102, 114–116
Sinus bradycardia, 183, *184–185*, 188
Sinus tachycardia, 183, *184–185*, 299
Snoring, 16
Sodium bicarbonate, 145, 147, 148, 149,
150–151
adverse effects of, 150, 307
AHA recommendations, 12
calculation of dose, 151
in exsanguination cardiac arrest, 302
in neonates, 289, 290
in pediatric resuscitation, 286
routes of administration, 129, 132
Sodium chloride solutions, *see* Saline
solutions
Sodium serum levels, 307
Spinal cord activity in brain death, 273
Spinal cord trauma, 116, **333**
see also Cervical spine trauma

Spine boards, *see* Backboards
Spine deformities, open-chest CPR in, 214
Spirometry, 142–143
Splinting of fractured extremities, 337
Stable side position, *18*, **19**, 124
Starch solutions, 175
Status asthmaticus, 300, **315–316**
  diagnosis, 315
  therapy for, 64, 158–159, 163, 315–316
Sternum, identification of pressure point for
    chest compression, 102–103, *104*,
    282, 284
Stethoscope, esophageal, 50, 178
Stokes-Adams syndrome, 158, 181, 182,
    187, 292
Stomach
  air in, during mouth-to-mouth
    ventilation, 75, 280, 296
  water in, in drowning victims, 311
Streptokinase, 253, 260
Stroke, 250
Stroma-free hemoglobin, 176, 327
Stylets for tracheal tubes, 47
Subarachnoid hemorrhage, 332
Subclavian vein cannulation, 130, 133, 134,
    135, 295
Subdural hematoma, 323–324, 332
Submersion accidents, *see* Drowning
Succinylcholine, 51, 168, 169
Suction
  catheters, size of, 42
  of obstructed airways, **32–33**, *32*, 287, 288
  of tracheobronchial tree, 32, 33, 50, 62,
    240
Suicide attempts, 318
Superior vena cava, catheterization of, 133
Superoxide dismutase (SOD), 253, 258
Supported supine aligned position, *18*, **19**,
    124
Supraventricular tachycardia, paroxysmal
    (PSVT) 183, *184–185*, 196
  treatment of, 160, 183, *185*, 186, 299
Suxamethonium, *see* Succinylcholine
SVC-CPR, *see* Simultaneous ventilation-
    compression cardiopulmonary
    resuscitation
Swan-Ganz catheterization, *see* Pulmonary
    artery catheterization

Tachycardia
  paroxysmal supraventricular, *see*
    Supraventricular tachycardia,
    paroxysmal
  sinus, 183, *184–185*, 299

ventricular, *see* Ventricular tachycardia
Teaching first aid and resuscitation,
    339–359
  certification of students, 354
  to health care personnel, 344–345
  to the lay public, 343–344
  methodology of, 344–354
  self-training systems, 350
  testing skills, 354–359
  training of instructors, 345
  what to teach to whom, 339–342
Teams
  disaster medical response, 375–376, 377
  resuscitation, 361–362
Telephone number for emergency medical
    services, 363
Temperature, body, control in neonates,
    289
Tension pneumothorax, *see* Pneumothorax,
    tension
Tetanus prophylaxis in trauma victims, 324
THAM (tris buffer), 152
Thiopental, 166–167
  in brain resuscitation, 249, 254–256, 258
  for control of seizures or restlessness,
    166–167, 246, 248
  for tracheal intubation in comatose
    patients, 51
Thoracic hemorrhage, open-chest CPR in,
    214
Thoracic trauma, 10, **333–335**
Thoracostomy tubes, insertion of 66–67
Thoracotomy, emergency, 11, *215*, 217,
    334
Thrombolytic therapy
  intracoronary, 299
  in pulmonary thromboembolism, 315
Thumb-jaw lift technique, *23*, 24
Tidal volume, *142*
Tongue, airway obstruction by, 15
Tongue-jaw-lift maneuver, *26*, 285
Topical anesthesia of upper airways, 51–52,
    53
Torsade de pointes, 196–197
Tourniquets, 119, **120**
  in acute pulmonary edema, 313
  in anaphylactic reactions, 320
Tracheal intubation, 11, 27, 31, **40–57**
  alternatives to, 59–61
  anatomical views for, *46*
  complications of, 57, 295
  in conscious patients, 40, **51–52**, 53
  difficulty with, 53–54
  during CPR, 40–1, 114
  equipment for, 41–47, *45*

external CPR steps A-B-C- after, 110, 112
extubation, 56
fiberoptic laryngoscopic, 55
in head trauma, 40, **51**, 52, 331
history, 3, 40
indications, 40
in infants and small children, 55, 281
muscle relaxants for, 51, 168
nasotracheal, *see* Nasotracheal intubation
in neonates, 288, 289
for open-chest CPR, 216
orotracheal, *see* Orotracheal intubation
post-resuscitation, 239
rapid sequence, 51
teaching proficiency in, 353, 358
techniques of, 48–55
Tracheal tubes, 41, 44–47
for infants and children, 41, 42, 44, 55
inflation of cuffs, 44–47, 240
obstruction of, 57
sizes of, 42
stylets for, 44
Tracheobronchial tree
instillation of drugs in, 132
suction of, 32, 33, 50, 62, 240
Tracheostomy tubes, sizes of, 42
Tracheotomy, 40, **62**, *63*
emergency mouth-to-stoma ventilation, 76
Training in first aid and resuscitation, *see* Teaching first aid and resuscitation
Transcutaneous carbon dioxide tension (tcPCO_2), 141–142
Transcutaneous oxygen tension (tcPO_2), 141–142
Transillumination orotracheal intubation, 54
Translaryngeal oxygen jet ventilation, 27, 31, **59–60**, *61*, 89
Transplantation, donation of organs for, 232, 272, 276
Transportation
of disaster victims, 373, 376
post-resuscitation, 238, 295–296, 362, 365
of trauma victims, 321–322, 323
see also Ambulances
Transthoracic wire pacing, 211
Transtracheal high-frequency jet ventilation HFJV), 90, *91*
Transvenous cardiac pacing, 187, 211, 212, 243
Trauma, 10–11, **320–337**
advanced trauma life support, *see* Advanced trauma life support
airway control in, 17, 75–76, 322, 323, 331

analgesia in, 337
of extremities, 337
extrication and positioning, 122–124
life supporting first aid in, *see* First aid, life supporting
primary survey, 124, 322–323
scale, 322
secondary survey, 124–125, 323–324
severe polytrauma, 324–325
tracheal intubation, 41
transportation to trauma centers, 321–322, 323
see also Abdominal trauma; Cervical spine traumas; Head trauma; Hemorrhage
Trendelenburg position, 124
Triage
critical care, 276, 277
in multicasualty incidents, 269, 377
Trimethaphan, 163, 164
Triple airway maneuver (jaw-thrust maneuver), 11, 15, 17, **22–24**, *23*
in trauma victims, 17, 322
Tris buffer (THAM), 152
Tuberculosis, risk of transmission of, 350–351
Tubocurarine, 168, 169
Tubular necrosis of kidneys, acute (ATN), 324
Two operator CPR, 11, **107–110**, *109*, **112**
transition from one operator, 113

Ulnar artery, assessing patency of (Allen's test), 136
Umbilical vessels, catheterization of, 289
Unconsciousness, *see* Coma
Urinary catheterization in trauma victims, 323

Vaccine proteins, anaphylactic reactions to, 319
Vagal maneuvers for supraventricular tachycardia, 183, 185, 186
Vascular resistances, systemic and peripheral, 241
Vasodilators, 163–164, 313
Vasovagal syncope, 181
Vecuronium, 169
Vegetative state, persistent (PVC), 249, 271
definition of, 272
diagnosis of, 277–278
'letting die' in, 276–278
Vena cava, superior, catheterization of, 133
Venous catheterization, central, *see* Central venous catheterization
Venous cut-down, 130, 326

Venous pressure, central, *see* Central venous
    pressure
Venous puncture and catheterization, *see*
    Intravenous cannulation, peripheral
Ventilation, alveolar, adequacy of, 94
Ventilation (artificial), 20–21, **68–97**
    assisted (AV), 21, 68, *71*
    history of, 88
    intermittent positive pressure, *see* IPPV
    muscle relaxants for, 169–170, 246, 248
    patterns, 68–69, *71*
    post-resuscitation, 239–240, 245–246, 248
    selection of techniques, 94–97
    weaning from 72, 96, 240
    see also CPPV; Exhaled air ventilation;
        IMV; PEEP; SB-PAP
Ventilation meters, 143
Ventilators, 117
    adjustable-pressure automatic oxygen-
        powered, 88
    automatic, 69, 95
    criteria for 'ideal', 88–89
    cuirass, 88
    field, 88
    manually triggered oxygen-powered, **86,**
        87
    tank, 88
Ventricular bigeminal rhythm, 193
Ventricular fibrillation (VF), 98, 178, **181,**
    197
    automatic external defibrillation for,
        209–210
    automatic internal (implanted)
        defibrillation, 210–211
    cough CPR in, 147, 291–292
    defibrillation in, 199–200, **204–207**
    diagnosis in open-chest CPR, 218
    drug treatment in, 145, **147,** 149, 152,
        154, 165, 199
    ECG patterns of, *182, 196*

electric shock causing, 308, 309
precordial thumping in, 147, 205–206,
    292–294
primary, 181, 296
prophylaxis, 146, 152, 153–154
recommended treatment of, 197, 294
secondary, 181
warning signs of sudden, 297
Ventricular tachycardia (VT), 178, **193–197**
    defibrillation in, 199, 204–205
    drug treatment in, 145, **147,** 149, 165, 299
    ECG patterns of, *195*
    precordial thumping in, 292–294
    prophylaxis, 146, 152
    recommended treatment of, 197, 294
Ventricular trigeminal rhythm, 193
Venturi mask, 94
Verapamil, 160, 161–162, 256, 257
Verbal responses of comatose patients, 264
Vital capacity (VC), *142, 143*
Vitamin C, 258
Vitamin E, 258
Volunteers, conscious human, teaching first
    aid and resuscitation on, 344–345,
    348–349

Waters tissue (ear) oximeter, 141
Wenckebach phenomenon (Mobitz type I
    AV block), 187, 188, *190–191*
Wheezing, 16
World Association for Emergency and
    Disaster Medicine (WAEDM), 371,
    375, 378
Wound care
    in burn injury, 328–329
    in trauma victims, 324

Xanthinoxidase inhibitors, 253, 258